Local and Regional Flaps in Head & Neck Reconstruction

Local and Regional Flaps in Head & Neck Reconstruction

A Practical Approach

Rui Fernandes, MD, DMD, FACS

Associate Professor & Associate Chair Department of Oral and Maxillofacial Surgery
Chief of Head and Neck Service
Director, Microvascular Fellowship
University of Florida College of Medicine – Jacksonville
Jacksonville, Florida, USA

WILEY Blackwell

This edition first published 2015

Editorial offices: 1606 Golden Aspen Drive, Suites 103 and 104, Ames, Iowa 50010, USA
The Atrium, Southern Gate, Chichester, West Sussex, PO19 8SQ, UK
9600 Garsington Road, Oxford, OX4 2DQ, UK

For details of our global editorial offices, for customer services and for information about how to apply for permission to reuse the copyright material in this book please see our website at www.wiley.com/wiley-blackwell.

Library of Congress Cataloging-in-Publication Data

Fernandes, Rui, author.
Local and regional flaps in head & neck reconstruction : a practical approach / Rui P. Fernandes.
p. ; cm.
Local and regional flaps in head and neck reconstruction
Includes bibliographical references and index.
ISBN 978-1-118-34033-2 (cloth)
I. Title. II. Title: Local and regional flaps in head and neck reconstruction.
[DNLM: 1. Head–surgery. 2. Neck–surgery. 3. Reconstructive Surgical Procedures. 4. Surgical Flaps. WE 705]
RD521
617.5′1059–dc23

2014025853

A catalogue record for this book is available from the British Library.

Wiley also publishes its books in a variety of electronic formats. Some content that appears in print may not be available in electronic books.

Cover image: © Craig Bowman
Cover design by Modern Alchemy LLC

Set in 9.5/12pt Palatino by Aptara Inc., New Delhi, India

MWEP410869051125

Contents

Preface

As a collector of medical books, I have found that the current emphasis of most texts on head and neck reconstructive surgery is on microvascular surgery. The impact of free tissue transfer on the surgeon's ability to repair difficult defects has been revolutionary, to say the least. For this reason, it is certainly tempting to focus our thought process chiefly on microsurgery for head and neck reconstruction. However, my own practice, travels, and experience have given me a greater appreciation for the relevance of regional pedicle flaps, and I believe that they play a bigger role in the practice of head and neck reconstruction than most surgeons give them credit for.

In planning for this project, I evaluated the merits of a textbook devoted entirely to local and regional flaps. When well planned and executed, these flaps often yield better results than those attained with microsurgery, offering patients better color, texture, and thickness matches by replacing like with like tissue. Local and regional flaps have great resource-sparing potential for the healthcare system in terms instrumentation and clinical resources, and offer a lower cost to the patient. Use of these flaps also provides more options for reconstruction for sicker patients who may not be well suited for the rigors of microsurgery.

In this book, I have sought to provide an "how to" approach for surgeons with and without specialized training in head and neck reconstruction. I have included my own clinical photos instead of sketches to demonstrate how useful local and regional flaps are in my own practice. Whenever beneficial, I have included videos to demonstrate the described techniques. My hope is that the reader, especially our younger colleagues who have grown up in the era of microsurgery, will realize that there is a definite role for regional and local flaps in head and neck reconstruction.

Acknowledgments

My deepest gratitude goes to all my family, especially my wife Candace and our children Gabriela and Alessandro. There were many nights and weekends spent working on this book, and I really appreciate their support and encouragement. Many thanks go out to Professor Robert Ord for the outstanding training he provided during my two-year fellowship at the University of Maryland. He gave me an inroad into head and neck surgery and has continued to support my academic career. I express my gratitude to Nelson Goldman, MD. When I joined the University of Florida College of Medicine in Jacksonville, he was a welcoming colleague that invested his time in mentoring me to become a better surgeon.

I believe that success in academic practice does not happen because of the efforts of an individual, but rather through the collaboration of colleagues. I have been extremely fortunate to have partners at the University of Florida that are unmatched in their dedication to excellent patient care and to moving our specialty forward. Thanks so much to each of you. The success of a department begins with a vision set by the chairman. I thank Dr. Tirbod Fattahi, our department chair, for his leadership and steadfast support of my academic goals and personal growth. His friendship is unquestionable. Lastly, many thanks to my fellows and residents who continue to challenge me to deliver my very best as they do on a daily basis.

About the companion website

This book is accompanied by a companion website:

www.wiley.com/go/fernandes/flapsreconstruction

The website includes:

- Powerpoints of all figures from the book for downloading
- Web-exclusive demonstration videos of surgical procedures featured in the book

Chapter 1
Introduction

Sir Harold Gilles is credited with the "Gilles concept"; he stated "the more adjacent the donor site is, the better the skin will match the recipient site."[1]

The overarching goal of all surgeons involved in reconstruction of head and neck defects is not only to reestablish the facial form and function but also to return the patient to a near pre-injury or pre-resection esthetics.

Today, the era of microvascular reconstructive surgery is well grounded in the vernacular of the reconstructive surgeon as well as the increasingly more educated and demanding public. One of the undisputed concepts in head and neck reconstruction is that whenever possible, one should strive to reconstruct the skin defects with tissues that more closely resemble the missing tissue not only in color but also in thickness and texture.

Equally important in the reconstructive discussion is to keep in mind the needs of our patients and their ability to undergo a more extensive reconstruction using free tissue transfer. In these cases as well as those where the free tissue transfer has failed, the use of pedicled local or regional flaps is an important aspect of the armamentarium of reconstructive surgeons.

The goal of this textbook is to provide readers with a practical guide on how to raise and inset a vast array of pedicle local and regional flaps to reconstruct various defects of the head and neck. The author uses actual clinical cases to depict each step in the process of raising a flap. The potential sites where the surgeon may encounter difficulties are discussed and ways to avoid potential problems are shared.

The book has four parts: the first is dedicated to fundamental concepts in flap reconstruction, the second to local flaps, the third is devoted to regional flaps, while the last part covers sites in the head and neck that are challenging to reconstruct.

Each chapter is structured to provide a "practical" description of the flap and a succinct description on how to raise the flap, sections on the anatomy of the flap and harvesting, and selected chapters also include a special circumstances section. Selected readings are given at the end of each chapter and comprise the author's choice of some important articles devoted to the flap being presented. Each chapter is well illustrated with clinical images of the flaps.

In addition to the text in the book, a set of CD-ROMs with selected videos is included, highlighting the key steps in raising flaps and how to use them in the head and neck.

The author and the publisher are very proud to present this book to help trainees, junior faculty, and practicing surgeons in disciplines such as dermatology, oral and maxillofacial surgery, otolarygology, and plastic surgery.

Reference

1. Gilles HD. The tubed pedicle in plastic surgery. *NY Med J* 1920; 111:1.

Local and Regional Flaps in Head & Neck Reconstruction: A Practical Approach, First Edition. Rui Fernandes.

Companion website: www.wiley.com/go/fernandes/flapsreconstruction

Chapter 2
Flap classification

Introduction

The literature is replete with descriptions and various classifications of flaps. This ample classification can be confusing. The intent of this chapter is to provide a brief clarification of the systems commonly consulted for classification of skin and muscle flaps. The chapter is not intended to be a treatise on flap physiology or classification but simply to define some of the terms, which will be used in the remainder of the book.

Our understanding and improved success with the use of local and regional flaps is a direct consequence of a better understanding of the physiology of skin perfusion.

The understanding of the arterial supply has been a continuous process that had its foundation in pioneering works from the likes of Manchot,[1] Cormack,[2] and Salmon[3] to Taylor[4] and most recently Saint-Cyr.[5] Continued advancements have been made in the entire reconstructive arena based on their work.

In general terms, we can classify flaps based on their vascularity, their composition, or their method of transfer.

Local flaps

Local flaps are flaps that are located adjacent to the defect site. They may be contiguous to the defect or a small amount of tissue may separate the flap from the defect. The surrounding tissue is transferred to repair the defect and therefore the flap tends to be similar in color and texture, and the thickness can often be tailored to the needs of the defect.

Local cutaneous flaps

Local flaps can also be classified based on the method of transfer. Broadly speaking, they can be pivot, advancement, or hinge flaps. The pivot flaps are further subdivided into: rotation, transposition, interpolated, and island flaps.

The rotational flap is a flap that is transferred to the recipient bed by pivoting around the base of the flap. The defect and the base of the flap have to be contiguous. Another form is to transpose a flap. This description entails the use of a flap with a geometric shaped design whereby the local tissue is undermined after elevation of the flap and then the flap is mobilized to fit the defect. At times, the design will include two shapes, as in a bilobed flap, so that the flap is transferred to the defect site and the smaller portion of the flap is transposed to the donor site. The area is closed after wide undermining.

The interpolated flap is where the defect is not intimately connected to the base of the flap. During transfer, the flap needs to cross over the intact portion of skin to reach the defect. There are two options for flap transfer. One is to develop a tunnel between the flap and the defect and then de-epithelialize the portion of the flap that will travel under the skin bridge and transfer the flap. The second and most commonly utilized method is to stage the reconstruction: transfer the flap over the tissue bridge, return after enough collateral blood supply to the flap has developed from the recipient bed, and then section the connecting portion of the flap between the recipient bed and donor site.

In the island flap design, the skin is circumferentially incised and the blood supply to the flap comes from the subcutaneous tissue or through the muscle or septum. A common design of the flap is with the pedicle composed mainly of the vasculature to the flap.

Regional flaps

Regional flaps are located at a significant distance from the donor site. Because of this distance, the flap

Local and Regional Flaps in Head & Neck Reconstruction: A Practical Approach, First Edition. Rui Fernandes.

Companion website: www.wiley.com/go/fernandes/flapsreconstruction

usually has its own blood supply in the form of a named vessel. There are several potential disadvantages of regional flaps. The first and perhaps the most important is the arc of rotation of the flap. The ability to use a particular regional flap will be dependent on the reach of the flap based on its arc of rotation. The reliability of regional flaps is improved when the flap can reach the defect and the inset is performed without tension. Other disadvantages for regional flaps are that the skin color match and texture may be slightly different from that found at the recipient site.

The discovery between 1965 and 1975 of axial pattern skin flaps, such as the deltopectoral flap, with their advantageous length-to-breadth proportions marked the next milestone in reconstructive surgery.[6] The term "axial pattern" was coined by McGregor and Morgan in 1973.[7] In that publication they defined the terms as:

> **Axial Pattern Flap** – A single flap which has an anatomically recognized arterio-venous system running along its long axias. Such a flap, because of the presence of its axial arterio-venous system, is not subject to many of the restrictions which apply to flaps in general.

> **Random Pattern Flap** – A flap which lacks any significant bias in its vascular pattern. Such a flap, because it lacks an axial arterio-venous system, is subject to the restrictions hitherto generally accepted in flap practice.

The physiological basis for the survival of axial pattern flaps was elucidated by Smith's rabbit study published in 1973.[8] In this study, Smith used flaps of varying length to width ratio and showed that the axial flaps survived as long as an 8#:#1 ratio. The ratio was limited to the flank length of the rabbit. In comparison, the random pattern flaps had a 1#:#1 ratio prior to developing distal tip necrosis.

Random pattern flaps can be classified according to their geometric configuration (rhombic, bilobed, V–Y, Z-plasties, or W-plasties) and by their method of transfer (rotation, advancement, interpolation, and island flaps).[9]

Distant (microvascular/free) flaps

The use of distant or free flaps will not be covered in this textbook in the procedure chapters. The use of various free flaps will be discussed in the site specific reconstruction found towards the end of the book. Unlike local or regional flaps, distant or microvascular free flaps require the detachment of the feeding vessels and transfer of the flap to the recipient site and anastomosing the vessels to a recipient artery and vein or veins. The advantage of this method of reconstruction is that the surgeon is no longer limited to the amount of tissue in the vicinity of the defect nor the art of rotation of the flap. It enables the use of small to large or simple to complex tissue transfer. The obvious disadvantage is that when the skin in the head and neck needs to be reconstructed, the color match and texture will be significantly different.

Flap classification (fasciocutaneous flap and muscle flap)

In 1984, Cormack and Lamberty, an anatomist and a plastic surgeon described a classification of fasciocutaneous flaps based on their vasculature. They described four different types.[10] They described the flaps as follows:

Type A – A pedicled fasciocutaneous flap dependent on multiple fasciocutaneous perforators at the base and oriented with the long axis of the flap in the predominant direction of the arterial plexus at the deep fascia.

Type B – A pedicled or a free flap depending on a single sizeable and consistent fasciocutaneous perforator feeding a plexus at the level of the deep fascia.

Type C – The support of the skin is dependent upon the fascial plexus that is supplied by multiple small perforators along the length which reach it from a deep artery by passing along the fascial septum between the muscles.

Type D – The osteo-myo-fasciocutaneous free tissue transfer. An extension of type C, the fascial septum is taken in continuity with adjacent muscle and bone which derive their blood supply from the same artery.

The most commonly utilized classification system for muscle flaps is that of Mathis and Nahai, published in 1984.[11] The classification was based on the vascular perfusion to the muscle. The classification had five types as follows:

- *Type I:* One dominant vascular pedicle.
- *Type II:* Dominant vascular pedicles and minor pedicles.
- *Type III:* Two dominant pedicles.
- *Type IV:* Segmental vascular pedicles.
- *Type V:* One dominant vascular pedicle and secondary segmental vascular pedicles.

The most recent addition to the reconstructive surgeon's armamentarium has been the perforator flaps. The perforator flap concept was first described by Koshima in 1989.[12] The basic premise of the technique was the harvest of a skin flap with dissection of the feeding vessels through the muscle down to the named source vessel. The Gent consensus defined a perforator as a vessel that has its origin in one of the axial vessels of the body and that passes through certain structural elements of the body, besides interstitial connective tissue and fat, before reaching the subcutaneous fat layer.[13] In the consensus paper, they defined five types of perforators:

- Direct perforators perforate the deep fascia only.
- Indirect muscle perforators predominantly supply the subcutaneous tissues.
- Indirect muscle perforators predominantly supply the muscle but have secondary branches to the subcutaneous tissues.
- Indirect perimysium perforators travel within the perimysium between muscle fibers before piercing the deep fascia.
- Indirect septal perforators travel through the intermuscular septum before piercing the deep fascia.

The chapters in this book will use the terms discussed here to describe various local and regional flaps utilized in head and neck reconstruction.

References

1. Manchot C. *The Cutaneous Arteries of the Human Body*. New York: Springer-Verlag; 1983.
2. Cormack GC, Lamberty BG. Fasciocutaneous vessels: their distribution on the trunk and limbs, and their clinical application in tissue transfer. *Anat Clin* 1984; 6:121–131.
3. Salmon M. *Arteries of the Skin*. London: Churchill Livingstone; 1988
4. Taylor GI, Palmer JH. The vascular territories (angiosomes) of the body: experimental study and clinical applications. *Br J Plast Surg* 1987; 40:113–141.
5. Saint-Cyr M, Wong C, Schaverien M, Mojallal A, Rohrich RJ. The perforasome theory: vascular anatomy and clinical implications. *Plast Reconstr Surg* 2009; 124:1529–1544.
6. Lamberty GH, Cormack GC. Progress in flap surgery: greater anatomical understanding and increased sophistication in application. *World J Surg* 1990; 14:776–785.
7. McGregor IA, Morgan G. Axial and random pattern flaps. *Br J Plast Surg* 1973; 26:202.
8. Smith PJ. The vascular basis of axial pattern flaps. *Br J Plast Surg* 1973; 26:150–157.
9. Maciel-Miranda A, Morris SF, Hallock GG. Local flaps, including pedicled perforator flaps: anatomy, technique, and applications. *Plast Reconstr Surg* 2013; 131:896e–911e.
10. Cormack GC, Lamberty BGH. A classification of fascio-cutaneous flaps according to their patterns of vascularization. *Br J Plast Surg* 1984; 37:80–87.
11. Mathes S, Nahai F. Classification of the vascular anatomy of muscles: experimental and clinical correlation. *Plast Reconstr Surg* 1981; 67:177–187.
12. Koshima I, Fukuda H, Utunomiya R, Soeda S. The anterolateral thigh flap; variations in its vascular pedicle. *Br J Plast Surg* 1989 May; 42(3):260–262.
13. Blondeel PN, Van Landuyt KHI, Monstrey SJM, et al. The "Gent" consensus on perforator flap terminology: preliminary definitions. *Plast Reconstr Surg* 2003; 112:1378–1383.

Chapter 3
Bilobed flap

Introduction

The bilobed flap is another form of a transposition flap; in fact, it is a double transposition flap and can also be used as a triple transposition flap. The flap dates back to 1918 when Esser[1] described its use for the repair of nasal defects. In that description, Esser used two flaps of equal size at 90 and 180 degrees from the axis of the defect. Since this time, the bilobed flap has remained a staple in the reconstructive arena, especially for its versatility in the reconstruction of defects in the facial region.

The use of the flap as described by Esser results in the formation of a dog-ear at the base of the flap. Zitelli modified the flap design by decreasing the angle of the flaps to about 45 degrees and from 90 to 110 degrees for the second flap with an elongation of the second.[2] This modification significantly improved the cosmesis of the flap.

The bilobed flap is extremely useful in the reconstruction of various head and neck defects, and is often used for small defects encountered by the surgeon, particularly in the nasal region, the forehead, or the cheek area. Note that the concept of the bilobed flap allows its use in larger defects, where the design of the flap is still the same.

The concept behind this flap is the successive transfer of a smaller quantity of tissue from the donor site into the defect site along a short arc of rotation.

The advantage of the bilobed flap is that it allows for the reconstruction of defects in the head and neck region with tissues that are immediately surrounding the defect site. Thus, the reconstruction is carried out with tissue of similar color, texture, and thickness to the missing tissue. The transposition of the flap allows for minimal donor site visibility and excellent cosmesis of both donor and recipient sites. Additionally, the bilobed flap can be performed with minimal time commitment and with few resource needs.

The main disadvantage of the bilobed flap is that the need to make additional incisions in the facial region may at times be less desirable.

Anatomy

The bilobed flap is a random pattern, single-stage flap that lacks a large caliber vessel at its base. A bilobed flap uses two adjacent lobes or flaps that are rotated around a pivot point. The primary lobe, usually the same size as the defect, is used to restore the defect. The secondary lobe is used to repair the donor site of the primary lobe. The donor site of the secondary lobe is closed primarily.[3]

As this is not an axial flap but rather a random-based flap, the most important decision will be the design and placement of the flap. The goal will be to minimize disturbance to the surrounding region, that is, not to alter the esthetics of the area while still moving an adequate amount of tissue to repair the defect.

Flap harvest

- The area of the defect site should be assessed to determine the size, depth, and contour of the defect.
- If the borders of the defect are not well defined and or the shape is too irregular, this should be addressed and the defect made into a well-contoured circular shape whenever possible.
- The surrounding tissues should be evaluated for tissue quality, texture, and pliability to design the flap in the most ideal location.
- The area should also be evaluated for esthetic zones that should not be altered; these zones would include the eyebrow, the hairline, etc.

Local and Regional Flaps in Head & Neck Reconstruction: A Practical Approach, First Edition. Rui Fernandes.

Companion website: www.wiley.com/go/fernandes/flapsreconstruction

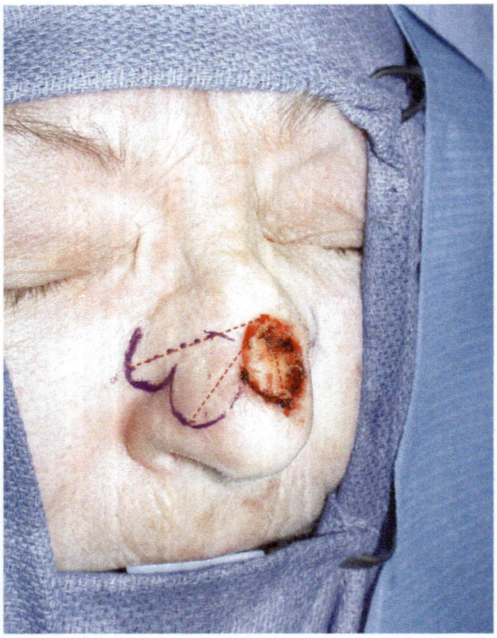

Fig. 3.1 Bilobed design after resection of a skin lesion on the dorsum of the nose.

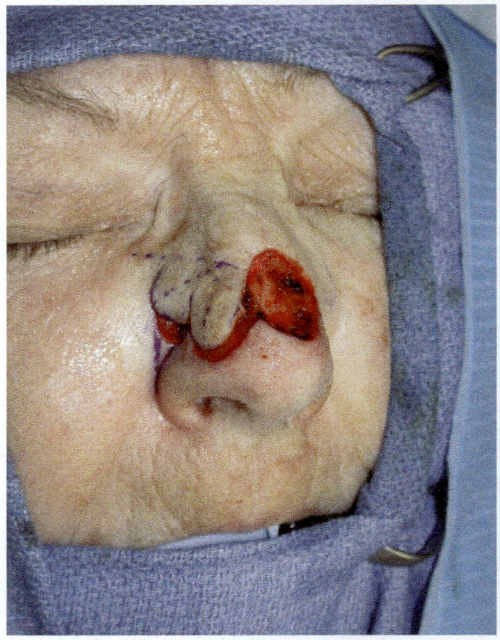

Fig. 3.2 Incision of the bilobed flap prior to transfer.

- The radius of the defect should be measured and transferred to a point inferior to the base of the defect.
- A line from both the lateral and medial aspect of the defect should be traced to the previously marked point.
- The resulting V-shaped tracing is the area of skin that will need to be excised to allow for rotation of the flap.
- Using the base of the new defect, two arcs should be drawn, one from the center of the defect and the other from the top of the defect.
- The smaller arc will correspond to the base of both of the two lobes to be transferred.
- Next, a line should be drawn from the center of the defect to the pivot point at the base. Another line, perpendicular to this should then be drawn.
- The perpendicular line represents the center of the second lobe while a line bisecting the 90 degree (i.e., 45 degrees) will be the center of the first lobe (Figure 3.1).
- The height of the first lobe will correspond to the second arch.
- The height of the second lobe should be twice that of the first lobe.
- The width of the first lobe should correspond to that of the defect while that of the second lobe should be slightly smaller than the first.
- Once the markings are drawn and confirmed to be in a good position, the base of the defect should be excised and the tissue discarded.
- The incisions for the first and second lobe should then be made and the flap raised.
- The surrounding areas should then be mobilized prior to insetting the flap.
- Any extra tissues should be excised to have the best esthetic reconstruction.
- The flaps are elevated and then rotated to the defect and inset (Figure 3.2 to Figure 3.7).

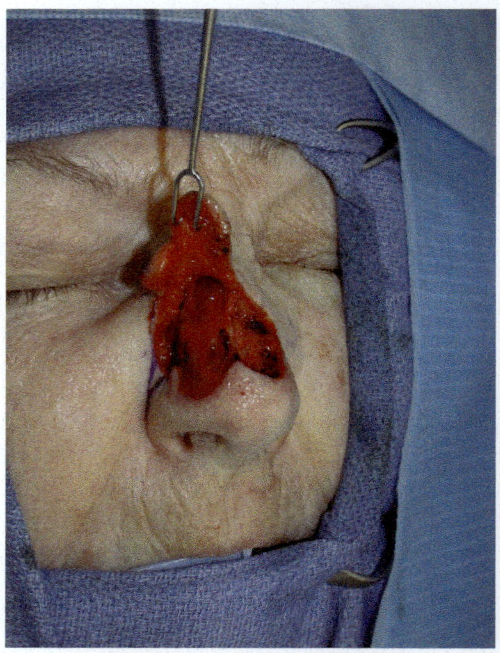

Fig. 3.3 Elevation of the bilobed flap.

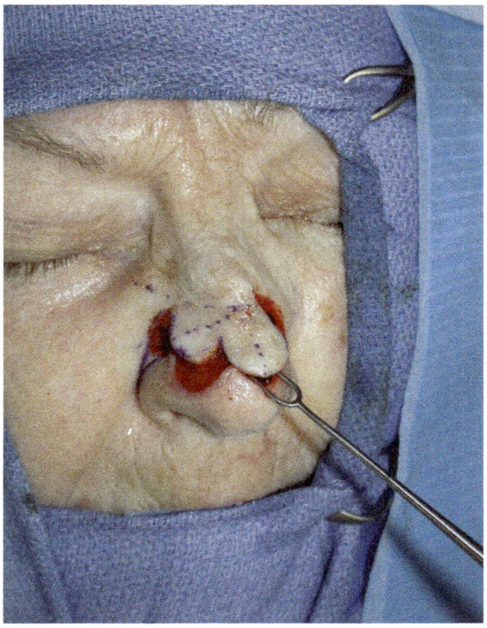

Fig. 3.4 Rotation of the flap into the defect prior to inset.

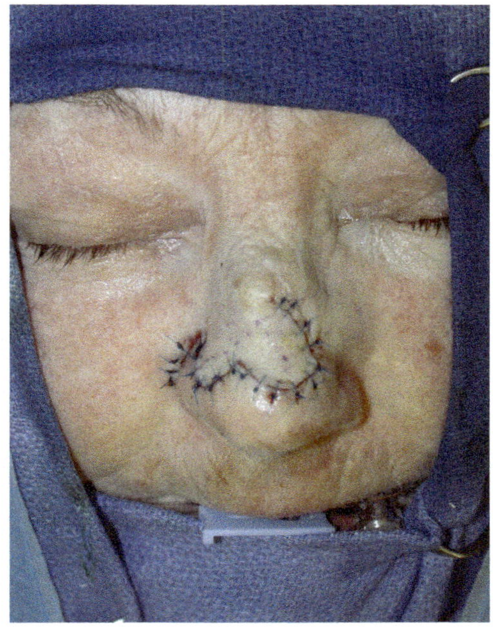

Fig. 3.6 Inset of flap into the nasal defect.

Case #1

A 74-year-old Caucasian female was referred to the clinic for evaluation and treatment of a biopsy-proven recurrent basal cell carcinoma of the nose. After discussion with the patient and review of the case, a decision was made to resect the lesion and reconstruct the defect with an immediate bilobed flap (Figure 3.8). The markings for the resection and reconstruction were made as well as plan for a small excision along the nasal cheek groove so as to minimize distortion of the final reconstruction (Figure 3.9). The lesion was resected (Figure 3.10). The flap was elevated and the small burrow's triangle was excised (Figure 3.11). The mobility of the flap

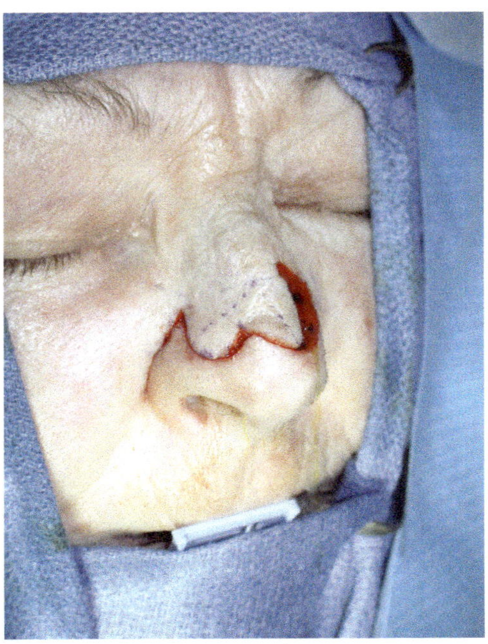

Fig. 3.5 Passive adaptation of the flap into the defect after excision of tissue in the lateral nasal wall.

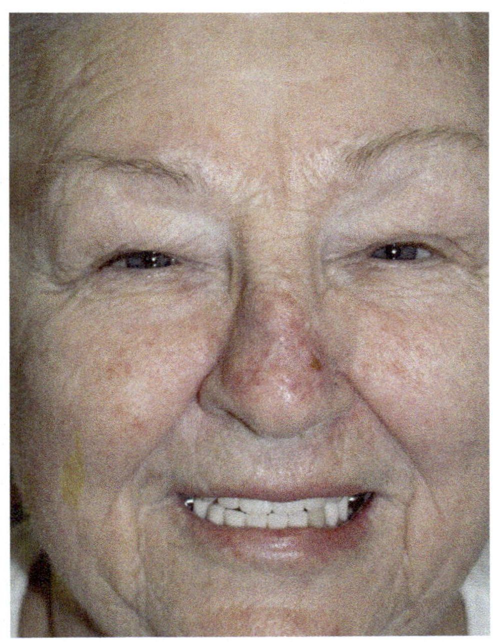

Fig. 3.7 Appearance of the reconstructed nasal defect.

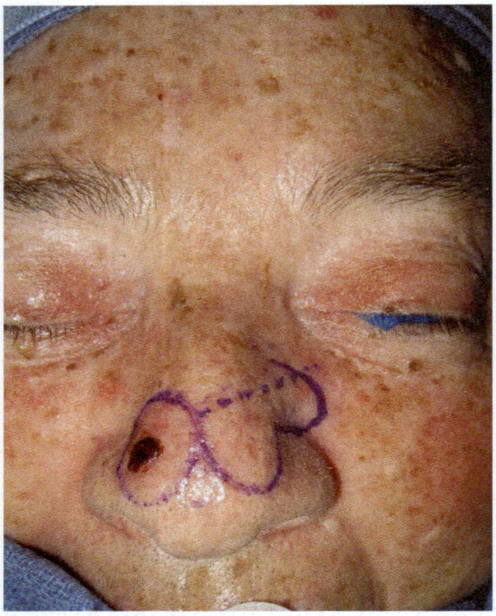

Fig. 3.8 Design of the planned excision and the bilobed flap.

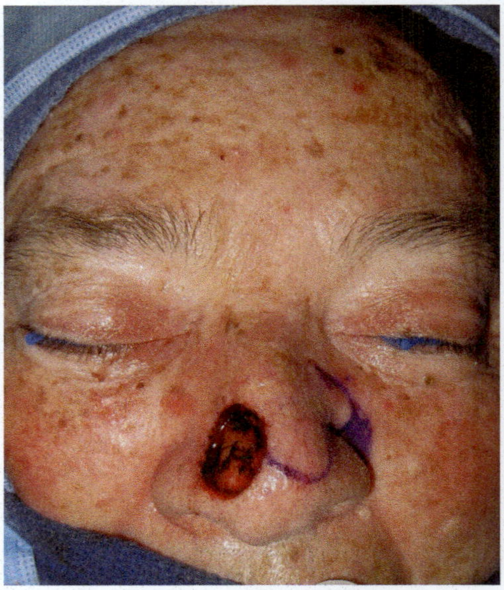

Fig. 3.10 Excision of the skin cancer.

was checked (Figure 3.12) and the flap was then inset (Figure 3.13).

Case #2

A 58-year-old Caucasian male presented with a biopsy-proven basal cell carcinoma approaching the medial canthal region of the left eye (Figure 3.14). A plan was made to reconstruct the eventual defect with a bilobed flap by transferring the tissue from the nasal dorsum and contralateral sidewall (Figures 3.15 and 3.16). The lesion was excised (Figure 3.17) and the flap was elevated (Figure 3.18) and wide undermining was performed (Figure 3.19). The rotation of the flap to the defect was checked and found to be adequate without tension (Figures 3.20 and 3.21. The flap was then inset with minimal distortion to the area (Figures 3.22 and 3.23).

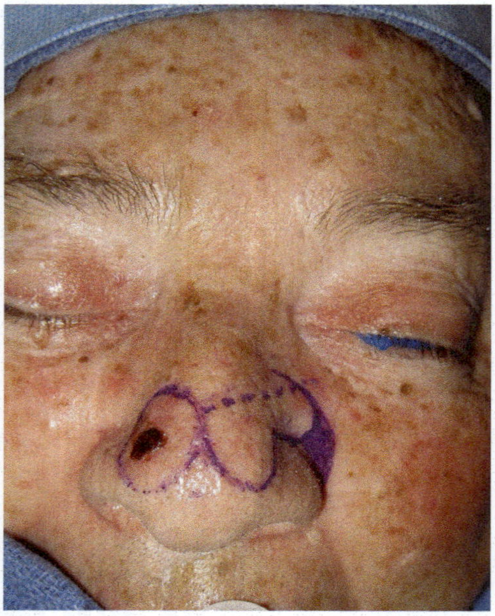

Fig. 3.9 Additional block out of tissue lateral to the nose for better final scar placement.

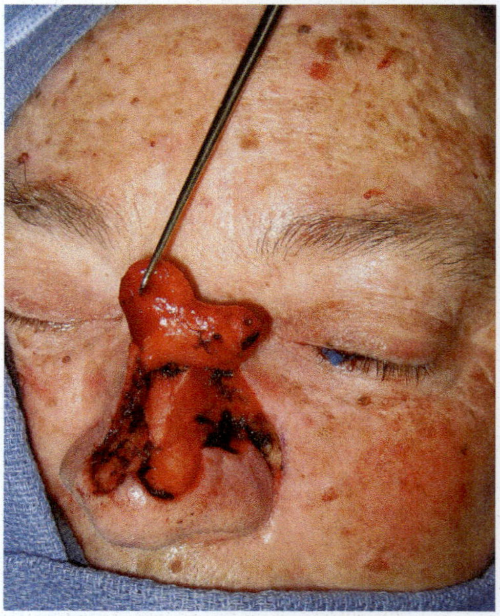

Fig. 3.11 Elevation of the bilobed flap prior to transfer.

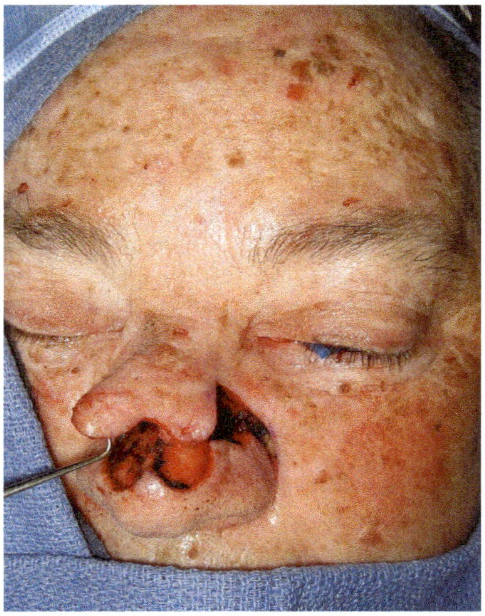

Fig. 3.12 Evaluation of the rotation of the flap into the defect.

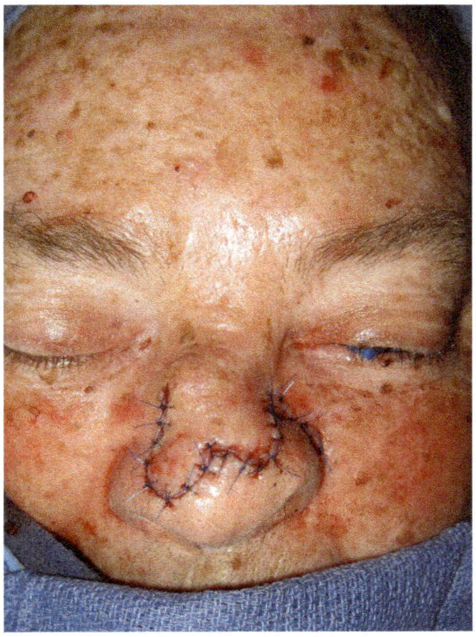

Fig. 3.13 Transfer and inset of the flap into the nasal defect.

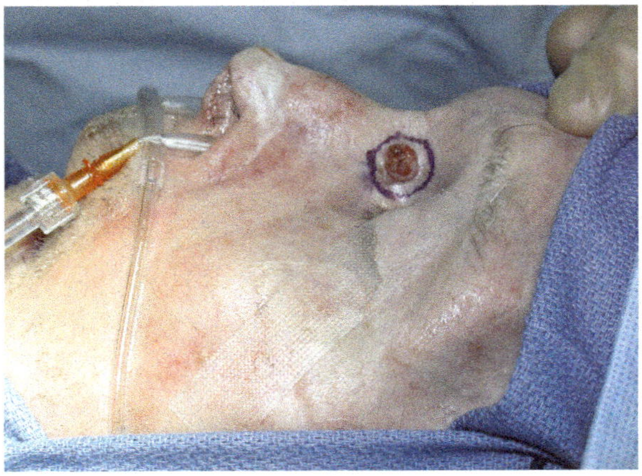

Fig. 3.14 Location of a skin cancer in the medial canthal region of the left eye.

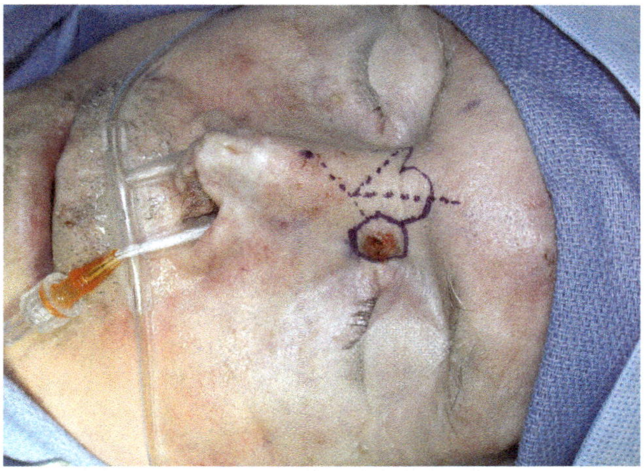

Fig. 3.15 Design of a bilobed flap after excision of the lesion.

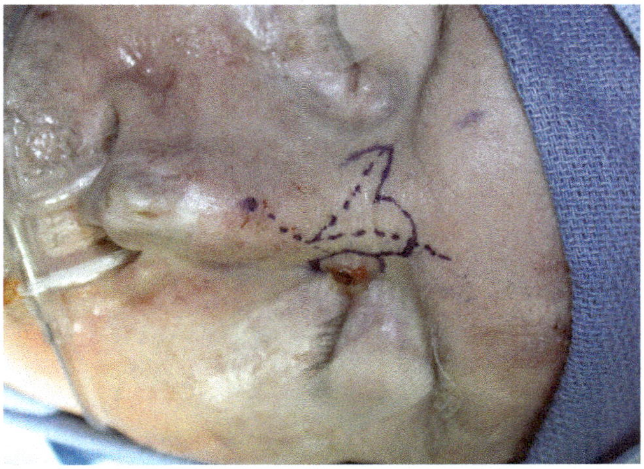

Fig. 3.16 View of the nasal dorsum from above showing planned transfer.

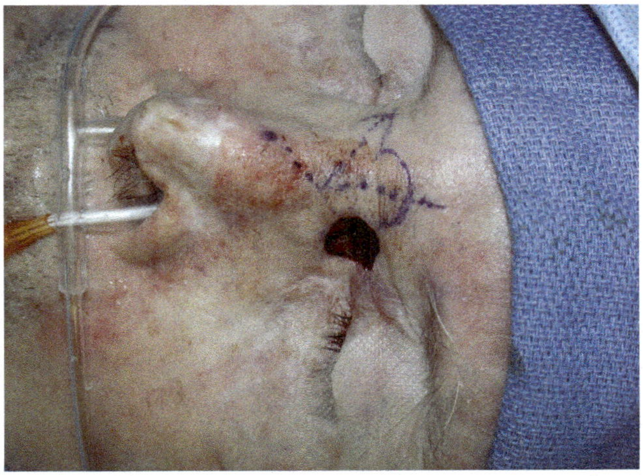

Fig. 3.17 Lateral view of the planned bilobed rotational flap.

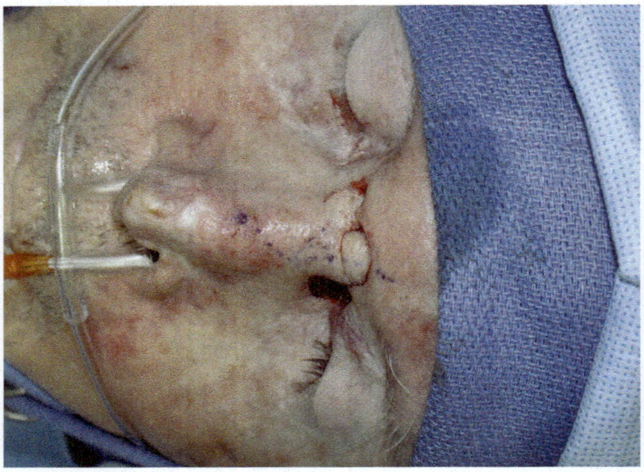

Fig. 3.18 Incision of the bilobed flap prior to transfer.

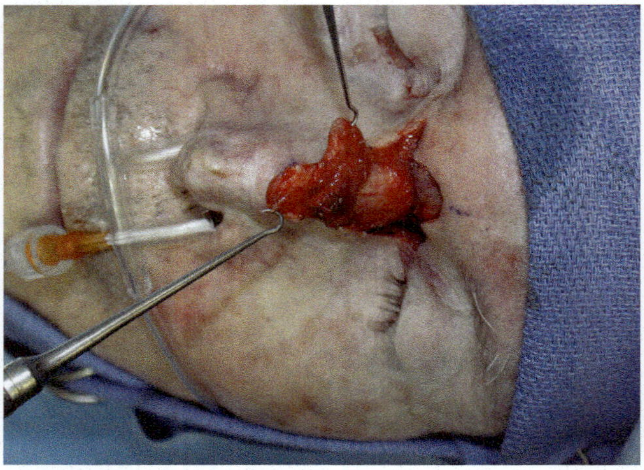

Fig. 3.19 Elevation of the flap prior to rotation into the defect.

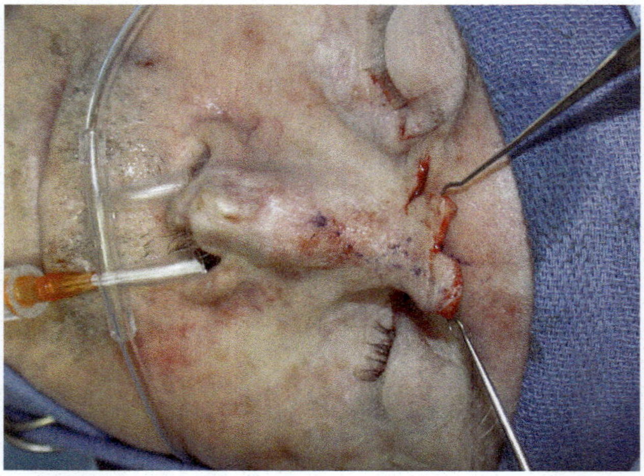

Fig. 3.20 Assessment of flap advancement after undermining.

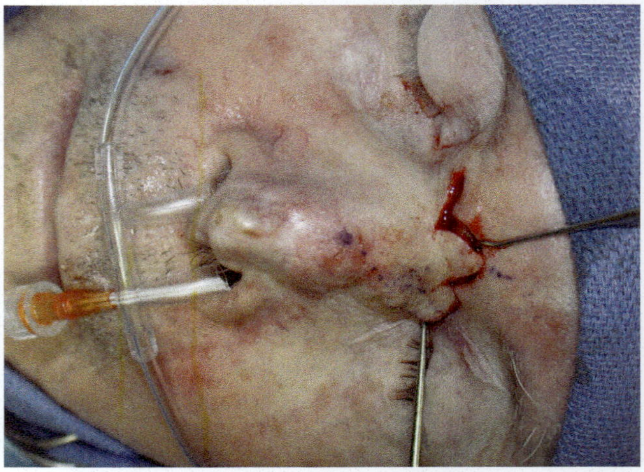

Fig. 3.21 Assessment of flap rotation to the defect.

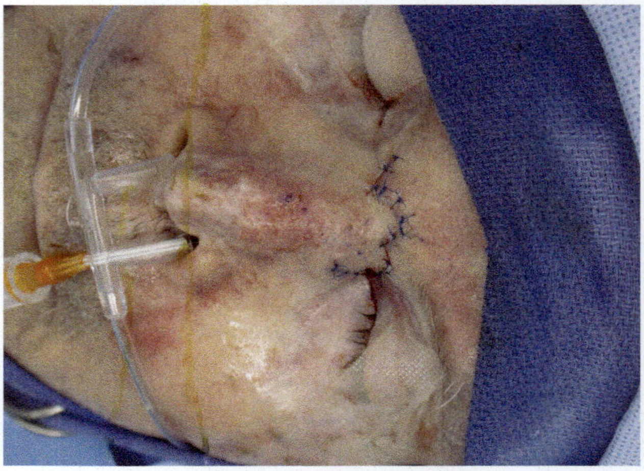

Fig. 3.22 View of inset of the flap into the defect.

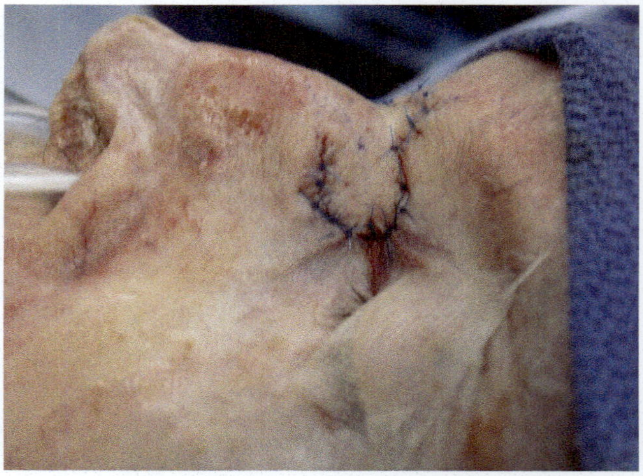

Fig. 3.23 Lateral view of the inset of the flap.

References

1. Esser JFS. Gestielte loakle Nasenplastik mit zweizipfligen Lappen, Deckung des sekundaren Defektes vom ersten Zipfel durch den Zweiten. *Dtsch Zschr Chir* 1918; 143:385–390.
2. Zitelli JA. The bilobed flap for nasal reconstruction. *Arch Dermatol* 1989; 125(7):957–959.
3. Zoumalan RA, Hazan C, Levine V, Shah A. Analysis of vector alignment with the Zitelli bilobed flap for nasal defect repair. *Arch Facial Plast Surg* 2008; 10(3):181–185.

Chapter 4
Rhomboid flap

Introduction

Limberg initially described the rhomboid flap in the 1940s,[1] and thus it is often referred to as the Limberg flap. The rhomboid flap was later modified by Lister and Gibson to encompass the classic angles of 60 and 120 degrees with equal lengths of all sides.[2] Several modifications of this flap have been described; however, most have been related to the mathematical principles of the flap rather than the clinical application.[3,4] In 1987, Quaba described a clinical modification of the rhomboid flap where he maintained the circular shape of the defect and the flap was kept nearly the same shape.[5] The modification allowed for an increased number of options for reconstruction of the defect rather than the conventional four flap options.

The rhomboid flap has long become one of the mainstay flaps for reconstruction of small to medium-sized head and neck defects. The benefits of this flap are many and the drawbacks few. The use of this flap revolves around the plasticity of the skin and its ability to be moved to adjacent locations without jeopardizing the blood supply to the flap or altering the appearance of the surrounding areas. This flap can be utilized to cover relatively small defects and with some modification of the base defect, one can use multiple rhomboids to cover a relatively large area. This makes the rhomboid flap indispensable for the head and neck surgeon, who needs to be able to perform the technique well.

Anatomy

The anatomy for the rhomboid flap is dependent on the area of the defect. The surgeon needs to be familiar with the local and regional anatomy of the facial region in order to be able to design the flap in what will be the most esthetically pleasing final result while at the same time not compromising or altering the local function of regional structures.

Like any other cutaneous flap, the rhomboid flap is also dependent on cutaneous perfusion. The cutaneous flap is based on the vascular anatomy of the skin, representing a continuum from small local random flaps based on the subdermal plexus to perforator flaps based on musculocutaneous or septocutaneous perforators of the deep fascia.[6]

Flap harvest

Single rhomboid flap

- The area to be excised is marked with the appropriate margins to render the patient disease-free from an oncologic standpoint.
- Once the marking is completed, the next step is to draw a rhomboid with the planned excision area inside this rhomboid. The internal angles formed by the sides of the rhomboid should be 60 degrees and 120 degrees (Figure 4.1).
- The next step is to determine the best area of tissue, which can be moved into the defect area without causing distortion to the surrounding area.
- The areas in the head and neck that are particularly important to consider would be areas in or around the eyebrows, the forehead hairline, the eyelids, upper and lower lips, and the nose (Figure 4.2).
- The marking is done by extending a line directly out from the 120 angle of the rhomboid to a length equal to the width of the defect.

Local and Regional Flaps in Head & Neck Reconstruction: A Practical Approach, First Edition. Rui Fernandes.

Companion website: www.wiley.com/go/fernandes/flapsreconstruction

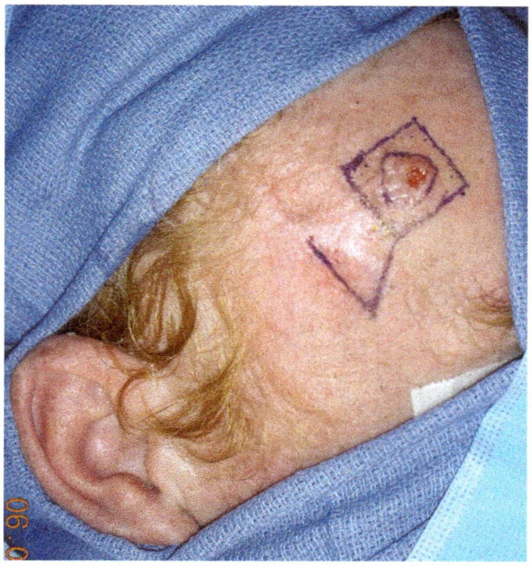

Fig. 4.1 View of the planned excision of a forehead lesion with plan for a rhomboid flap.

- Next, another line is drawn from the end of the previously drawn line parallel to the side of the rhomboid and equal in length to the side of the rhomboid.
- This area will be the tissue that will be moved onto the defect site.
- The marked area is incised down to the connective tissue (Figure 4.3).
- The flap is elevated and the area is undermined in a wide area so as to allow for the transposition of the flap into the defect (Figure 4.4).

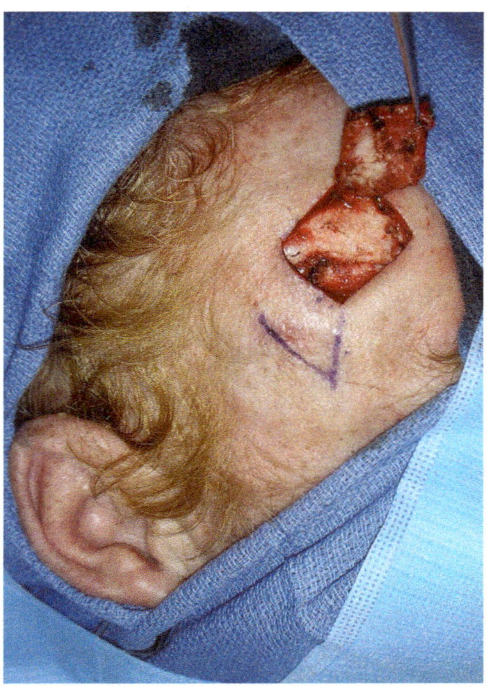

Fig. 4.2 Excision of the lesion prior to flap elevation.

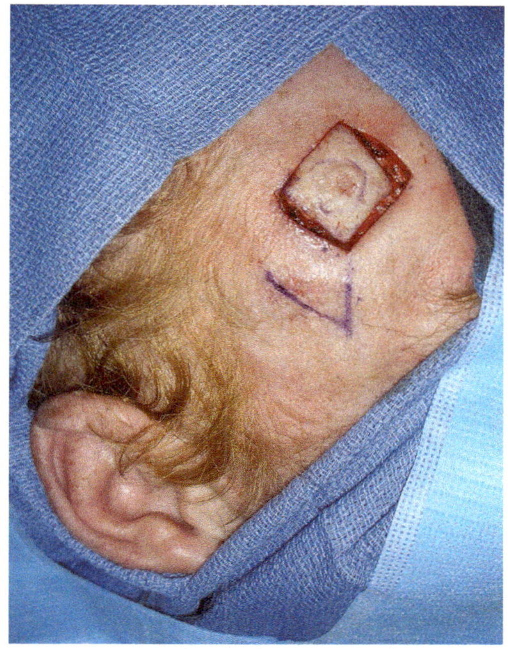

Fig. 4.3 Completed excision prior to removal of the lesion.

- The flap is inset by placing key anchoring sutures at the sites of maximal tension (Figure 4.5).
- Dermal sutures are placed to reapproximate the tissues and the skin is closed according to surgeon's preference (Figure 4.6).

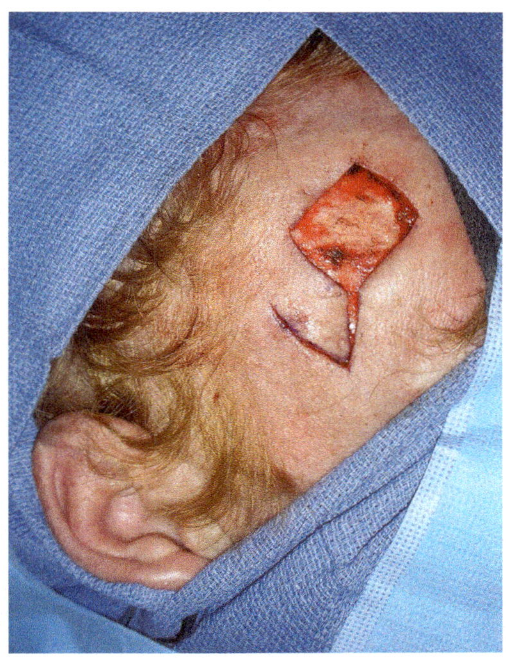

Fig. 4.4 Incision of the planned rhomboid flap, note the position of the flap is done so as to minimize disruption to the position of the eyebrow and forehead.

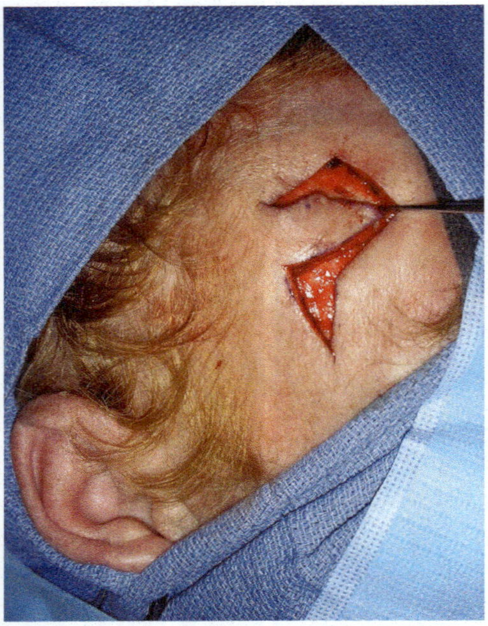

Fig. 4.5 Rotation of the flap into the defect after appropriate undermining.

Multiple rhomboid flaps

- For larger defects, where a single rhomboid may be deemed unsuitable for coverage, the use of multiple rhomboids to close the defect can be considered.
- The key difference between using single or multiple rhomboid flaps is the design of the defect area.

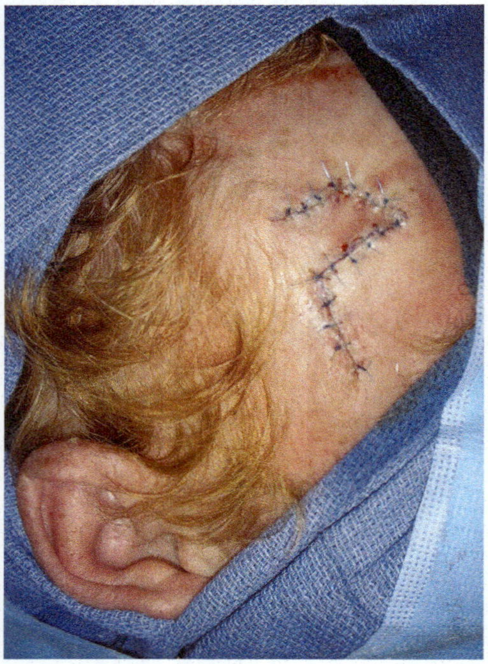

Fig. 4.6 Inset of the flap into the defect.

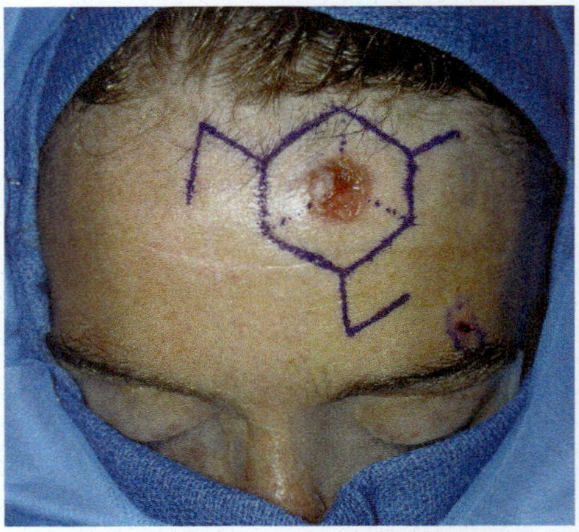

Fig. 4.7 Design of multiple rhomboid flap for a planned resection of a large forehead lesion.

- The site to be excised should be viewed as multiples of rhomboids within the defect area (Figure 4.7).
- In cases where the use of multiple rhomboids is contemplated, the number of rhomboids required to repair the defect needs to be decided.
- The excision of the tumor is carried out followed by raising the respective flaps with wide undermining and transposition of the flaps (Figure 4.8).
- The flaps are then closed as per routine by first placing dermal stitches along the areas of maximum tension (Figure 4.9).

Case #1

A 77-year-old male was referred for excision of a biopsy-proven squamous cell carcinoma of the right cheek region

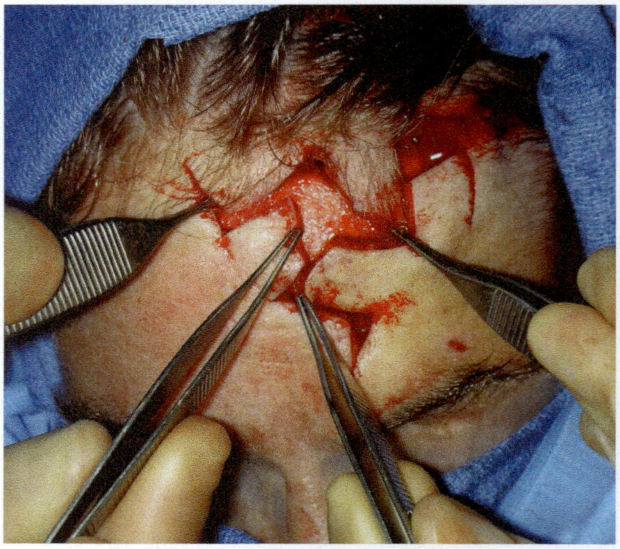

Fig. 4.8 Assessment of the flap rotation into the defect prior to inset.

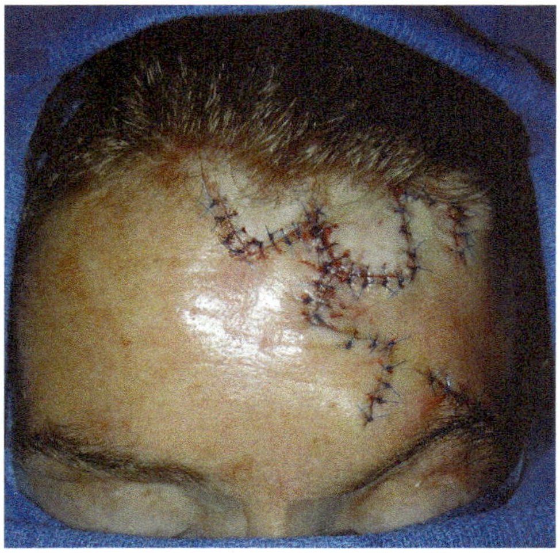

Fig. 4.9 Inset of the flaps, note that the hairline has not been altered.

with close approximation to the periorbital region (Figure 4.10). The area was excised in a rhomboid fashion and the markings for the rhomboid flap were made to move the tissues further away from the orbital region to prevent distortion of the eyebrows and eyelids and displacement of the hairline (Figure 4.11). The area was mobilized and the tissue was transferred to the defect with minimal distortion of the eyelid or the surrounding tissues (Figure 4.12). The final outcome early on the postoperative course showed minimal distortion of the area with very pleasing esthetics (Figure 4.13).

Case #2

An 84-year-old Caucasian female was referred to the practice for excision of a skin malignancy located on the left forehead region approximating the hairline (Figure 4.14). A decision was made to perform a wide local

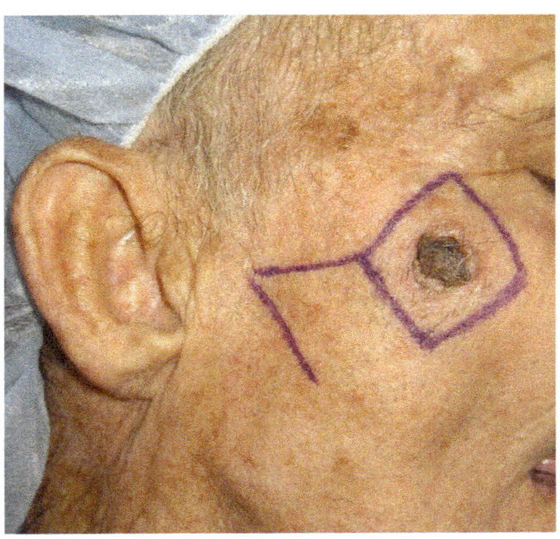

Fig. 4.10 Marking for excision of a cheek lesion.

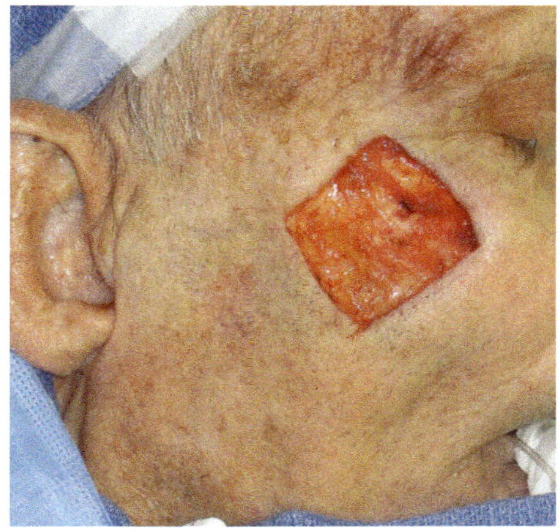

Fig. 4.11 Excised lesion prior to elevation of a rhomboid flap.

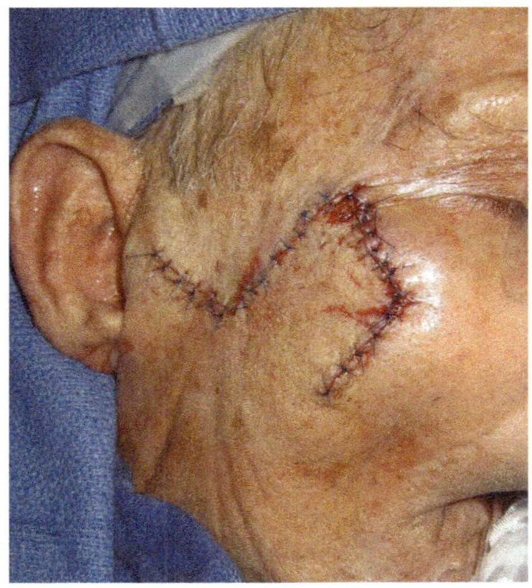

Fig. 4.12 Inset of flap into the cheek without deforming the lower eyelid.

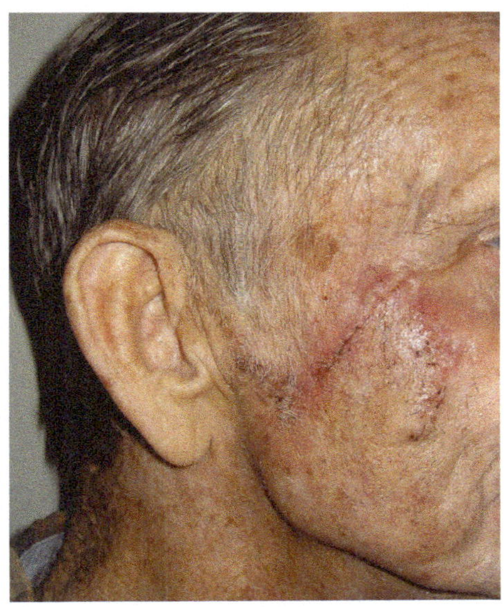

Fig. 4.13 Early appearance of the healing reconstruction.

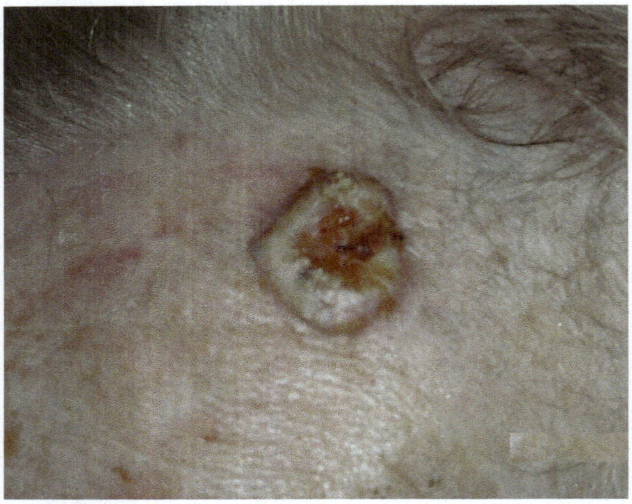

Fig. 4.14 Large forehead skin malignancy.

excision with immediate reconstruction with a rhomboid flap. The markings for the flap were made to include two possible transpositions which would not result in the distortion of the hairline (Figure 4.15). The lesion was excised (Figure 4.16). After evaluating the options, the right superior flap option was chosen and elevated (Figure 4.17). The flap was then inset into the defect with minimal distortion of the hairline (Figure 4.18).

Case #3

An 86-year-old Caucasian female was referred for excision of a longstanding scalp lesion, which had recently been confirmed to be a squamous cell carcinoma (Figure 4.19). The workup prior to excision revealed that

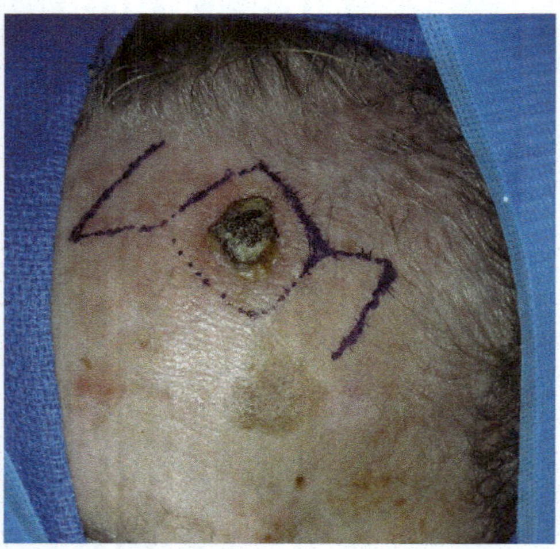

Fig. 4.15 Surgical planning for excision of lesion and reconstruction with rhomboid flap.

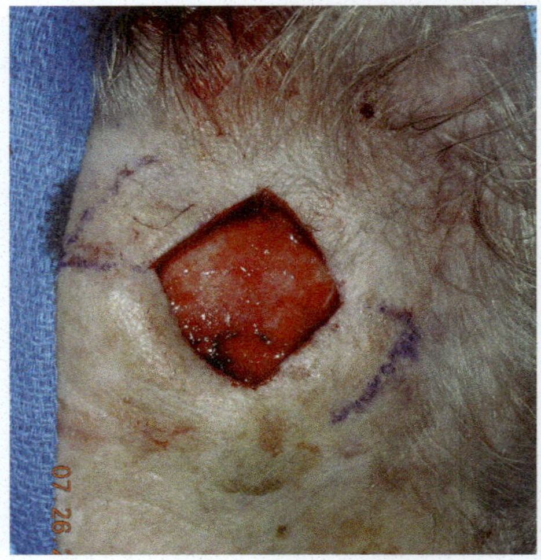

Fig. 4.16 Excised lesion prior to elevation of the flap.

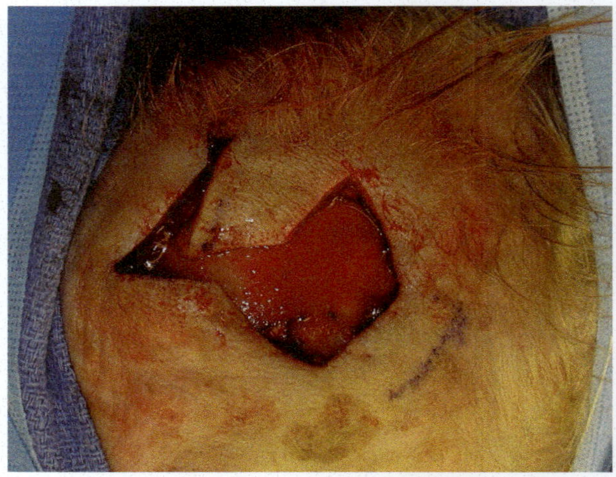

Fig. 4.17 Elevation of the rhomboid flap with its base towards the hairline

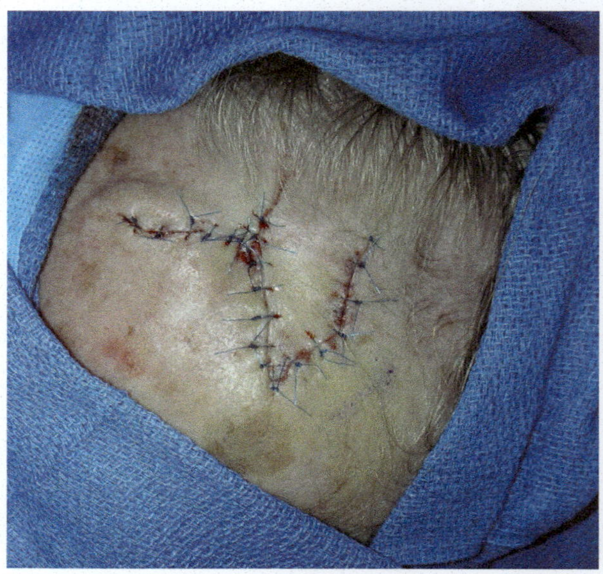

Fig. 4.18 Inset of the flap into the defect.

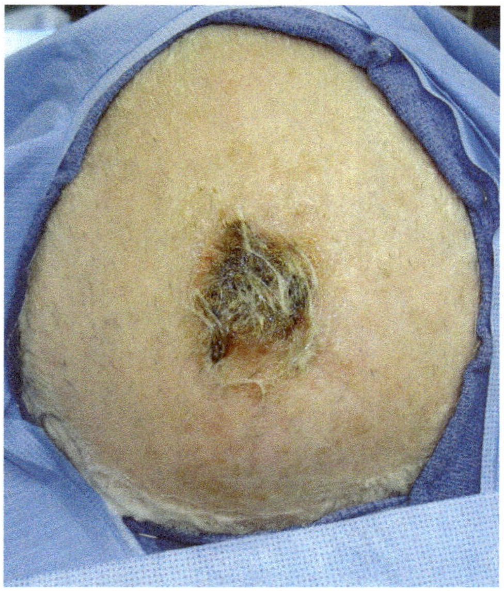

Fig. 4.19 Appearance of a midline scalp lesion.

the tumor did not invade the calvarium and therefore was amenable to a conservative excision and reconstruction (Figure 4.20). Due to the patient's numerous comorbidities, it was deemed that they would be better served with an immediate tissue rearrangement using multiple rhomboid flaps. The excision was carried out as if there were three rhomboid flaps fused together to make one large defect (Figure 4.21). The lesion was excised and confirmed that there was an intact calvarium and therefore amenable for the reconstruction with the rhomboid flaps (Figure 4.22). The patient went on to have an uneventful recovery and healing (Figure 4.23).

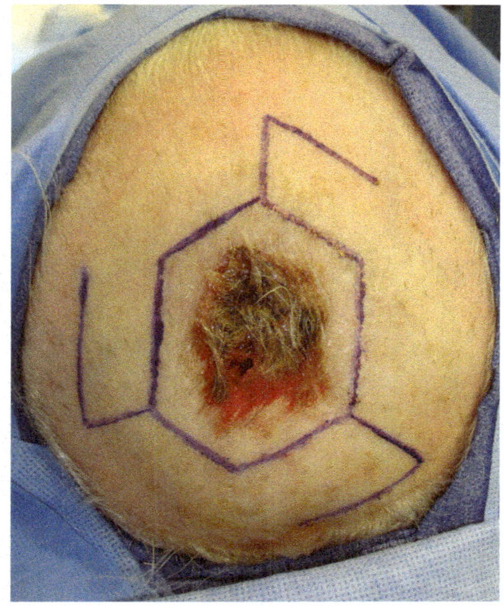

Fig. 4.21 Design of multiple rhomboid flaps based on a design of the resection in the shape of three independent rhomboids next to each other.

Case #4

A 63-year-old Caucasian male was referred for resection of a biopsy-proven melanoma of the left temporal region. A plan was made to carry out resection of the lesion with

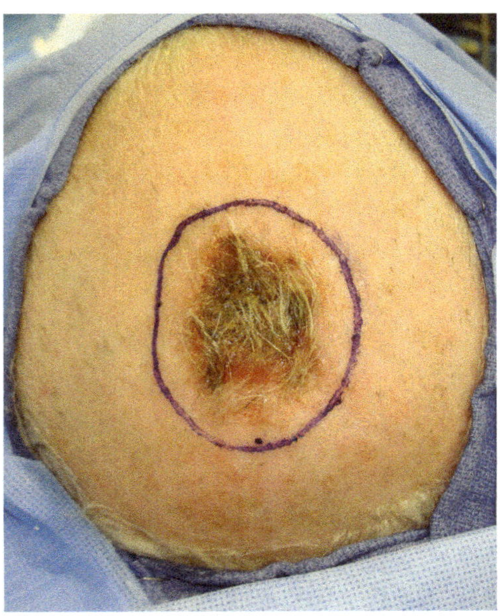

Fig. 4.20 Planned excision of the lesion, note that this will create a very large defect.

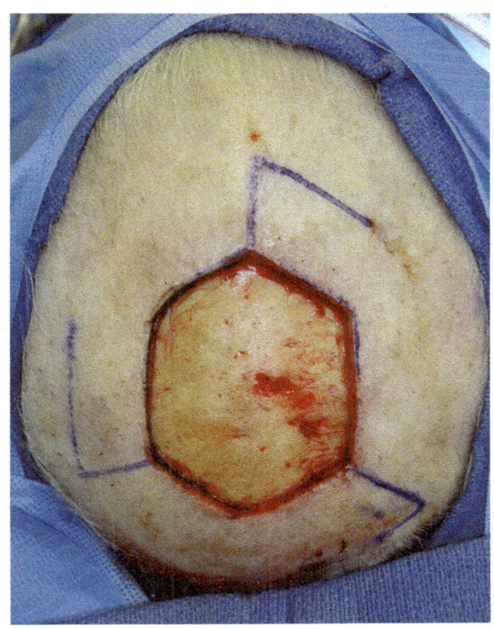

Fig. 4.22 Excised lesion with its resultant defect prior to flap elevation.

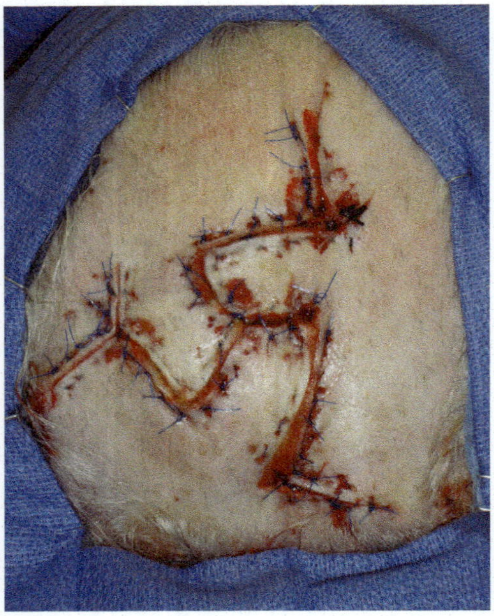

Fig. 4.23 Elevated and transferred flaps into the defect.

simultaneous sentinel node biopsy and reconstruction of the acquired defect with a rhomboid flap (Figure 4.24). The area was excised after the sentinel node dissection had been performed (Figures 4.25 and 4.26). Because the location of the lesion was immediately adjacent to the left brow, the reconstruction necessitated the transposition of the flap from the superior aspect (Figure 4.27). The area was undermined and the advancement of the flap was checked to insure that it would not result in the displacement of the brow (Figure 4.28). The flap was inset and the area repaired without distortion (Figure 4.29).

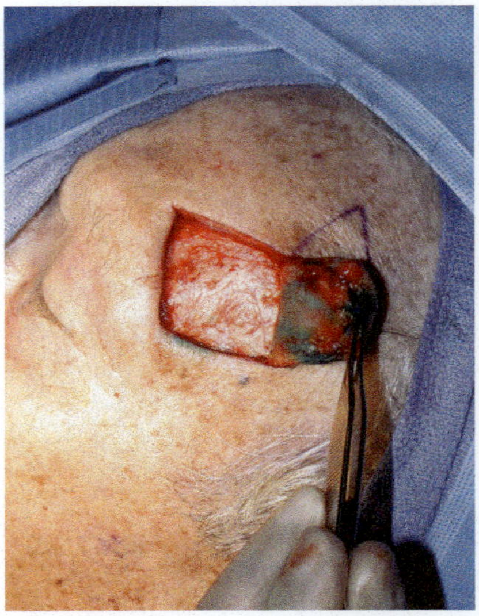

Fig. 4.25 Excision of the melanoma.

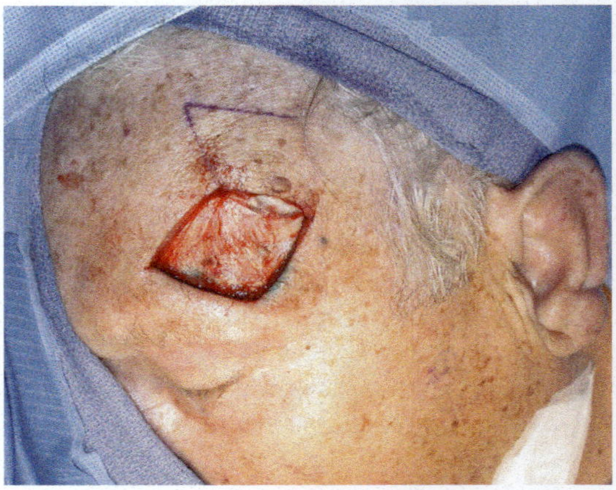

Fig. 4.26 Defect after excision of the melanoma, markings for the rhomboid flap so as not to alter the hairline nor the eyebrow.

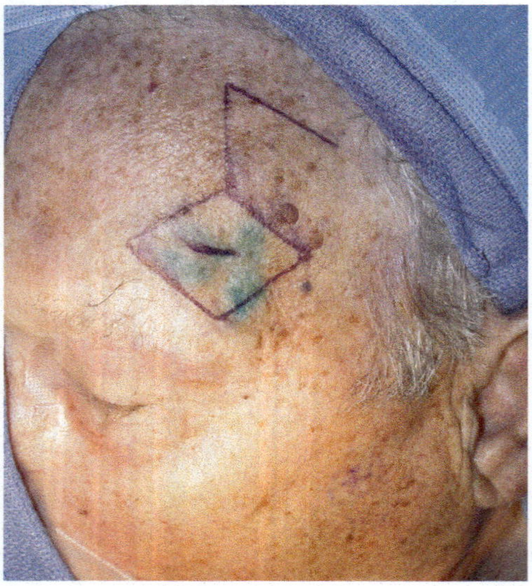

Fig. 4.24 Markings for excision of a melanoma of the forehead region.

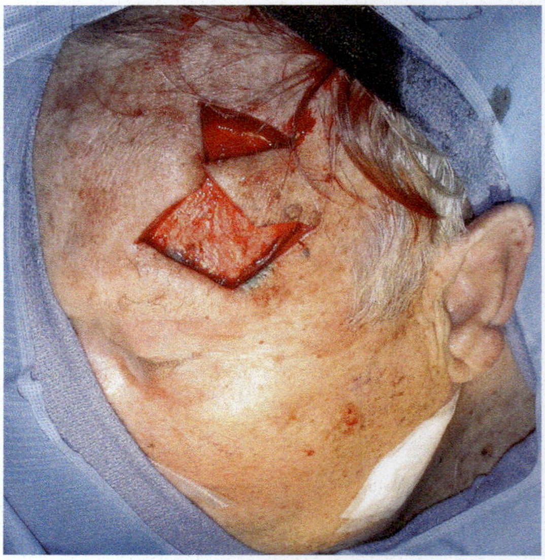

Fig. 4.27 Elevation of the flap with undermining prior to transfer.

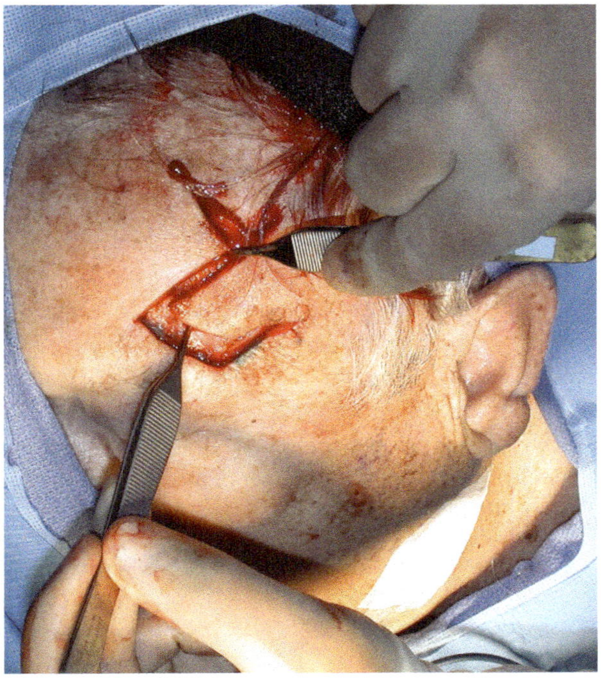

Fig. 4.28 Assessment of the degree of advancement achieved with the flap.

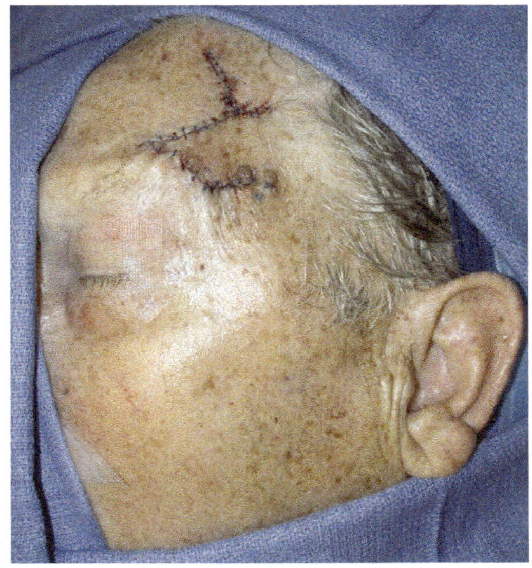

Fig. 4.29 Inset of the rhomboid flap into the defect.

References

1. Limberg A. *Mathematical Principles of Local Plastic Surgery Procedure on the Surface of the Human Body*. Leningrad: Medgis, 1946.
2. Lister G, Gibson T. Closure of rhomboid skin defects: the flaps of Limberg and Dufourmentel. *Br J Plast Surg* 1972; 25:300–314.
3. Becker F. Rhomboid flap in facial reconstruction. *Arch Otolaryngol* 1979; 105:569–573.
4. Dufourmentel C. An L-shaped flap for lozenge-shaped defects. Transactions of the Third International Congress of Plastic Surgery, p722, Amsterdam: Excerpta Medica Foundation, 1963.
5. Quaba A, Sommerlad B. A square peg into a round hole: a modified rhomboid flap and its clinical application. *Br J Plast Surg* 1987; 40:163–170.
6. Maciel-Miranda A, Morris S, Hallock G. Local flaps, including pedicled perforator flaps: anatomy, technique, and applications. *Plast Reconstr Surg* 2013; 131:896e–911e.

Chapter 5
Crescentic flap

Introduction

Webster published the first description of the crescentic perialar flap in 1955.[1] Since then the crescentic flap technique has been used in many forms and with various descriptors.[2–4] The basic rationale for this flap is the removal of tissue in the form of a crescent in the perialar or chin region, which then allows for the advancement of the surrounding tissues to repair an adjacent defect. This technique finds a unique niche in the repair of both upper and lower lip defects. The crescentic flap enables reconstruction of defects that would otherwise require the use of cross-lip flaps or other less elegant options.

The main advantage of using the crescentic flap is that it enables repair of the defect with minimal tissue distortion. The placement of the incision gives a less conspicuous final scar.[5] Further, the use of the perialar crescentic flap to repair either upper or lower lip defects, preserves the oral sphincter.

The repair of the lip is addressed in detail in Chapter 22.

Anatomy

The anatomy as it relates to the use of the crescentic flap depends on the site where the defect is located.

The most common sites for crescentic flap repair are the upper lip or the lower lip. In cases where the defect is located in the lower lip, the anatomical area of interest will be the perialar tissues and the upper lip itself. The area of the perialar zone is an intricate anatomical region. The subtleties of the area of the nasal sill and the upper lip allow for an easy cosmetic alteration and therefore the potential for a less than ideal result. The blood supply for a flap in the alar region (i.e., the perialar crescentic flap) is the superior labial artery and the facial artery. The veins are the accompanying veins. The mobilized flap will be a portion of the upper lip supplied by the superior labial artery and vein as well as a portion of the cheek, which will be advanced medially to restore the missing tissue; thus, the facial artery and vein are the blood supply to this portion of the flap.

In cases where the flap is being used to repair of lower lip defects, the anatomical area of interest will be the area lateral to the labiomental crease. The blood supply to the portion of the lip to be mobilized is the inferior labial artery and vein and the tissues lateral to the defect site are supplied by branches from the facial artery and vein as well as the mental and submental arteries and veins.

Flap harvest

Perialar crescentic flap

- The area of the upper lip defect is measured to determine the width for the excision (Figure 5.1).
- The width is then drawn along the floor of the nose and laterally along the ala of the nose in the shape of a crescent (Figure 5.2).
- The greatest width of the crescent is equal to the width of the defect. If the width is determined to be too large, the width is divided in half and distributed to either side of the perialar region.
- The design of the perialar crescentic flap enables advancement of the cheek into the missing upper lip defect without distorting the nose.
- In cases where the defect extends below the ala of the nose to potentially undermine the support of the nose, this is taken into account when excising the crescentic

Local and Regional Flaps in Head & Neck Reconstruction: A Practical Approach, First Edition. Rui Fernandes.

Companion website: www.wiley.com/go/fernandes/flapsreconstruction

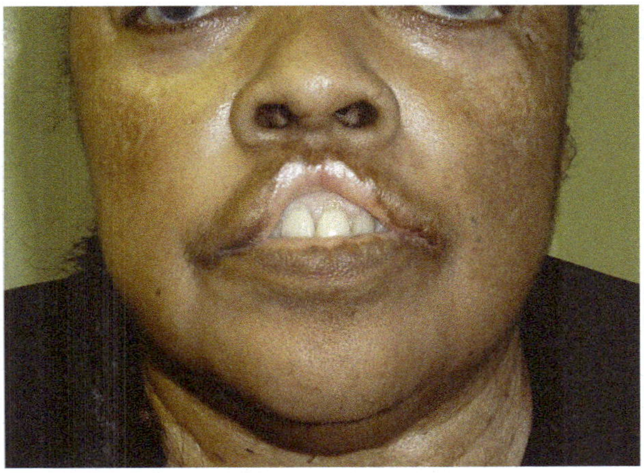

Fig. 5.1 Appearance of the upper lip after loss of the central/philtral unit.

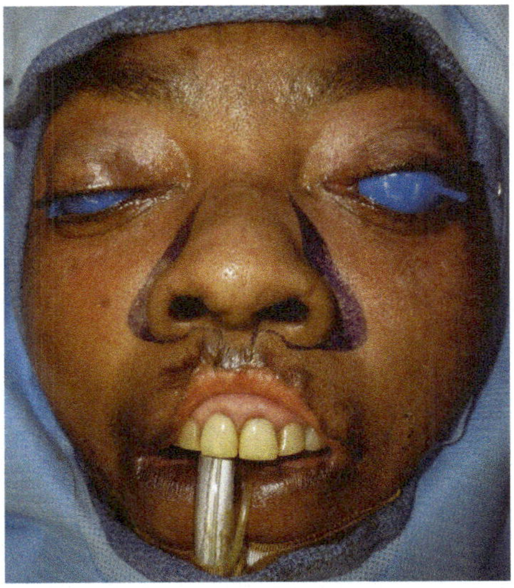

Fig. 5.2 Markings for bilateral crescentic flaps.

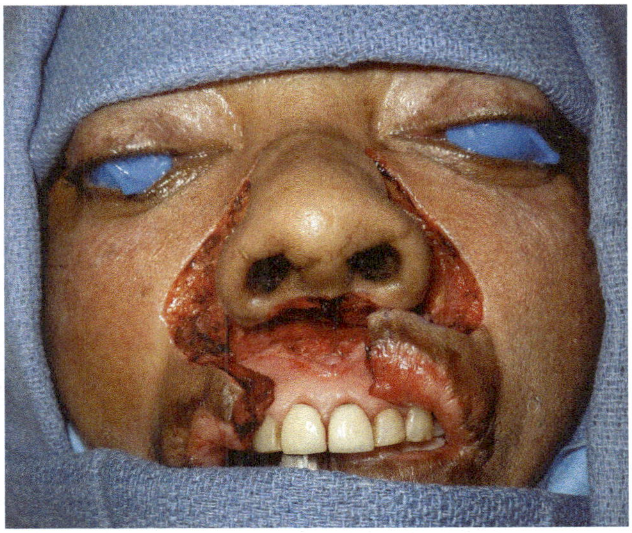

Fig. 5.4 Closer view of the excised tissue and developed flaps.

area and only the skin in this area is removed, so support is provided under the nose and ala.

- Once the crescent is drawn, a full thickness excision of the area crescent is performed (unless nasal ala support is needed) (Figures 5.3 to 5.6).
- The mucosa is incised along the buccal vestibule and the path of the predicted advancement.
- The remaining lip and cheek is then advanced into the defect.
- The area is then closed in layers with first reapproximation of the orbicularis muscle (Figure 5.7).
- The mucosa is closed along the vestibule and the lip.

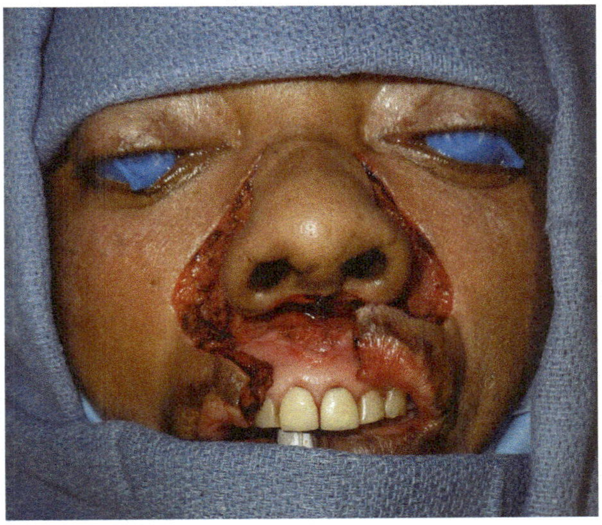

Fig. 5.3 Excision of bilateral perialar tissue to allow for advancement of bilateral upper lip flaps.

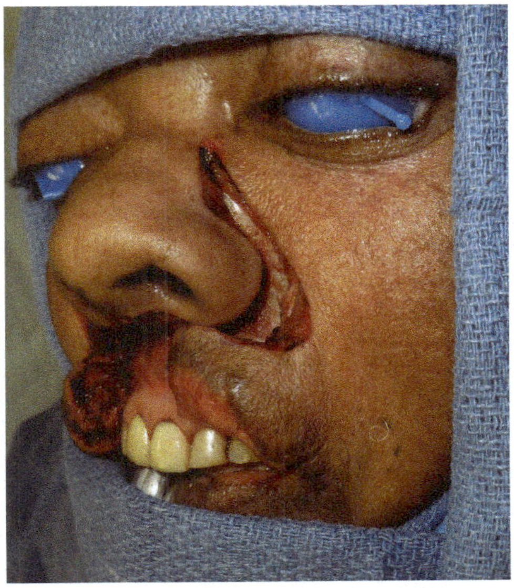

Fig. 5.5 Lateral view of the flap. Note that the excision is extended to the anterior wall of the maxilla.

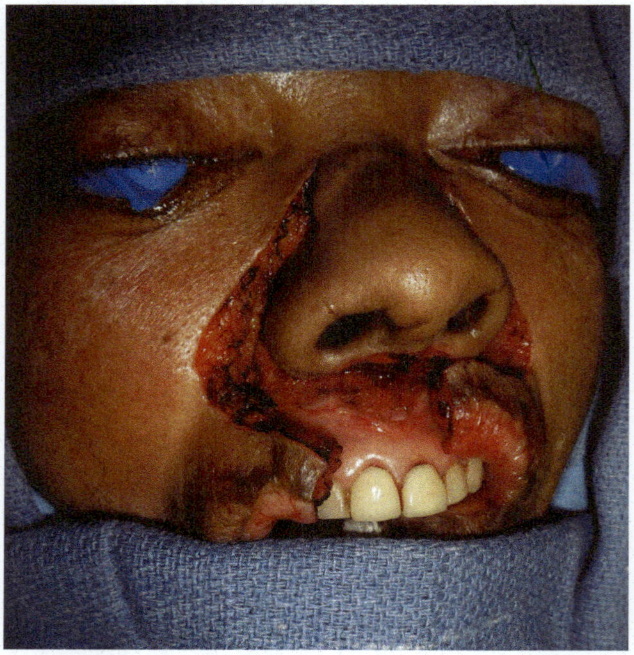

Fig. 5.6 Contralateral view of the flap.

- Deep sutures are placed along the ala of the nose and the nasal sidewall.
- The final closure is that of skin.
- The final outcome is often very pleasing with minimal evidence of the donor site while preserving the oral sphincter (Figures 5.8 to 5.11).

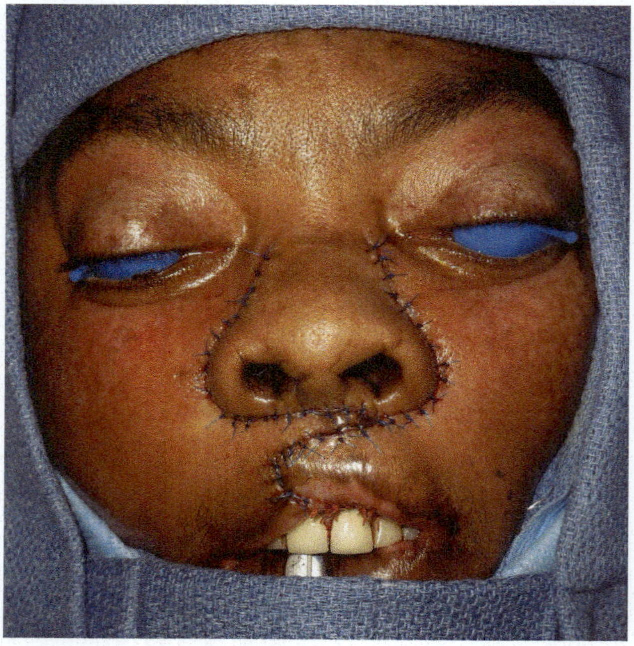

Fig. 5.7 View after bilateral advancement of the flaps.

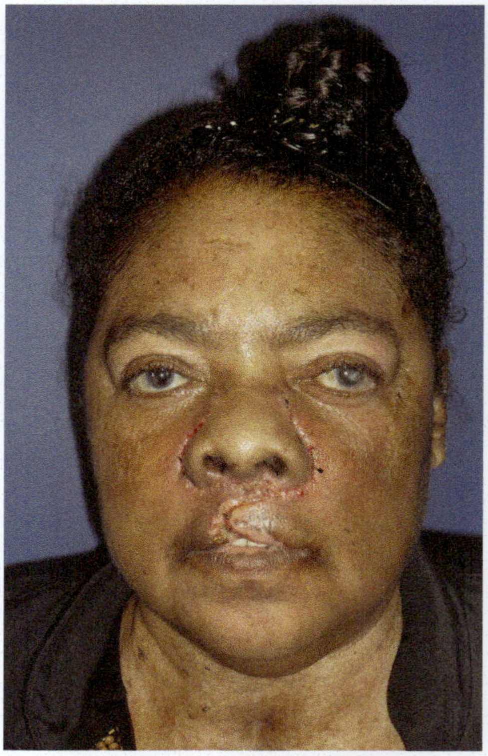

Fig. 5.8 Early postoperative view. Note that the central defect has been eliminated.

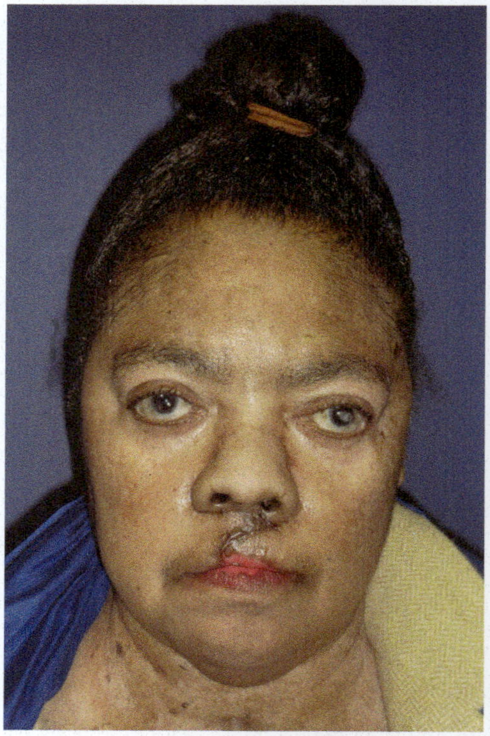

Fig. 5.9 Late view of the healed upper lip after bilateral crescentic flaps.

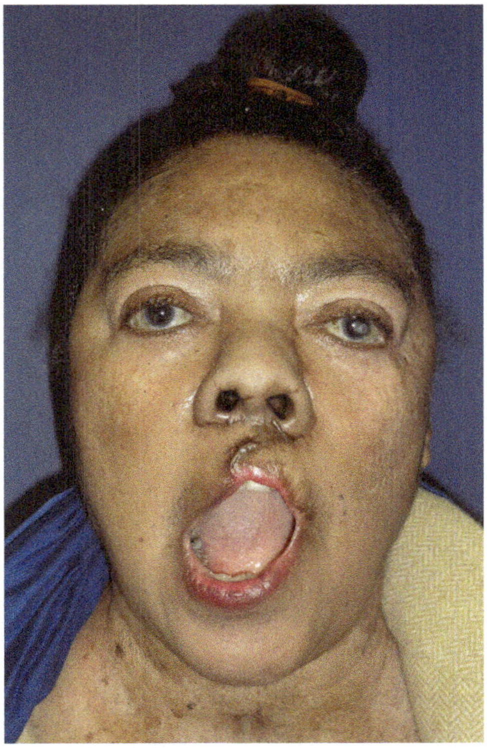

Fig. 5.10 Note that there is no restriction in mouth opening.

Crescentic flap for lower lip

- The area of the planned defect in the lower lip is marked and measured to determine the width of the expected defect.

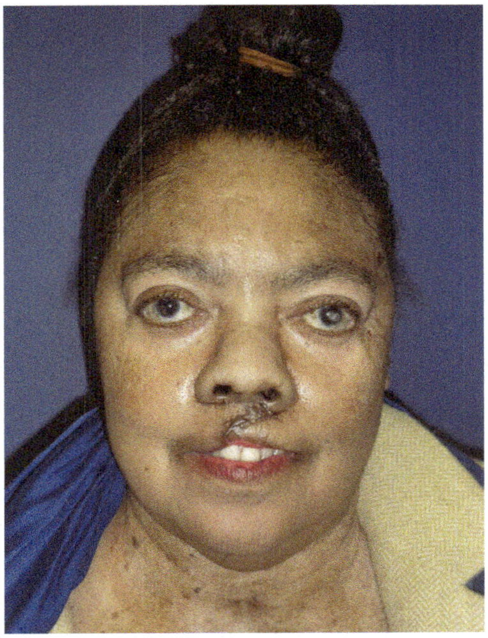

Fig. 5.11 Patient has good lip movement with animation.

- The measurement should be made prior to excision of the defect to obtain the most accurate measurement.
- If the measurement is made after excision of the tumor, the measurement will be greater than the true defect due to muscle contracture.
- The area of the crescentic excision for lower lip reconstruction is along the labiomental crease. The area where the lip meets the chin (i.e., the labiomental crease) is traced from the midline to the lateral aspect of the chin as it begins to curve inferiorly towards the submental area.
- A line is carried out laterally from the labiomental crease at the midline to extend at least half the width of the defect lateral to the previously marked labiomental crease and then parallel to the marking in a crescent shape.
- A full thickness excision of the marked crescent is then carried out.
- A mucosal excision may also be extended along the labial sulcus at the depth of the vestibule.
- The lip and cheek is then advanced towards the midline to repair the defect.
- The muscle is first approximated, followed by the mucosa, and finally the skin.

Case #1

A 30-year-old Caucasian male presented with a biopsy-proven squamous cell carcinoma of the left upper lip (Figure 5.12). Given the size of the lesion and the anticipated defect size (Figure 5.13), a decision was made to reconstruct the defect with a crescentic flap (Figure 5.14). Once the lesion was excised, the crescentic perialar tissue was also excised (Figure 5.14) and the lateral tissue advanced

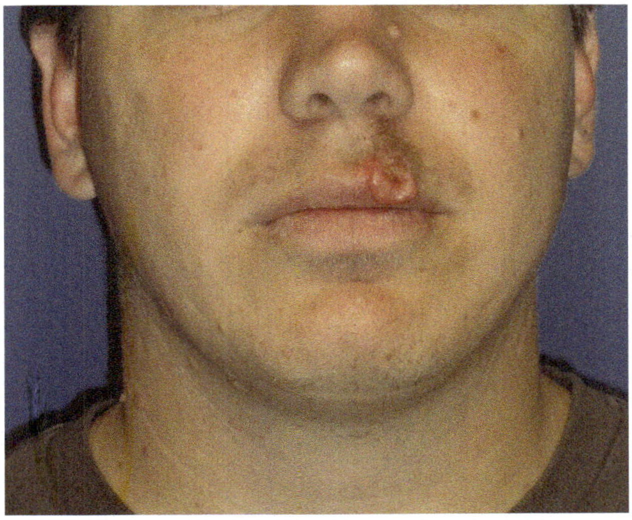

Fig. 5.12 View of large squamous cell carcinoma on the left upper lip.

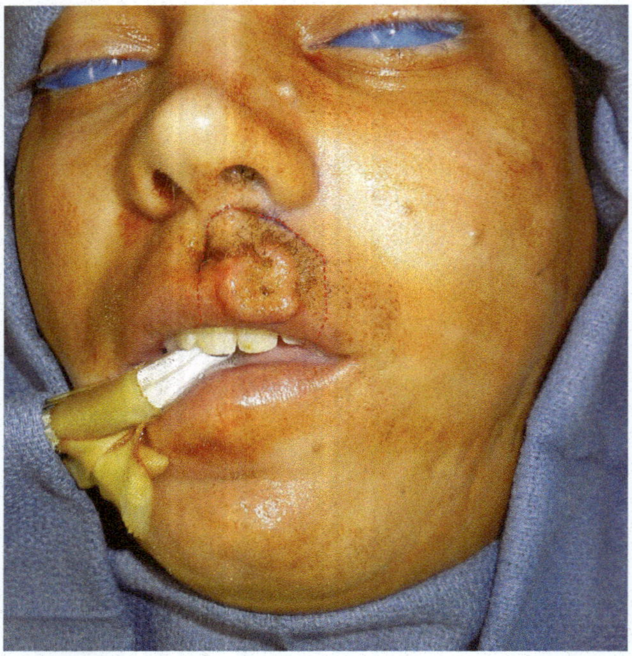

Fig. 5.13 Markings for the excision of the lesion.

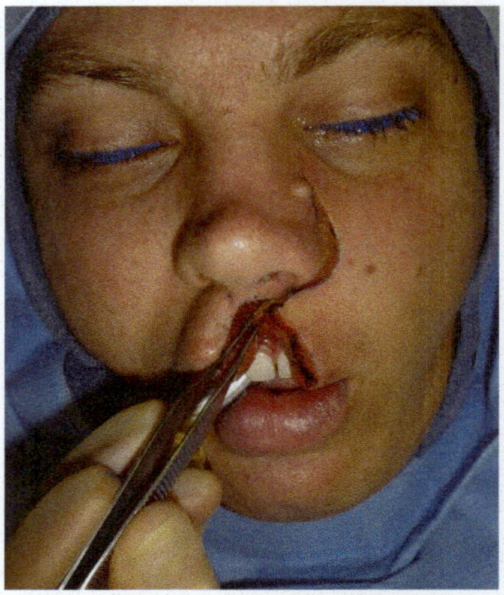

Fig. 5.15 Assessment of advancement of the flap into the defect.

to ensure that it would reach the other side of the defect without tension (Figure 5.15). The flap was advanced and inset to repair the defect while restoring the oral sphincter (Figure 5.16). Early postoperative appearance shows the reconstruction of the defect with good cosmetic appearance and oral opening (Figures 5.17 and 5.18).

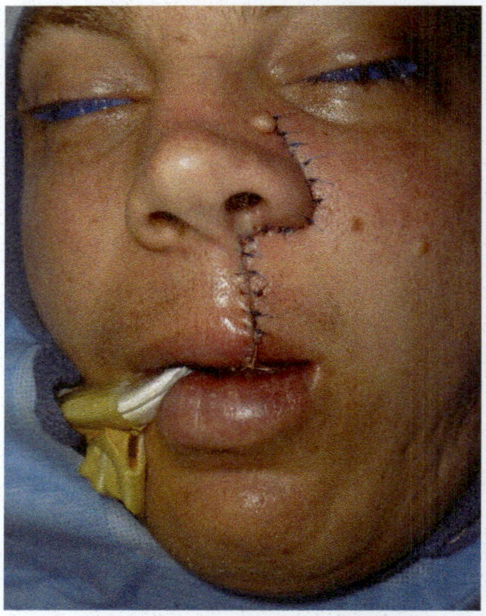

Fig. 5.16 Inset of the flap into the defect. Note that the lip vermellion has been reestablished.

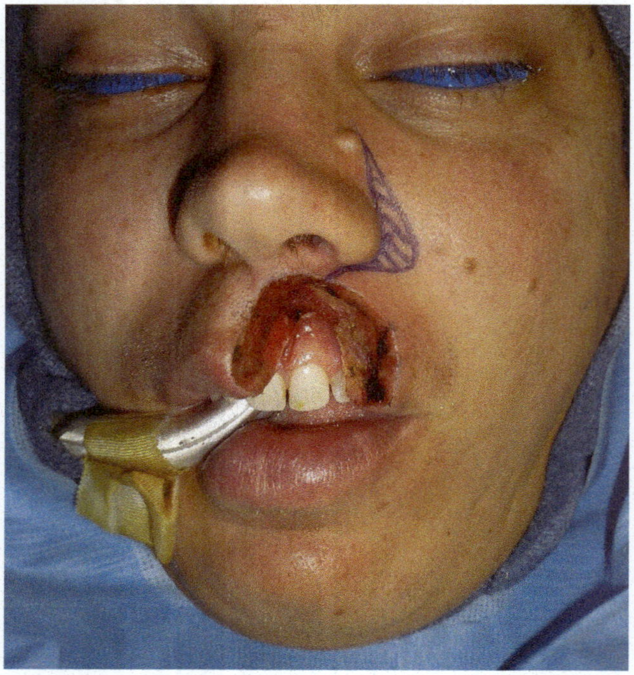

Fig. 5.14 The lesion has been excised the planned excision was marked.

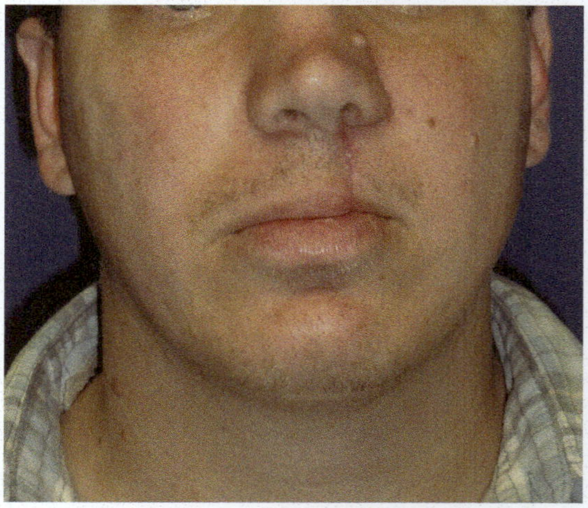

Fig. 5.17 Early postoperative view of the healed reconstruction. Note the good lip form.

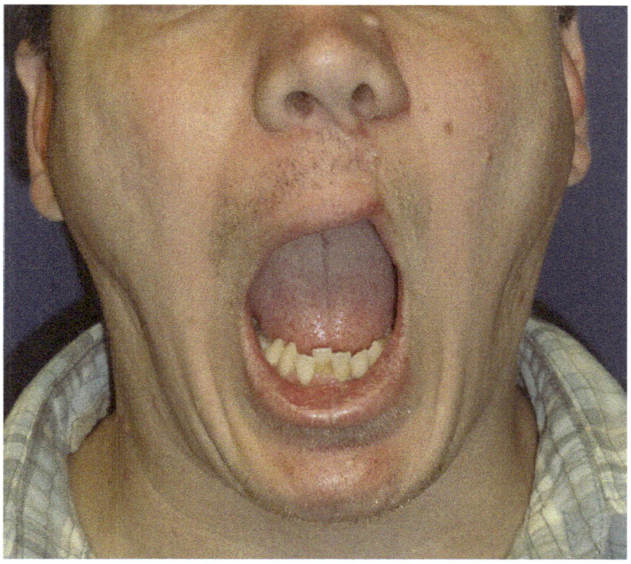

Fig. 5.18 The mouth opening was not restricted.

Case #2

A 61-year-old Caucasian female was referred for treatment of a biopsy-proven squamous cell carcinoma of the left upper lip (Figure 5.19). The planned excision would result in a defect approaching half the length of the upper lip (Figures 5.20 and 5.21). The decision was made to reconstruct the defect by performing bilateral crescentic advancement flaps (Figure 5.22). The size of the defect was divided into equal halves and distributed to either

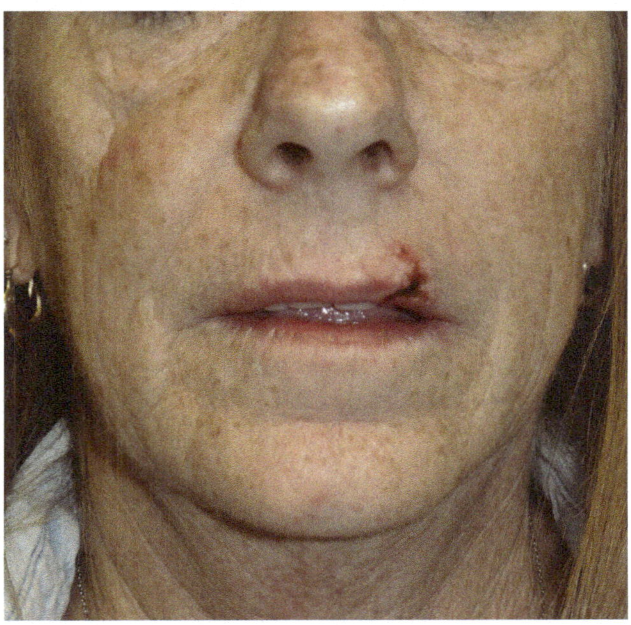

Fig. 5.19 Upper lip lesion with subcutaneous extension.

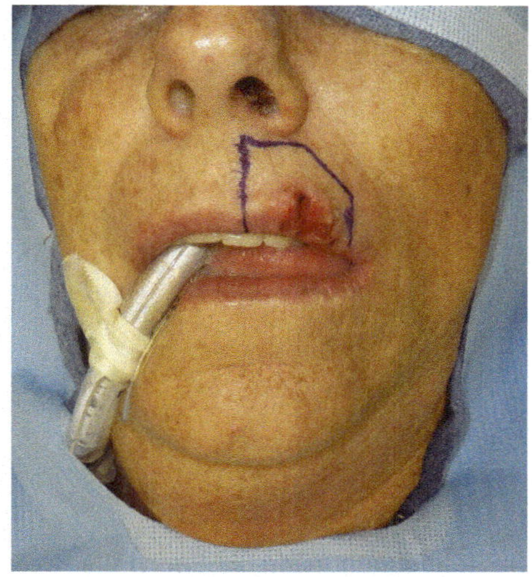

Fig. 5.20 Markings for the resection to obtain negative margins.

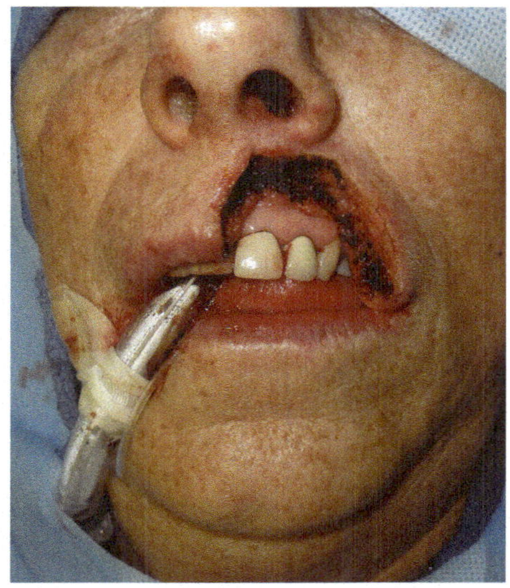

Fig. 5.21 Defect after resection of the lesion; note the significant size of the defect.

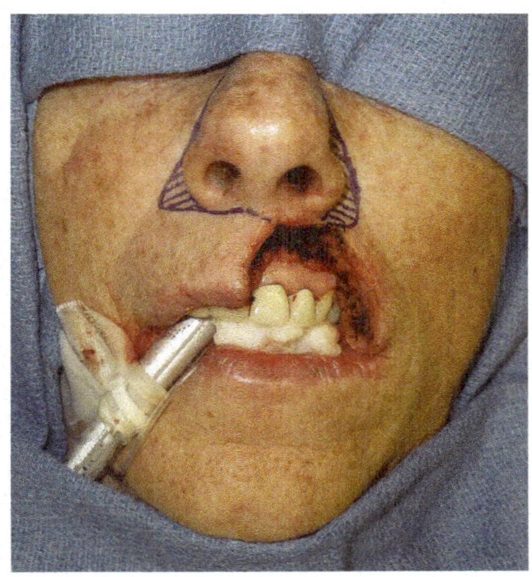

Fig. 5.22 Planned for bilateral excisions and advancement flaps.

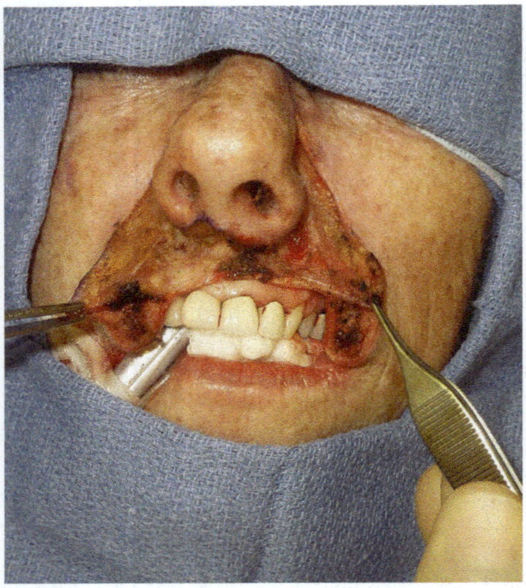

Fig. 5.23 Confirmation of the flap mobility prior to advancement.

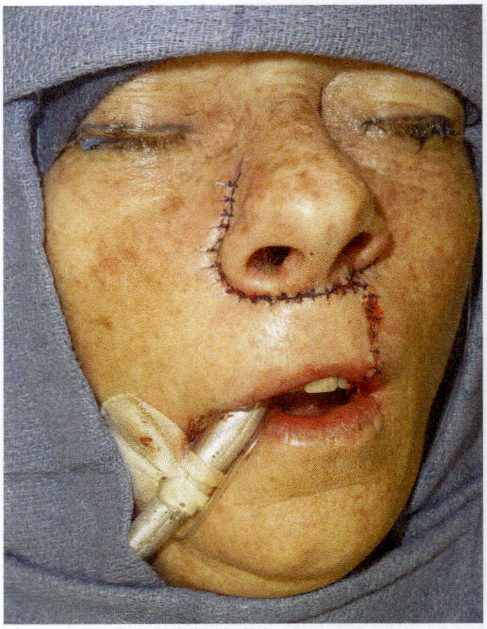

Fig. 5.25 Lateral view of the inset.

side of the nasal region (Figure 5.23). The tissues were resected and the defect was repaired in layers (Figure 5.24 and 5.25). Early postoperative views showed good lip length and cosmetic result (Figures 5.26 and 5.27). Late postoperative view showed a good final outcome with acceptable cosmesis and perioral sphincter without compromise in mouth opening (Figures 5.28 to 5.30).

Case #3

A 65-year-old African American male was referred with a neglected squamous cell carcinoma of the lower lip (Figures 5.31 to 5.33). After discussion with the patient and the recommendation of the multidisciplinary tumor board, a decision was made for resection of the lip tumor

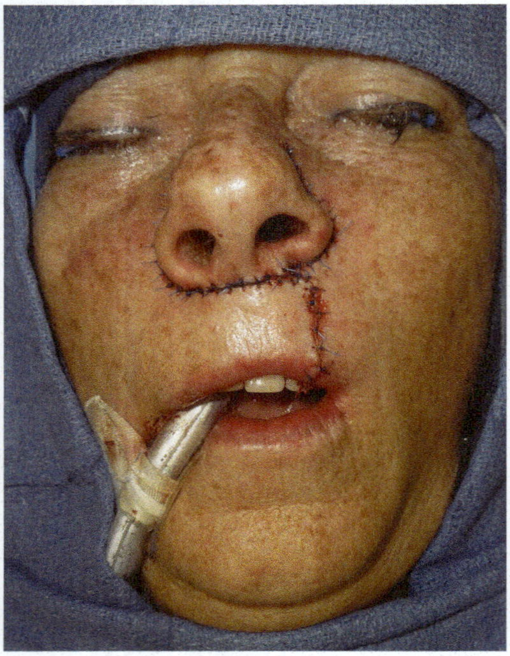

Fig. 5.24 Inset of the flap after bilateral advancements.

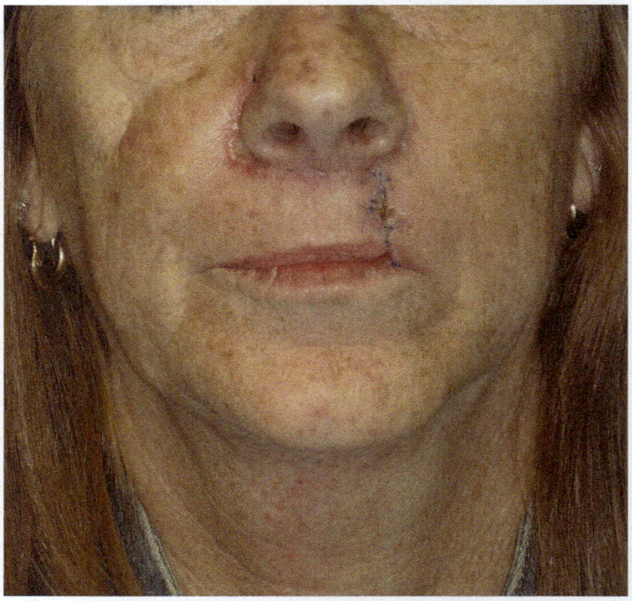

Fig. 5.26 Early postoperative view of the healing reconstruction. Note softening of the lip.

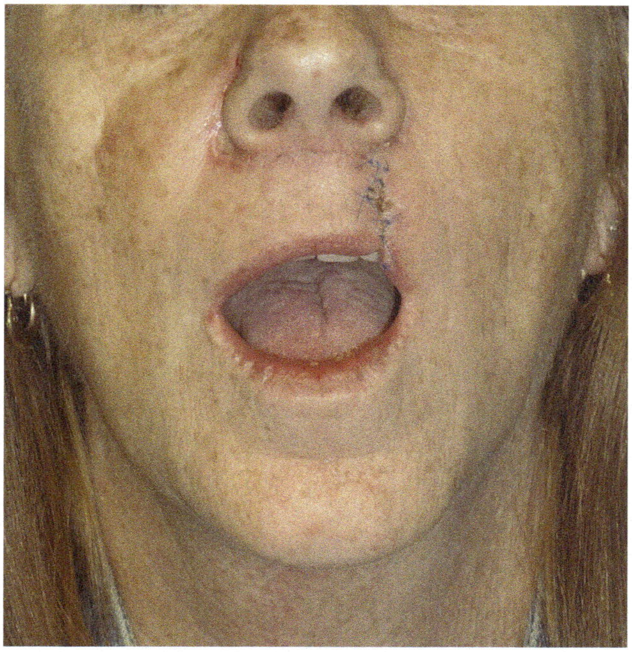

Fig. 5.27 Early postoperative view of the mouth opening.

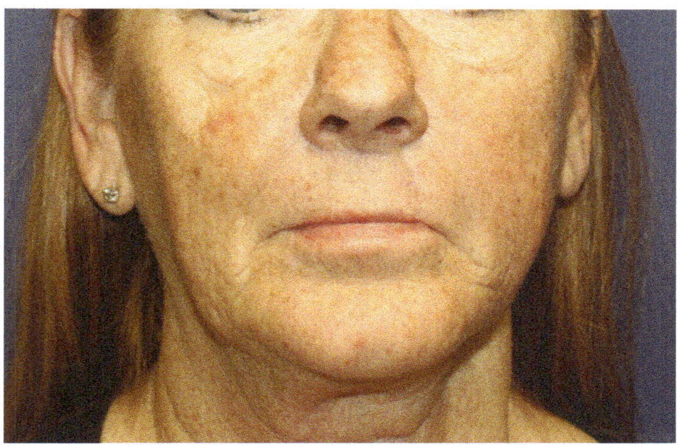

Fig. 5.28 Late postoperative view of the reconstructed lip in repose.

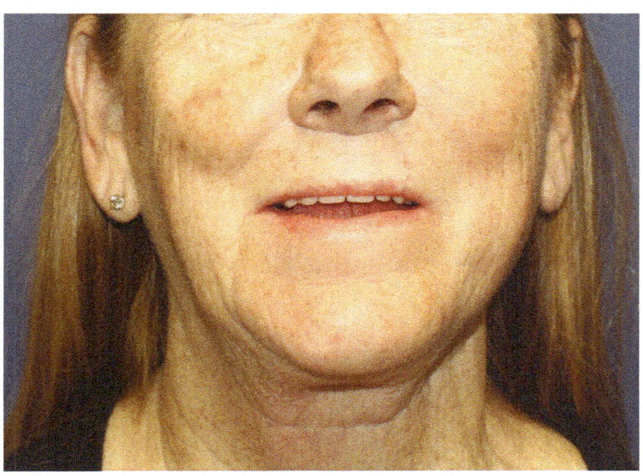

Fig. 5.29 Late postoperative view of the reconstructed lip with mouth slightly open to reveal overall pleasing lip form.

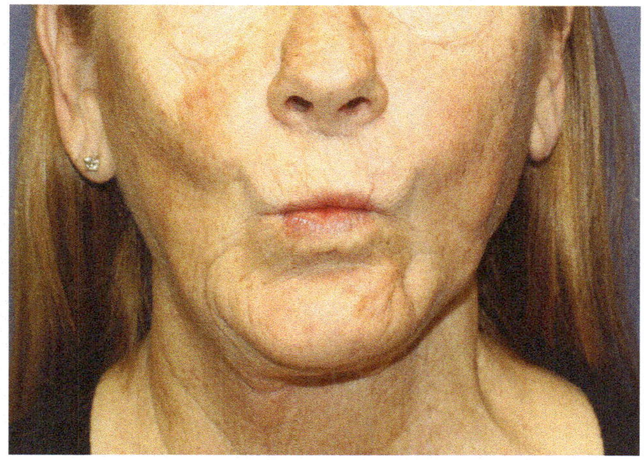

Fig. 5.30 Late postoperative view of the reconstructed lip showing preservation of oral sphincter tone.

with vermillionectomy and bilateral neck dissection (Figure 5.34). The resected specimen of the lip was fairly extensive (Figure 5.35). The reconstruction of the defect was planned with a lower crescentic flap (Figure 5.36). The resected crescentic tissue was carried out and including the muscle (Figure 5.37). The lateral flap was then advanced to check if the defect could be closed without tension (Figure 5.38). The defect was then closed in layers (Figure 5.39). The final outcome of the reconstruction was deemed satisfactory without a noticeable scar and with preservation of oral competence (Figures 5.40 and 5.41).

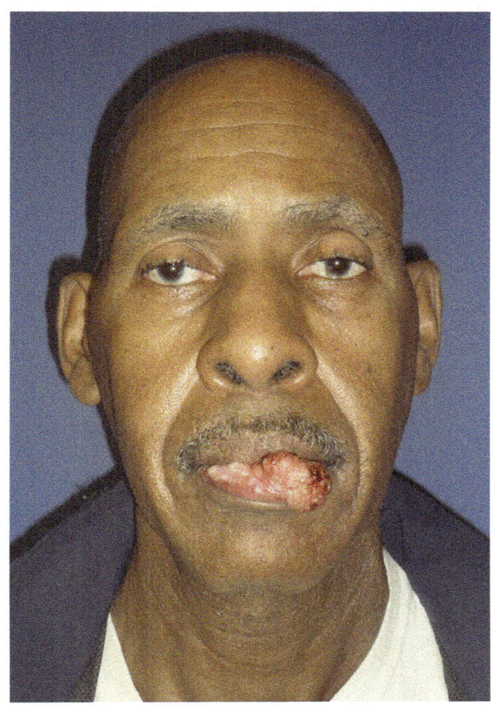

Fig. 5.31 View of patient with large neglected lip malignancy.

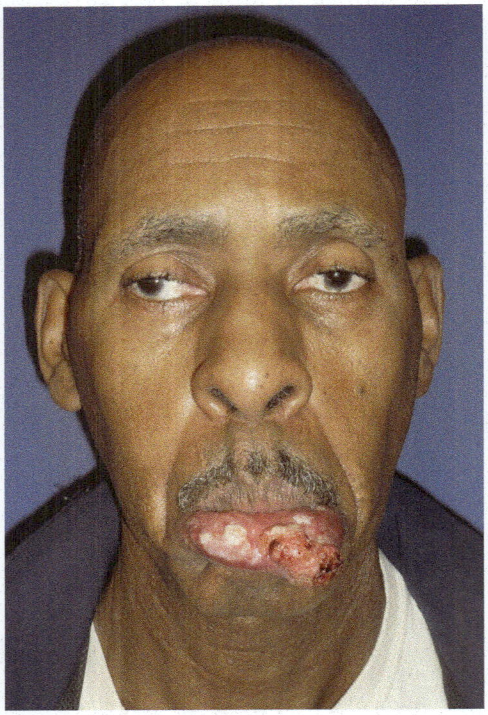

Fig. 5.32 View of lip revealing extent of tumor as a multifocal in appearance.

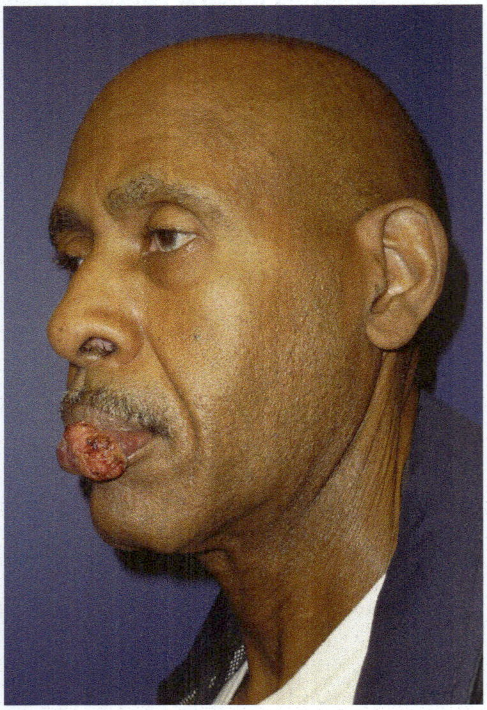

Fig. 5.33 Lateral view of the lip and chin.

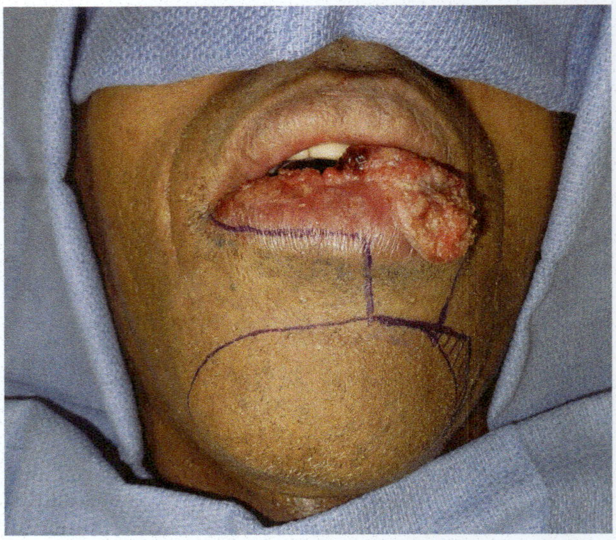

Fig. 5.34 Surgical plan for excision of lip with immediate crescentic advancement flap.

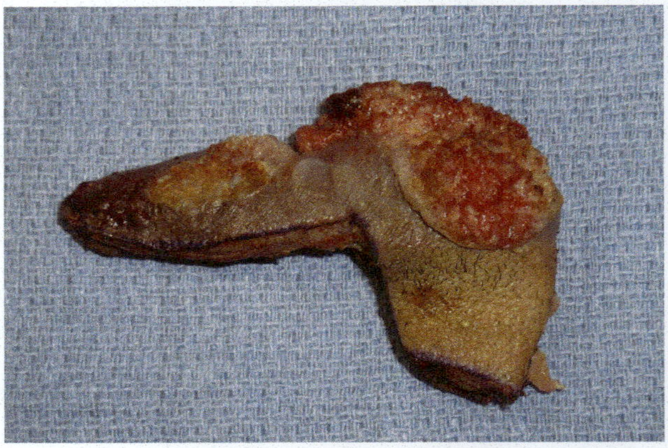

Fig. 5.35 View of the resected lip specimen. Patient also underwent bilateral neck dissection due to nodal enlargement.

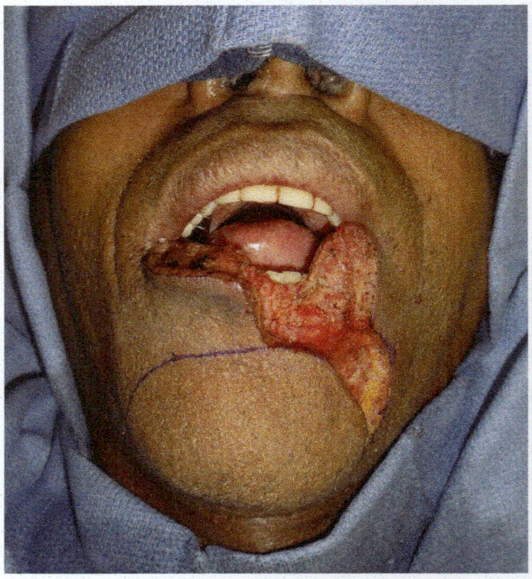

Fig. 5.36 Appearance of lip after resection of tumor and plan for advancement flap.

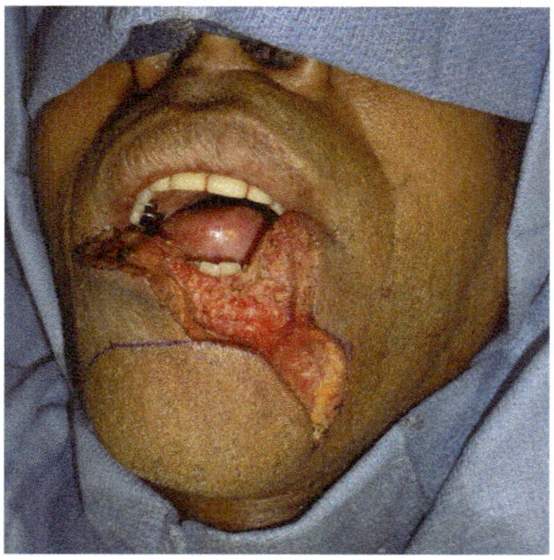

Fig. 5.37 Lateral view showing the resected tissue and plan for the advancement. Note the amount of tissue removed, which will allow for the advancement of the lateral tissues along the labiomental crease.

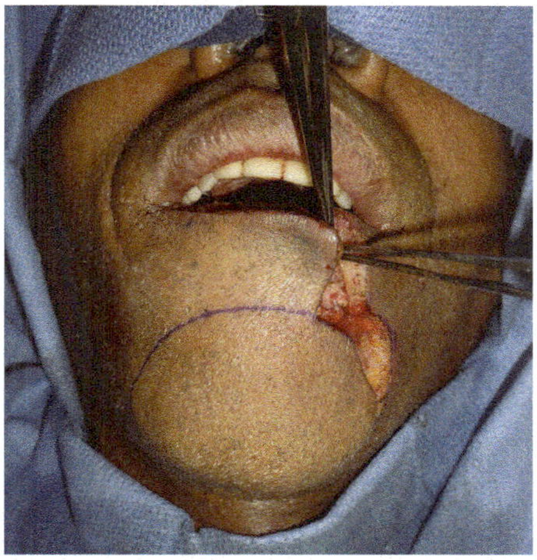

Fig. 5.38 Confirmation of the advancement of the flap to check for passive repair of the defect.

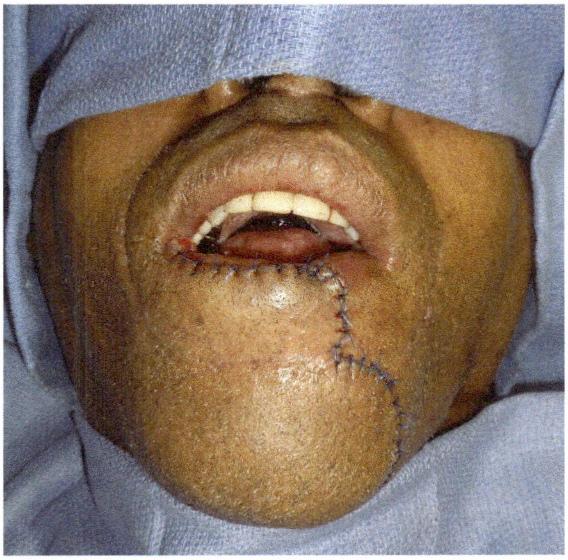

Fig. 5.39 Repair of the defect with crescentic flap, and mucosal advancement flap to repair the mucosal defect.

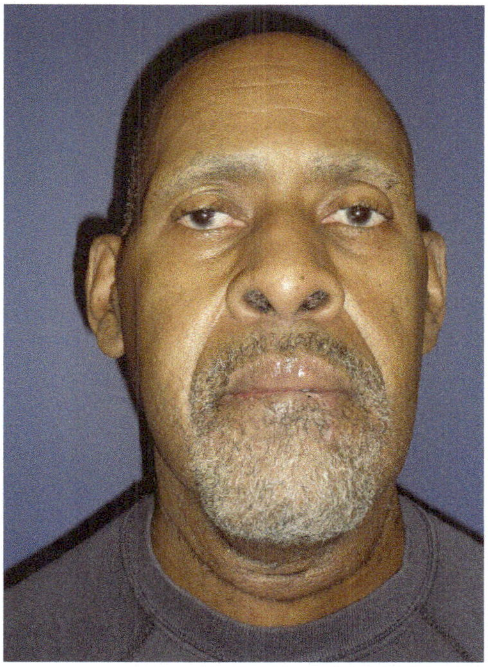

Fig. 5.40 View of healed lip reconstruction, note the good form and nearly imperceptible labiomental scar.

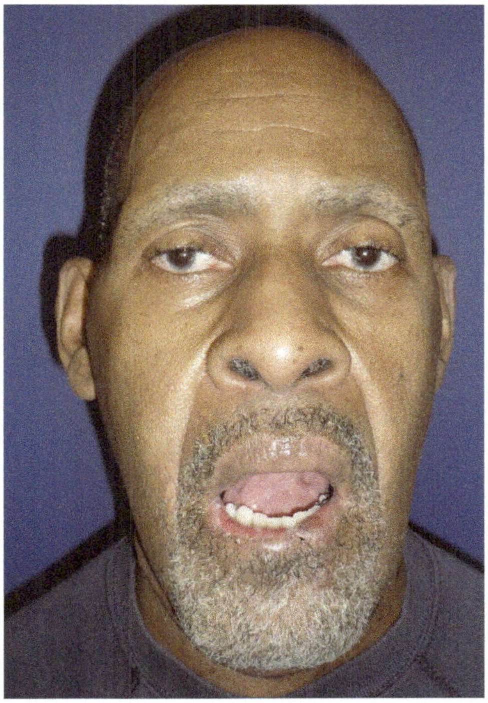

Fig. 5.41 View of the reconstructed lip in action;note the good form.

References

1. Webster JP. Crescentic peri-alar cheek excision for upper lip flap advancement with a short history of upper lip repair. *Plast Reconstr Surg* 1955; 16:434–464.
2. Nakajima T, Tokiwa N, Obata K. Primary reconstruction of defects in the upper and lower lips following tumor excision. *Int J Oral Surg* 1979; 8:186–193.
3. Wang SQ, Behroozan DS, Goldberg LH. Perialar crescentic flap for lip defects. *Dermatol Surg* 2005; 31(11 Pt 1):1445–1447.
4. Tirone L, Moscatiello F, Molea G. Reconstruction of the upper lip and philtrum. *J Plast Reconstr Aesthet Surg* 2006; 59:865–866.
5. Pirgousis P, Fernandes R. Reconstruction of subtotal defects of the lower lip: a review of current techniques and a proposed modification. *J Oral Maxillofac Surg* 2011; 69:295–299.

Chapter 6
Septal flap

Introduction

The septal flap is a commonly used flap due to its arc of rotation and the quantity of tissue available for use as a lining in nasal reconstruction. In cases where there is a full thickness defect of the nose, the reconstruction of the defect should attempt to restore each of the missing layers and, whenever possible, matching tissues. In these cases, a septal pivot flap or mucoperichondrial flap is exceptionally useful in providing good tip support and a well-vascularized nasal lining for reconstruction after major resection of the nasal tip.[1]

The use of the septal flap is often carried out in stages. The flap is rotated to reconstruct the defect, but by doing this it obliterates the nasal airway. In the second stage, carried out several weeks later, the nasal passage is opened by separating the mucosa from its pivot point in the septum.

In cases where the defect is limited to the nasal lining, raising the flap is technically more demanding due to the confined space. The challenge centers on diminishing the likelihood of perforations to the mucoperichondrial flap. In these cases, it is recommended that the surgeon be facile with endonasal procedures, preferably with endoscopic harvest.

This nasoseptal flap has become one of the most utilized flaps in the reconstruction of anterior skull base defects. The technique for endoscopic harvest of the flap was described by Hadad and Bassagasteguy in 2006 and is named after them.[2] This technique will not be discussed in this chapter.

The septal pivot flap is a modification that transfers both mucosal septal components as well as the interpositioned cartilage. This flap is most commonly used in situations where the anterior nasal tip and columella are missing. These defects are often encountered secondary to trauma, principally gunshot wounds, or due to oncologic resection. These acquired defects pose a significant challenge to the reconstructive surgeon charged with rebuilding the nasal complex.

The septal pivot flap enables the restoration of the projection of the nose as well as the support of the reconstructed nose. When an adequate quantity of the septum and the perfusion is intact, use of this flap obviates the need for alloplastic implants and their associated risk of extrusion.

Anatomy

The anatomy of the nasal septum is simple, yet with several critical nuances that are of significant importance to raising the septal mucoperichondrial and septal pivot flaps.

The septum is composed of cartilage anteriorly and bone posteriorly. The bony part of the septum is the perpendicular plate of the ethmoid bone. The septal mucosa on either side is separated by the cartilage, which is covered by the perichondrium. The septum gives the nose support and is responsible for dorsal as well as tip support and the projection of the nose.

The arterial perfusion to the septum consists of an array of vessels. The anterior portion of the septum (i.e., the cartilage) obtains its blood supply from the septal branch of the superior labial artery. The superior labial artery is a branch from the facial artery and it gives off the septal branch lateral to the philtrum and columella.

Branches of the sphenopalatine artery, mainly the posterior septal branch, perfuse the posterior aspect of the septum. The superior aspect is perfused by branches from the anterior and posterior ethmoidal arteries.[3]

The survival of the cartilaginous portion of the septum is dependent on the perfusion from the mucoperichondrium. The cartilage can survive as long as one of the mucoperichondrial sides is intact.

Local and Regional Flaps in Head & Neck Reconstruction: A Practical Approach, First Edition. Rui Fernandes.

Companion website: www.wiley.com/go/fernandes/flapsreconstruction

A flap of septal mucoperichondrium, either unilateral or bilateral and with or without a cartilage component, will survive if based on a 1.3-mm pedicle located in the zone between the anterior plane of the upper lip and the lower edge of the piriform aperture—the zone containing the septal branch of the superior labial artery.[4]

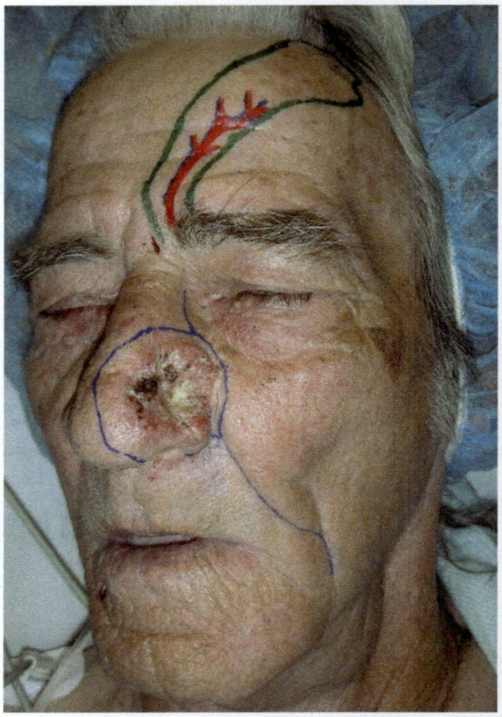

Fig. 6.1 Appearance of a large nasal skin cancer with markings for immediate reconstruction.

Flap harvest

Septal mucosal flap

First stage

- In cases where the septal mucosal flap is being used for lining defects in full-thickness nasal defects, access to the septum is often unimpeded.
- The nasal cavity is packed with Afrin-soaked cotonoids to shrink the mucosa while at the same time diminishing the potential bleeding caused by surgical intervention.
- The area to be incised will be dependent on the amount of tissue needed.
- The superior incision is normally carried out along the plane of the nose and parallel to the planned inferior incision.
- The inferior incision is made about 5 mm above the nasal floor and as far posterior as possible.
- The superior incision is then connected to the inferior incision by dropping a perpendicular incision from superior to inferior incision.
- The flap is then elevated by dissecting between the septal mucosa and the cartilage; care should be taken to not perforate the mucosa.
- The elevation is continued posteriorly, avoiding any trauma to the tissues. The flap is then elevated and rotated to the defect.

Second stage

- Approximately 3 weeks after the first stage surgery, the flap should have enough collateral circulation to tolerate the division of the pedicle without compromise of the transferred tissue.
- The takedown of the flap is achieved by making an incision near the septum along the width of the flap.
- The mucosal end of the flap used to line the nose is inset using chromic gut sutures.
- The septal mucosa is also transferred to the septal area and secured with trans-septal sutures.
- Alternatively, a nostril former or nasal packing can be used to keep the flaps in place until adhesion to the transferred bed.

Figures 6.1 to Figure 6.11 depict the steps in raising the septal mucoperichondrial flap.

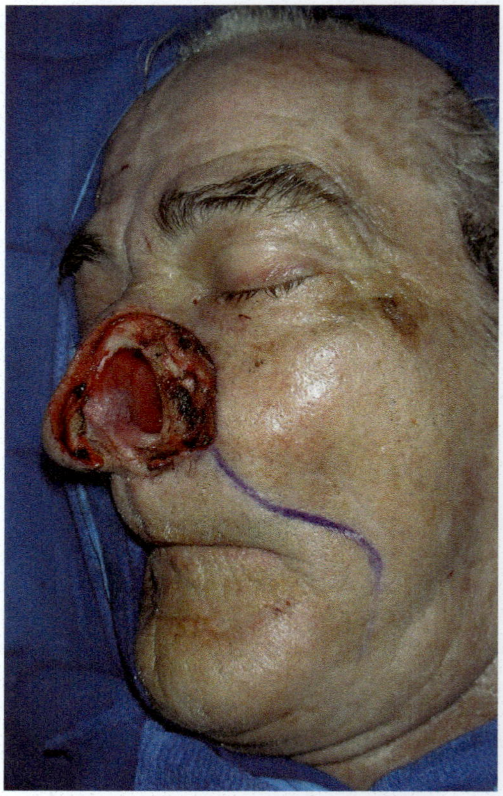

Fig. 6.2 View of the resected nasal lesion in the form of a hemirhinectomy.

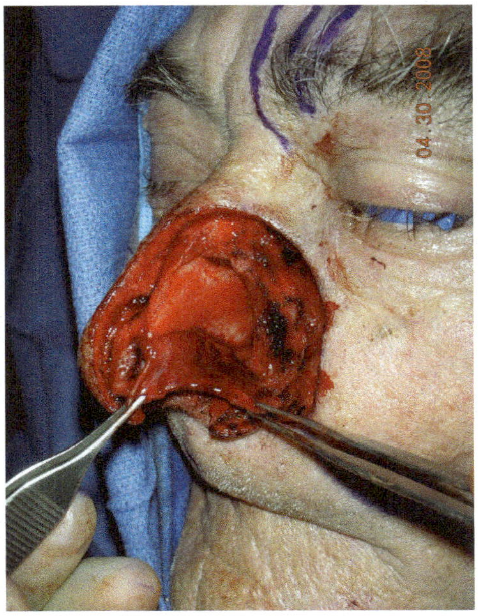

Fig. 6.3 Elevated left septal flap.

Septal pivot flap

- The septal pivot flap is used to transfer the entire septal complex, i.e., mucosa on both sides as well as the septal cartilage.
- Prior to making the incision, the defect is analyzed to determine the amount of cartilage support needed to reestablish nasal projection and tip support.
- Equally, the remaining septum is evaluated to determine the amount of residual tissue and potential for transfer.

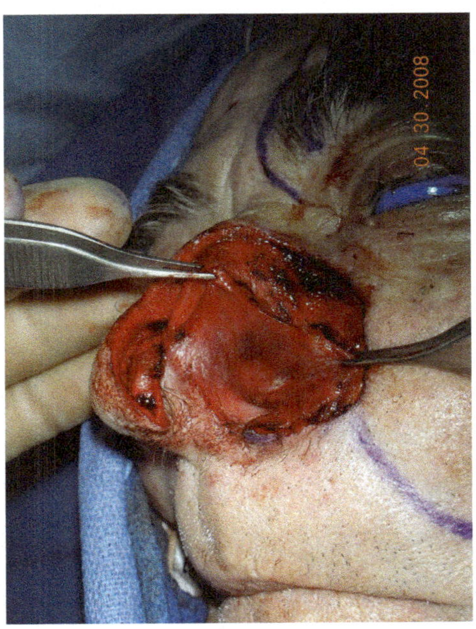

Fig. 6.4 View of the septal mucosal flap from inferior.

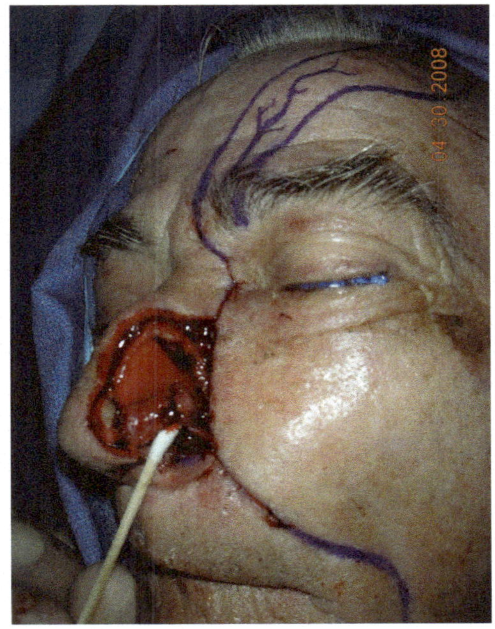

Fig. 6.5 Inset of the septal flap to recreate the inner lining of the nasal reconstruction.

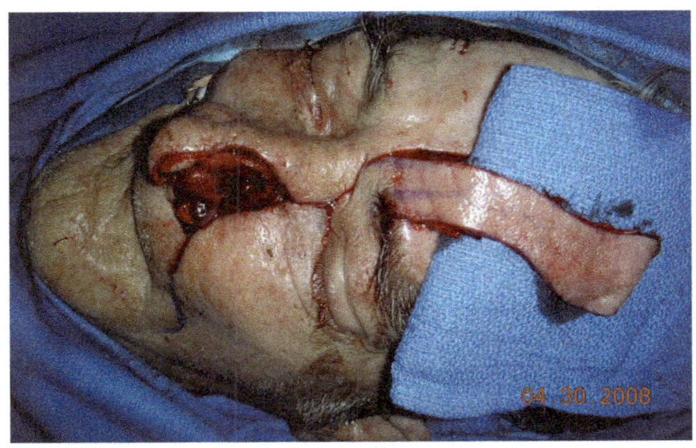

Fig. 6.6 View of the elevated paramedian flap after cheek advancement flap and inset of the septal flap.

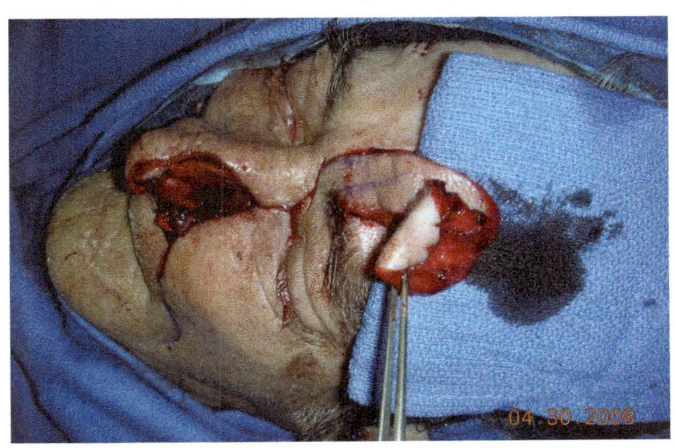

Fig. 6.7 Folded paramedian flap prior to transfer.

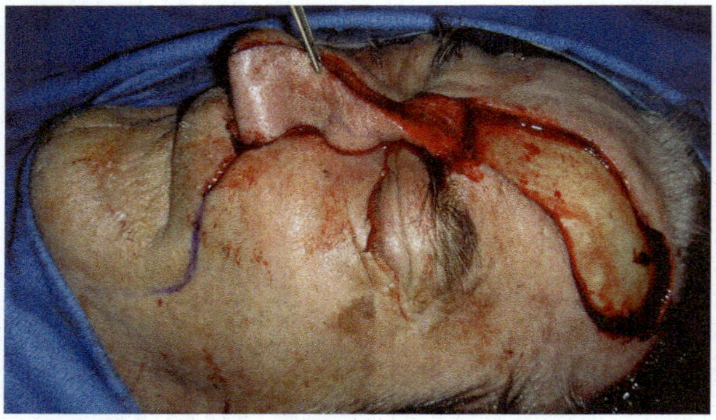

Fig. 6.8 Inset of the paramedian flap into the nasal defect.

- The base of the septum along the anterior nasal spine and upper lip must be intact to ensure that the superior labial artery and septal artery remain intact.
- The superior incision should be made about 1 cm inferior to the nasal dorsum to preserve the integrity of the residual nasal dorsum without compromising its support.
- The incision is a through-and-through incision beginning on the mucosa on one side, progressing through the cartilage, and through the opposite mucosa.
- The inferior incision is made parallel to the base of the septum in the same manner as the superior incision but staying approximately 8 mm posterior to the anterior nasal septum to maintain an intact blood supply to the flap.
- The posterior incision is made from superior to inferior to connect the two previous incisions.

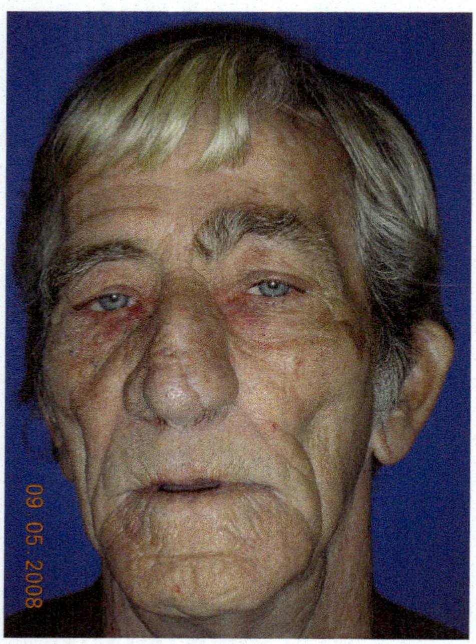

Fig. 6.9 View of the reconstructed hemirhinectomy with a septal flap, cheek advancement flap, and paramedian forehead flap.

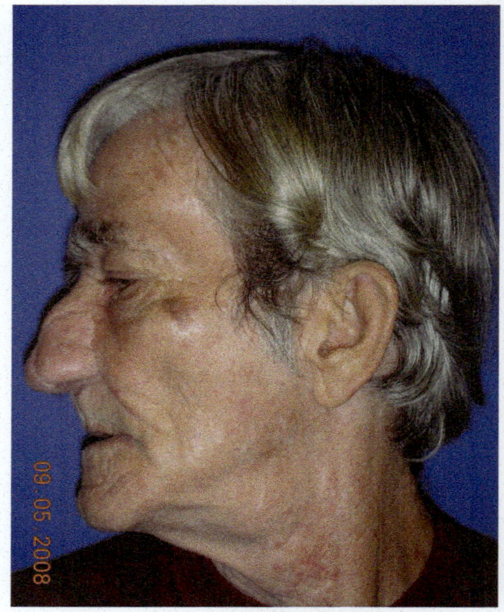

Fig. 6.10 Profile view of the reconstructed nose.

- The septal flap is then mobilized based on its anterior inferior attachment and pivoting out of the nasal cavity. This maneuver enables the septum to protrude out of the nose.
- The mucosa is reflected from both sides to expose the septal cartilage and this is trimmed to the desired height to match the nasal profile and inferiorly to create the columella support.
- In cases where there is extra mucosa, this can be reflected and used as an inner lining for the nose.

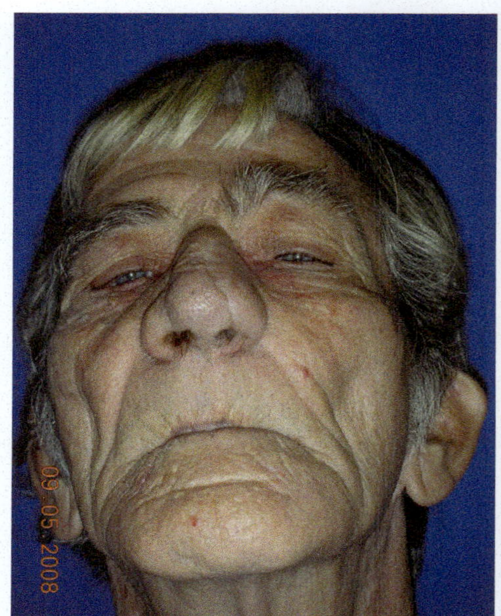

Fig. 6.11 Inferior view of the nasal reconstruction.

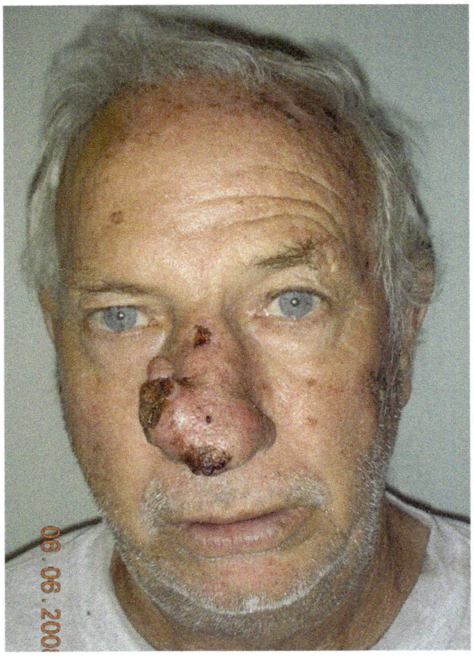

Fig. 6.12 View of a patient with a very large, neglected nasal skin carcinoma.

Case #1

A 68-year-old male was referred for treatment of a long-standing, neglected squamous cell carcinoma of the nasal sidewall (Figures 6.12 and 6.13). The surgical plan was for a hemirhinectomy and reconstruction of the acquired defect in stages. The initial reconstruction would include the use of a septal mucoperichondrial flap for lining, reestablishing support with cartilage grafts, and skin cover with a paramedian forehead flap (Figures 6.14 and 6.15). The resection was completed and the defect was greater than a hemirhinectomy defect, but the septum and mucosa were intact allowing for the continuation of the surgical plan (Figures 6.16 and 6.17). A septal mucoperichondrial flap was elevated to restore part of

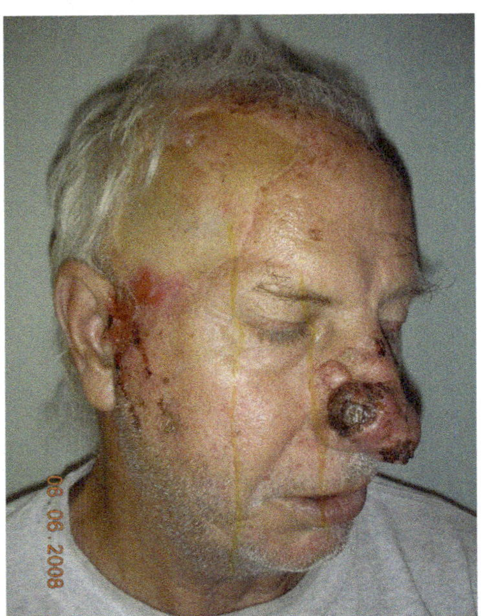

Fig. 6.13 Lateral view of a large skin cancer affecting the entire right hemi nose.

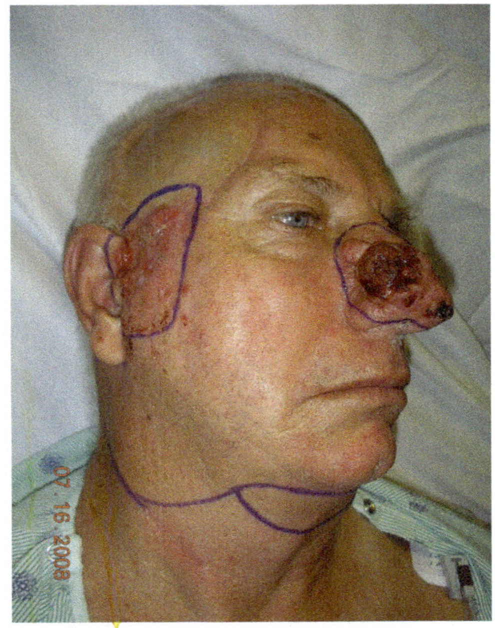

Fig. 6.14 Surgical planning for the resection of the nasal lesion.

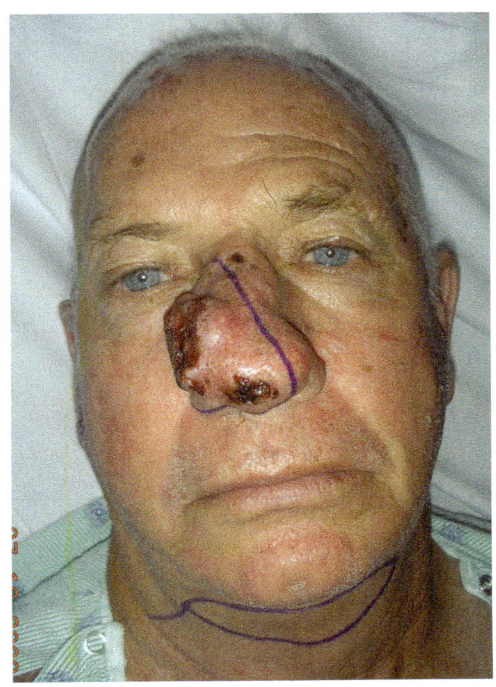

Fig. 6.15 Frontal view of the extended nasal resection.

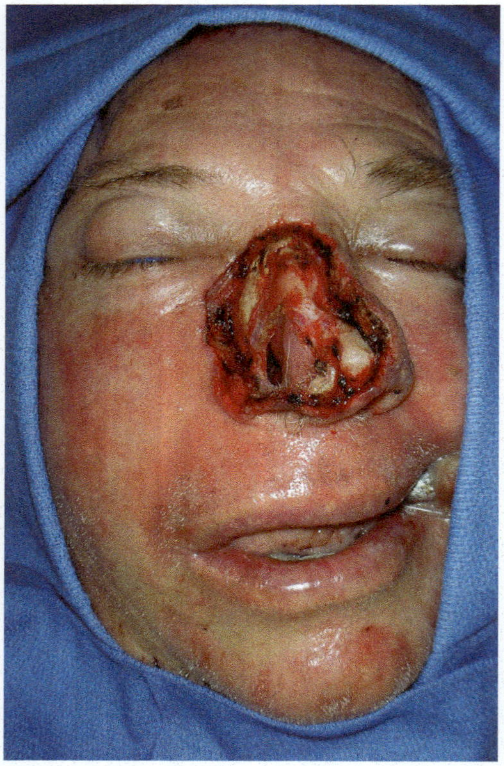

Fig. 6.16 View of the resected nasal lesion. Note the large composite defect.

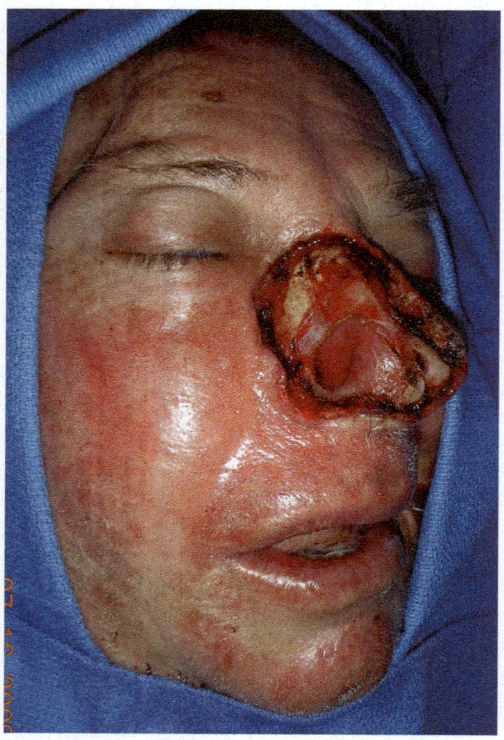

Fig. 6.17 Lateral view of the nasal defect.

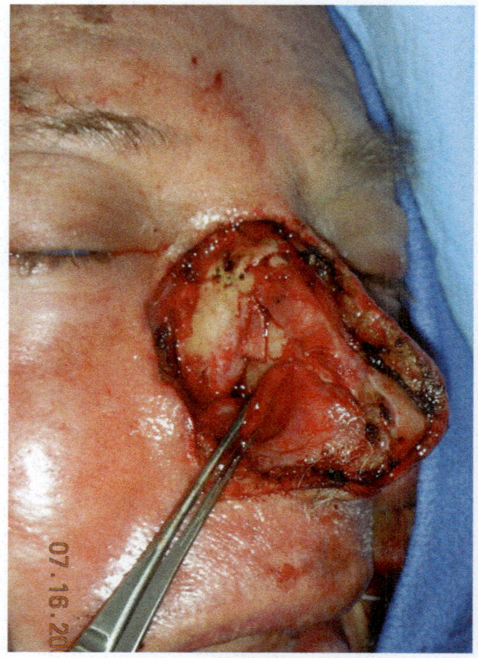

Fig. 6.18 Elevated right septal mucosal flap to create the inner lining.

the nasal lining (Figures 6.17 and 6.18). The remainder of the surgical plan was executed as planned (Figures 6.19 to 6.21). The appearance of the patient nearly 6 months after surgery was acceptable although he had some retraction of the ala on the ipsilateral side (Figure 6.22). An offer was made for further reconstruction but the patient

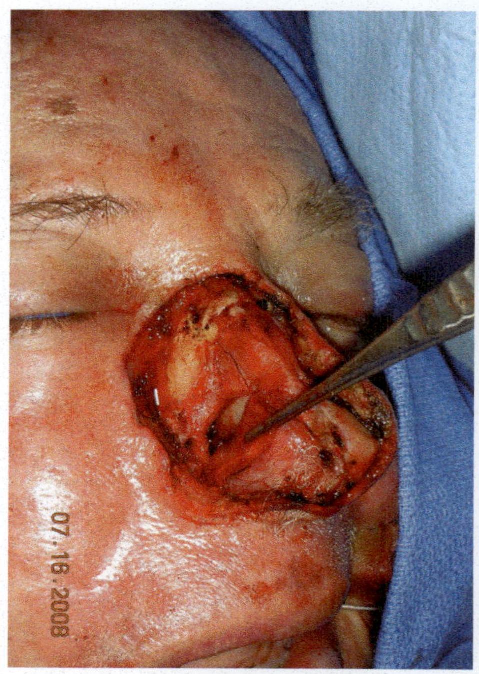

Fig. 6.19 View of elevated septal flap.

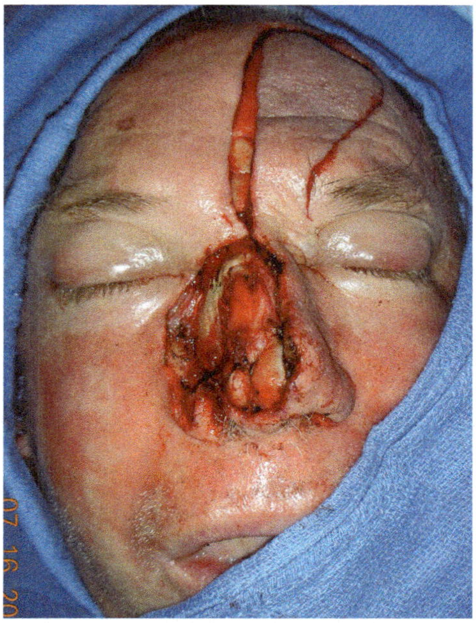

Fig. 6.20 Inset of the septal mucosal flap.

was pleased with the appearance and declined further revision.

Case #2

This 27-year-old male had a history of a gunshot wound to the facial region which had occurred nearly 5 months earlier. He had undergone multiple major procedures to reconstruct his mandibular defect as well maxillary defects with microvascular tissue transfer. These reconstructions had restored his mandibular and maxillary form allowing separation of the oral cavity from the nasal and sinus cavities. He had also undergone surgical correction of significant tissue loss of both the upper and lower lips. Currently, his major deficit remained the amputation of his nose. After long discussion with the patient, a staged reconstruction was planned. The reconstruction would entail a septal pivot flap to reestablish support and projection of the nasal dorsum and tip (Figures 6.23 and 6.24). A mucoperichondrial septal pivot flap was performed and the septum was adjusted to the desired projection height and tip projection (Figures 6.25 to 6.27). Once the lining and cartilage support was completed, a paramedian forehead flap was raised and inset (Figures 6.28 and 6.29). The second stage was carried

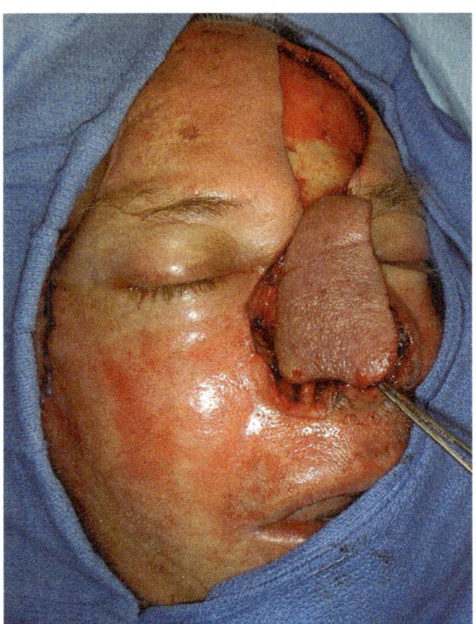

Fig. 6.21 Assessment of the reach of the paramedian forehead flap.

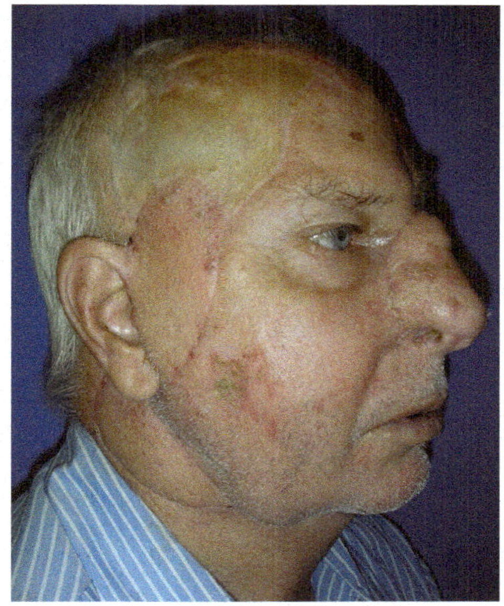

Fig. 6.22 Appearance of the reconstructed nose without revision.

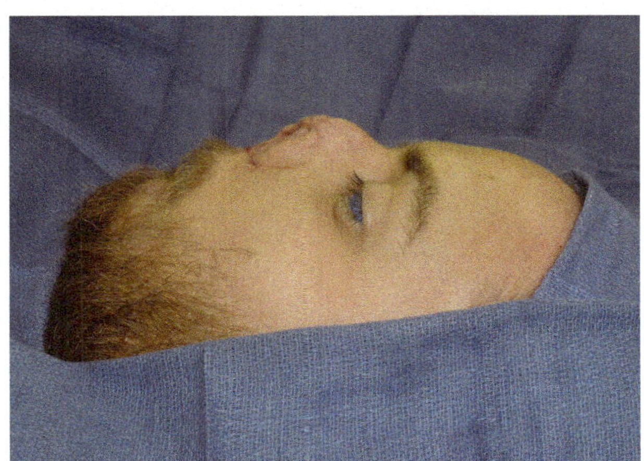

Fig. 6.23 View of a large complex nasal defect secondary to a gunshot injury.

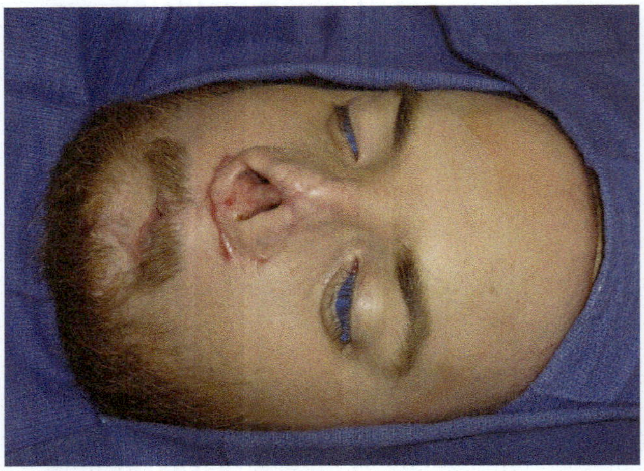
Fig. 6.24 Frontal view of the nasal defect.

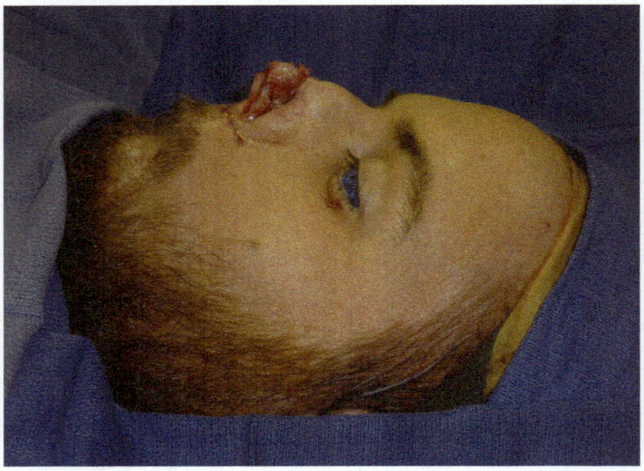
Fig. 6.25 Lateral view of a septal pivot flap to recreate the nasal projection.

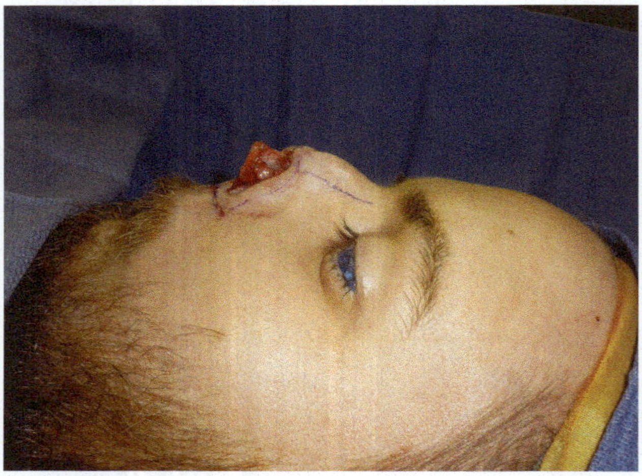
Fig. 6.26 View of the trimmed septal pivot flap.

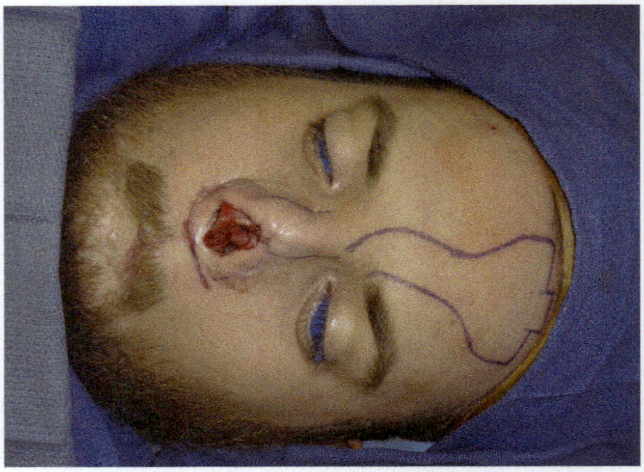
Fig. 6.27 View of the planned paramedian forehead flap.

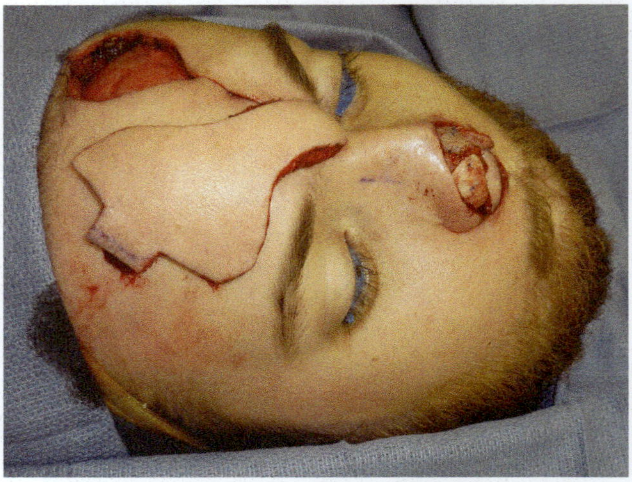
Fig. 6.28 Elevated paramedian forehead flap prior to transfer.

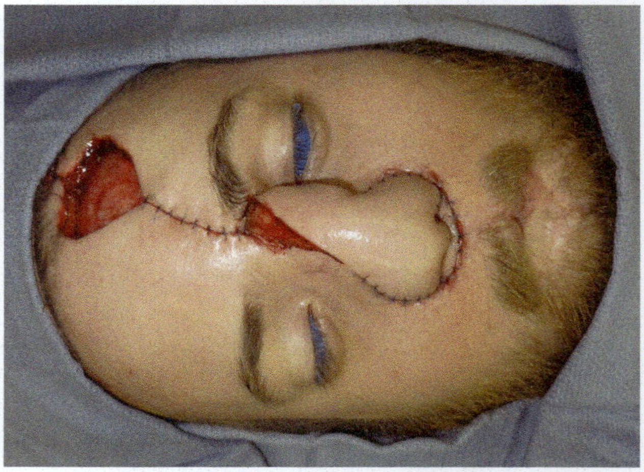
Fig. 6.29 Transfer of the paramedian forehead flap after the inset of the septal flaps and cartilage reconstruction.

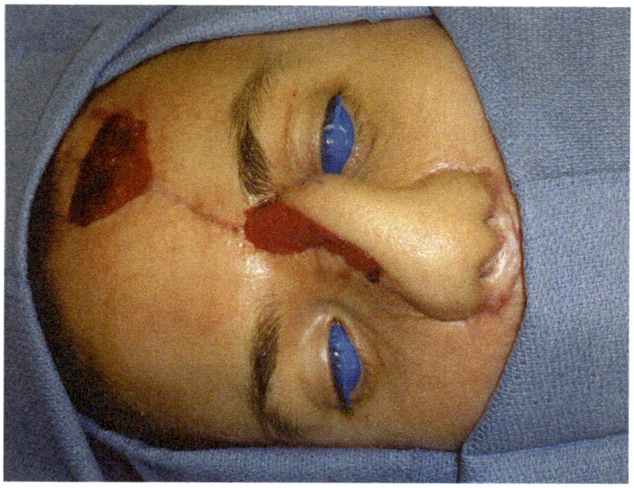

Fig. 6.30 View of the nasal appearance prior to sectioning of the paramedian flap.

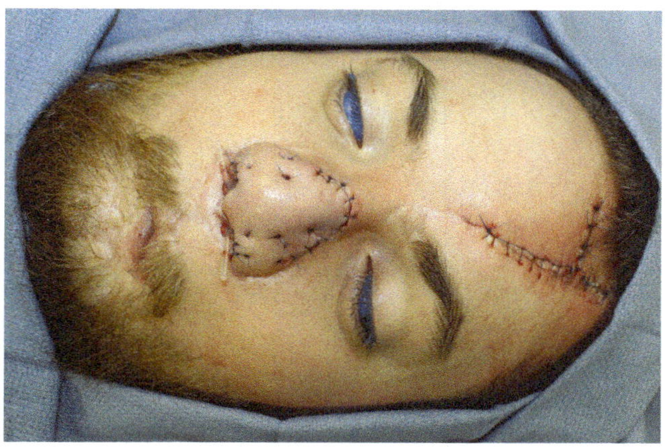

Fig. 6.31 Thinning of the paramedian flap and placement of quilting suture to aid in nasal form.

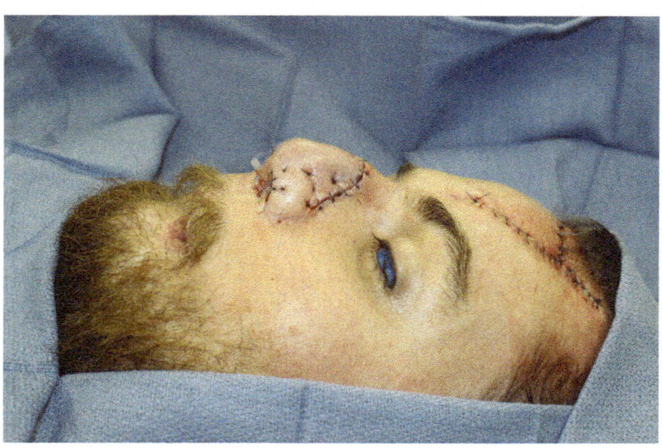

Fig. 6.32 Lateral view of the nasal projection after takedown of the paramedian forehead flap.

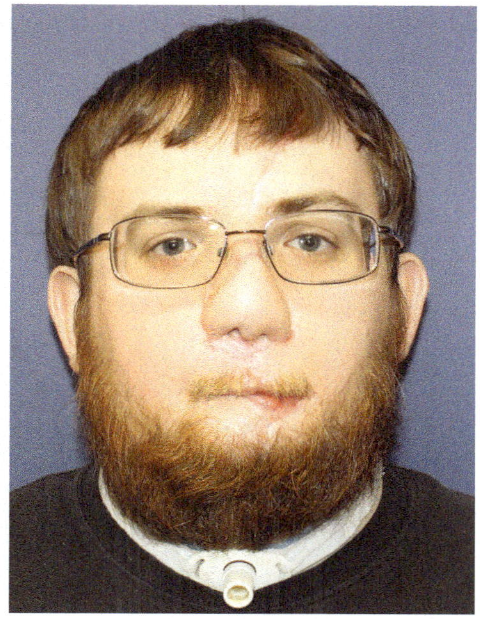

Fig. 6.33 Early view of the reconstructed nose prior to secondary reconstruction.

out approximately 4 weeks later and some thinning and quilting sutures were done at the same time (Figures 6.30 to 6.32). The patient had an acceptable appearance with good projection after the second stage, which could be appreciated on both frontal and profile views (Figures 6.33 to 6.35).

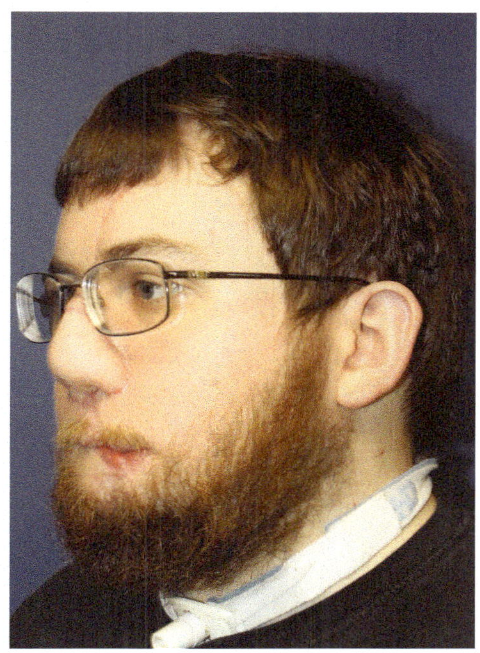

Fig. 6.34 Lateral view of the nasal reconstruction. Note the projection obtained from the septal pivot flap.

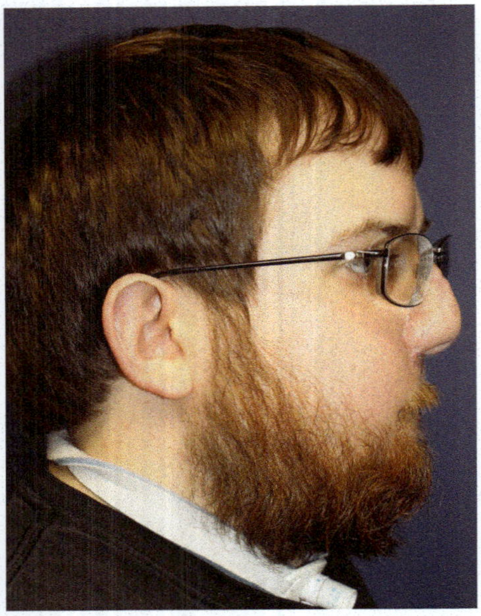

Fig. 6.35 Contralateral view of nasal projection.

References

1. Aneeshkumar MK, Chueng K, Hart R, Trites J, Taylor M. Pivoted composite nasal septal flap for reconstruction of the nose. *Eur Arch Otorhinolaryngol* 2013; 270:244–2450.
2. Hadad G, Bassagasteguy L, Carrau RL et al. A novel reconstructive technique after endoscopic expanded endonasal approaches: vascular pedicle nasoseptal flap. *Laryngoscope* 2006; 116:1882–1886.
3. Lessard ML, Daniel RK. Surgical anatomy of septorhinoplasty. *Arch Otolaryngol Head Neck Surg* 1985; 111: 25–29.
4. Burget GC, Menick FJ. Nasal support and lining: the marriage of beauty and blood supply. *Plast Reconstr Surg* 1989; 84(2):189–203.

Chapter 7

Nasolabial flap

Introduction

The nasolabial flap is a hardy flap that finds its use in the everyday reconstruction of various defects in the head and neck. The flap may be superiorly or inferiorly based. The choice between the two will depend on the location of the defect and the arc of rotation needed to reach it with the least amount of tension.

The use of the nasolabial flap varies. In broad terms, it is commonly used as a superiorly based flap to reconstruct nasal defects and oral defects located in the upper sulcus or palate. When it is raised as an inferiorly based flap, it is used most commonly to address lower lip defects or intraoral defects such as floor of mouth, lower gingival sulcus, and buccal mucosa defects.[1] The nasolabial flap has found a unique role as one of the go-to flaps in the reconstruction of buccal defects such as those encountered after the excision of scar bands and or fibrosis secondary to betel nut chewing.[2] Prior to the establishment of microvascular transfer as a routine option in the reconstruction of head and neck defects, the nasolabial flap was very popular for the repair of floor of mouth defects created after excision of squamous cell carcinomas.

The main advantages of using the nasolabial flap for reconstruction of external skin defects are the color and texture match to the defect site.[3] Because of the proximity of the donor site to the defect site, the use of this flap allows for a near imperceptible reconstruction for these two factors.

The main disadvantage of the nasolabial flap is the scar at the donor site. The location of the scar renders its use less than favorable to many patients. In some cases, when the flap is utilized in younger patients and only on one side, there is a potential for postoperative facial asymmetry. Lastly, in cases where the flap is needed for the reconstruction of floor of mouth defects, the remaining dentition needs to be evaluated to see if it will traumatize the flap when the patient is chewing and the reconstruction is carried out in stages.

Anatomy

The regional anatomy relevant to the nasolabial flap extends from about 5 mm inferior to the medial canthus and extends inferiorly towards the inferior border of the mandible.

The bulk of tissue available for use in a nasolabial flap is found along the area of the nasolabial fold as it extends lateral to the ala of the nose to a few millimeters below the lateral aspect of the oral commissure. The common design of the nasolabial flap would include the tissues in the nasolabial fold and lateral to it and as it extends inferiorly, it would include a small quantity of tissue just medial to the fold but with a greater quantity on the lateral aspect.

The vascular anatomy of the periorbital and perinasal region comes mainly from the facial artery, angular artery, and the nasal arteries.

The facial artery travels in a superior oblique direction once it emerges above the mandible. Along its path it gives off a number of branches, those being the inferior and superior labial arteries, and the lateral nasal artery before it becomes confluent with the angular artery.[4]

The angular artery is a branch of the ophthalmic artery that joins the facial artery as it descends inferiorly along the superior lateral aspect of the nose.

In the superior aspect of the nose, the ophthalmic artery also gives off the dorsal nasal artery.

Local and Regional Flaps in Head & Neck Reconstruction: A Practical Approach, First Edition. Rui Fernandes.

Companion website: www.wiley.com/go/fernandes/flapsreconstruction

All of these arteries give off perforators to the skin, which are responsible for the perfusion to the nasolabial flap. The main perfusion to the flap comes from the perpendicular vessels originating from the facial artery and angular artery.

The venous supply to the flap is based on the accompanying veins.

The nasolabial flap may be raised as an axial flap, a random flap, or as an island flap.[5] An inferiorly based nasolabial flap has been raised in patients where the ipsilateral facial artery has been ligated either at the time of surgery or in a previous surgical encounter[5].

Flap harvest

Superiorly based flap

- Once the decision has been made to raise a superiorly based flap, the next decision is to determine its width and length, and therefore the reach of the flap.
- The flap should be designed so that the inferior tip of the flap narrows down to a point. This design will allow for the closure of the donor site with the least amount of undermining and excision of dog ear. Equally, the flap design should place the final scar within the nasolabial groove. The placement of the scar within this region will give the least conspicuous evidence of the surgery.
- The flap is elevated from the distal tip towards the base by first making an incision deep to the dermis along the marked width of the flap.
- The flap is elevated in a plane superficial to the muscles.
- Care should be taken to identify and avoid injury to the perpendicular branches of the facial artery as they penetrate the muscle on their way to perfuse the overlying skin.
- The surrounding area is undermined to improve the rotation of the flap without causing distortion of the tissues around the base of the flap.
- In cases where the flap is to be used along the nasal sidewalls, the flap is rotated to insure the reach is adequate and without tension.
- The flap is contoured to the defect and inset by placing one to two deep sutures along the base to recreate the groove and the rest of the flap is inset in the usual fashion as per the surgeon's routine.

Inferiorly based flap

- The inferiorly based flap is designed with the superior medial border of the flap running in the nasolabial fold and widening to incorporate the desired width of the flap laterally along the cheek.
- In the inferior region of the flap, around the upper lip and towards the commissure, the medial incision should extend about 4 mm medial to the crease.
- The inferior width of the flap should be about 1.5 cm in order to capture enough of the perforating vessels and to allow for adequate perfusion to the distal tip of the flap.
- The incision is made superiorly around the flap design and then carried deep to the dermis.
- The terminal branches of the facial artery as it becomes the angular artery may be encountered depending on the superior extent and depth of the flap.
- If the vessel is encountered, it is ligated and then divided. The dissection continues in an inferior direction toward the base of the flap along the plane above the muscle.
- In cases where the flap is to be used for the reconstruction of oral cavity defects, an incision is made in the muscle bed and through the oral mucosa to develop the tunnel for transfer of the flap to the oral cavity.

Oral cavity defects

- For defects located in the oral cavity, access must be created in order to transfer the flap.
- With the flap elevated, the rotation is checked to see where the best access to the oral cavity should be placed in order to maintain the length of the flap as well as to minimize kinking or compression of the flap.
- The entry to oral cavity is achieved by making an incision in the buccinator muscle and then proceeding to the buccal mucosa.
- The tunnel should be wide enough to allow for passive transfer of the flap into the oral cavity. It should be anticipated that the width of the tunnel will narrow significantly with postoperative edema.
- In cases where the flap is to be used in the reconstruction of floor of mouth defects, the flap should be checked to insure that there is no interference with the dentition. Care should be taken to minimize trauma to the flap from the opposing dentition.
- The ideal patients for reconstruction of floor of mouth defects are older and edentulous patients. These patients have redundancy of the skin and laxity that will tolerate the harvest of a wider flap as well as a minimal possibility of trauma due to occlusion.
- Prior to insetting the flap, the skin along the base of the flap should be de-epithelialized in order to allow for primary closure of the skin.
- If the flap is to be carried out in a two stages, the takedown of the flap should be performed about 3 weeks after the transfer.
- See Figures 7.1 to 7.8.

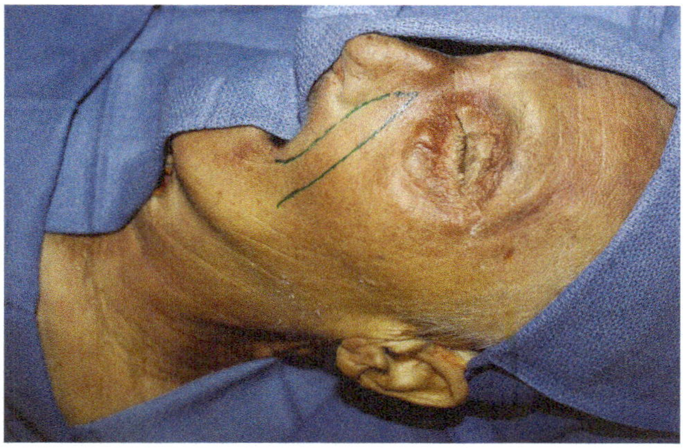

Fig. 7.1 Design of an inferiorly based nasolabial flap.

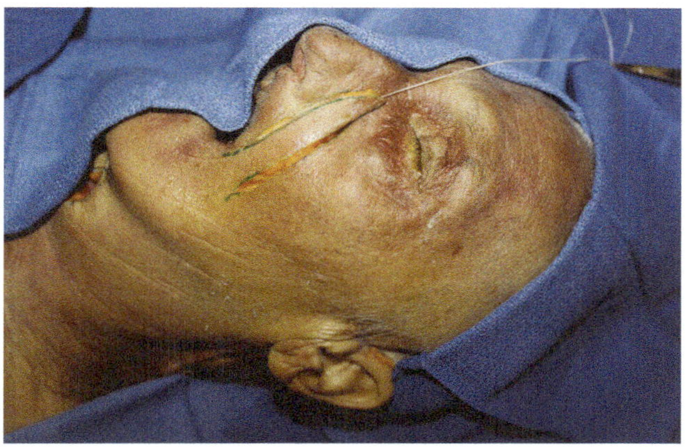

Fig. 7.2 View of the incised flap with suture holding the superior tip.

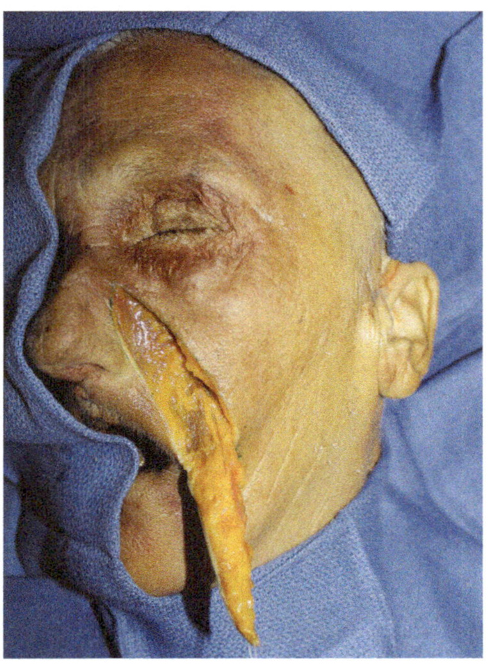

Fig. 7.3 Elevated flap prior to transfer.

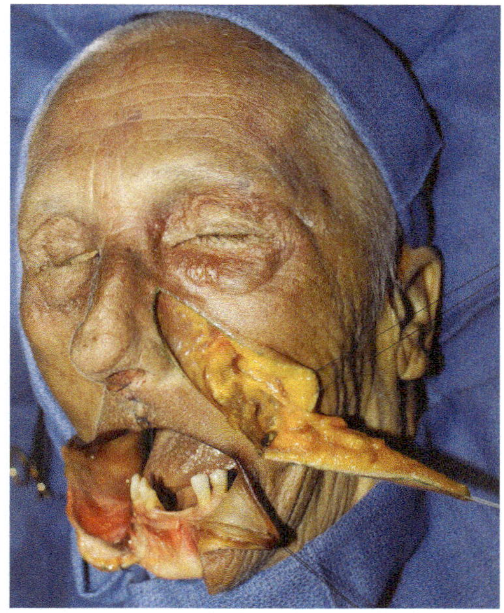

Fig. 7.4 View of the elevated flap with preservation of the vascular pedicle prior to transfer into the oral cavity; cadaveric dissection.

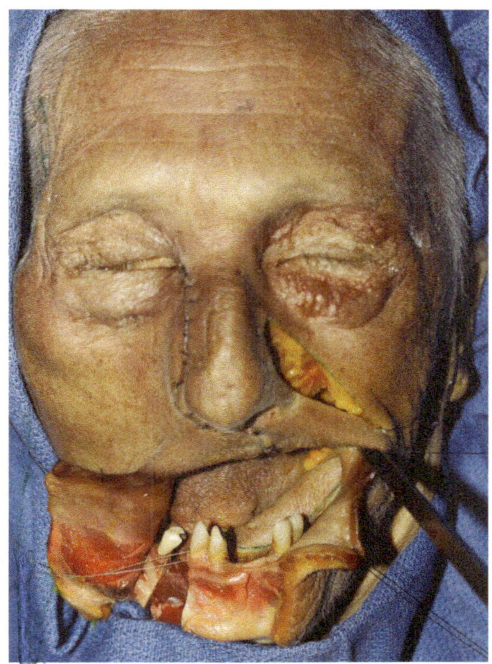

Fig. 7.5 View of the transferred flap into the oral cavity after developing a tunnel into the oral cavity.

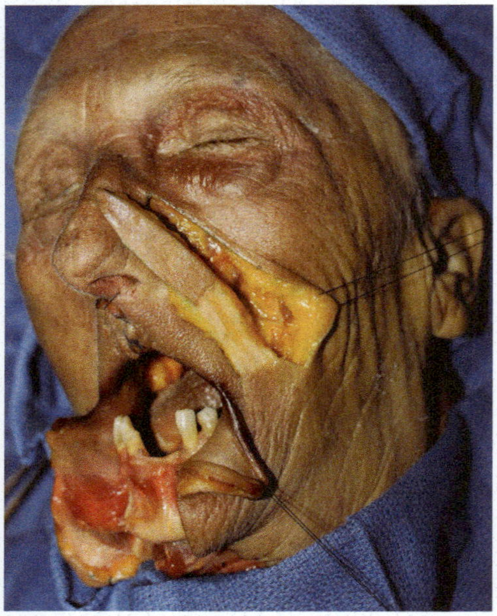

Fig. 7.6 View of the de-epithelialized flap prior to transfer.

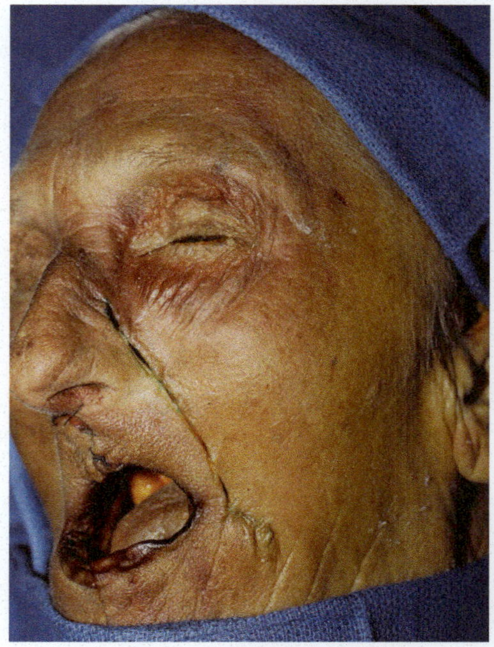

Fig. 7.8 Closure of the donor site along the nasolabial groove.

Case #1

A 73-year-old male was referred for surgical resection of a biopsy-proven squamous cell carcinoma of the right ala of the nose (Figure 7.9). The surgical plan involved resection of the lesion and immediate reconstruction of the defect with a superiorly based nasolabial flap (Figure 7.10). The lesion was removed with a resultant defect that did not include the resection of the cartilage or nasal lining (Figure 7.11). Once the resection was completed, marking was made for the elevation of the nasolabial flap with the correct width to repair the defect (Figure 7.12). A thin superiorly based nasolabial flap was elevated (Figure 7.13) and Figure 7.14). The rotation of the flap was checked to be sure that the reach would be adequate, it was then inset into the defect (Figures 7.15 and 7.16). The final appearance of the patient soon after a few weeks later, no revision to the flap had been done (Figure 7.17).

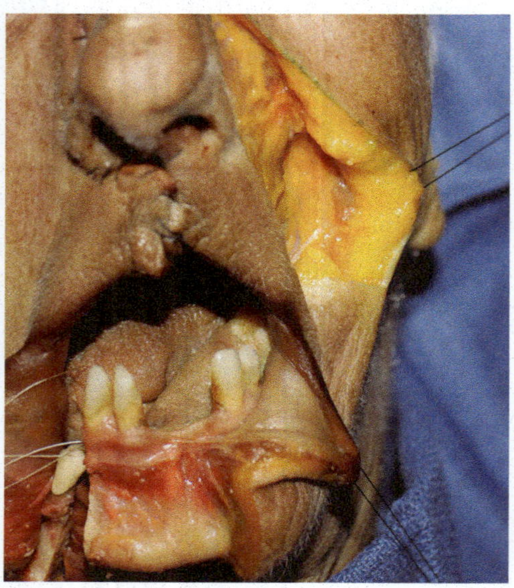

Fig. 7.7 View of the flap transfer to the tunnel.

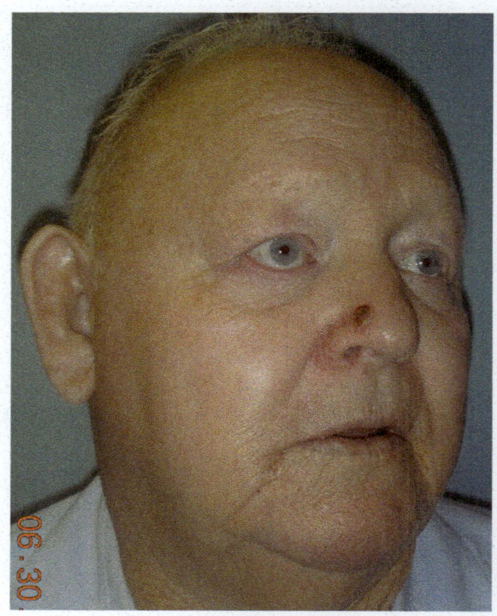

Fig. 7.9 View of a lateral nasal skin cancer.

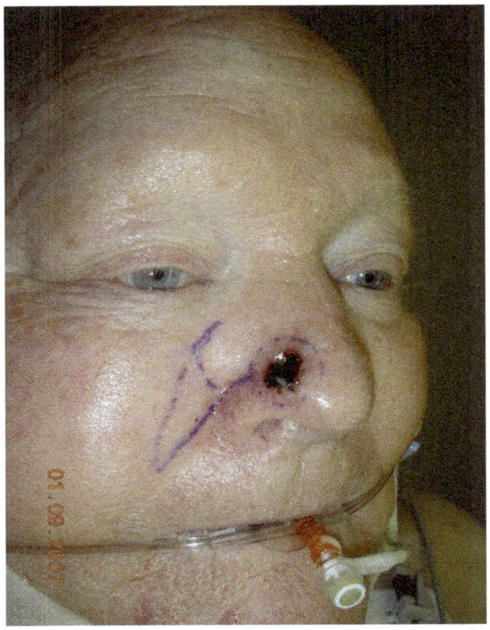

Fig. 7.10 Design of the flap as a superiorly based nasolabial flap to reconstruct the nasal defect.

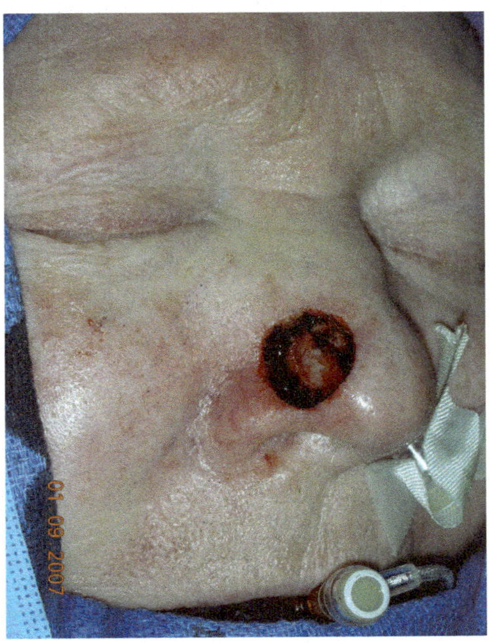

Fig. 7.11 View of the defect prior to reconstruction.

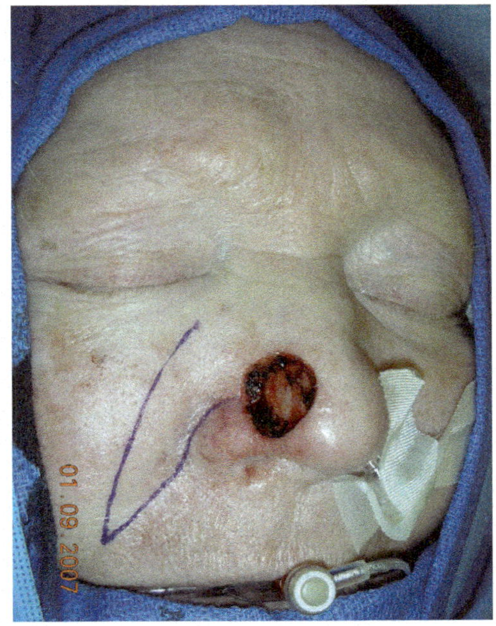

Fig. 7.12 Design of the superiorly based nasolabial flap.

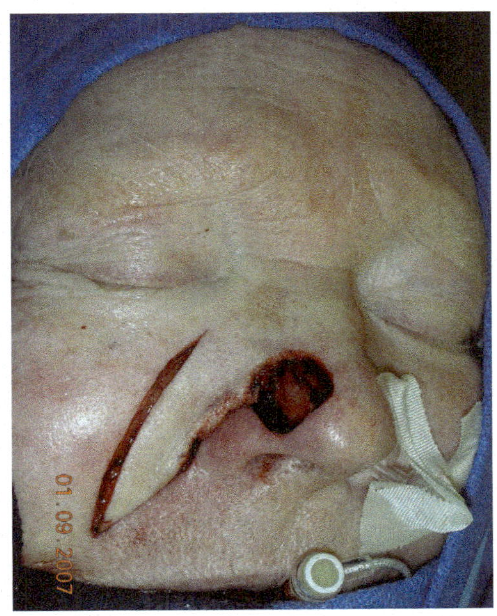

Fig. 7.13 Incised flap prior to transfer.

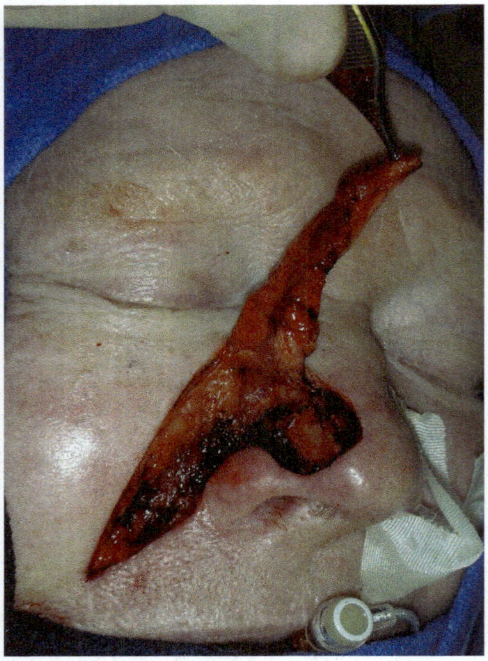

Fig. 7.14 Elevated superiorly based nasolabial flap.

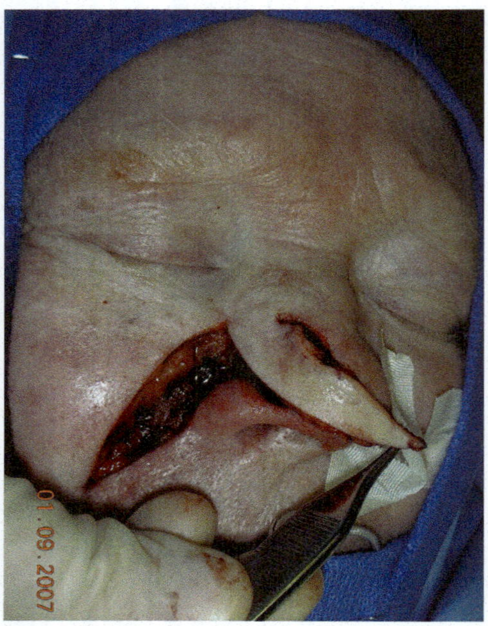

Fig. 7.15 Assessment of the arc of rotation and reach of the flap into the nasal defect.

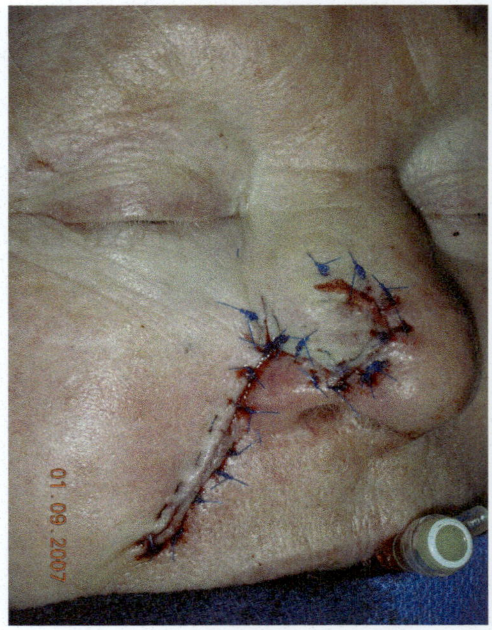

Fig. 7.16 Inset of the flap to reconstruct the defect. Note the closure of the donor site along the nasolabial groove in order to better camouflage the scar.

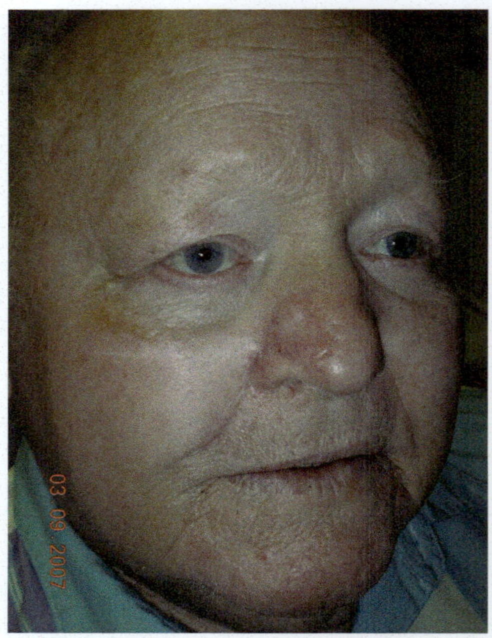

Fig. 7.17 Early view of the healed reconstruction, note that the donor site is not readily apparent.

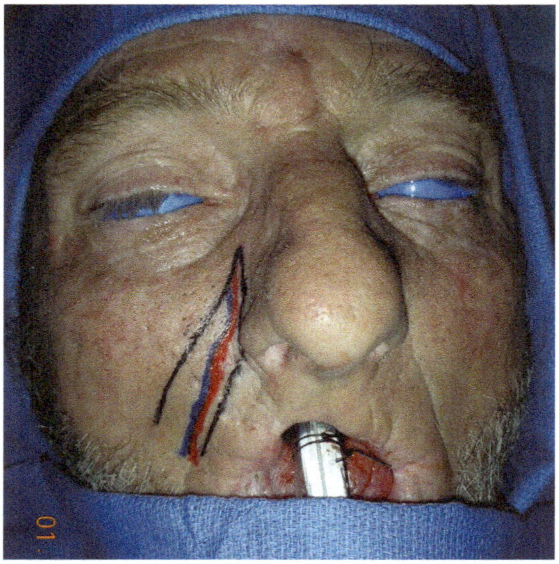

Fig. 7.18 View of a design for an inferiorly based nasolabial flap.

Case #2

A 64-year-old male with long history of multiple excisions of skin cancer from the face as well as the lip was referred for evaluation of an oral nasal fistula that had developed after the completion of his radiation therapy for a lip squamous cell carcinoma. Given the location of the fistula, a decision was made to repair the defect with an inferiorly based nasolabial flap (Figures 7.18 and 7.19). A thick flap was raised and dissected inferiorly to allow

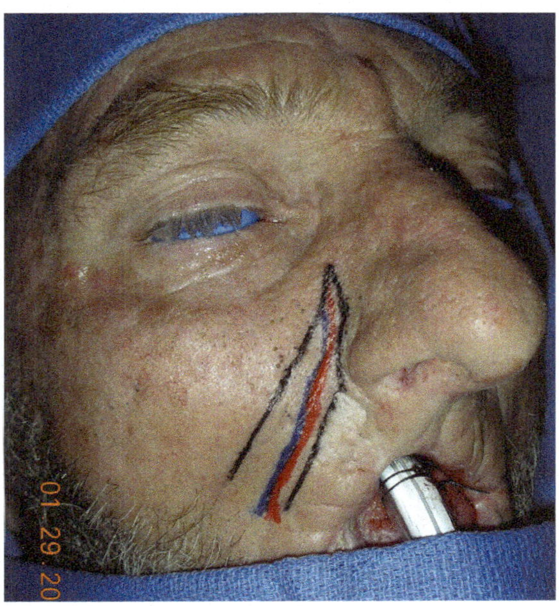

Fig. 7.19 Lateral view of the planned nasolabial flap.

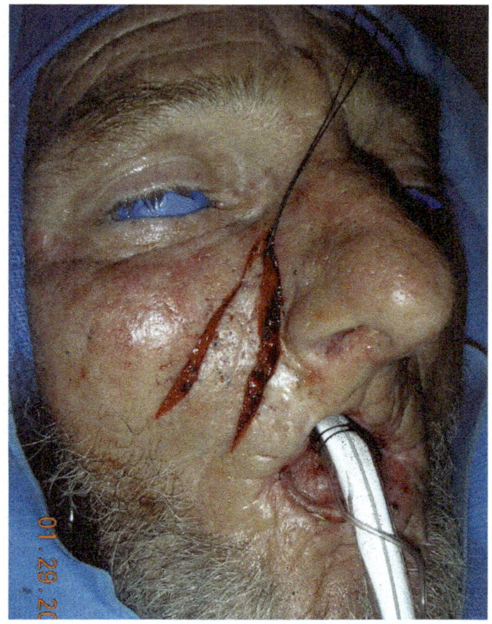

Fig. 7.20 Elevated, inferiorly based flap prior to transfer.

for adequate rotation (Figures 7.20 to 7.22). A small area of the skin was de-epithelialized to allow for the tunneling of the flap into the oral cavity (Figures 7.23 to 7.25). The flap was then inset into the defect and the donor site was closed (Figures 7.26 and 7.27).

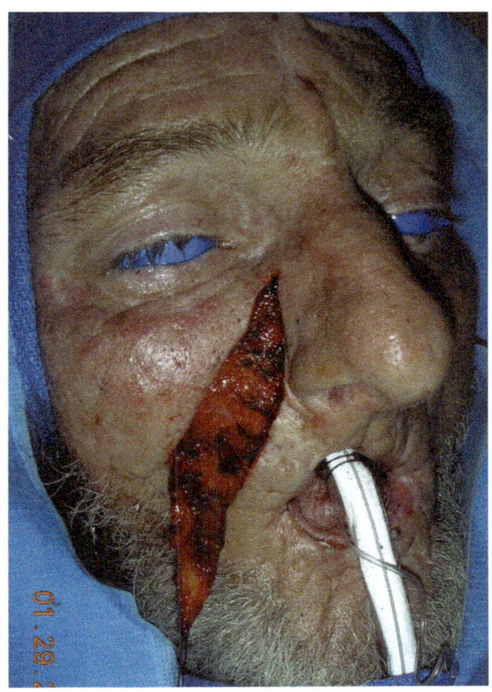

Fig. 7.21 View of the elevated flap prior to transfer to the oral cavity.

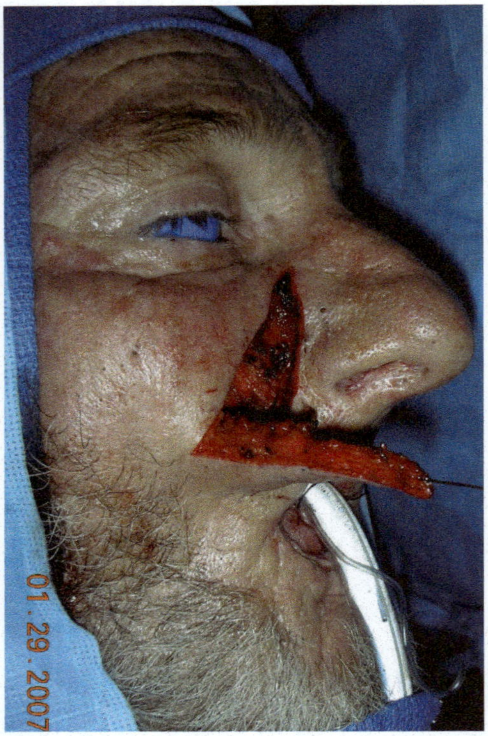

Fig. 7.22 Lateral view of the elevated flap; note the thickness of the flap.

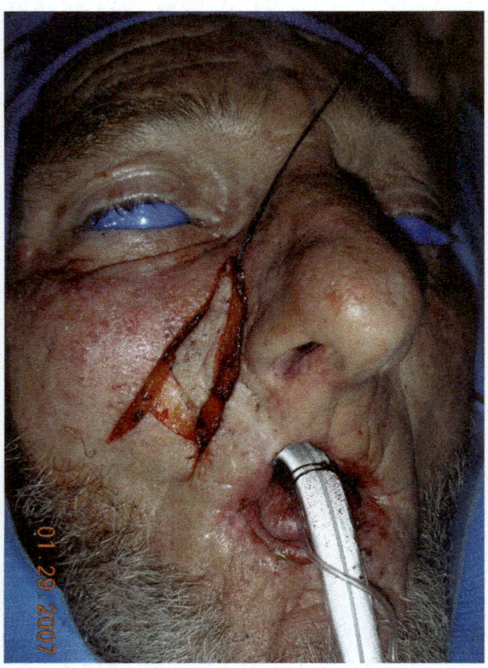

Fig. 7.23 De-epithelialized flap segment prior to transfer.

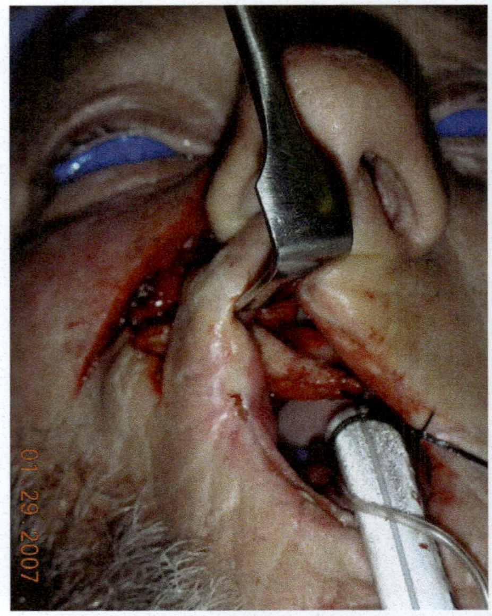

Fig. 7.24 View of transfer of the flap into the defect after development of the transfer tunnel.

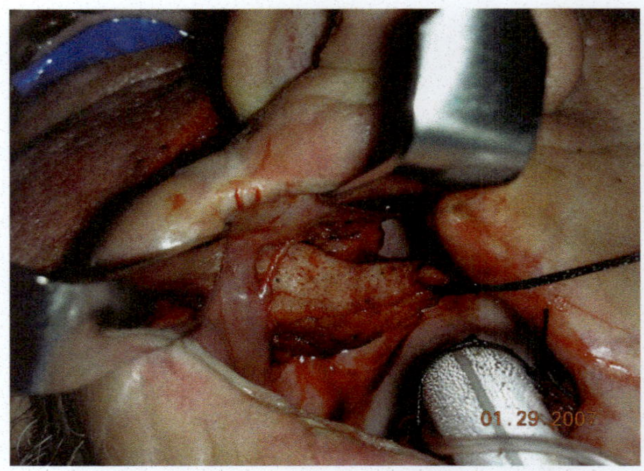

Fig. 7.25 View of the flap; note the good vascularity of the flap.

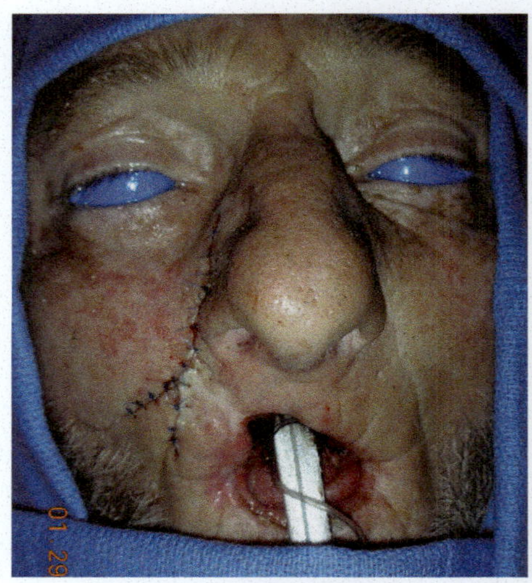

Fig. 7.26 Closure of the donor site after transfer to the oral cavity.

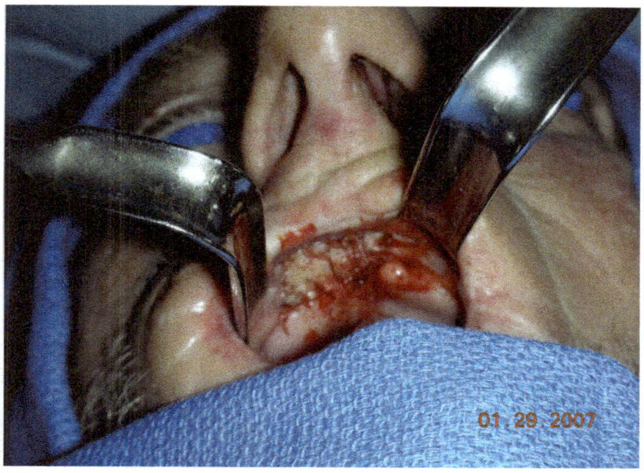

Fig. 7.27 View of the flap in the oral cavity to repair an oral nasal fistula.

References

1. Ducic Y, Burye M. Nasolabial flap reconstruction of oral cavity defects: a report of 18 cases. *J Oral Maxillofac Surg* 2000; 58:1104–1108.
2. Agarwal M, Gupta DK, Tiwari AD. Extended nasolabial flaps in the management of oral submucous fibrosis. *J Maxillofac Oral Surg* 2011; 10(3):216–219.
3. Karsidag S, Ozcan A, Sumer O, Ugurlu K. Single stage ala nasi reconstruction: lateral nasal artery perforator flap. *J Craniofac Surg* 2010; 21:1887–1889.
4. Guero S, Bastian D, Lassau JP, Csukonyi Z. Anatomical basis of a new naso-labial island flap. *Surg Radiol Anat* 1991; 13:265–270.
5. Lazaridis N, Tilaveridis I, Karakasis D. Superiorly or inferiorly based "islanded" nasolabial flap for buccal mucosa defects reconstruction. *J Oral Maxillofac Surg* 2008; 66:7–15.

Chapter 8
V to Y advancement flap

Introduction

The V to Y advancement flap has many uses in the reconstruction of skin defects at various head and neck sites. This advancement flap is commonly used in the reconstruction of defects located in the cheek region[1] or in the upper lip.[2] The technique can be used in various other sites within the head and neck, and its use seems to be gaining popularity, particularly for reconstructing scalp defects.[3–5]

One advantage of the V to Y advancement flap is the ability to use tissue that is located adjacent to the defect site and which therefore possesses similar quality skin color and texture. Another advantage of the use of this flap is that the placement of the incision sometimes camouflages the final scar as it is in a less conspicuous area.[6]

The V to Y advancement flap is excellent for reconstruction of superficial defects of the upper lip skin. The location of these defects makes reconstruction challenging, often leading the less experienced surgeon to convert them to a full thickness defect and advancing the lip or undermining and closing the lip. Either of these two options leads to a less than desirable esthetic outcome.

Anatomy

The use of the V to Y advancement flap is dependent on the random perfusion to subcutaneous tissues and ultimately to the skin. Because the design of the flap is often in the reconstruction of small defects, its transposition is not dependent on a named source vessel. The main perfusion to the flap comes from the dermal plexus and from the subdermal plexus from the perforating arteries.[7]

The venous drainage of the flap is equally random and depends on the integrity of the vascular bed of the flap to its underlying bed.

The survivability of the flap is generally dependent on the maintenance of the perforating vessels from the underlying tissues. The reliance on the perfusion from the perforators requires a broad subcutaneous bed under the cutaneous portion of the flap to be transposed.

Flap harvest

- The most important step when raising a V to Y advancement flap is the location and design of the flap.
- The location of the defect needs to be well understood as it relates to the potential movement of the surrounding skin in a V–Y advancement.
- An understanding of the pliability of the skin over its underlying tissue bed is essential in the design of the flap.
- The location of the donor site should take into account where the final scar will be placed and whether the movement will cause distortion of the surrounding tissues or structures.
- Once the location is determined, the donor site is marked and the flap is designed taking into consideration the size and shape of the defect to be reconstructed.
- The shape and size of the defect is drawn to fit within the design of a large V-shaped flap.
- The flap is elevated by making the skin incision deep to the dermis and into the subcutaneous fat.
- The adjacent tissues are undermined in a broad front on both sides of the V as well as inferiorly along the point of the V. This undermining should be in the subcutaneous layer along the same depth of the incision of the flap.
- The area along the front of the V (at the opening) is slightly undermined, usually just superficial to the muscle.

Local and Regional Flaps in Head & Neck Reconstruction: A Practical Approach, First Edition. Rui Fernandes.

Companion website: www.wiley.com/go/fernandes/flapsreconstruction

- This area under the flap, along the shape of the V, should not be undermined as this is where the flap gains its vascularity from the perforating vessels that come from below.
- The mobility of the flap is checked to see if it will reach the defect site without tension.
- If the flap doesn't reach the defect site, further undermining is carried out and the process rechecked until the desired mobility is achieved, and the flap is mobilized to cover the defect site.
- The flap is then contoured to fit the shape of the defect and to achieve a harmonious fit.
- The donor site is closed and the amount of advancement is noted by the area from the tip of the V at its new location compared to its location at the time of incision.
- The difference between the two points is the amount of advancement achieved with the flap advancement.
- The wound is closed by first placing a few sutures deep in the dermal layer and then the skin is closed with non-resorbable sutures.
- See Figures 8.1 to 8.6.

Case #1

A 51-year-old African American female was referred for the management of a biopsy-proven keratoachantoma of the left upper lip region. A surgical plan was devised

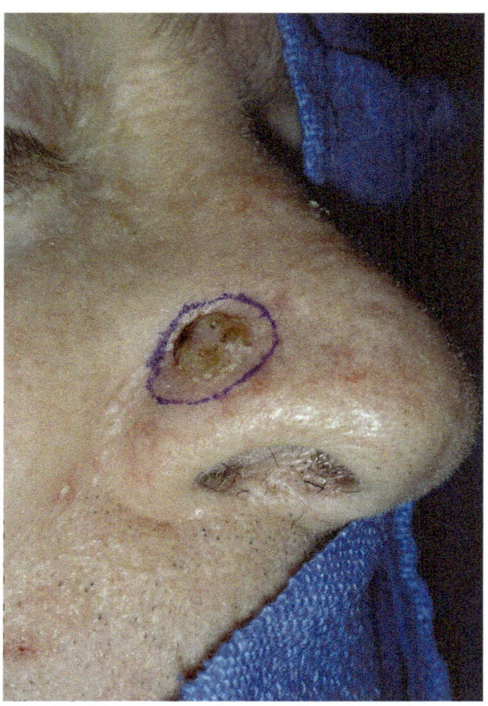

Fig. 8.1 View of a lateral nasal lesion prior to excision.

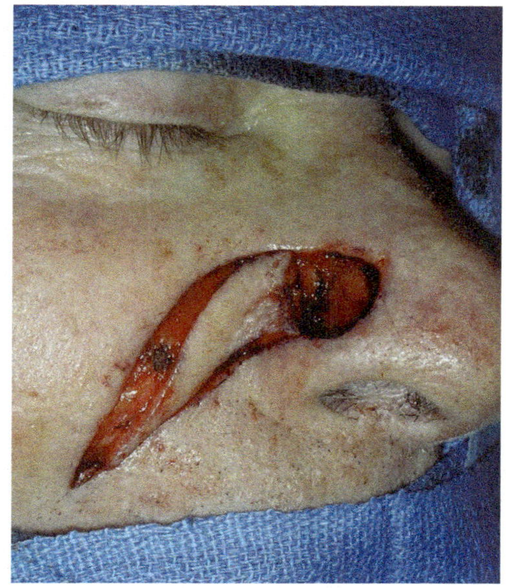

Fig. 8.2 incision of the V–Y flap with lateral undermining prior to advancement.

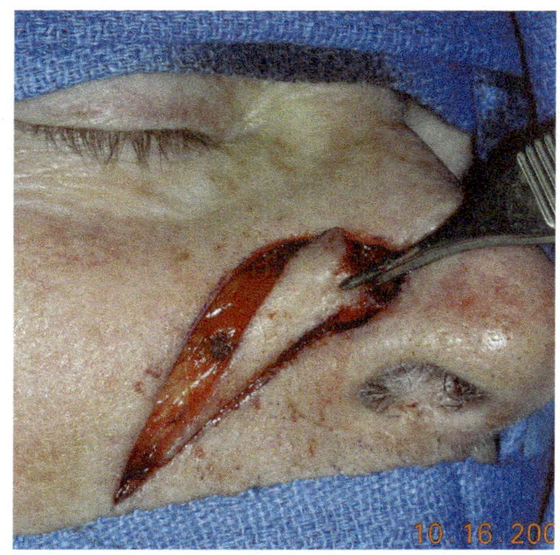

Fig. 8.3 Confirmation of passive advancement of the flap into the defect.

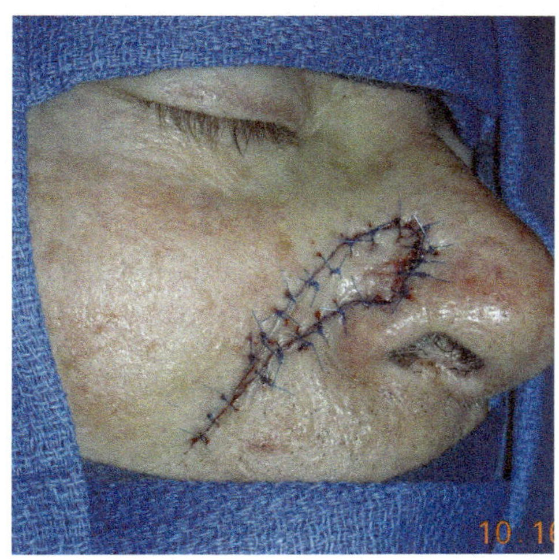

Fig. 8.4 Inset of the flap with scar placement along the nasolabial groove.

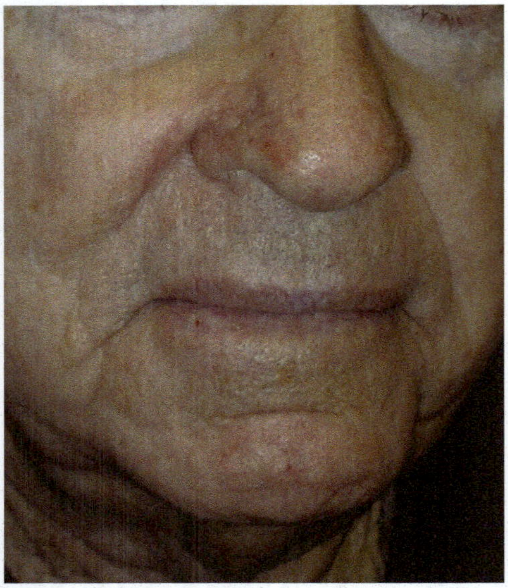

Fig. 8.5 Early view of the reconstructed nasal defect with excellent appearance of both the donor as well as recipient site.

which included resection of the tumor followed by reconstruction of the acquired defect. The markings for the resection were outlined as well as the area for the V to Y advancement (Figure 8.7). The excision was performed and margins assessed with frozen sections. The excision was extended along the nasoalar crease in anticipation of cheek advancement in conjunction with the V to Y advancement flap (Figure 8.8). The excision was made at the perialar region to prevent the formation of a dog-ear at the junction of the nose, cheek, and upper lip. The flap was developed taking care to maintain a wide sub-

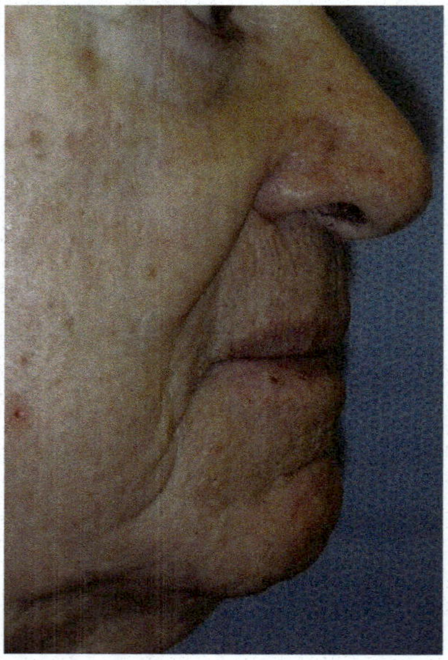

Fig. 8.6 Lateral view of the reconstructed nasal defect with a V–Y flap.

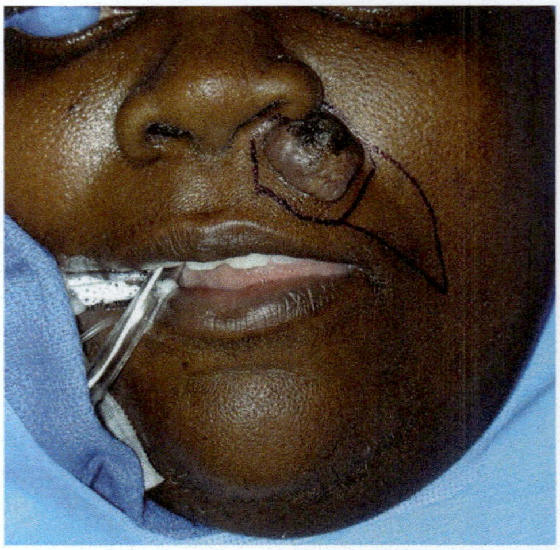

Fig. 8.7 View of a large upper lip carcinoma prior to excision.

cutaneous bed and freeing the fascia to allow for ease of advancement without much tension (Figure 8.9). The flap was inset with several dermal sutures and a subcuticular closure was then performed (Figure 8.10). The final appearance of the patient was satisfactory with minimal distortion of the lip and alar base (Figure 8.11).

Case #2

A 56-year-old Caucasian female was referred for the management of a biopsy-proven squamous cell carcinoma of the left cheek, which had been recently excised, but with

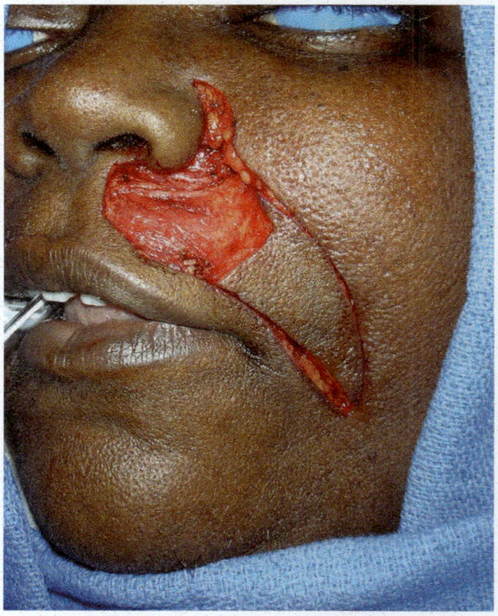

Fig. 8.8 View of the resected upper lip cancer and incision for a V–Y flap. Note the small excision along the lateral nasal wall to accommodate a cheek advancement and better overall final appearance.

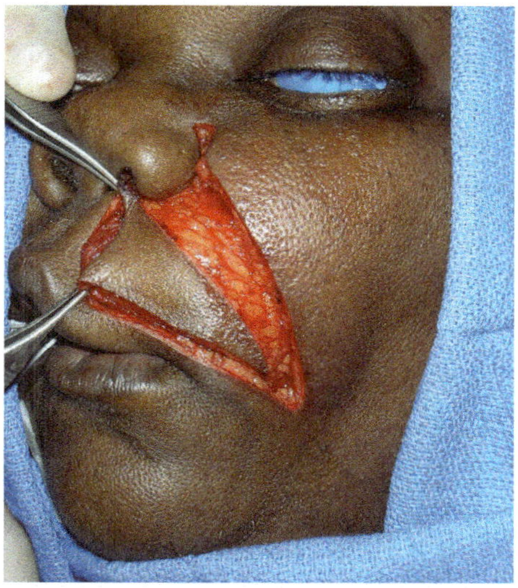

Fig. 8.9 Confirmation of flap advancement after lateral undermining of the flap.

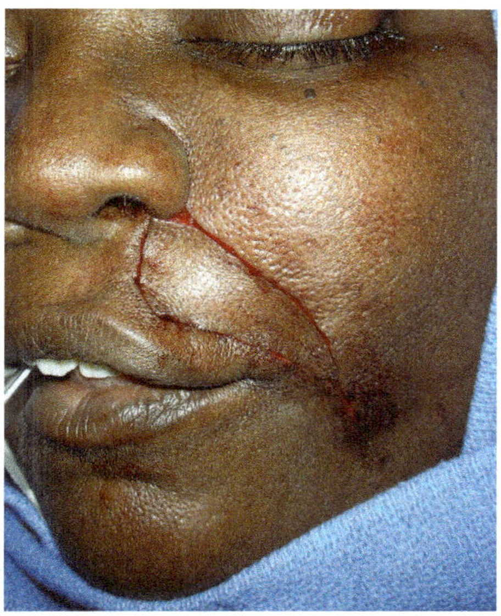

Fig. 8.10 Inset of the flap. The reconstruction of the lip shows good lip contour without deformation of the lip.

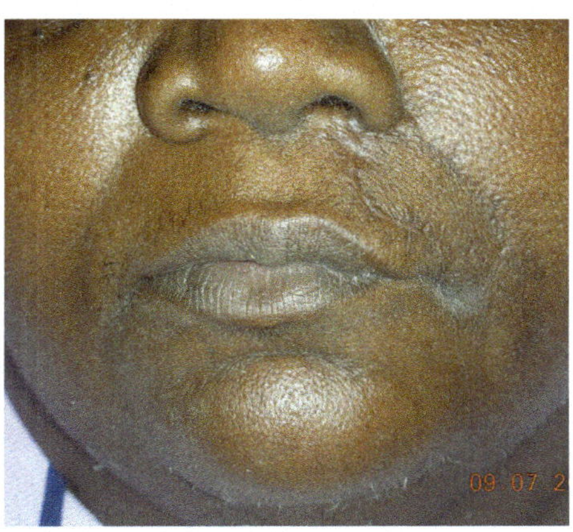

Fig. 8.11 Appearance of the lip after the V–Y reconstruction.

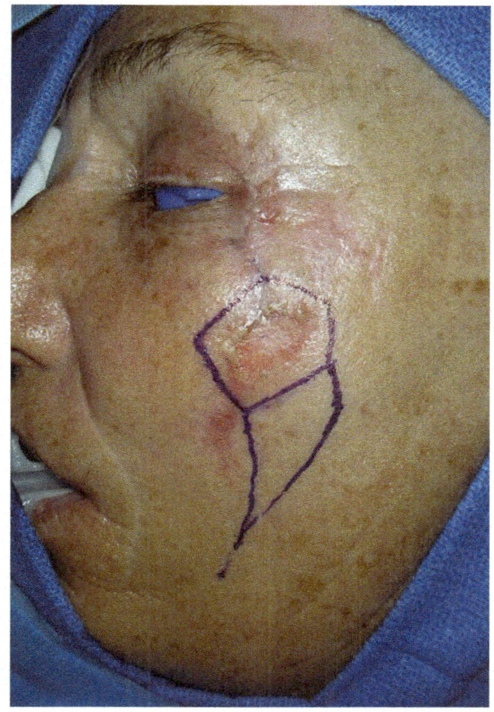

Fig. 8.12 View of a skin malignancy originating in a long standing traumatic lesion.

persistent positive margins. The plan was made for re-excision of the bed and confirmation with frozen section followed by immediate reconstruction of the defect with a vertical V–Y advancement flap (Figure 8.12). The excision was performed and the incision for the V–Y flap was also carried out (Figure 8.13). Following the incision, wide undermining was performed to diminish the likelihood of the downward pull of the cheek resulting in a possible ectropion (Figure 8.14). The mobility of the flap was checked and noted to be adequate to repair the defect without tension; the flap was then inset (Figures 8.15 and 8.16).

Case #3

A 53-year-old Caucasian female was referred for evaluation and treatment of a basal cell carcinoma of the right upper lip with extension towards the ala of the nose (Figure 8.17). A surgical plan was made for resection of the lesion and confirmation with frozen section margins followed by a V–Y advancement flap (Figure 8.18). The excision was completed with a resultant moderately sized defect involving the upper lip, the base of the right nose, and a portion of the cheek (Figure 8.19). A V–Y advancement flap was designed to be transferred to the defect with minimal distortion of the lip and nose (Figures 8.20 and 8.21). The flap was then inset, first by placement of

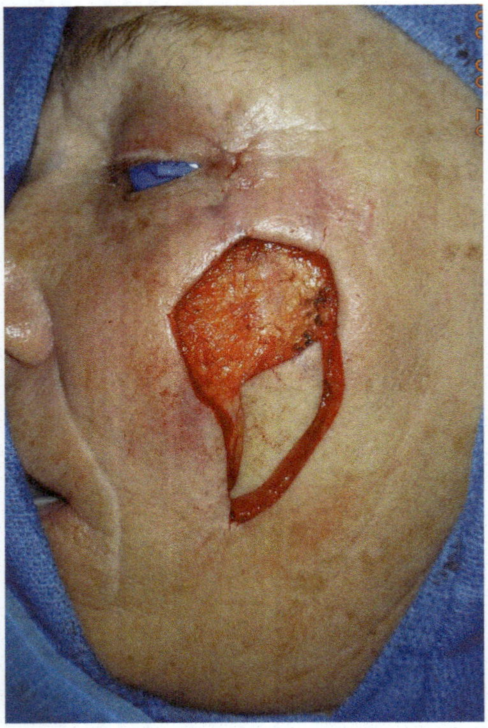

Fig. 8.13 Appearance of the defect after excision of the lesion and incision for the advancement flap.

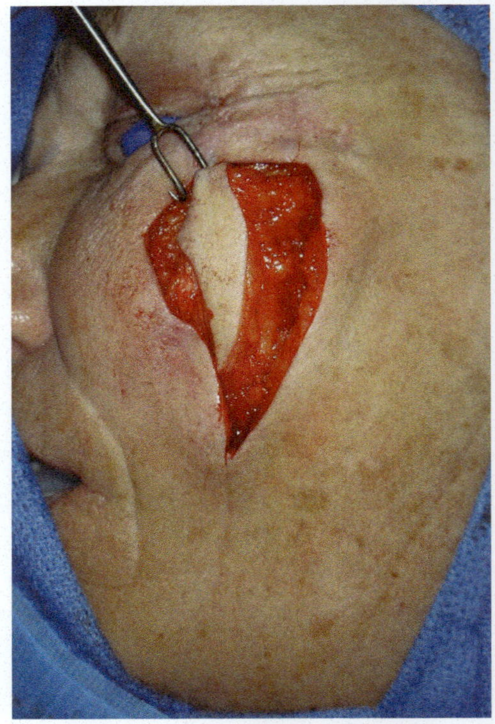

Fig. 8.15 Ensuring passive advancement of the flap to the defect site.

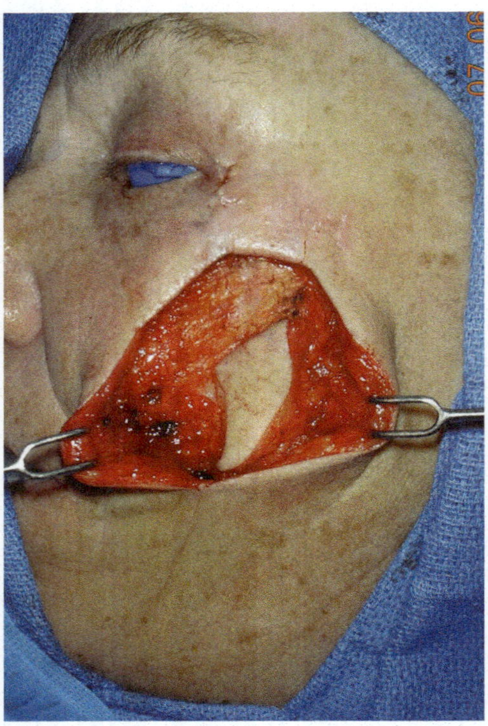

Fig. 8.14 Note the wide undermining of the flap prior to advancement.

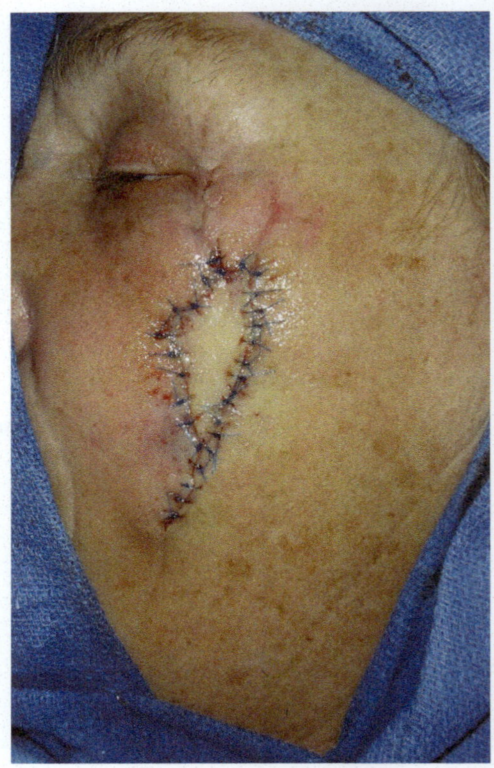

Fig. 8.16 Inset of the flap into the defect.

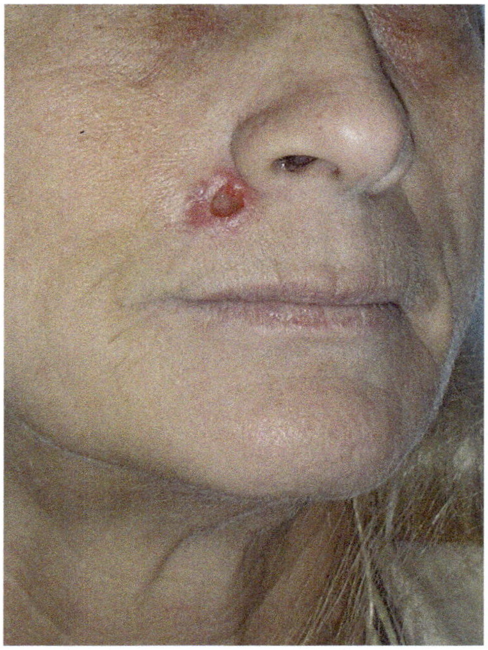

Fig. 8.17 Appearance of a large upper lip skin malignancy.

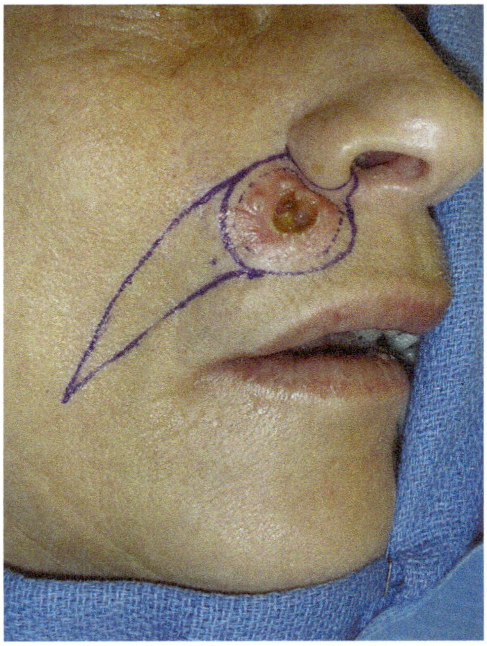

Fig. 8.18 Design for the excision of the lesion with immediate reconstruction of the defect with a V–Y advancement flap; Note the subtle detail for excision along the nasal sill.

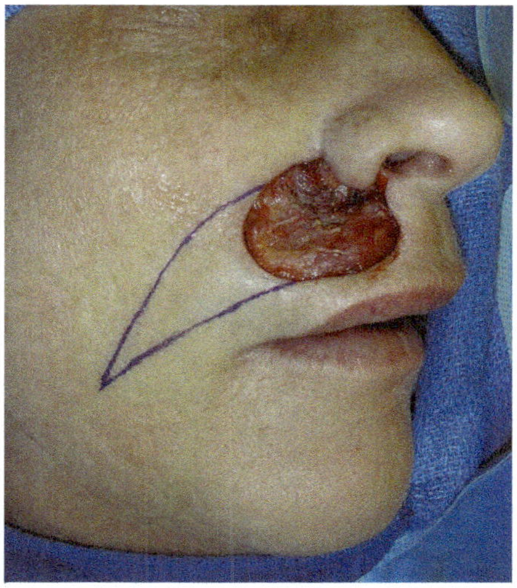

Fig. 8.19 Defect site after excision and prior to the reconstruction.

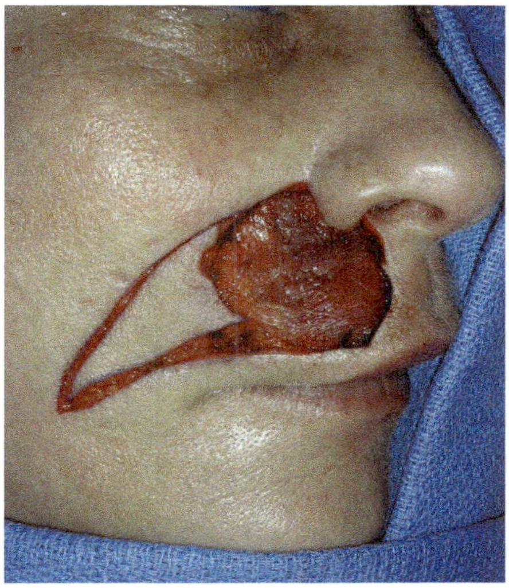

Fig. 8.20 Incision for V–Y advancement flap.

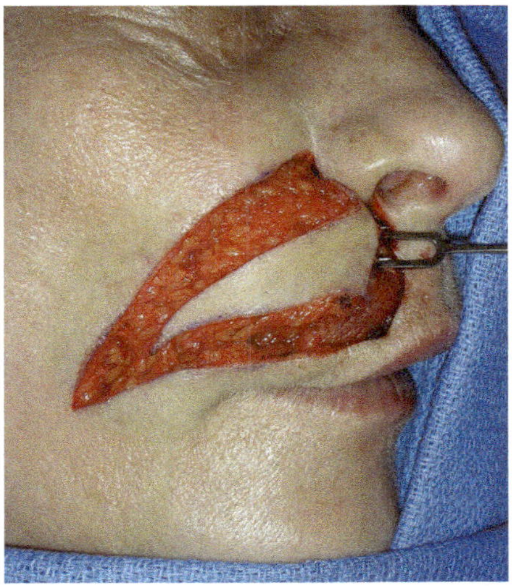

Fig. 8.21 Confirmation of the advancement of the flap to repair the lip defect.

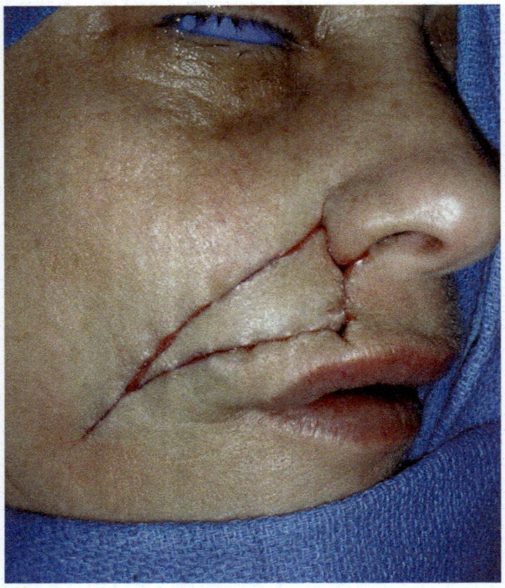

Fig. 8.22 Inset of the flap into the defect with deep sutures; note that there is no deformation of the lip.

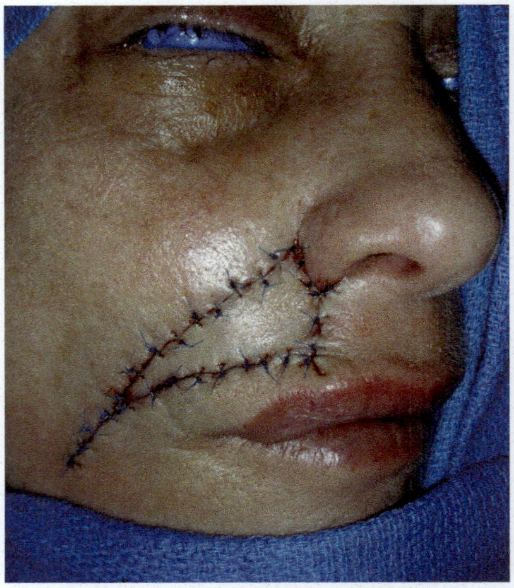

Fig. 8.23 Final inset of the flap into the defect.

dermal sutures and then closure of the epidermis (Figures 8.22 and 8.23). Note that even for this moderately sized defect, the proper planning and transfer of a V–Y advancement flap, in this case based on the facial artery perforators, there is minimal distortion of the lip and nose. The appearance on the table was very acceptable.

References

1. Kim JY, Chung S, Chung YK. Croissant shaped V–Y advancement flap with 2 horns for repair of small and medium sized facial defects. *J Craniofac Surg* 2011; 22:1781–1784.
2. Griffin GR, Weber S, Baker SR. Outcomes following V–Y advancement flap reconstruction of large upper lip defects. *Arch Facial Plast Surg* 2012; 14(3):193–197.
3. Onishi K, Maruyama Y, Hayashi A, Inami K. Repair of scalp defect using a superficial temporal fascia pedicle VY advancement scalp flap. *Br J Plast Surg* 2005; 58:676–680.
4. Sharma KR, Tuli P. Occipital artery island V–Y advancement flap for reconstruction of posterior scalp defects. *J Plastic Reconstr Aesthetic Surg* 2010; 63(3):410–415.
5. Sharma R, Sirohi D, Sinha R, Menon PS. Reconstruction of a large posterior scalp defect using occipital artery based pedicled island V–Y advancement flap: a case report. *J Maxillofac Oral Surg* 2011; 10(3):262–265.
6. Brunetti B, Tenna S, Aveta A, Segreto F, Persichetti P. Freestyle local perforator flaps: versatility of the V–Y design to reconstruct soft tissue defects in the skin cancer population. *Plast Reconstr Surg* 2013; 132:451–460.
7. Kwon KH, Lee DG, Koo SH, Jo KM, Shin H, Seul JH. Usefulness of V–Y advancement flap for defects after skin tumor excision. *Arch Plast Surg* 2012; 39:619–625.

Chapter 9
Keystone flap

Introduction

Dr. Felix Behan first introduced the keystone flap in the literature in 2003 as a new method for closing skin defects following skin cancer resection.[1] The flap was described as a curvilinear-shaped trapezoidal design flap forming essentially two V–Y advancement flaps in an end to side arrangement. Since this first description, several other publications have demonstrated the reliability of this reconstructive method for several areas of the body.[2,3]

Although the use of the keystone flap has yet to gain widespread popularity, it is still a very useful option for both small and large defects in the head and neck region.

The keystone was described in the initial manuscript as having several variances.

The *Type I* flap is a standard flap design where the curvilinear flap is transferred to the defect and the donor site is closed primarily. This can be done in defects up to 2 cm in width.

The *Type IIA* flap is a modification where the reconstruction is over a muscular compartment and the deep fascia on the outer compartment is divided in order to facilitate mobility.

The *Type IIB* is when the flap is transferred and the donor site is repaired with a split thickness skin graft.

The *Type III* is the use of a double Keystone flap to repair larger defects.

The *Type IV* incorporates the use of a rotation component in the flap. In order to perform this maneuver, a maximum of 50% of the flap is elevated and then rotated to close the defect.

Surgeons from the Sydney Melanoma Unit described a modification of the keystone flap.[4] The modification enables preservation of the central portion of the outer skin bridge along the outer arc. This modification increases the vascularity of the flap.

The main advantage of the flap is that it transfers adjacent tissues to repair the defect therefore taking the advantage of tissue color, pliability, and texture. The final esthetic result obtained using this flap is very pleasing. This advantage puts this flap in the same category as the V–Y advancement flap as well as other flaps already described in this book.

The final result of the reconstruction when using a keystone flap is one that shows a reconstructed defect with a flap, yet the donor site remains an enigma to all except the surgeon who performed the reconstruction.

The disadvantage of the keystone flap is that the main attraction of the flap, i.e. the ability to repair a defect without evidence of donor site harvest, is restricted to smaller defects. In cases where large defects need to be repaired, the use of the standard Type I keystone becomes more limited and the alternative Type III or IV can be contemplated.For larger defects, other flap options may often be considered.

Anatomy

The vascular anatomy of the keystone flap varies with its location. The flap is based as a random flap, which receives its blood supply from perforating vessels emerging from the fascia to profuse to the dermal and subdermal layers via small capillaries. The venous drainage of the flap is based on a similar system with larger deep veins draining the flap.

Flap harvest

- Once the resection is completed, the shape of the defect should resemble that of an ellipse or a shape similar to it.

Local and Regional Flaps in Head & Neck Reconstruction: A Practical Approach, First Edition. Rui Fernandes.

Companion website: www.wiley.com/go/fernandes/flapsreconstruction

- The width of the excision is measured then transferred to the adjacent tissue to be moved to the defect.
- A curvilinear mark is made parallel to the shape of the ellipse while maintaining the same width.
- At each end of the ellipse, the connecting point between the edge of the ellipse and the marked line should form a 90 degree angle.
- The ratio between the defect and the width of the flap should be one to one.
- An incision is made circumferentially around the marked flap and carried down deep to the dermis and to the subcutaneous fat.
- The fascia along the outer aspect of the flap may be incised to gain mobility if needed.
- Minimal undermining is done just along the edge of the flap but preferably no undermining should be attempted underneath the flap as the perfusion to the flap is gained from the perforating vessels penetrating the fascia and perfusing the skin.
- Closure of the defect can begin once the flap mobility and reach to the defect has been checked and confirmed.
- The closure is done by placing the first suture in the central portion of the inner aspect of the flap and mobilizing it to meet the outer aspect of the opposing defect site.
- The second and third sutures are placed at two points in the outer aspect of the flap and the donor site, thus simultaneously beginning the closure of the donor site.
- The next two sutures should be placed at each end of the flap in a V–Y advancement of the edges.
- This maneuver allows for migration of the flap centrally, therefore bringing more tissue for the remainder of the closure.
- The rest of the flap is closed with interrupted sutures and if redundant tissues are noted, they can be trimmed to allow for a passive and esthetic fit of the flap.

Case #1

An 82-year-old Caucasian male was referred for the management of a large preauricular lesion which had been recently biopsied and proven to be a squamous cell carcinoma (Figure 9.1). Given the location of the lesion, and the medical status of the patient, a decision was made for a conservative resection with immediate reconstruction of the defect with a keystone flap. The decision to use a keystone flap was made because of the immediate location of the lesion in the preauricular area without any tissue posterior to it. The lesion was excised and the margins assessed and found to be negative based on frozen section analysis (Figure 9.2). Markings were made for a large keystone flap to transpose the tissues anterior to the defect (Figure 9.3). The marked area was incised (Figure 9.4). The flap was transferred by first placing the keystone suture and advancing the flap to the defect (Figure 9.5). The remainder of the flap was inset as described earlier (Figure 9.6). The initial follow-up showed a healing flap with excellent reconstruction of a potentially difficult site (Figure 9.7).

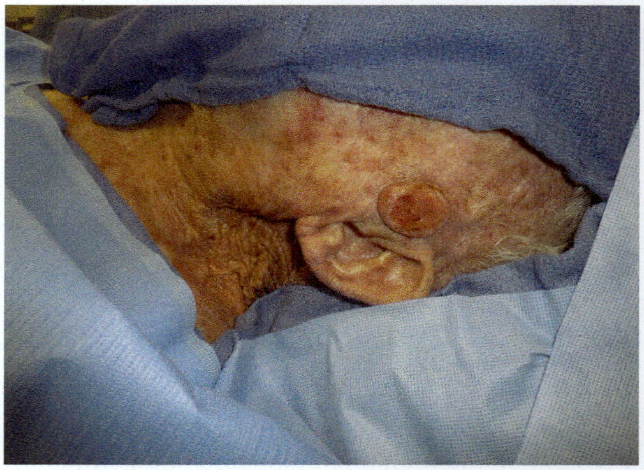

Fig. 9.1 Appearance of a large preauricular lesion prior to excision.

Case #2

An 84-year-old Caucasian male was referred to the practice for evaluation of a lesion on the right upper neck region. The area was raised, ulcerated, and within an area of multiple previous excisions of squamous cell carcinomas (Figure 9.8). A decision was made to excise the lesion and perform immediate reconstruction of the resultant defect with a keystone flap. The lesion was excised and

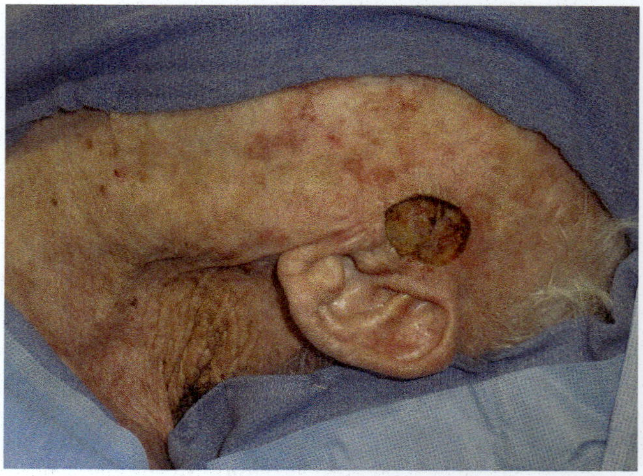

Fig. 9.2 View of the defect prior to flap reconstruction.

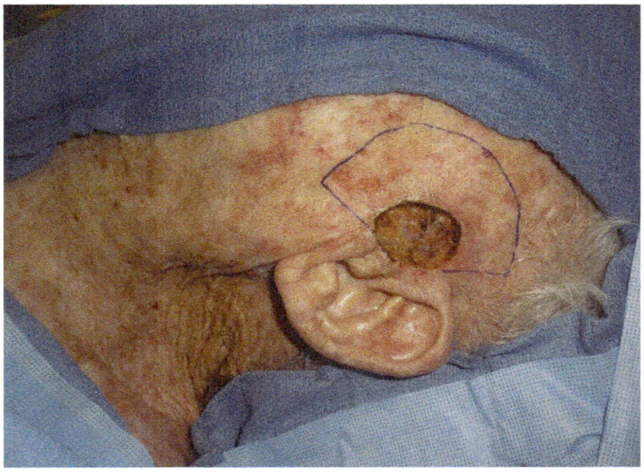

Fig. 9.3 Design for a keystone flap to repair the defect.

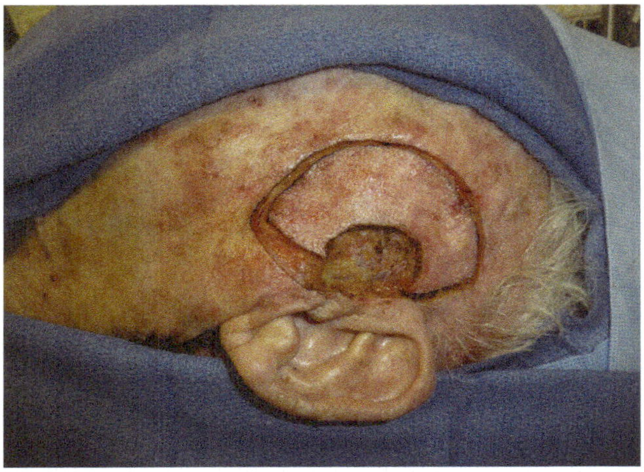

Fig. 9.4 Incision of the flap prior to inset.

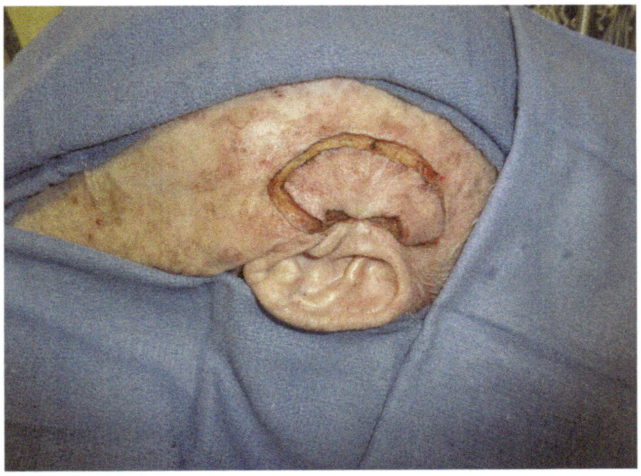

Fig. 9.5 Insetting of the flap into the defect.

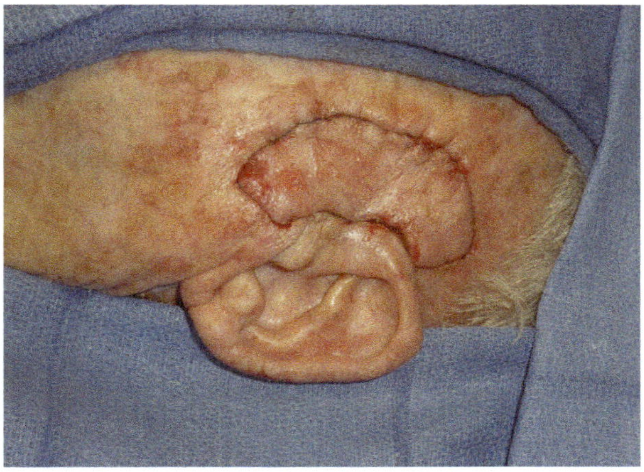

Fig. 9.6 Final inset of the flap.

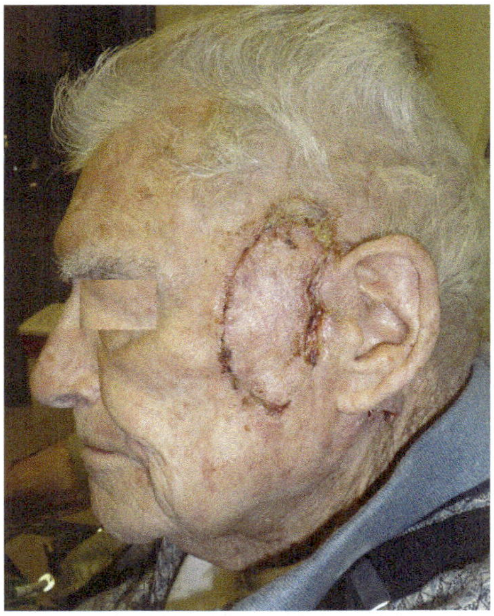

Fig. 9.7 Early postoperative view of the reconstruction, with good healing and appearance of the flap.

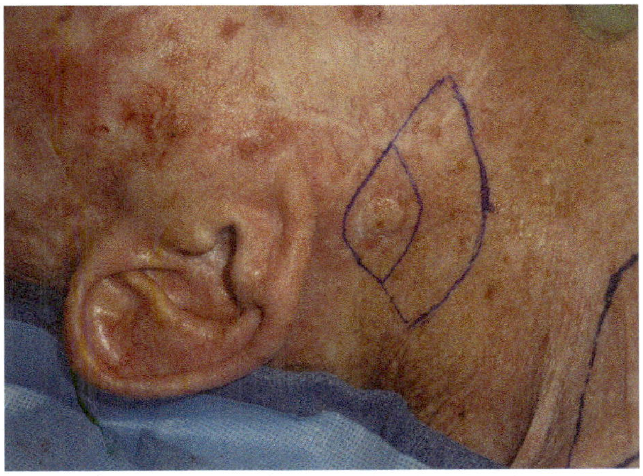

Fig. 9.8 View of a neck lesion prior to excision and reconstruction with a keystone flap.

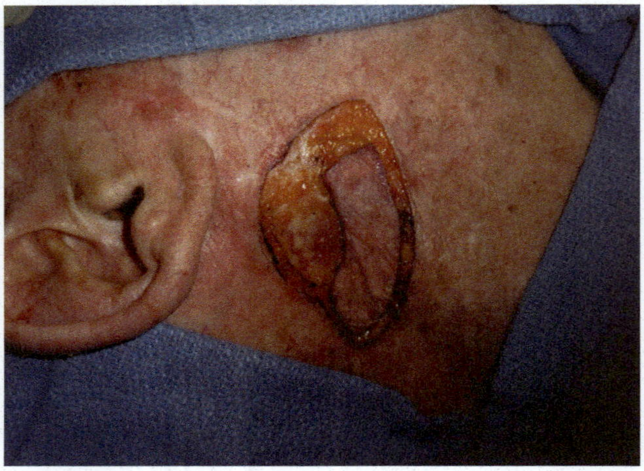

Fig. 9.9 The lesion has been excised and the flap incisions have been made.

the margins cleared by frozen section analysis. The keystone flap was developed by incising the inferior area, which had been previously marked (Figure 9.9). The flap was then mobilized and inset using the previously described method of insetting a keystone flap (Figure 9.10). The patient did very well, and early post-operative evaluation showed a well-healed flap without a "donor site" (Figure 9.11).

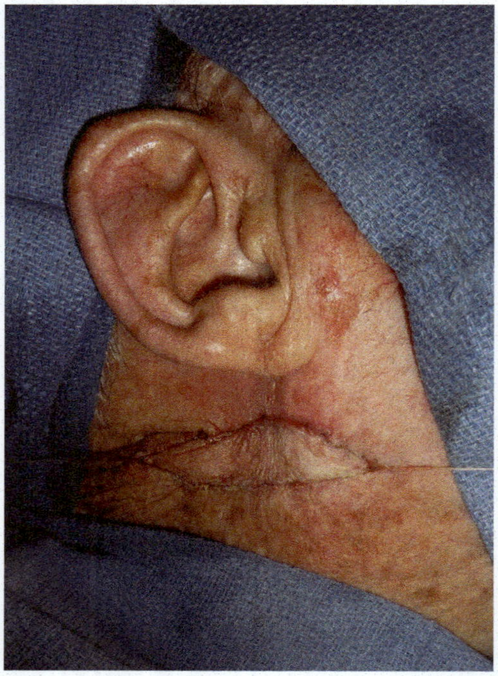

Fig. 9.10 View of the inset of the flap. Note that the reconstruction gives the illusion of transferred flap without an obvious donor site.

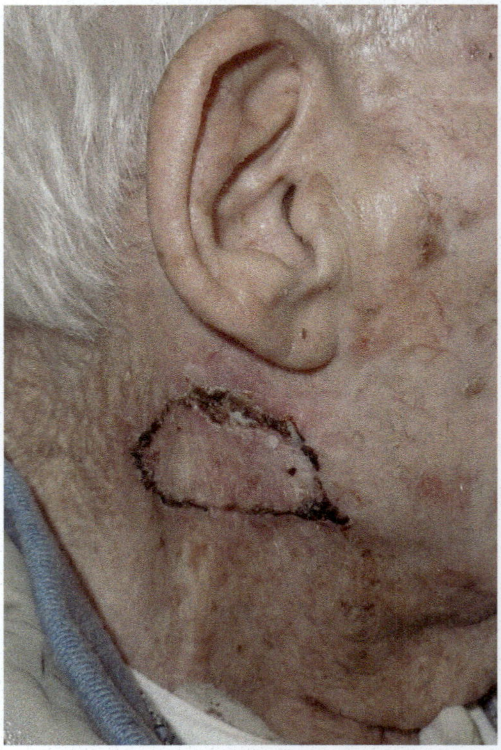

Fig. 9.11 Early postoperative appearance of the reconstructed defect.

Suggested reading

Felix Behan, The keystone design perforator island flap in reconstructive surgery. Australian New Zealand Journal of Surgery, 2003; 73: 112–120.

This was the original publication of the use of the keystone flap. The author eloquently describes the various uses of this reconstructive technique as well as several permutations of the flap, which he categorizes as Type I through IV. In the description the author details the closing methods for these varied options.

Marc D. Moncrieff, et al., Keystone flap reconstruction of primary melanoma excision defects of the leg – The end of skin graft? Annals of Surgical Oncology 2008; 15(10):2867–2873.

This publication describes the Sydney Melanoma Unit modification of the keystone flap whereby the central portion of the outer incision of the flap is left intact. This modification allows for the maintenance of a skin bridge between the flap and the donor site. Using scissors, the fascia along the entire arc of the outer arc may be incised to increase the mobility. This incision is carried out under the skin bridge. The remaining portions of the flap are as was described by Behan. Although this modification was described in the reconstruction of defects of the lower extremity, its use can also be employed in the head and neck.

Philipe Pelissier, Max Santoul, Vincent Pinsole, et al., The keystone design perforator island flap. Part I: Anatomic Study. Journal of Plastic, Reconstructive & Aesthetic Surgery, 2007; 60:883–887.

This first part of a two part series by Dr. Behan's group describes the vascularity of the flap as well as the anatomical changes in the skin paddle as a result of the traction forces placed on the skin.

Pelissier P[1], Gardet H, Pinsolle V, Santoul M, Behan FC. The keystone design perforator island flap. Part II: Clinical Applications. J Plast Reconstr Aesthet Surg. 2007; 60(8):888–891. Epub 2007 May 9.

References

1. Behan FC, The keystone design perforator island flap in reconstructive surgery, *ANZ J Surg* 2003; 73:112–120.
2. Martinez JC, Cook JL, Otley C. The keystone fasciocutaneous flap in the reconstruction of lower extremity wounds. *Dermatol Surg* 2012; 38:484–489.
3. Behan F, Sizeland A, Porcedu S, Somia N, Wilson J. Keystone island flap: an alternative reconstructive option to free flaps in irradiated tissue. *ANZ J Surg* 2006; 76: 407–413.
4. Moncrieff MD, Bowen F, Thompson JF, et al., Keystone flap reconstruction of primary melanoma excision defects of the leg – the end of the skin graft ?. *Ann Surg Oncol* 2008; 15(10): 2867–2873.

Chapter 10
Paramedian forehead flap

Introduction

The paramedian forehead flap may be one of the oldest flaps in use for the reconstruction of facial defects. Its use in nasal reconstruction dates as far back as 1500 BC as it was used to reconstruct nasal amputation defects.[1,2] The classic Indian forehead flap became popular in the United States when Blair[3] in 1925 and Kazanjian[4] in 1946 described the median forehead flap for nasal repair. Several years later, Millard revised the flap by narrowing the base and rendering the perfusion based solely on the supratrochlear vessels.[5] The modification allowed for an increase in the length of the flap to be harvested and ease of rotation of the flap due to the narrower pedicle width. The modification increased the reliability of the flap by diminishing the torsion on the vessels and therefore allowing for better perfusion and diminished likelihood of congestion.[6]

The main use of the paramedian forehead flap has been in the reconstruction of partial to total nasal defects. Its use is not limited to nasal reconstruction; the flap may be used to reconstruct any defect within the reach of its arc of rotation. This fact allows for its use in reconstructing defects in the forehead, and the periorbital region.

The main advantages of this flap rest on its texture, thickness, and color match to the surrounding skin, making it an indispensable option in reconstructing a vast range of nasal defects.

The drawback of the paramedian forehead flap is the need for multiple stage surgery. Typical use requires first a transfer then sectioning of the pedicle and inset of the flap several weeks later. In order to keep the positives of this flap while removing the main drawback, some authors have advocated its use as a single stage flap.[7,8]

Anatomy

The anatomy of the forehead is relatively simple in terms of tissue composition. The layers of the forehead consist of the skin, the subcutaneous skin, the frontalis muscle, areolar tissue, and the pericranium. The skin of the forehead region is of similar color, texture, and thickness to many of the surrounding areas within the reach of the paramedian forehead flap.

The vascular supply to the forehead comes from the paired supraorbital arteries, which divide into a superficial and a deep branch, and the paired supratrochlear arteries. Both the supraorbital and the supratrochlear arteries are branches of the ophthalmic artery, which in turn is a branch of the internal carotid artery. The glabellar region of the forehead also receives terminal branches from the angular artery, which is a branch from the facial artery. The latter is a branch from the external carotid artery. The forehead region in fact receives its arterial supply from both the internal and external carotid system. The venous drainage of the forehead region is carried out by the accompanying venae comitantes of the supraorbital and supratrochlear vessels. The sensory innervation of the forehead is by the supraorbital nerve and the supratrochlear nerve, while the motor innervation to the frontalis muscle comes from the frontal branch of the facial nerve.

The blood supply of the paramedian forehead flap is based on the supratrochlear artery and vein as its axial

Local and Regional Flaps in Head & Neck Reconstruction: A Practical Approach, First Edition. Rui Fernandes.

Companion website: www.wiley.com/go/fernandes/flapsreconstruction

and random blood supply from the anastomosing vessels from the terminal branches of the angular artery and the contralateral. The artery can be located as it emerges from the foramen and travels in a cephalad direction in the forehead region between the medial brow and the lateral aspect of the nasal dorsum. The path of the artery and the venae commitantes is in a more or less vertical direction, thus resulting in an axial flap.

In the caudal aspect, as the artery begins its cephalad travel, it is located above the pericranium. As it travels, it migrates towards the subcutaneous plane. In the forehead region near the hair line, the vessel branches are found in the subcutaneous plane.

The frontalis muscle is found in the location of this flap, especially at the most superior portion of the flap.

Flap harvest

First stage

- The path of the supratrochlear artery is marked as it travels in a cephalad direction in the forehead.
- The size of the defect to be transferred is measured and the location of the defect is noted.
- The outline of the defect can be retraced with a marking pen. Using a small piece of paper from the surgical glove packing, the imprint of the defect is picked up onto the paper by pressing down over the marking.
- The template is trimmed and transferred to a good position on the forehead.
- With a suture string, a pivot point along the brow is marked and the string is then rotated to the most inferior point of the defect.
- The string is then rotated along this pivot point to the forehead and the point is marked. This will be the most cephalad portion of the flap.
- The defect shape is then transferred to the forehead, taking care to center it along the axial path of the artery.
- The elevation of the flap is begun on the most superior portion of the flap and is extended to a depth superior to the frontalis muscle.
- The incision is made along the marked flap and dissection is carried out in a caudal direction towards the nasal bridge and medial canthus along the main axial direction of the artery.
- The depth of the dissection is extended to the subperiosteal layer about 3 cm superior to the brow region. This depth offers a layer of protection to the vascular pedicle.
- Once the dissection nears the brow region, care should be taken not to injure the main pedicle.
- The medial portion of the pedicle should be extended in a curvilinear fashion towards the medial canthus, leaving at least a 1 cm bridge of skin overlying the vascular pedicle.
- The dissection in the brow region should be made with care not only to maintain the integrity of the vascular pedicle but also to release the periostium in this area, therefore aiding rotation of the flap to reach the defect site passively.
- Once the flap dissection is completed, the rotation and reach of the flap is assured to be in a passive fashion. The flap may be thinned if the defect warrants it.
- If thinning is needed, this is carried out using thernotomy scissors only in the area of the flap to be inset into the recipient site.
- The flap is inset in the recipient site from the most caudal area to the most cephalad region. The most superior portion of the flap will not be sutured into the defect because of the axial extension of the skin and vascular pedicle. The area is, however, in tight contact to the underlying defect site.
- The forehead defect is undermined widely and advanced towards the midline.
- The closure of the defect is begun from the inferior aspect and extended in a superior direction. In cases where primary closure is not possible, the area is then left to heal in a secondary intention.
- See Figures 10.1 to 10.13.

Second stage

- The flap is allowed to heal and develop collateral circulation for a period of no less than 3 weeks.

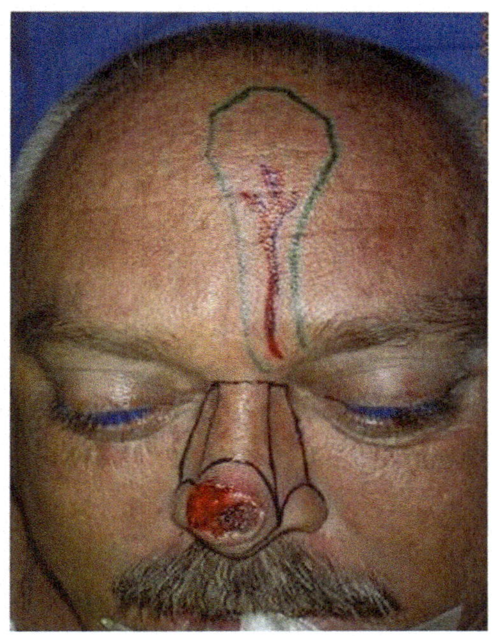

Fig. 10.1 Markings for the resection of the nasal lesion and reconstruction of the planned defect with a paramedian forehead flap.

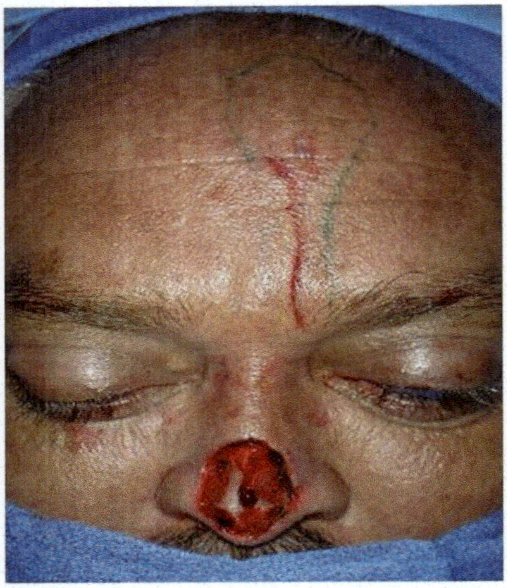

Fig. 10.2 View of the defect after resection of the nasal lesion.

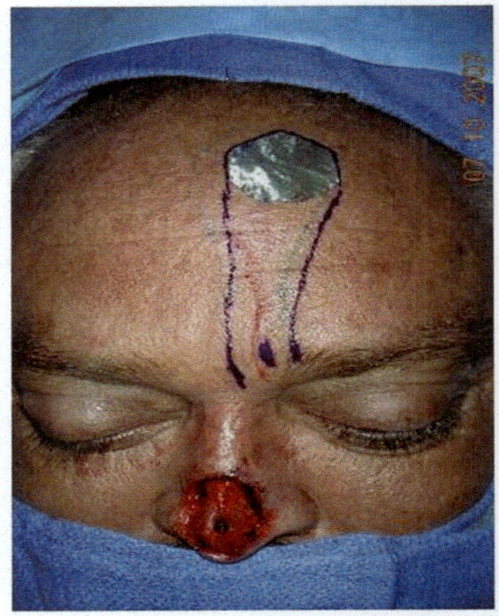

Fig. 10.4 Transfer of the template to the forehead.

- The flap can then be sectioned and the superior aspect of the defect closed along with insetting of the donor site in the brow region.
- In cases where there is a question about the amount of collateral blood supply, the flap pedicle can be constricted with a rubber band for a few minutes to evaluate the color and perfusion of the flap.
- Once satisfied, the flap is pedicle is sectioned.
- The donor side of the flap is addressed by elevating a portion of the flap from the recipient bed and then thinning it by taking a wedge from the flap. The base of the wedge should be the cephalad portion. This will allow the flap to lie at the same depth as the superior portion of the surrounding area of the defect site. The flap is then inset.
- The donor area is then addressed by first opening the tube of the pedicle and laying it down in a cephalad direction along the previous forehead incision. The flap is then incised as a triangle shape to be inset to the donor site and allow for the medial brow to be returned to its normal position (in those cases with a

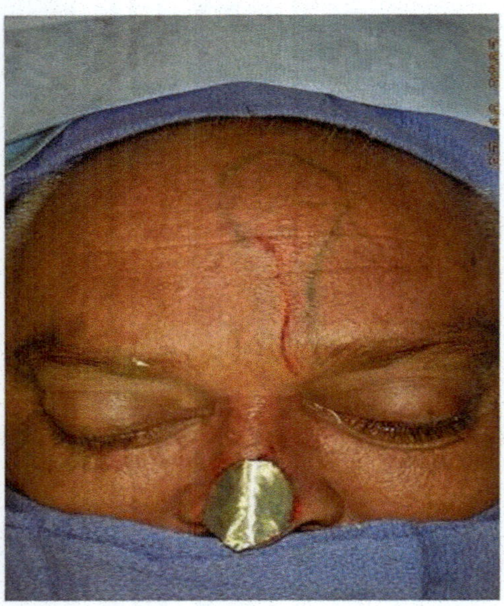

Fig. 10.3 Assessment of the donor site defect to be used as a template for the reconstruction.

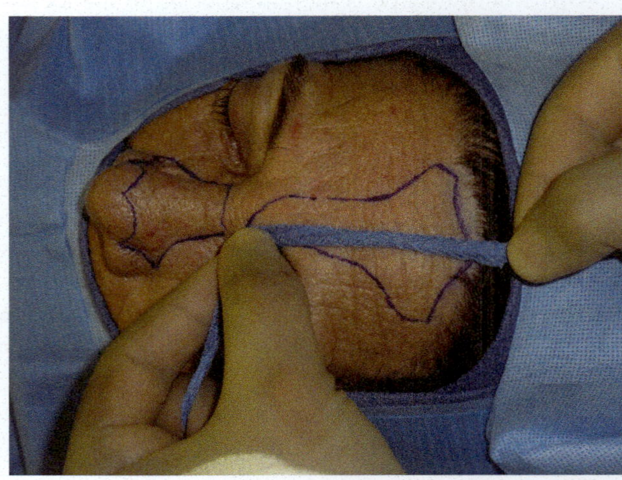

Fig. 10.5 Measurement of the flap to confirm reach of the flap to the defect site.

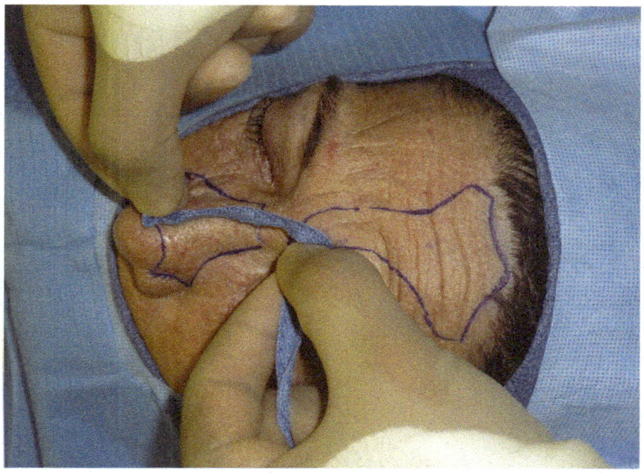

Fig. 10.6 Rotation of the measurement to the planned defect from the pivot point.

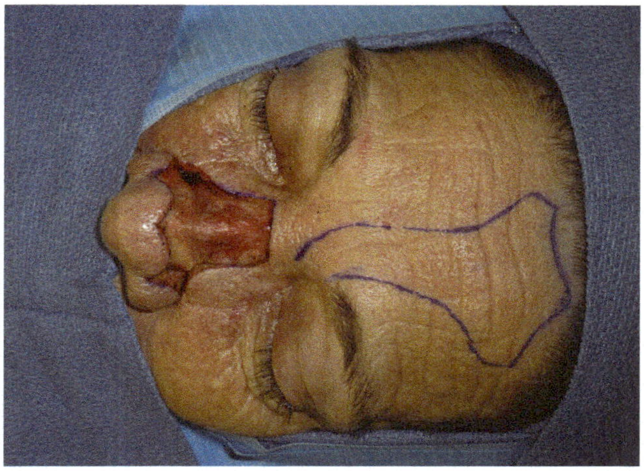

Fig. 10.7 Nasal defect prior to the reconstruction.

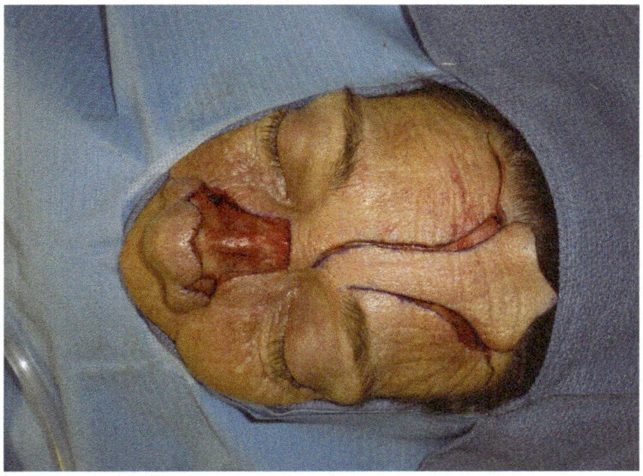

Fig. 10.8 Elevation of the flap prior to transfer to the nasal defect.

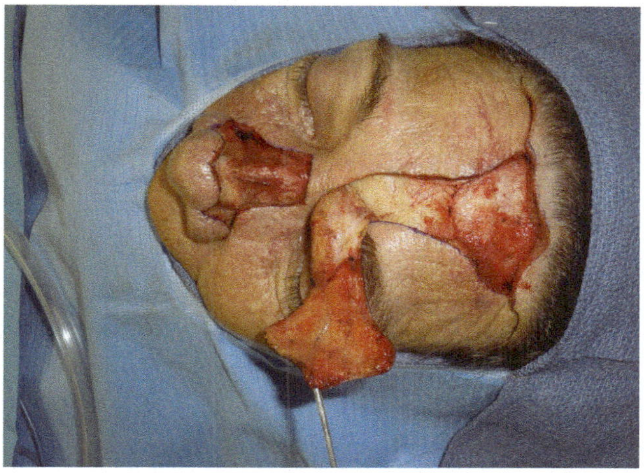

Fig. 10.9 Elevated flap. Note that the depth is changed to a subperiosteal plane in the region of the brow.

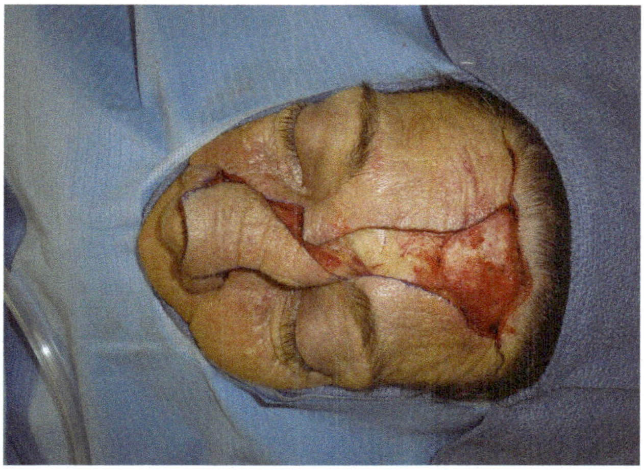

Fig. 10.10 Assessment of the reach of the flap to the defect.

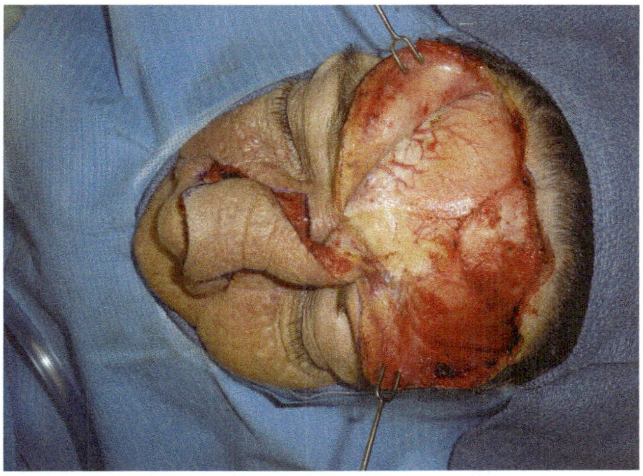

Fig. 10.11 Elevation of the forehead to diminish the defect size; the incision was made along the hairline.

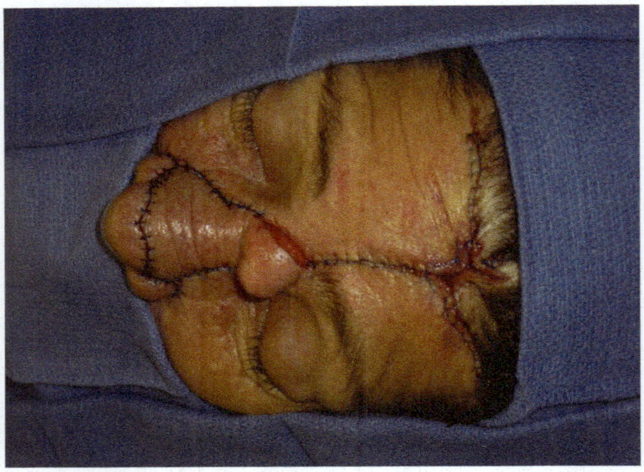

Fig. 10.12 Closure of the forehead donor site.

medial displacement of the brow) (Figures 10.14 and 10.15).

Quilting/shaping of the flap

- In cases of nasal reconstruction or where there is a need to further shape the flap to contour to the defect, the flap is thinned and quilting sutures are placed in the desired areas to mold the shape of the flap to create the necessary concavities and convexities.
- The quilting sutures are removed about 5 days later and the flap.

Single stage forehead flap

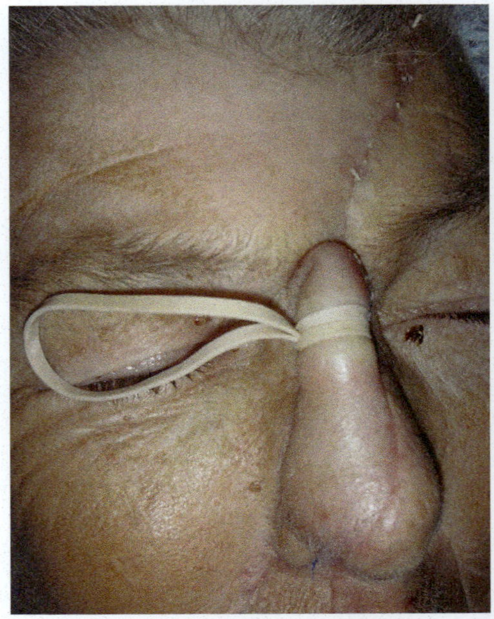

Fig. 10.14 Assessment of the perfusion to the flap prior to takedown. This illustrates the evaluation by using a rubber band along the pedicle.

The paramedian forehead flap can also be used as a single stage or island flap in certain situations.[9,10] In cases where the flap is being used as a rotational flap to directly cover adjacent defects without an intact bridge of skin between the pedicle and the flap, the forehead may be used as a single stage. Other situations where the flap is being transferred to a defect distant from the donor site with an intact bridge of skin between the recipient site and the donor site, it can be used as a single stage. In these rare cases, a subcutaneous tunnel is developed between the two sites which would allow the passive transfer of the flap to the recipient site without constriction of the pedicle. Next, the area of the flap that will be in the

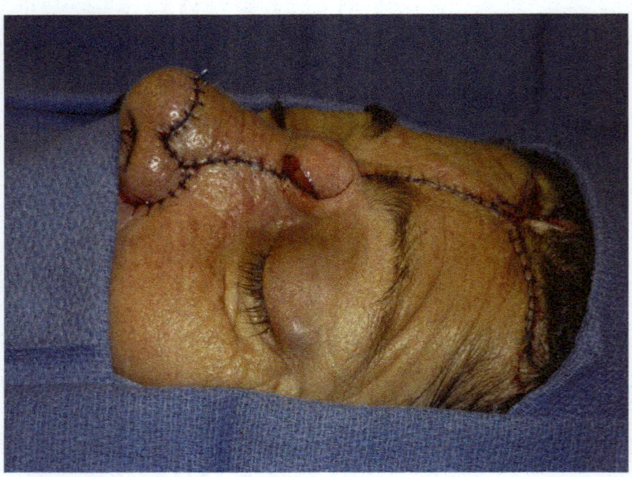

Fig. 10.13 Lateral view of the nasal reconstruction.

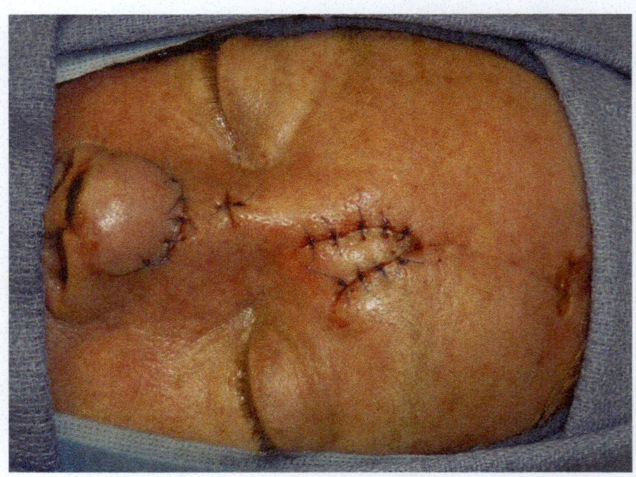

Fig. 10.15 View after takedown of the paramedian forehead flap.

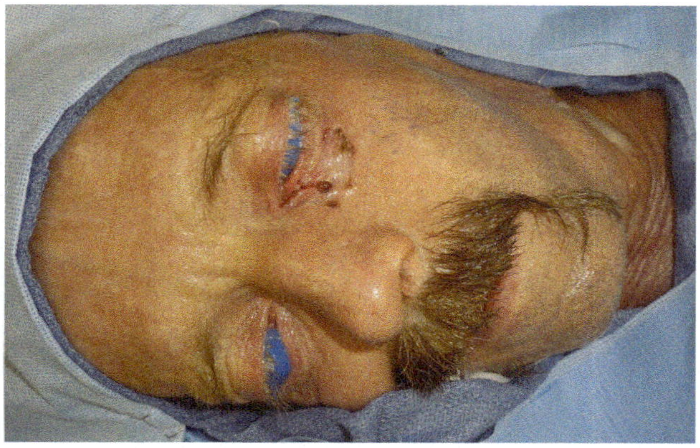

Fig. 10.16a View of a large left infraorbital lesion.

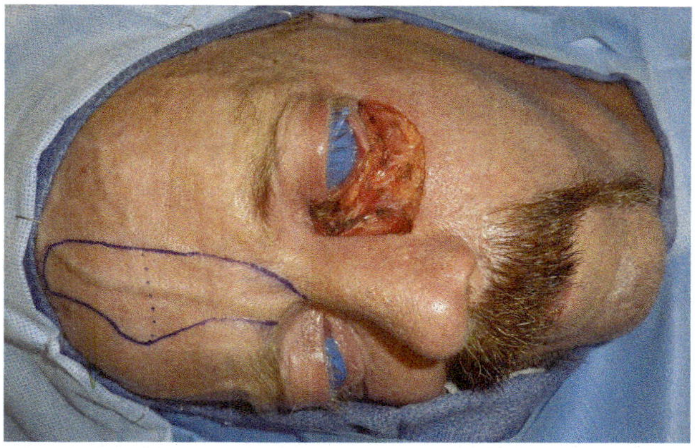

Fig. 10.17 Defect size after excision of the lesion.

subcutaneous tunnel is de-epithelialized, taking care to not injure the underlying vascular pedicle.

The main disadvantage of this technique is the resultant bulk along the nasal bridge at the site where the flap is turned into the defect. This bulk may be of significant prominence which will detract from the final esthetic outcome, thus rendering this method a less desirable technique.

Case #1

A 48-year-old male was referred to the service for evaluation and treatment of a longstanding morpheaform basal cell carcinoma of the left infraorbital region. The resection and reconstruction was discussed with the patient. Given the location of the lesion and concern for ectropion and significant color mismatch, it was decided that a good option would be for resection and immediate reconstruction of the defect with local tissue repositioning and a paramedian forehead flap (Figure 10.16a and b). Prior to resection of the lesion, a template was made and the planned defect was transferred to the forehead and designed over the supratrochlear vessels which were very apparent on this patient (Figure 10.17). The flap was elevated and the arc of rotation and reach was confirmed to be sure that there would be minimal tension on inset (Figures 10.18 and Figure 10.19a and b). Approximately 3 weeks later, the patient was brought to the operating room where the take down of the pedicle was performed and the remaining flap was inset to the defect (Figure 10.19c and d). The second stage was carried out as per routine and the early appearance of the reconstruction was deemed satisfactory by the patient (Figure 10.20a and b).

Case #2

A 67-year-old female was referred for the reconstruction of a Mohs' defect of the nasal dorsum and tip

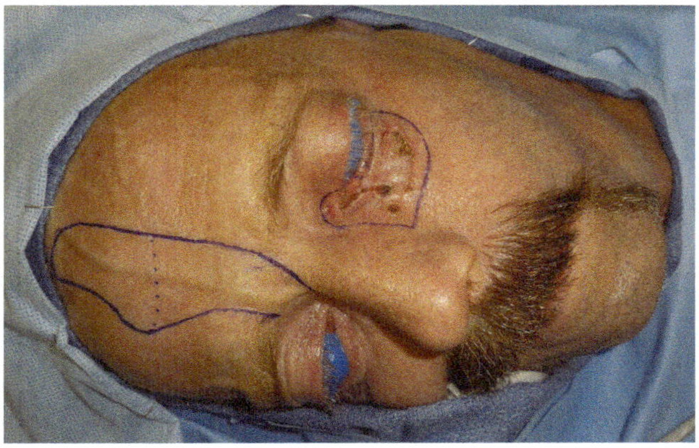

Fig. 10.16b Design of the planned resection area and forehead flap.

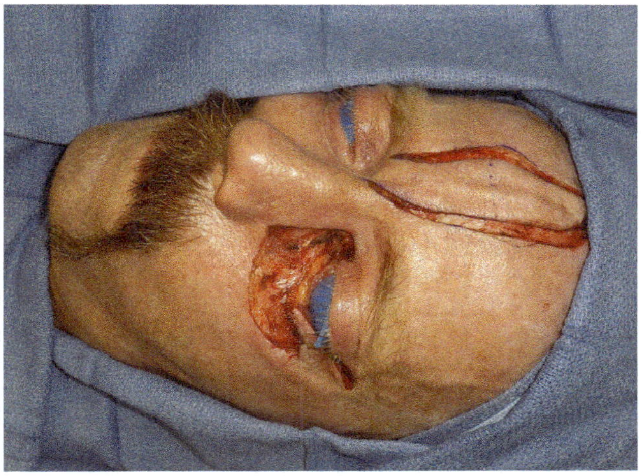

Fig. 10.18 Elevation of the paramedian forehead flap prior to transfer.

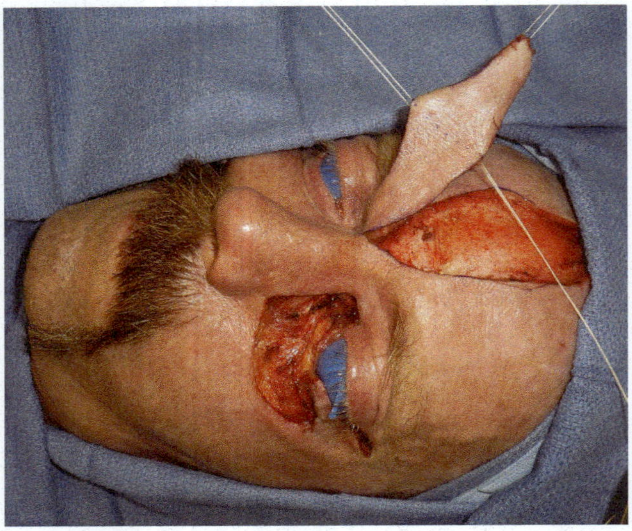

Fig. 10.19a Elevated flap prior to transfer to the defect site.

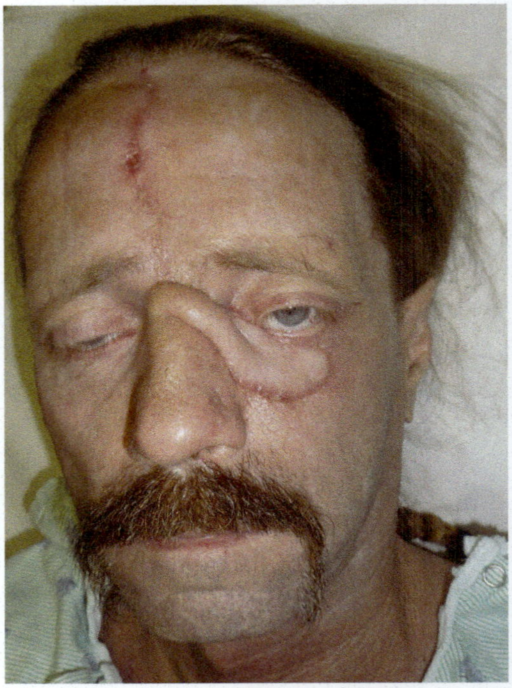

Fig. 10.19c Early post operative healing prior to takedown of the flap.

secondary to resection of a skin squamous cell carcinoma (Figure 10.21). She was taken to the operating room where a template was made of the defect and transferred to the forehead region along the axis of the trochlear vessels (Figure 10.22). The flap was marked with a narrow pedicle that would extend beneath the eyebrow (Figure 10.23). The flap was raised and rotated to the defect site (Figures 10.24 and 10.25). The flap was then inset and then allowed to heal for about 3 weeks (Figures 10.26 and 10.27). The patient was very satisfied with the outcome but a decision was made to carry out a debulking procedure with placement of quilting sutures to better outline the nasal form (Figures 10.28 to 10.31). The final profile view showed a natural form of the nasal dorsum without bulge in the reconstructed area (Figure 10.32).

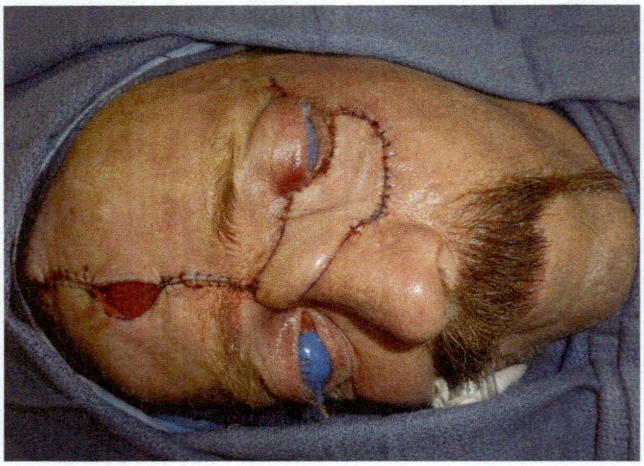

Fig. 10.19b Inset of the flap into the left infraorbital defect.

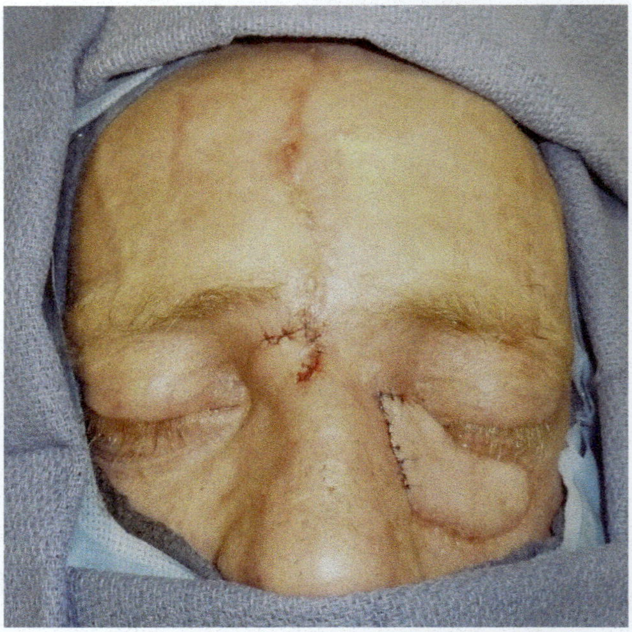

Fig. 10.19d Appearance after the takedown of the flap.

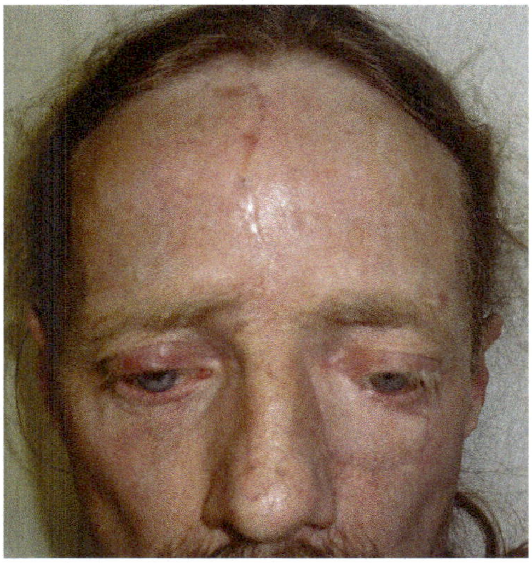

Fig. 10.20a Late view of the appearance of the reconstruction of the infraorbital region with the use of the paramedian forehead flap.

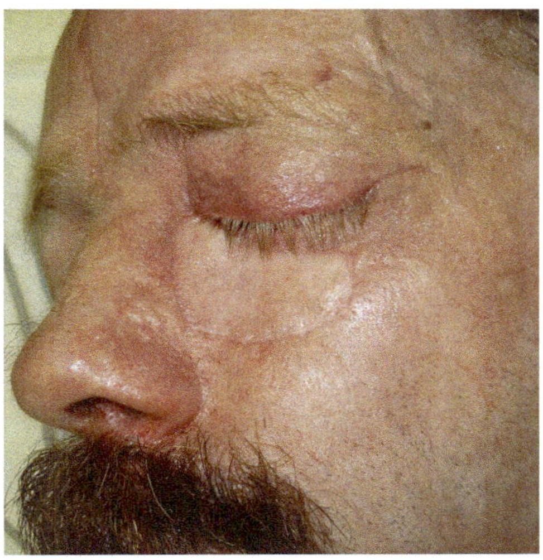

Fig. 10.20b Lateral view of the reconstructed infraorbital defect.

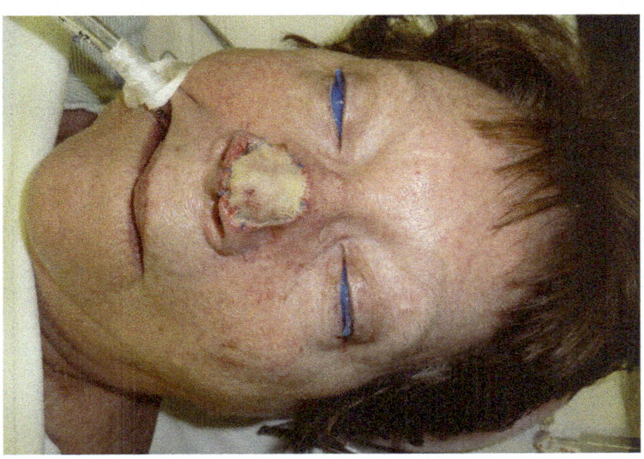

Fig. 10.21 View of a nasal defect after a Mohs' resection.

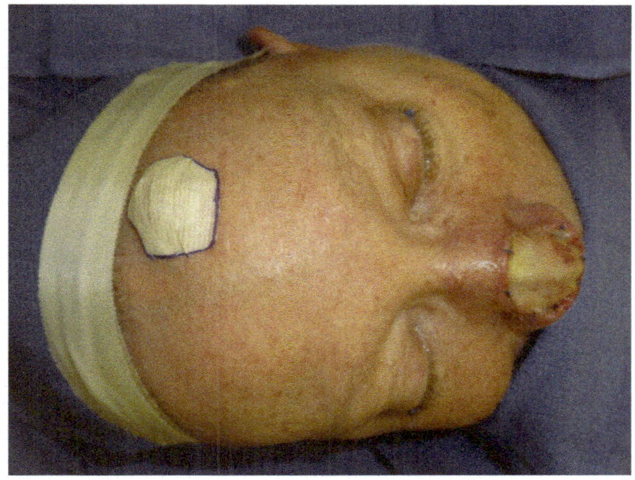

Fig. 10.22 Transfer of the defect template to the forehead donor site.

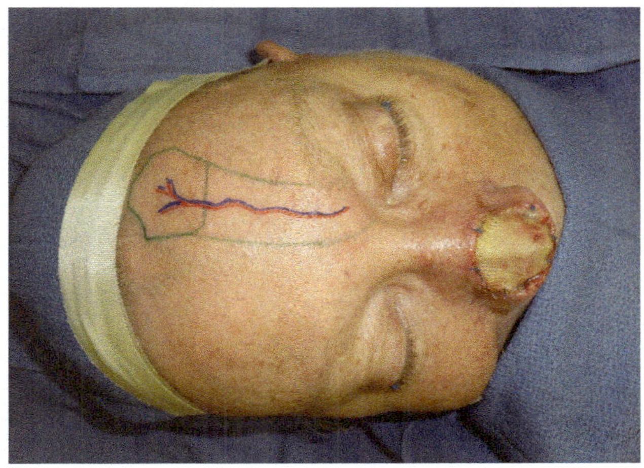

Fig. 10.23 Appearance of the markings for the flap.

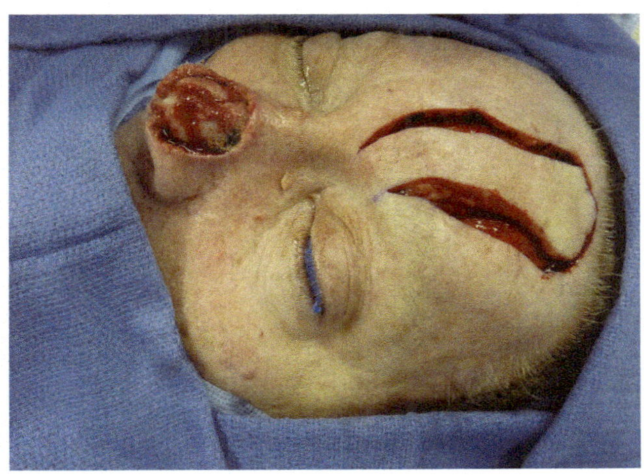

Fig. 10.24 Elevated forehead flap prior to transfer.

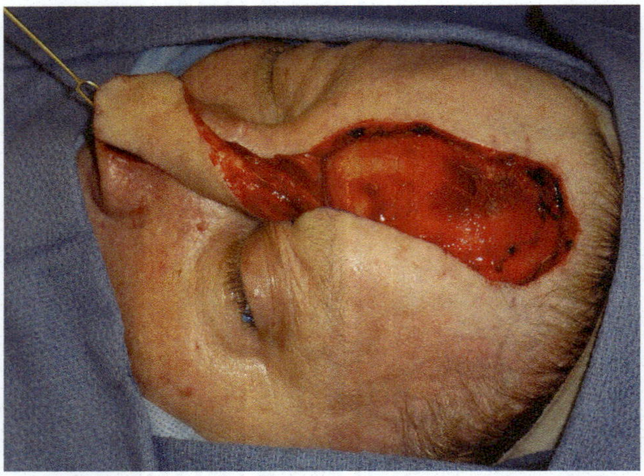

Fig. 10.25 Assessment of the arc of rotation of the flap into the defect.

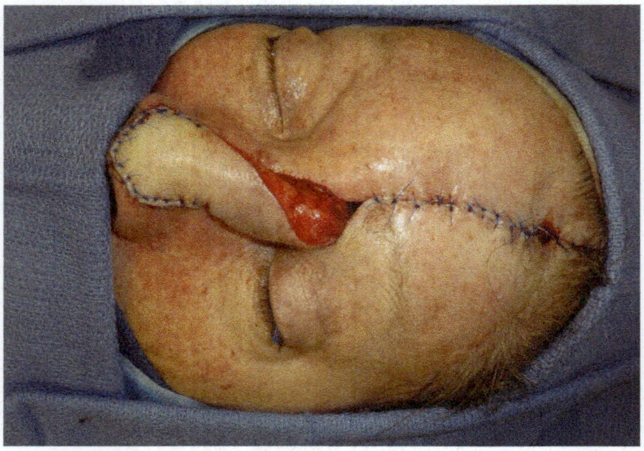

Fig. 10.26 Inset of the flap into the defect.

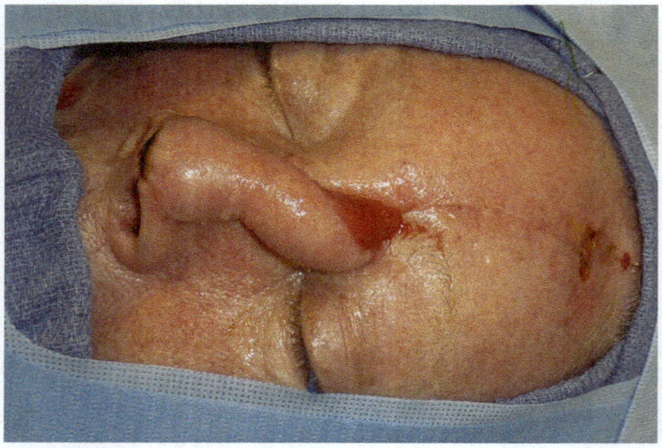

Fig. 10.27 Appearance of the flap immediately prior to the second stage.

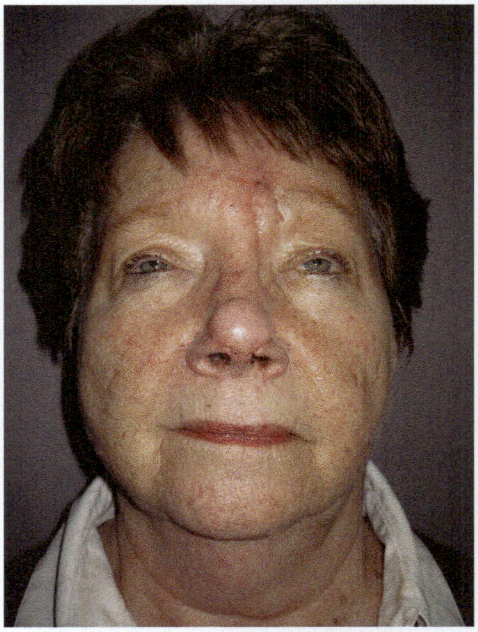

Fig. 10.28 Early appearance of the reconstruction of the nasal defect prior to debulking.

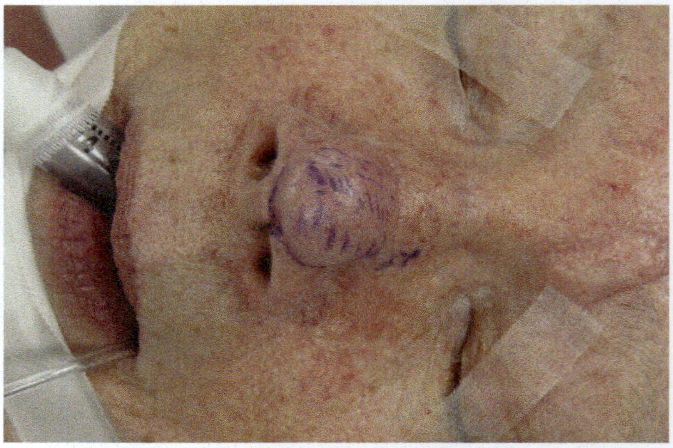

Fig. 10.29 View of the reconstruction prior to debulking.

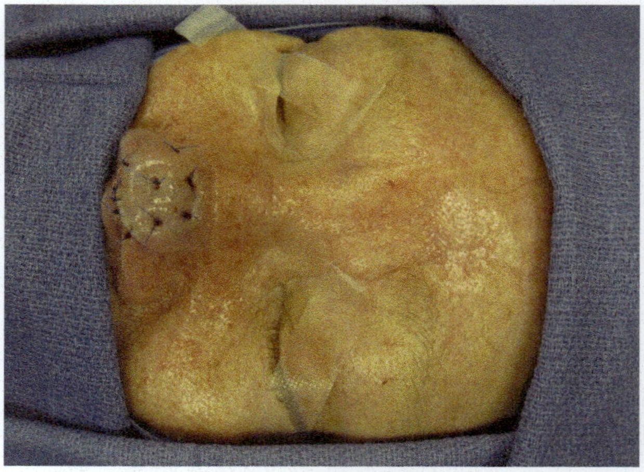

Fig. 10.30 Debulked flap with placement of quilting sutures.

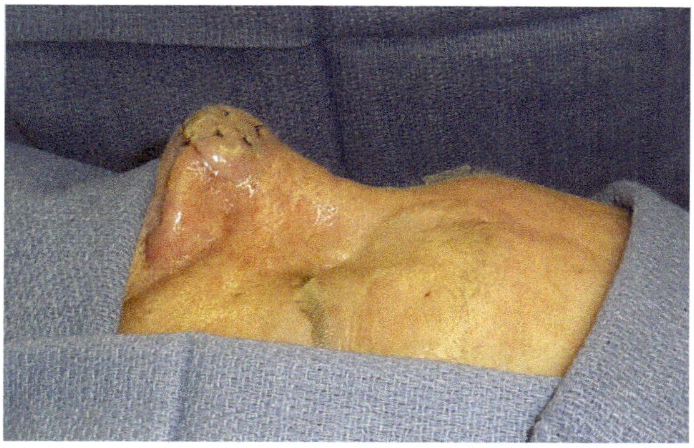

Fig. 10.31 Profile view of the reconstructed defect. Note the confluence between the native tissue and the reconstructed site.

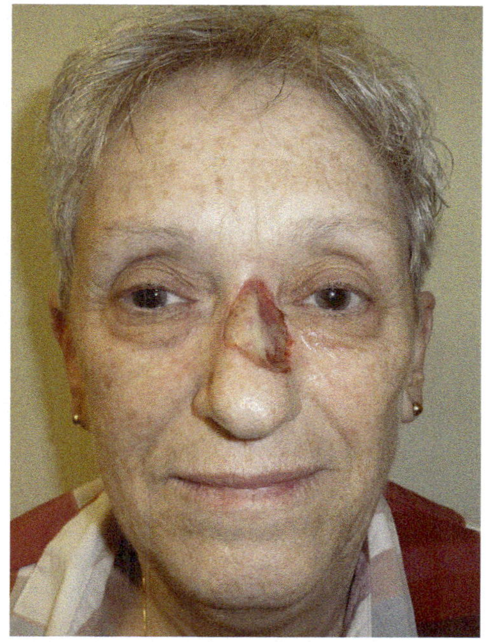

Fig. 10.33 View of a large nasal defect after Mohs' resection.

Case #3

A 70-year-old female was referred by her Mohs' surgeon for the reconstruction of a nasal dorsum and sidewall defect secondary to resection of a skin malignancy (Figures 10.33 to 10.35). She was taken to the operating room where the defect was measured and a template was used to transfer the dimension and shape to the forehead (Figure 10.36). The flap was raised and transferred to the defect site and inset (Figure 10.37). The patient was allowed to heal for a period of at least 3 weeks before she was taken back to the operating room where the pedicle was taken down and the flap partially thinned for a better inset to the intact nasal walls (Figures 10.38 to 10.42). The final appearance of the patient without further debulking or quilting was very satisfactory for the patient and she did not wish to have any further revisions (Figure 10.43 to 10.45).

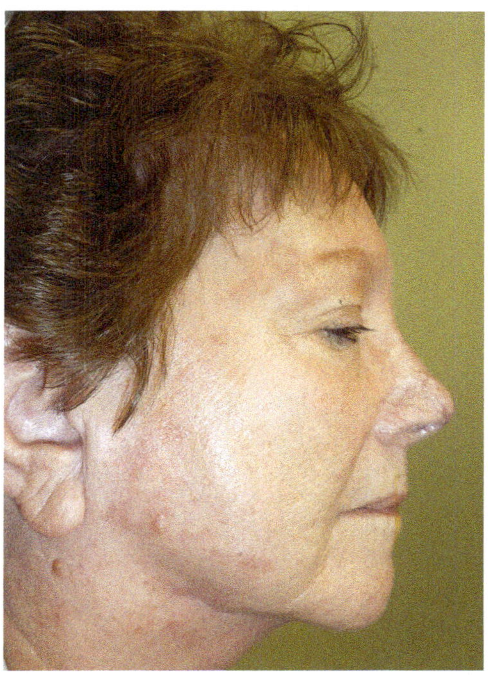

Fig. 10.32 Late view of the reconstructed nose, note the pleasing profile.

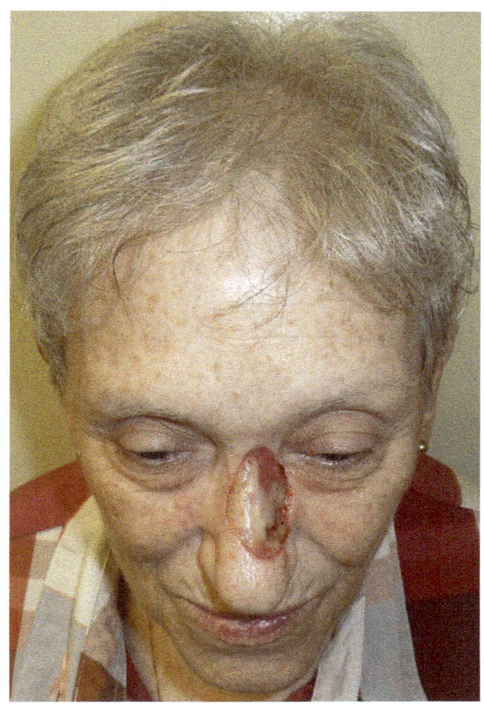

Fig. 10.34 Superior view of the defect.

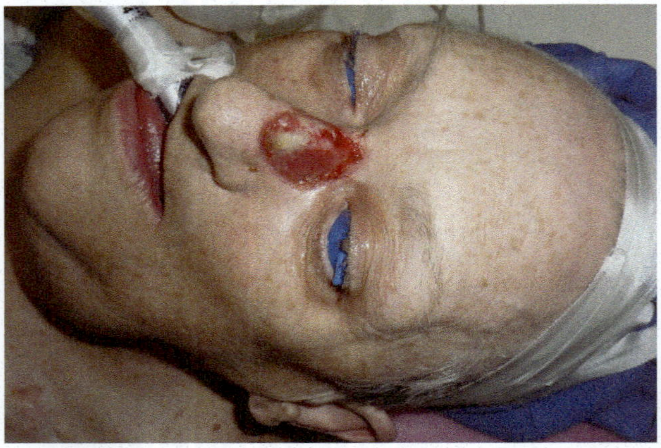

Fig. 10.35 View of the defect prior to reconstruction.

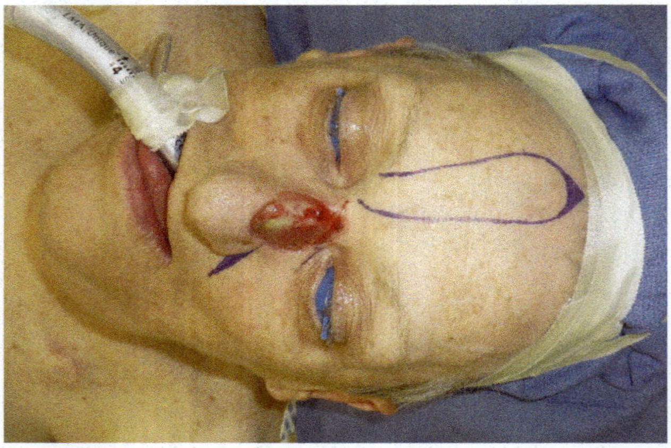

Fig. 10.36 Planned for a paramedian forehead flap to reconstruct the acquired defect.

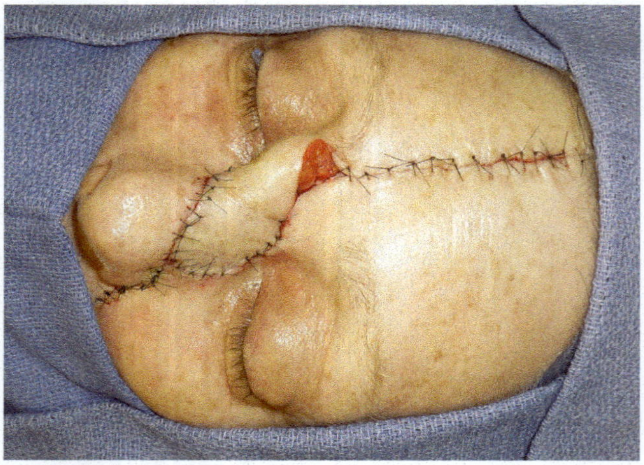

Fig. 10.37 Inset of the flap into the defect.

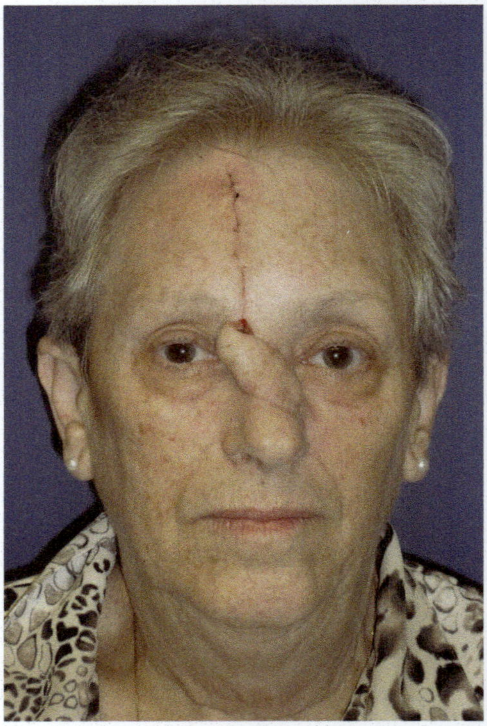

Fig. 10.38 Early appearance prior to takedown of the flap.

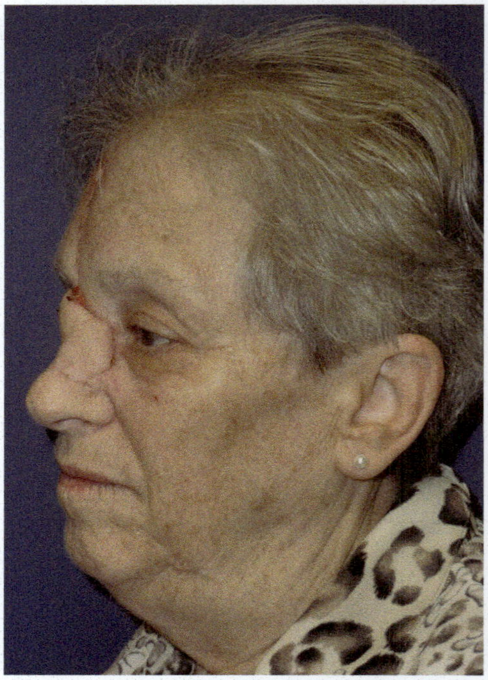

Fig. 10.39 Lateral view of the inset flap.

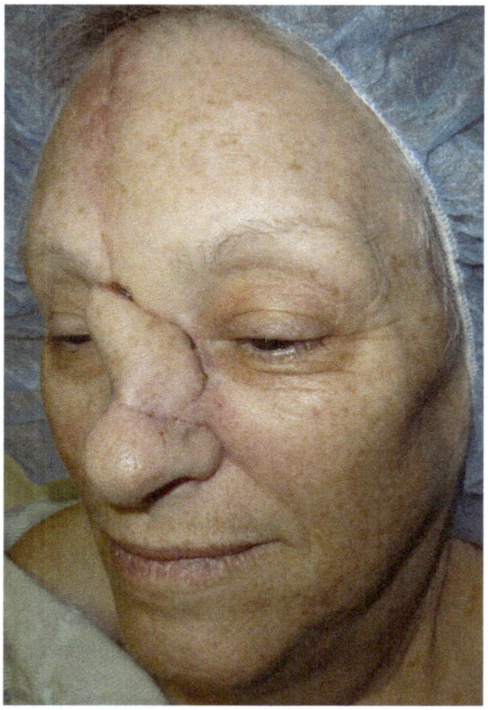

Fig. 10.40 View of the flap prior to takedown.

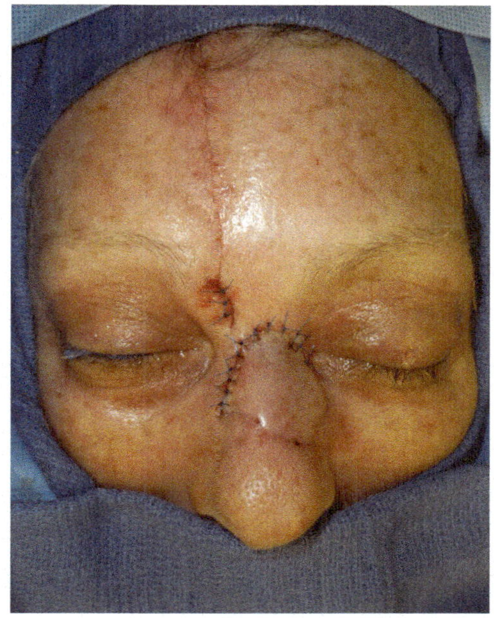

Fig. 10.42 View of the reconstruction after the takedown of the pedicle.

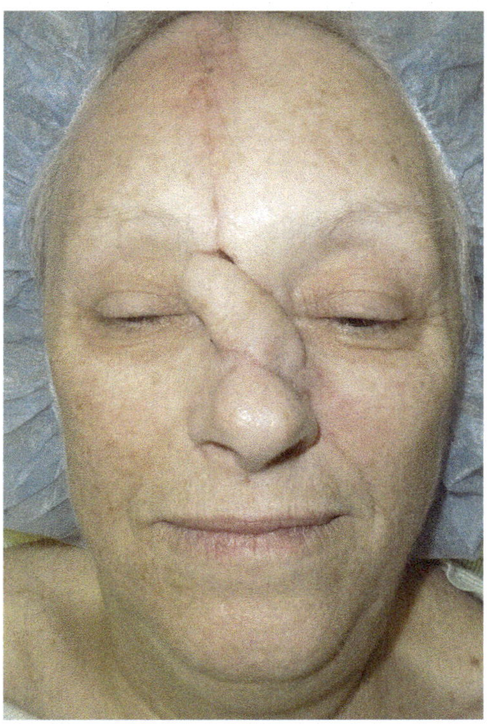

Fig. 10.41 Frontal view of the flap prior to takedown.

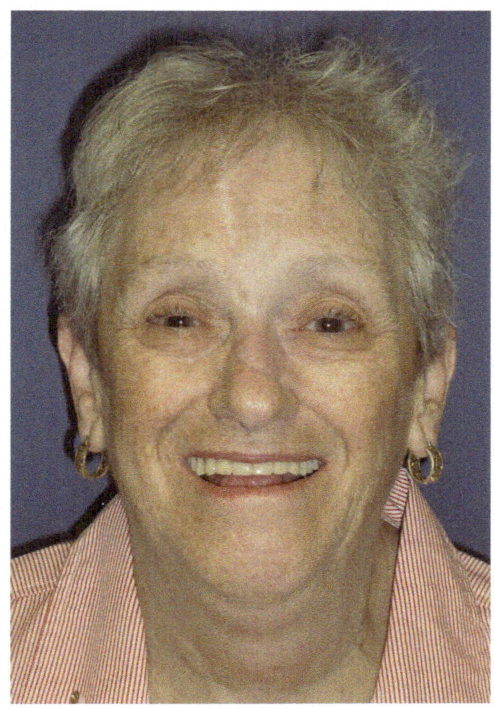

Fig. 10.43 View of the reconstruction after several weeks post takedown of the flap.

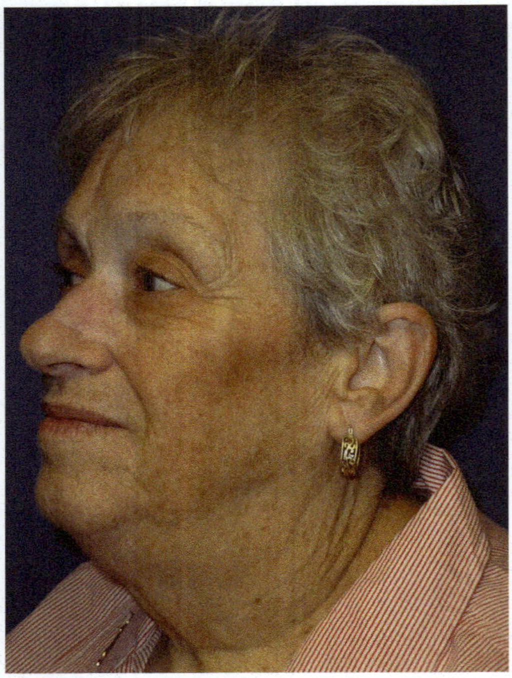

Fig. 10.44 Lateral view of the final reconstruction.

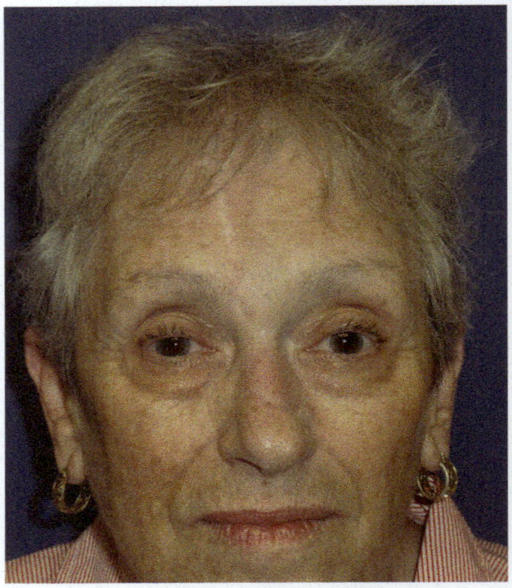

Fig. 10.45 Close up view of the reconstructed nose.

References

1. Almast S. History and evolution of the Indian method of rhinoplasty, in *Transactions of the Fourth International Congress of Plastic and Reconstructive Surgery,* edited by G Sanvenero-Rosselli, 49. Rome, Amsterdam: Excerpta Medica Foundation, 1969.
2. Alford EL, Baker SR, Shumrick KA. Midforehead flap, in *Local Flaps in Facial Reconstruction,* edited by SR Baker and NA Swanson, 197–223. St. Louis, MO: Mosby, 1995.
3. Blair VP. Total and subtotal restoration of the nose. *JAMA* 1925; 85:1931.
4. Kazanjian VH. The repair of nasal defects with the median forehead flap: primary closure of the forehead wound. *Surg Gynecol Obstet* 1946; 83:37–40.
5. Millard DR Jr. Total reconstructive rhinoplasty and a missing link. *Plast Reconstr Surg* 1966; 37:167–183.
6. Millard DR Jr. Hemirhinoplasty. *Plast Reconstr Surg* 1967; 40:440–445.
7. Converse JM, Wood-Smith D. Experiences with the forehead island flap. *Clin Plast Surg* 1963; 31:521–537.
8. Park SS. The single stage forehead flap in nasal reconstruction. *Arch Facial Plast Surg* 2002; 4:32–36.
9. Argamaso RV. Island forehead skin flap, in *Grabb's Encyclopedia of Flaps*, Vol 1 (2nd edn), edited by B Strauch, LO Vasconez and EJ Hall-Findlay, 197–199. Philadelphia, PA: Lippincott-Raven, 1998.
10. Har-El G. Single-stage paramedian forehead flap for nasal reconstruction. *Oper Techn Otolaryngol Head Neck Surg* 1999; 10(2) (Jun):127–130.

Chapter 11

The temporoparietal fascia flap

Introduction

The temporoparietal fascia flap is one of the most versatile flaps in head and neck reconstruction. Monks described the flap at the end of the nineteenth century for the use of reconstruction of eyelid defects as well to reconstruct auricular defects.[1] The flap was slow to gain popularity until the 1980s and 1990s. Since this time, the flap has gained a solid place in the armamentarium of head and neck reconstructive surgeons.

The slow adoption of the temporoparietal fascia flap (TPF) was likely due to the inherent difficulty in raising this flap. The surgeon raising the TPF flap has to be very familiar with the anatomy of the region. He or she also has to be able to carry out the meticulous dissection needed to ensure that the elevation of the scalp flap remains in the right plane. A misstep in elevation of the scalp flap will lead to violation of the TPF and potentially result in the compromise of the flap.

The main advantages of the TPF flap are the width, length, thickness, and pliability. All of these properties render the TPF a good option for use in lining various defects. The flap is also a first option in the coverage of prosthetic ear implants without the loss of details. This fact is one of the reasons why the TPF is widely used in the reconstruction of auricular defects.

The TPF can be used in several variations. The TPF can be elevated with a portion of the forehead skin or scalp in cases where the eyebrow needs to be reconstructed. Additionally, the fasciocutaneous TPF is often used to reconstruct an upper lip defect in males. Less often, the flap can be raised with bone to transfer a vascularized split calvarium bone.

The disadvantages of the TPF are the difficulty in flap elevation and the associated postoperative alopecia that can be seen in and near the area of the scalp incision site.

Anatomy

The temporoparietal fascia lies immediately deep to the skin and subcutaneous tissue of the scalp overlying the temporal fossa. It is continuous with the superficial musculoaponeurotic system inferior to the zygomatic arch and with the galea aponeurotica above the superior temporal line. It is also continuous with the orbicularis oculi and frontalis muscle anteriorly and the occipitalis muscle posteriorly.[2] The temporoparietal fascia is approximately 2–3 mm thick over the parietal region.[3] An area approximately 10 cm wide and 14 cm long can be safely harvested. It can be harvested as a fascial, fasciocutaneous, or osseofascial flap and is classified according to the Mathes and Nahai classification system as a Type A fasciocutaneous flap.[4] The dominant blood supply is the superficial temporal artery, a terminal branch of the external carotid artery. The artery ascends behind the ramus of the mandible and becomes superficial, piercing through the substance of the parotid gland 5 mm in front of the tragus.[5] The artery has a tortuous course and divides into an anterior (frontal) and posterior (parietal) branch 2–4 cm above the zygomatic arch. The mean diameter of the superficial temporal artery is 2 mm.[6] Prior to its division the middle temporal artery arises and enters the temporalis muscle. The anterior branch anastomoses with the supraorbital and supratrochlear vessels over the forehead, while the posterior branch anastomoses with the posterior auricular and occipital arteries. The superficial temporal vein is found anterior and superficial to the artery within the subdermal fat. It generally runs with the artery but can be found as far as

Local and Regional Flaps in Head & Neck Reconstruction: A Practical Approach, First Edition. Rui Fernandes.

Companion website: www.wiley.com/go/fernandes/flapsreconstruction

3 cm away. The sensory innervation arises from the third division of the trigeminal nerve via the auriculotemporal nerve. The frontal branch of the facial nerve is known to course obliquely 1.5 cm lateral to the eyebrow and not more than 2 cm above the brow, therefore limiting the anterior extent of the dissection to avoid inadvertent injury to the facial nerve.[7]

Flap harvest

- The patient is placed in a supine position with the head slightly elevated and rotated to the donor side.
- Alternatively, the head may be placed in a Mayfield headrest and then rotated to the donor side.
- A small strip of hair may be shaven along the intended path of incision (alternatively, the head can be shaven, this allows for ease of prep, dissection, and closure of the defect). Typically the incision begins at the superior aspect of the pre-auricular area and is extended towards the vertex of the head.
- The incision is made just through the dermis with caution so the superficial temporal vessels are not injured as they are in close proximity in the pre-auricular site of incision.
- In the scalp area, a very thin flap is elevated just under the hair follicles. The surgeon should be able to see the follicles on the underside of the scalp flap in order to be assured that the TPF is not being elevated with the scalp reflection.
- The dissection should be done with elevation and tension to facilitate the view of the dissection plane.
- The direction of dissection is continued superiorly towards the vertex of the scalp. In some circumstances, particularly when a large width of flap is needed, the superior incision is converted to a V shape to allow for easier reflection of the anterior scalp flap and therefore visualization of the TPF.
- Once the anterior scalp elevation is completed, the posterior elevation is carried out in a similar fashion. Due to the close proximity to the hair follicles when elevating the scalp flap, electrocautery should be used sparingly.
- The desired length of the flap should be checked using a suture or string from the lap sponge with the fixed point in the pre-auricular area and rotated to the furthest point of the defect. The length is then transferred superiorly to the distal end of the TPF flap, which corresponds to the region of the scalp vertex.
- Once the desired width and length of the flap is measured, the flap may be elevated by first incision the fascia and staying superficial to the temporalis muscle fascia.
- The flap is elevated in a fan-shaped manner with the narrow end being the pre-auricular area in front of the ear. The dissection typically stops in front of the tragus.
- At this point, the rotation and passive reach of the flap to the defect is confirmed.
- A subcutaneous tunnel is developed to transfer the flap to the defect site.
- The tunnel should wide enough to allow for ease of transfer of the flap while at the same time not compressing the pedicle along its path to the defect site.
- The flap is inset into the defect and the path of the pedicle is evaluated to ensure that the vessels are not twisted or kinked.
- The scalp is closed in layers over a suction drain.

Fasciocutaneous flap

- In some cases, the TPF flap can be elevated with a portion of the skin of the forehead or scalp depending on the needs of the defect.
- In these cases, exact reconstruction of the defect is facilitated by the construction of a template.
- The template design is transferred to the scalp or forehead and checked based on the arc of rotation as well as the reach to be sure that the orientation of the flap will be as intended.
- A Doppler ultrasound can be used to trace the anterior branch of the superficial temporal artery to aid in the placement of the template over a well-vascularized region of the flap.
- Once the anterior scalp flap is raised, the path of the anterior branch of the superficial temporal artery is confirmed to be as previously dopplered and that it will carry the skin or scalp component.
- At this point, the incision made around the template design and the flap is elevated as per routine.
- See Figures 11.1 to 11.5.

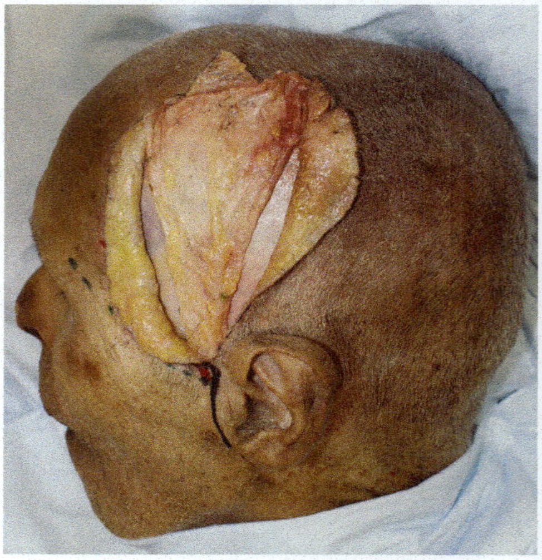

Fig. 11.1 Elevated temporoparietal fascial flap prior to rotation.

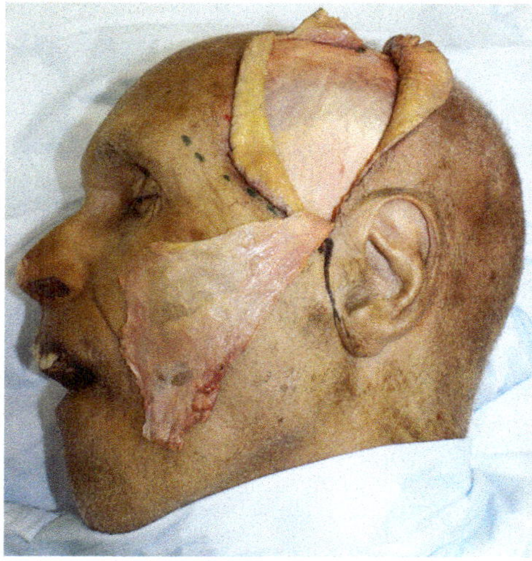

Fig. 11.2 Arc of rotation of the flap towards the oral cavity region.

Temporoparietal fascia with vascularized split cranial bone flap

- Once the scalp flap are elevated and reflected, the desired width of the flap is marked.
- The superior aspect of the flap is incised and the desired length of the bone to be elevated is marked.
- The anterior and posterior incisions are made in the TPF and the periostium is reflected in these three areas, i.e., superior, anterior, and posterior.
- A trough is created on these three sides to facilitate the elevation of a split-thickness calvarium graft.
- Multiple drill holes are placed along the bone and then the fascia is sutured to the bone to prevent shearing.
- At this point, the TPF is elevated inferiorly away from the underlying temporalis muscle fascia.

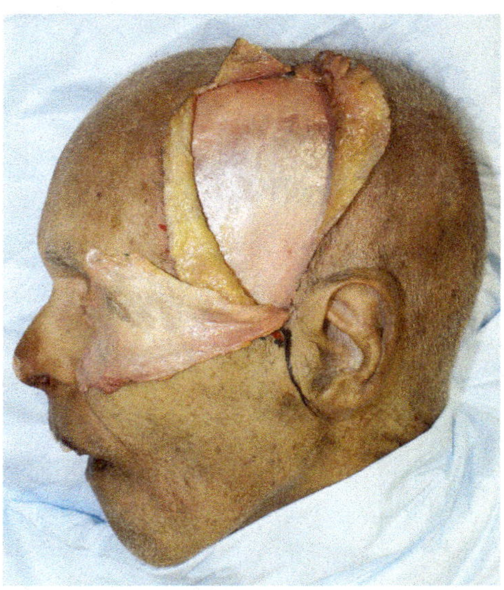

Fig. 11.3 Arc of rotation of the flap towards the orbital region.

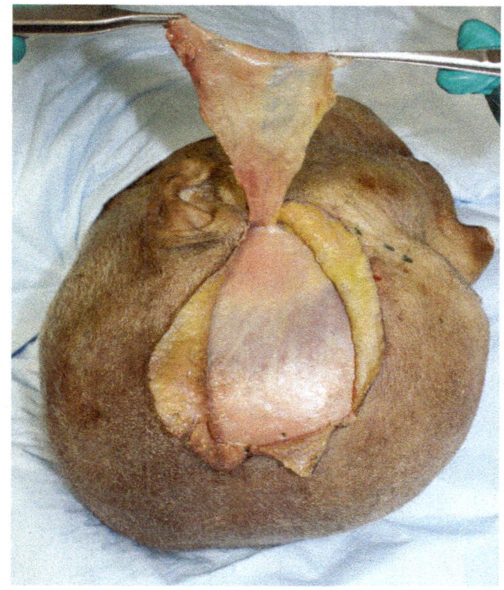

Fig. 11.4 Superior view of the flap showing the transparency of the flap.

- The dissection is carried up to the inferior aspect of the bone graft. Care should be taken to not elevate the flap too far superiorly so as not to reflect it off of the bone.
- At this time, the inferior periostium is incised and the inferior bone cut is done in the tunnel created by the elevated TPF.
- With all of the ostectomies completed, a spatula osteotome is used to elevate the bone while keeping gentle finger pressure on the overlying flap and bone.
- Once the bone is split, the flap is elevated towards the pre-auricular area.
- The perfusion of the bone is confirmed by checking for bleeding points in the bone.
- The flap is transferred to the defect and secured as desired.

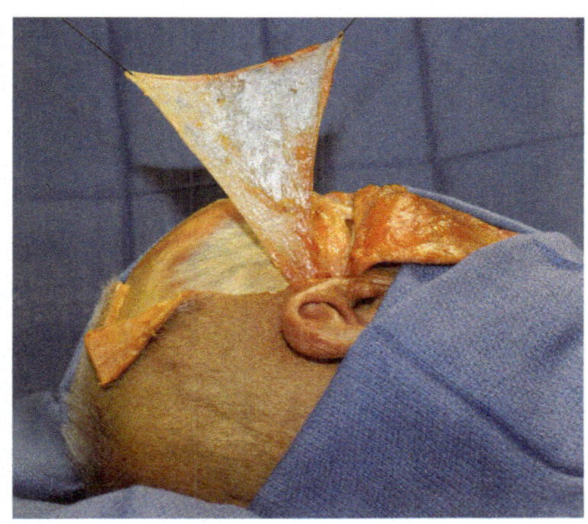

Fig. 11.5 View of the elevated flap from an inferior aspect.

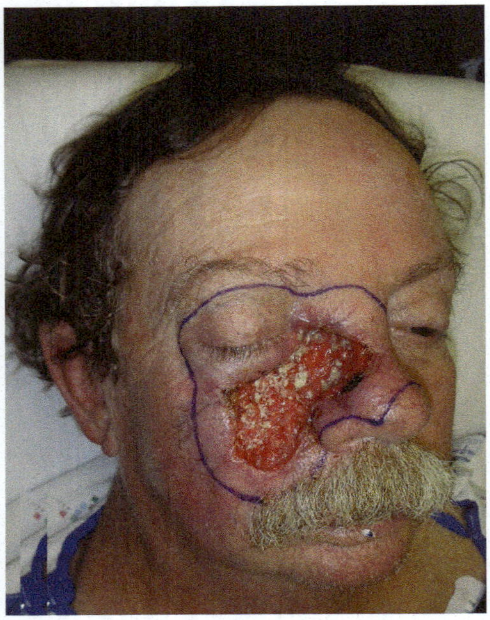

Fig. 11.6 View of a patient with a very large, neglected basal cell carcinoma of the face with extension to the orbit.

Case #1

A 67-year-old male presented with a longstanding, neglected basal cell carcinoma of the right cheek. Over the past several months he began to experience visual problems progressing to significant diminution of vision. He was also concerned because of the persistent drainage and increasing malodorous scent (Figure 11.6). A discussion was had with the patient and after workup and presentation at the multidisciplinary head and neck tumor board, it was recommended that he undergo a wide local resection to include a maxillectomy, orbital exenteration, and partial rhinectomy (Figures 11.7 and 11.8). Given the complexity of the defect, multiple flaps were used to restore the facial form. The cheek was reconstructed with titanium mesh and a radial forearm free flap, while the hemirhinectomy defect was reconstructed with a bone graft, septal mucosal flap, and a paramedian forehead flap. The orbital cavity was relined with a TPF flap (Figures 11.9 to 11.11). The final reconstruction on the day of

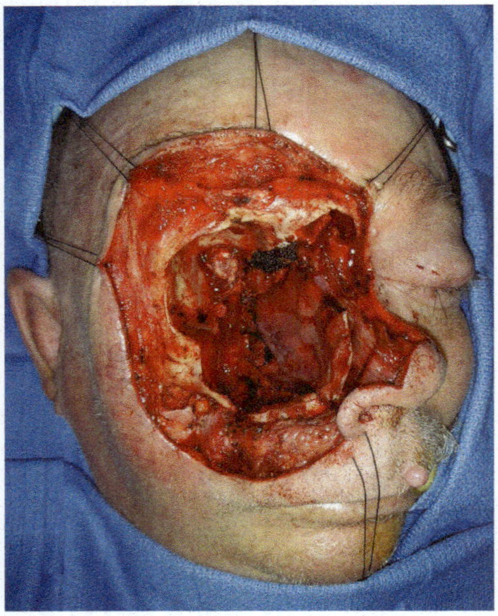

Fig. 11.7 View of the defect after completion of the resection.

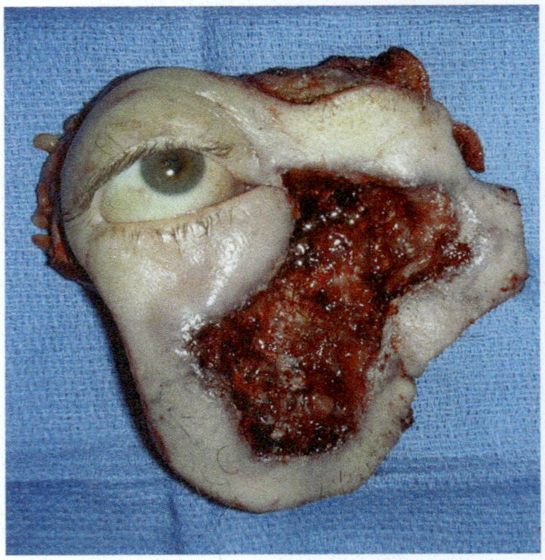

Fig. 11.8 View of the resected specimen.

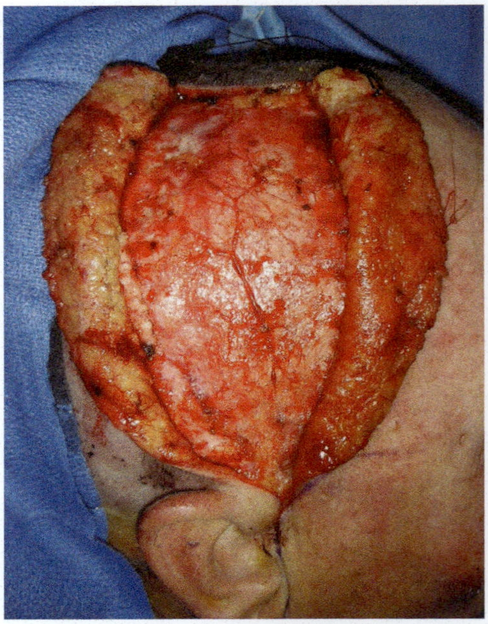

Fig. 11.9 View of the elevated scalp flaps prior to the flap elevation, note the path of the superficial temporal artery.

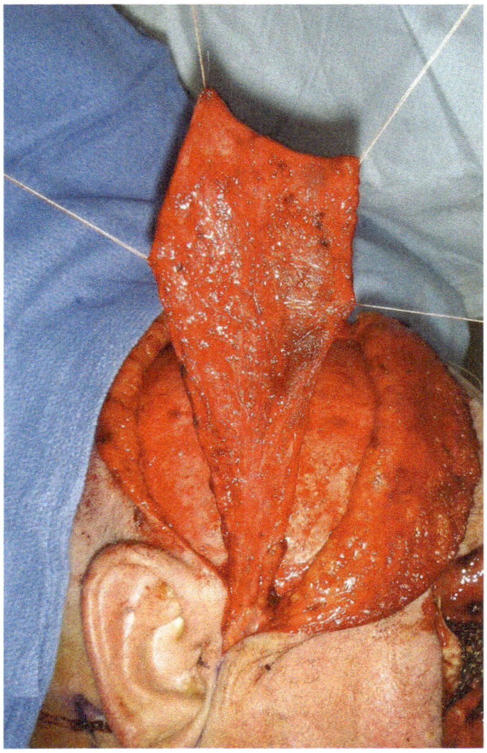

Fig. 11.10 Elevated temporoparietal fascial flap prior to transfer to the orbital cavity.

surgery was satisfactory (Figure 11.12). Early postoperative results remained adequate (Figure 11.13).

Case #2

A 37-year-old Caucasian female was referred for evaluation for the reconstruction of a right ear defect. She had a history of a motor vehicular accident where she suffered loss of the right auricle (Figure 11.14). She wanted to have reconstruction of the defect with restoration of her ear to near pre-injury form. A decision was made to reconstruct her defect in a staged fashion with the aid of a Medpor ear implant (Stryker, USA) and the TPF flap to wrap the implant and then skin graft the defect (Figures 11.15 to 11.19). The patient returned to the operating room for one

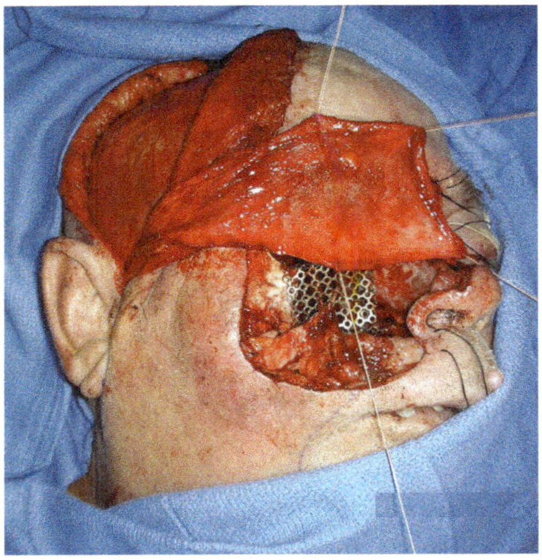

Fig. 11.11 Assessment of the arc of rotation of the flap to the orbital cavity.

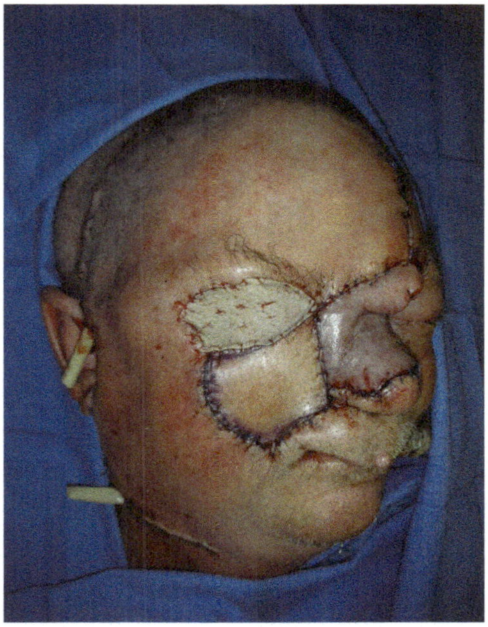

Fig. 11.12 Immediate view of the inset of the flaps to reconstruct the large defect.

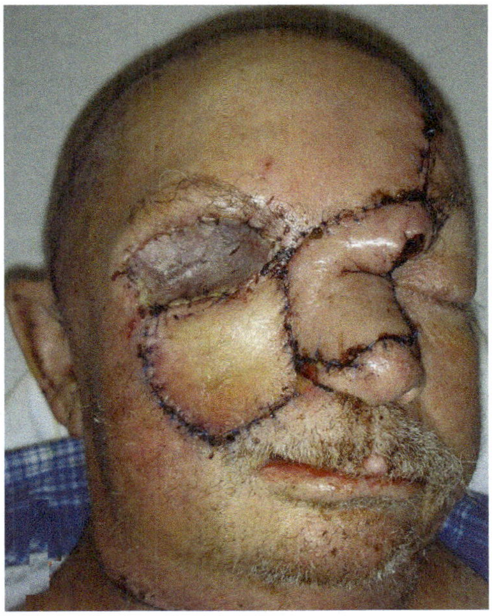

Fig. 11.13 Postoperative view of the reconstruction.

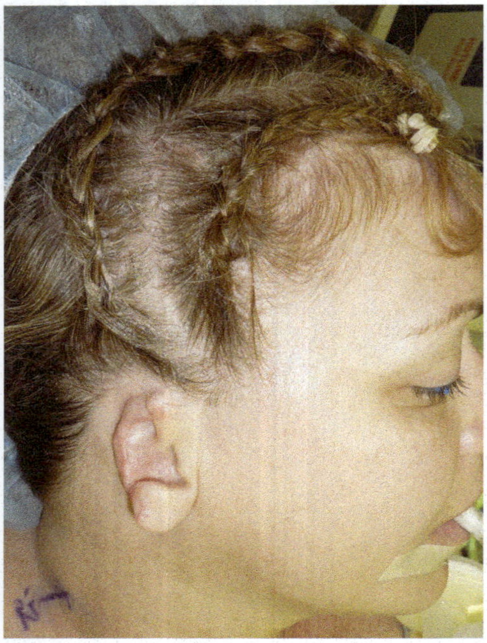

Fig. 11.14 View of the auricular defect and donor site for a temporoparietal fascial flap prior to elevation.

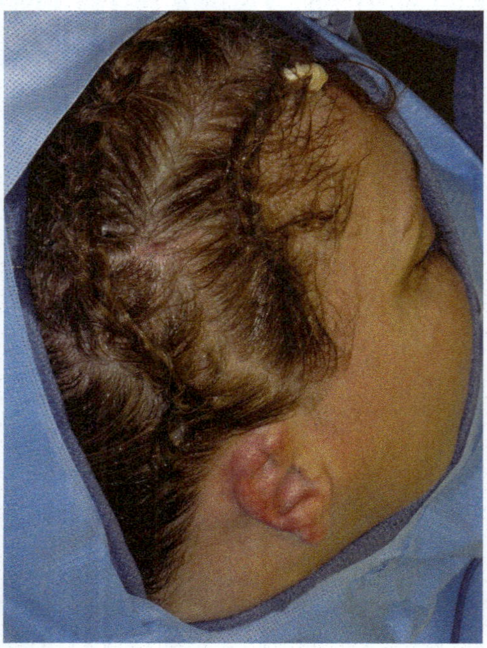

Fig. 11.15 Superior view of the scalp prior to elevation of the flap.

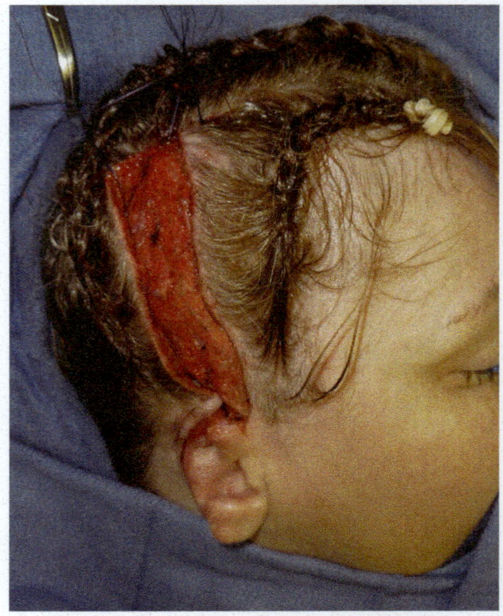

Fig. 11.16 Initial elevation of the scalp prior to raising the temporoparietal fascia flap.

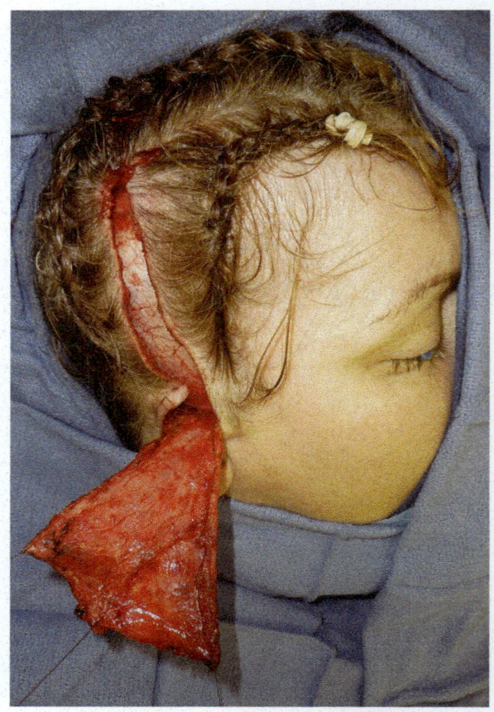

Fig. 11.17 View of the elevated flap, note that the inferior portion is just wider than a centimeter. The vascular pedicle enters the flap in this region.

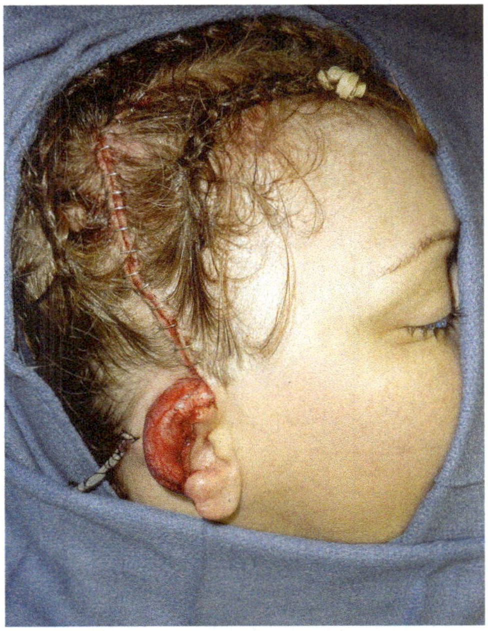

Fig. 11.18 Closure of the donor site and use of the flap to reconstruct the auricular defect.

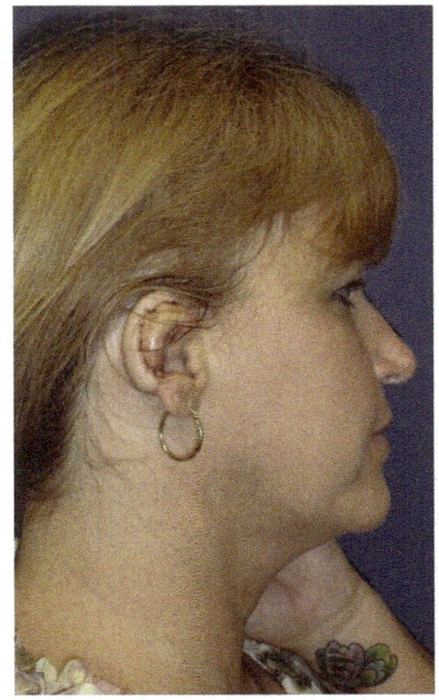

Fig. 11.20 View of the reconstructed ear after debulking.

further revision and was pleased with the outcome and did not wish to have further revisions (Figure 11.20).

Case #3

A 32-year-old Caucasian male was brought to the trauma bay after suffering from a self-inflicted gun shot wound to the face in a suicide attempt. The patient needed a number of free tissue transfers including a fibula free flap to the mandible, a radial forearm free flap to the maxilla, and advancement of the tissues in the upper lip to recreate oral competence. The tissues in the right midface adjacent to the upper lip and nasal sidewall were found to be lacking. A decision was made to replace the tissue with a TPF with overlying skin. The markings for the flap were made (Figure 11.21). The scalp was elevated, leaving the TPF intact with clear visibility of the arterial supply to the flap (Figure 11.22). The flap was elevated and the arc of rotation checked to be sure that it would reach the desired location (Figures 11.23 to 11.25). The site was then

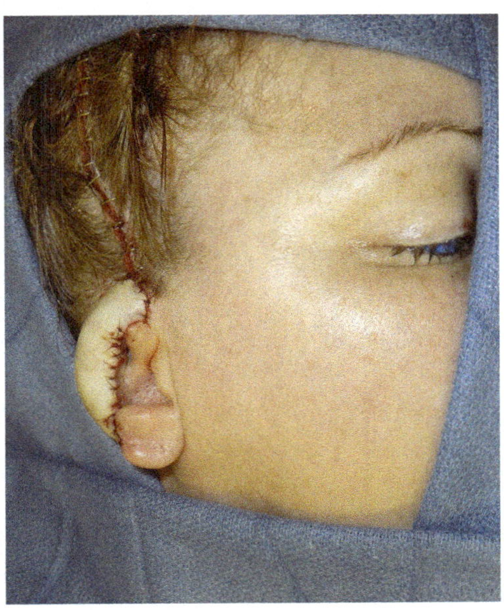

Fig. 11.19 A skin graft has been placed over the temporoparietal fascial flap.

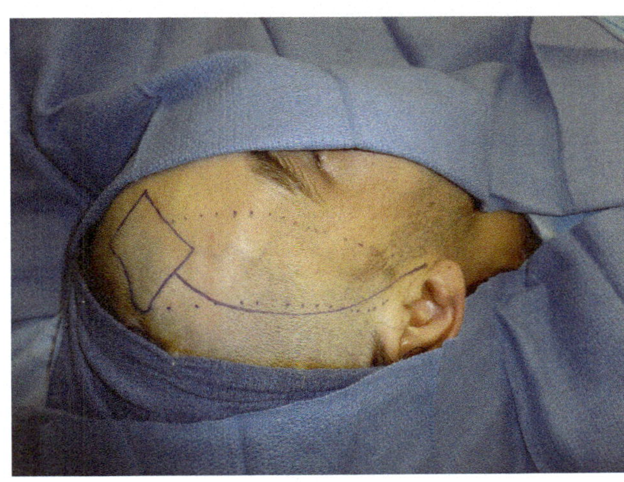

Fig. 11.21 Markings for a temporoparietal fascial flap with a skin component.

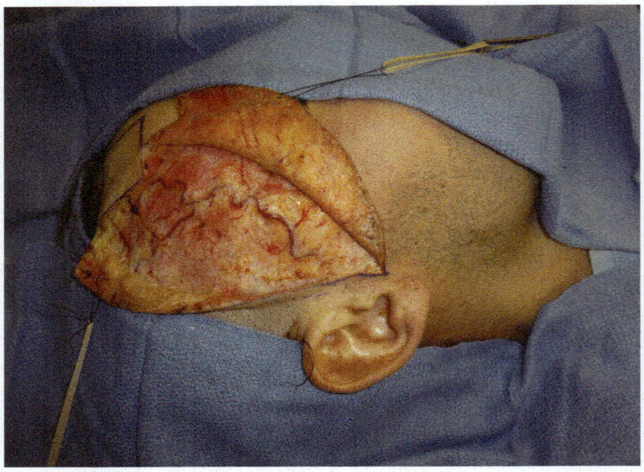

Fig. 11.22 Initial elevation of the scalp prior to elevation of the flap, note the path of the superficial temporal artery.

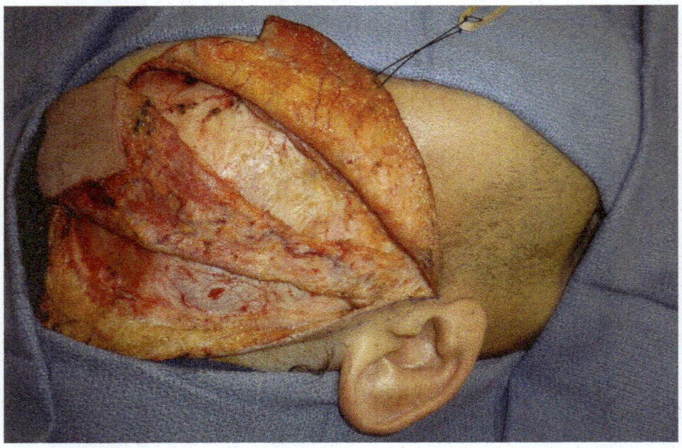

Fig. 11.23 Elevated temporoparietal flap with skin component.

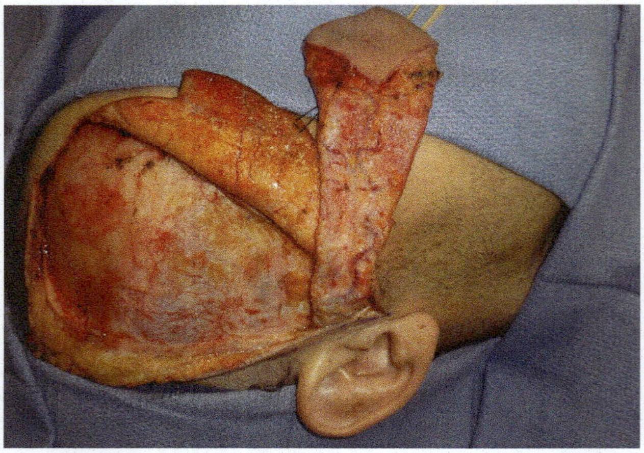

Fig. 11.24 Assessment of the arc of rotation of the flap to confirm adequate reach of the flap.

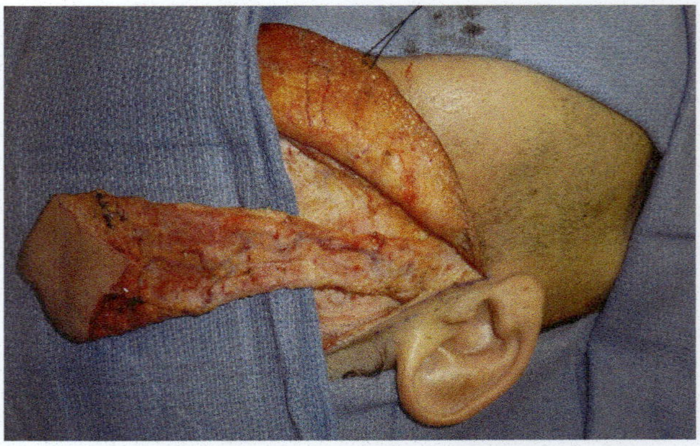

Fig. 11.25 Temporoparital fascial flap with skin component, elevated and ready for transfer.

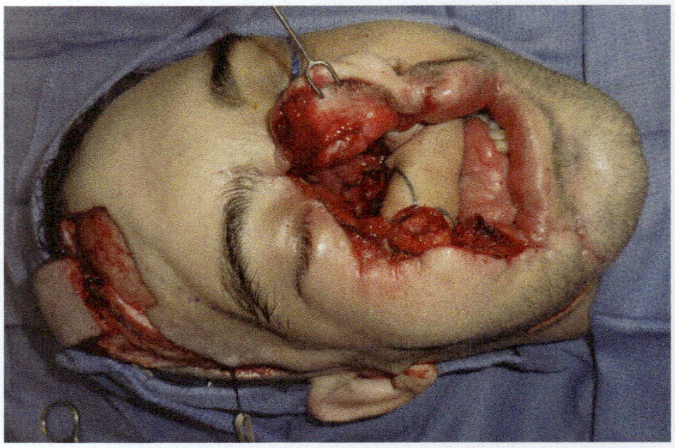

Fig. 11.26 View of the recipient site prior to transfer of the flap.

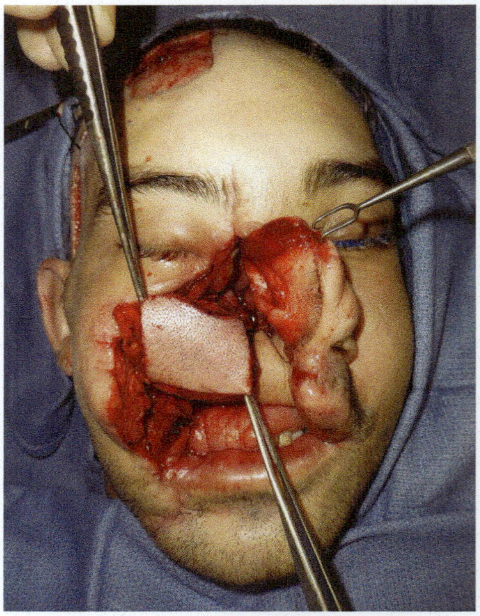

Fig. 11.27 Transfer of the flap into the defect prior to insetting.

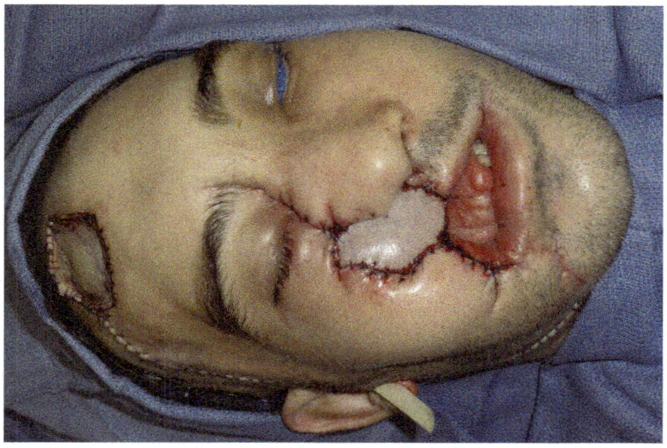

Fig. 11.28 Inset of the flap into the defect.

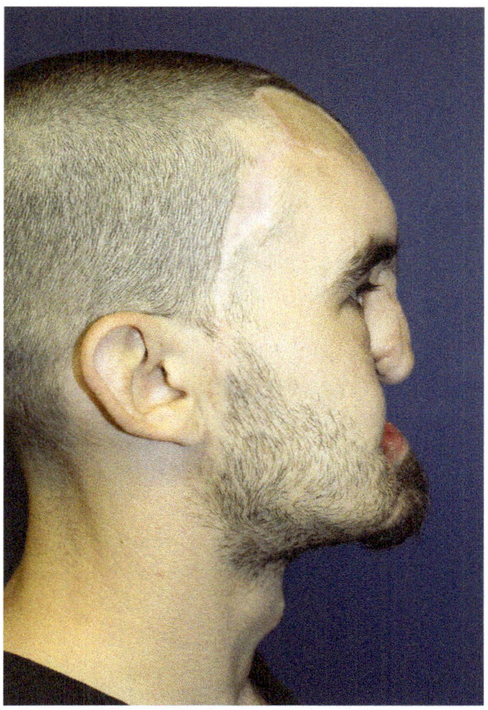

Fig. 11.29 View of the donor site after transfer of the fasciocutaneous temporoparietal fascial flap.

prepared and a subcutaneous tunnel created (Figure 11.26). The flap was transferred to the defect and rotated and inset in the proper orientation (Figures 11.27 and 11.28). The healing at the donor site was found to be very acceptable (Figure 11.29).

References

1. Cesteleyn L. The temporoparietal galea flap. *Oral Maxillofacial Surg Clin N Am* 2003; 15(4):537–550.
2. Tellioglu AT, Tekdemir I, Erdemli EA, Tuccar E, Ulusoy G. Temporoparietal fascia: an anatomic and histologic reinvestigation with new potential clinical applications. *Plast Reconstr Surg* 2000; 105:40–45.
3. Cheney ML, Varvares MA, Nadol JB. The temporoparietal flap in head and neck reconstruction. *Arch Otolaryngol Head Neck Surg* 1993; 119: 618–623.
4. Mathes S, Nahai F. *Reconstructive Surgery: Principles, Anatomy and Technique*. London: Churchill Livingstone, 1997.
5. Cesteleyn L. The temporoparietal galea flap. *Oral Maxillofacial Surg Clin N Am* 2003; 15:537–550.
6. David SK, Cheney ML. An anatomic study of the temporoparietal fascial flap. *Arch Otolaryngol Head Neck Surg* 1995; 121:1153–1156.
7. Zide BM, Jelks GW. Forehead, temporal region and cheek, in *Surgical Anatomy of the Orbit*, edited by BM Zide and GW Jelks, 13–19. New York, NY: Raven, 1988.

Chapter 12
Temporalis muscle flap

Introduction

The temporalis muscle flap has limited utility in the routine reconstruction of head and neck defects. The use of this flap has been commonly associated with the reconstruction of maxillectomy defects. The use of the temporalis for these defects has significantly diminished over the past two decades as the role of microvascular flaps have become the mainstay for reconstruction of maxillectomy defects. The temporalis flap remains as one of the reconstructive options for patients with facial paralysis. In these cases, the muscle may be employed to restore dynamic function to the paralyzed face.

The advantage of the temporalis muscle flap is the ease of access to the muscle, the moderate quantity of muscle that can be harvested, and the ability to transfer the muscle to the oral cavity. Because of the limited length of the muscle, and the arc of rotation needed to reach the maxilla, the flap can be brought into the oral cavity by two routes. The first route travels over the zygomatic arch and the other travels under the arch. If the path to the oral cavity is chosen to travel over the arch it will result in a diminished reach of the muscle due to the longer path needed to travel to reach the defect. The alternative route, i.e., under the arch, improves the reach of the muscle but requires an osteotomy of the zygomatic arch and reposition of the arch after the muscle is transferred.

The main disadvantage of the temporalis muscle flap is the resultant hollowing associated with the use of the muscle. In cases where the majority of the muscle is used to reconstruct the defect, the temporal defect can be addressed at the time of surgery with the placement of a temporal implant. One commonly used implant is the Medpor (Stryker, USA) temporal implant. The surgeon can modify the implant to fit the patient's defect and therefore minimize the hollowing that would otherwise result.

Anatomy

The temporalis muscle is a fan-shaped muscle that originates along the temporal lines of the parietal bone of the skull. The muscle lies within the temporal fossa, is covered by a strong fibrous aponuerotic sheath, the temporalis fascia, and passes medial to the zygomatic arch. Insertions of the muscle are onto the anterior and medial surfaces of the coronoid process and along the anterior ascending ramus of the mandible. The muscle thickness varies from 5 mm along its periphery to 15 mm at the level of the zygomatic arch.[1] The area of muscle that can be harvested measures 10 cm wide and 20 cm long. The temporalis muscle is classified as a Type III[2] muscle receiving its main vascular supply from the anterior and deep temporal arteries, branches from the second portion of the internal maxillary artery. Both deep temporal arteries have a mean vessel diameter of 1 mm. The minor pedicle to the temporalis muscle is via the middle temporal artery, a branch from the superficial temporal artery that has a mean vessel diameter of 0.5 mm.[3] In 1996, Chueng demonstrated the increased vascular contribution of the middle temporal artery to the temporalis muscle.[4] Paired venae comitantes accompany the named arteries. The innervation to the temporalis muscle, like the other muscles of mastication, arise from the anterior division of the mandibular branch of the trigeminal nerve via the anterior and posterior deep temporal nerves.[5] The temporalis muscle functions in retraction (posterior horizontal fibers) and elevation (anterior vertical fibers) of the mandible.

Local and Regional Flaps in Head & Neck Reconstruction: A Practical Approach, First Edition. Rui Fernandes.

Companion website: www.wiley.com/go/fernandes/flapsreconstruction

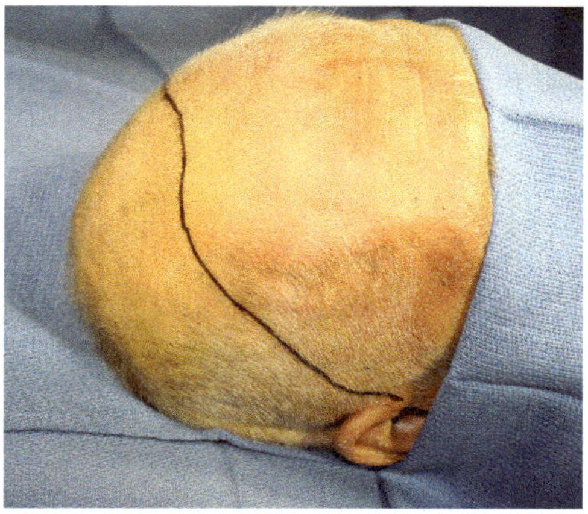

Fig. 12.1 Incision planning for raising a temporalis muscle flap.

Flap harvest

- The patient is positioned with the head rotated to expose the donor side towards the surgeon.
- A decision to shave a strip of the hair along the path of the incision or to shave the entire head will often depend on the gender of the patient. In males, the head is more commonly shaven while in females only a strip of the hair along the path of the planned incision is shaven.
- The incision for the harvest of the temporalis muscle is designed from the pre-auricular area and extends superiorly towards the vertex of the head (Figure 12.1).
- Incision is made along the marked incision line and carried deep to the dermis in the pre-auricular area and deep to the temporoparietal fascia along the scalp.
- The scalp flap is then elevated superficial to the temporalis muscle fascia. This fascia is easily identified by its very white appearance.

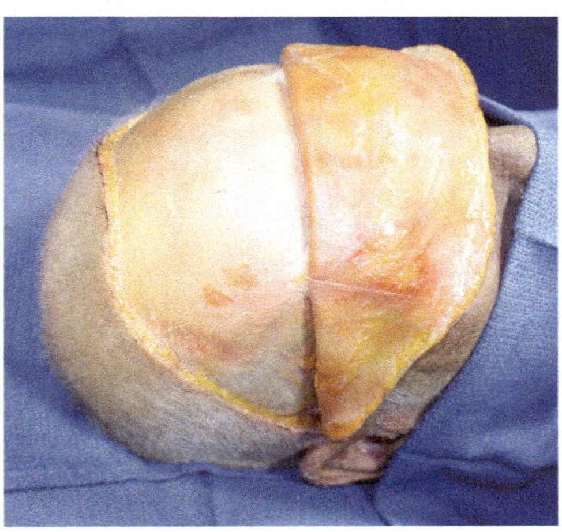

Fig. 12.2 Elevation of a coronal flap revealing the left temporalis muscle.

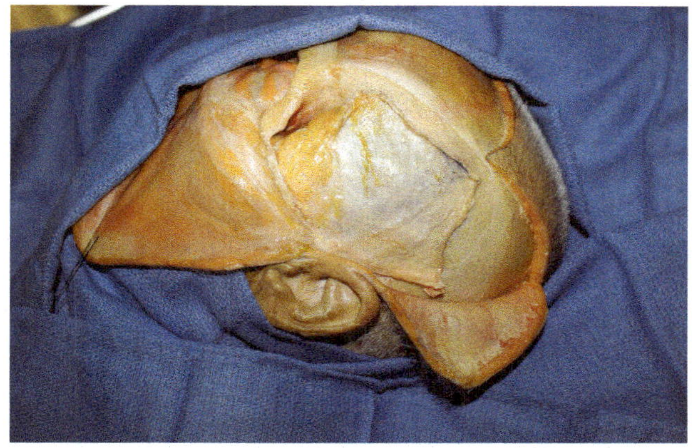

Fig. 12.3 View of the elevated temporalis muscle flap prior to rotation.

- Once the anterior and posterior scalp flaps are elevated, the muscle is exposed up to the temporal crest and as far anteriorly as possible towards the muscle attachment in the anterior temporal crest (Figure 12.2).
- An anterior incision is then made in the muscle and carried down to the bone (Figure 12.3).
- The muscle is elevated from its temporal crest and the posterior incision is made based on the desired width needed to repair the defect.
- The dissection is directed inferiorly towards the pre-auricular area and the insertion of the muscle in the coronoid process and anterior ramus of the mandible. Care should be taken as dissection is carried deep to not traumatize the muscle and injure the deep temporal vessels as they penetrate the muscle near the level of the zygomatic arch.

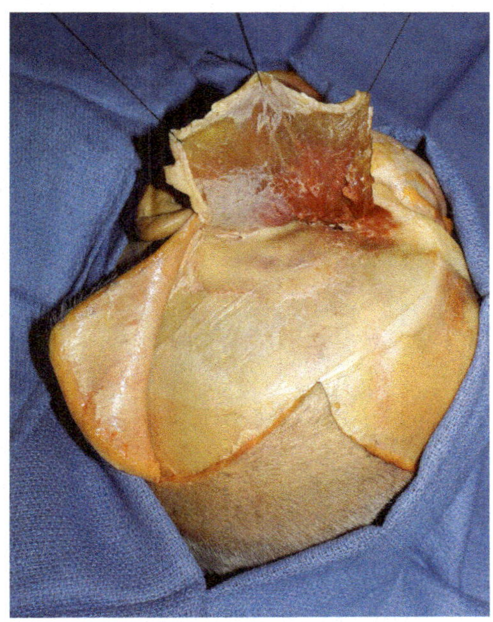

Fig. 12.4 View of the raised temporalis muscle off of the temporal bone and deep to the zygomatic arch.

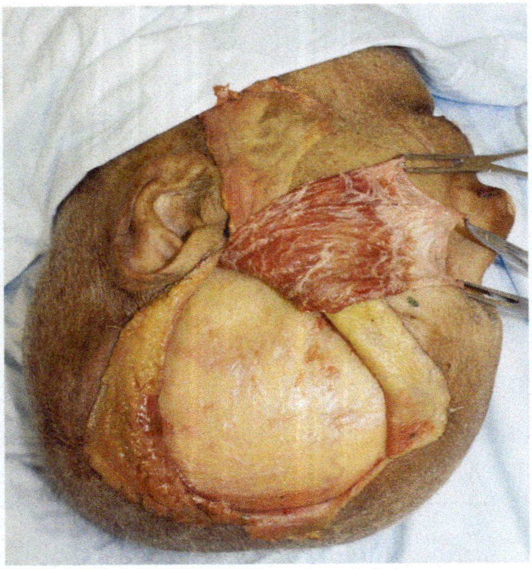

Fig. 12.5 Assessment of the arc of rotation and reach of the temporalis muscle flap.

- Several stay sutures are then placed at the distal end of the muscle to facilitate the rotation of the muscle and minimize trauma to the muscle (Figure 12.4).
- The arc of rotation can be checked to insure reach to the desired defect. In cases where the intent is to reconstruct orbital defects, the rotation can be checked and a subcutaneous tunnel developed to reach the site (Figures 12.5 and 12.6).
- In cases where the muscle is to be transferred into the oral cavity to reconstruct a maxillectomy, the surgeon needs to decide how the muscle transfer will be carried out, i.e., over or under the arch. This can be done after checking the arc of rotation and potential reach (Figure 12.7a–c). A tunnel will need to be created from

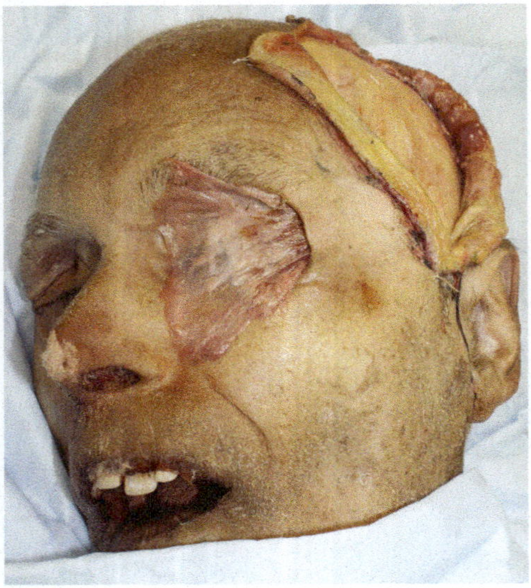

Fig. 12.6 Transfer of the flap into an orbital defect. Note that the reach is adequate to repair the orbit.

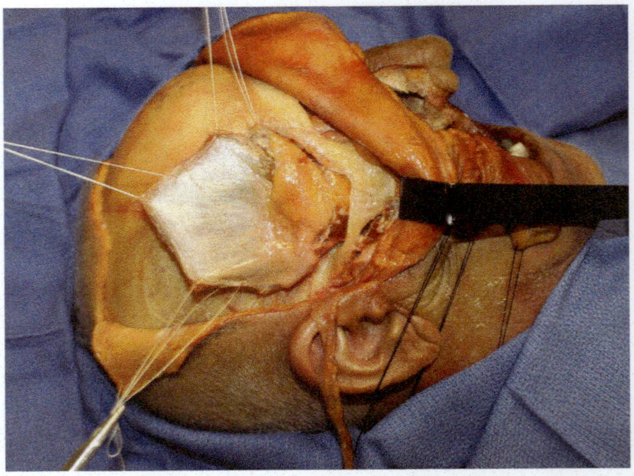

Fig. 12.7a View of the elevated temporalis flap with a view towards the insertion in the coronoid.

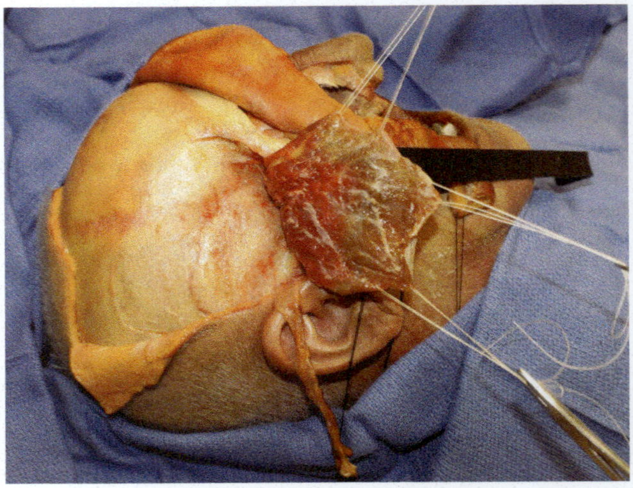

Fig. 12.7b Rotation of the flap over the arch.

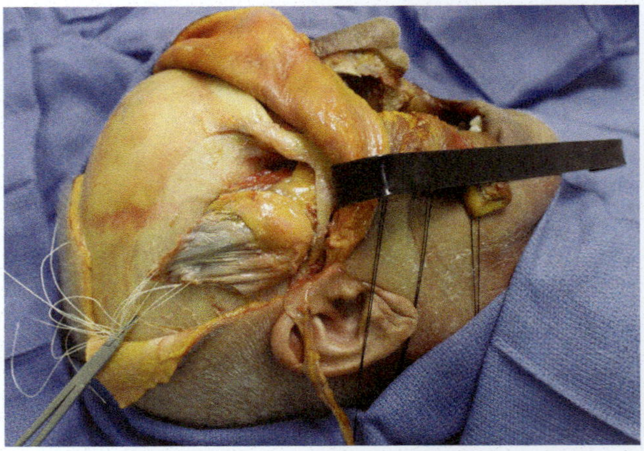

Fig. 12.7c Prior to transfer of the temporalis muscle into the oral cavity, the sutures are gathered into one hemostat and readied for transfer into the oral cavity.

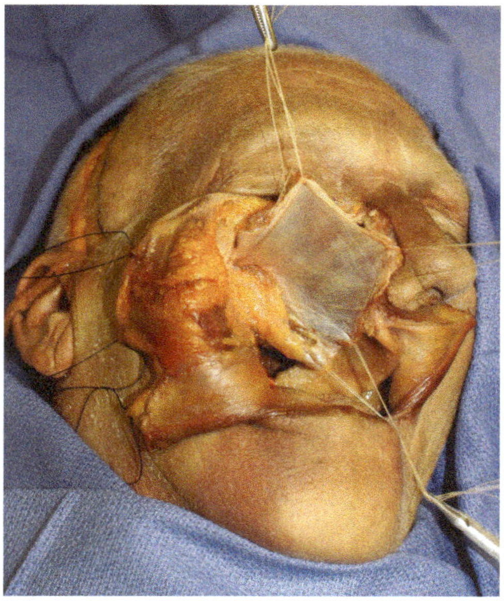

Fig. 12.8 Transferred muscle in the oral cavity; note the reach to the oral cavity.

the defect to the temporal area. Using a curved clamp, dissection is extended from the oral defect towards the temporal region. The tunnel dissection is easier when done under the zygomatic arch (Figure 12.8).

- The flap is then inset based on the defect. In cases where it is being used to reconstruct a maxillectomy defect, the edge of the muscle is advanced to reach the medical defect of the orbit and palate (Figures 12.9 and 12.10).

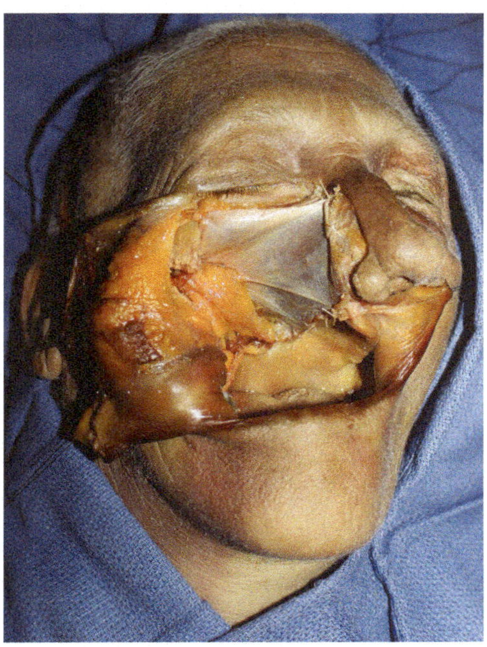

Fig. 12.9 Inset of the flap into the maxillectomy defect.

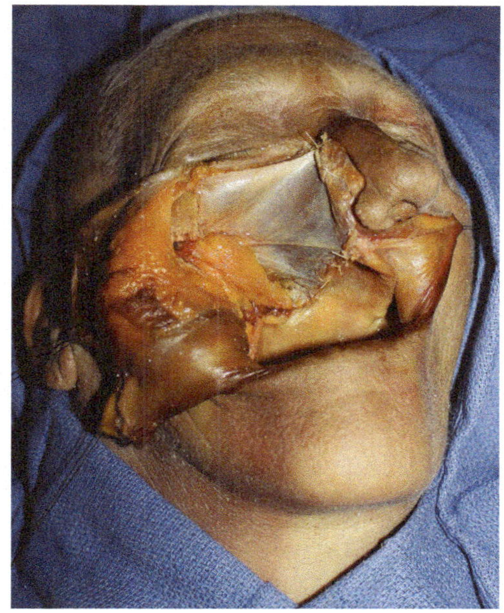

Fig. 12.10 Inferior view of the inset of the flap into the maxillectomy cavity.

Special circumstances

Facial reanimation

- The elevation of the flap is as described earlier with the modification that only the central segment of the muscle is raised rather than the entire muscle.
- The muscle reach can be augmented by using a fascial extension. The fascia is reflected from the inferior aspect of the muscle towards the temporal crest. The area of remaining attachment of the muscle and fascia can be strengthened by placing a few sutures to minimize dehiscence when the muscle contracts.
- When reanimating the mouth, the fascial extension is split into two. One is inserted in the upper lip and the other in the lower lip. The area of division of the fascia is sutured to the commissure. The vector of pull from the muscle contraction would allow for elevation of the corner of the mouth when the patient wishes to animate the face.
- The correction should be slightly exaggerated anticipating a slight postoperative relapse.

Temporal hollowing

A known shortcoming of the use of the temporal muscle flap is the resultant temporal hollowing. The appearance is very conspicuous and leads to significant complaints by the patients, especially female patients.

Several methods exist to counteract this shortcoming. One option is to take advantage of the segmental

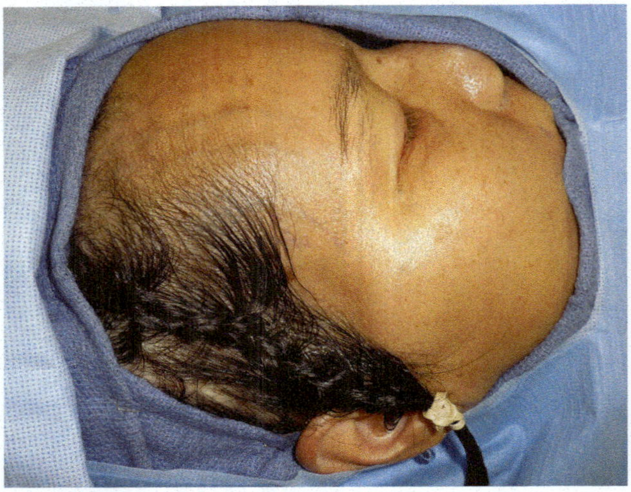

Fig. 12.11 View of a right temporal hollowing.

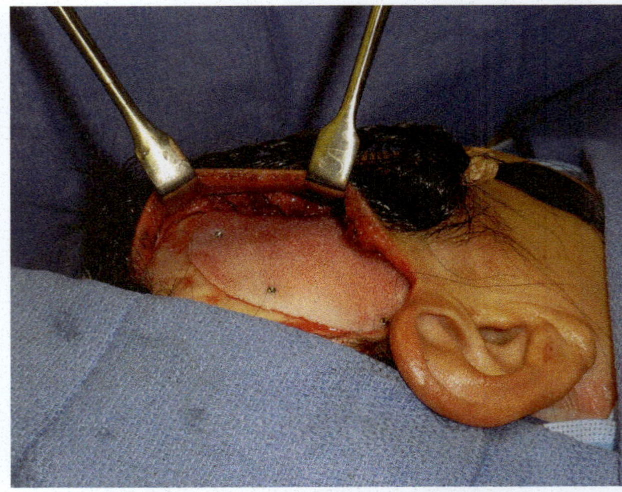

Fig. 12.13 View of the temporal implant used to restore the form.

blood supply to the muscle. Given that the muscle has an anterior, middle, and posterior blood supply, it allows for potential segmentation of the muscle. The temporalis muscle can be divided into three different segments corresponding to anterior, middle, and posterior leaflets.

If the defect can be reconstructed with a smaller muscle, then one can take advantage of the ability to segmentalize the muscle. In these cases, if the anterior segment is used, the middle segment may be advanced to the anterior position therefore preventing the hollowing.

In cases where the reconstruction demands the use of the entire muscle, the use of a temporal implant can be used to combat the hollowing. In these cases, a Medpor (Stryker, USA) implant can be modified to fit the patient and prevent the hollowing (Figures 12.11 to 12.13).

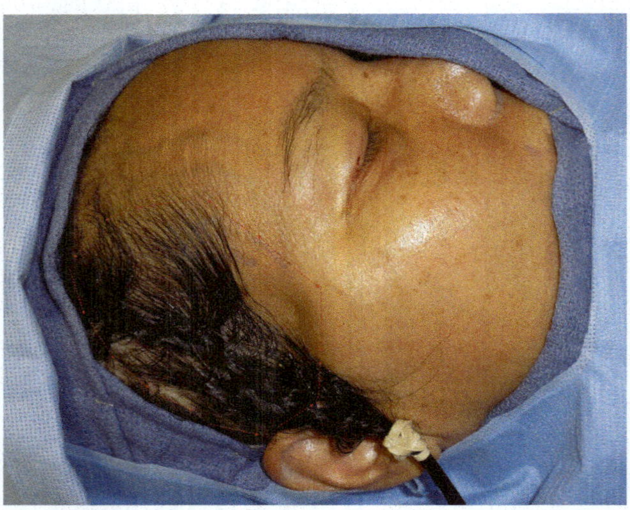

Fig. 12.12 Outline of the area of hollowing prior to reconstruction.

Case #1

A 66-year-old African American male was referred for treatment of a longstanding left maxillary sinus squamous cell carcinoma. The patient described a long history of sinus trouble, which had been medically managed without resolution. He was eventually referred to a head and neck surgeon who performed an incision biopsy, which provided the diagnosis. The workup of the patient

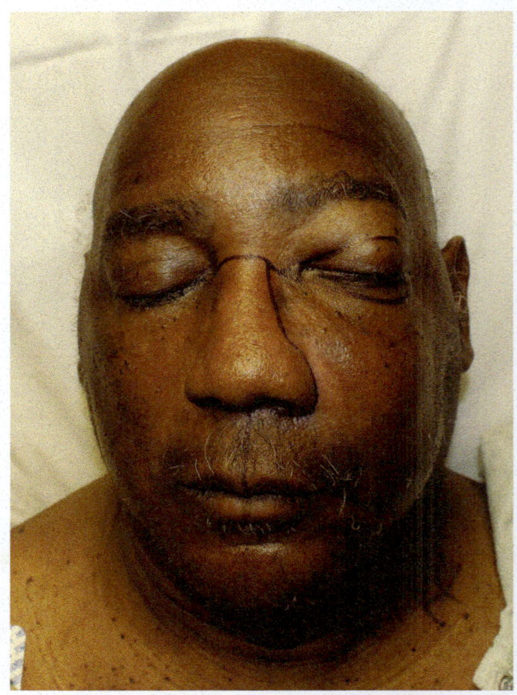

Fig. 12.14 Facial appearance of a patient prior to craniofacial resection with plans for immediate reconstruction of the skull base defect with a temporalis muscle flap.

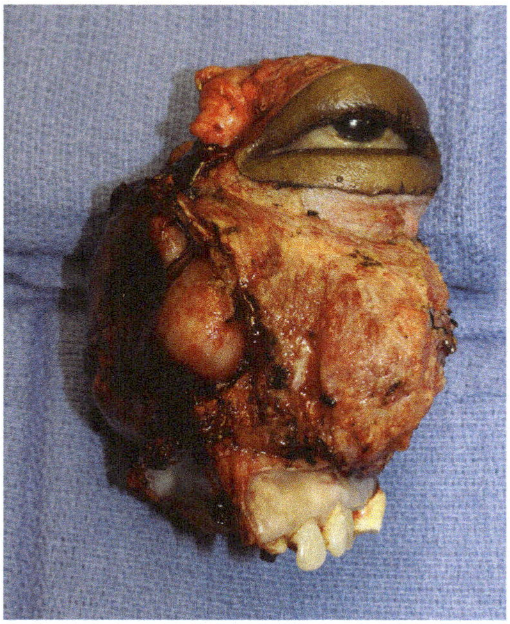

Fig. 12.15 View of the resected tumor.

revealed the sinus tumor extending into the left orbit and infiltrating the orbital contents as well as extending to the ethmoid sinuses. The formulated treatment plan was for a maxillectomy with orbital extension and ethmoidectomy with evaluation of the cranial base involvement by neurosurgery (Figure 12.14).

The ablative procedure was performed with confirmation of frozen section margin assessment providing some assurance of complete resection (Figure 12.15). The access to the surgery was done by a Weber–Ferguson approach (Figures 12.16 and 12.17).

Because of the patient's multiple co-morbidities, a decision was made to perform the reconstruction with a

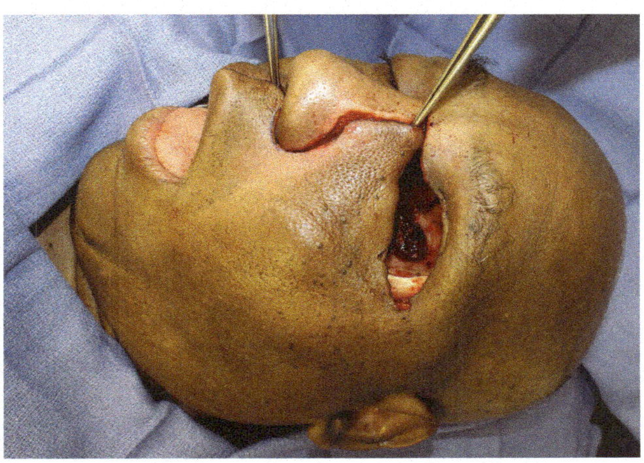

Fig. 12.16 Reapproximation of the Weber Ferguson flap revealing the orbital defect.

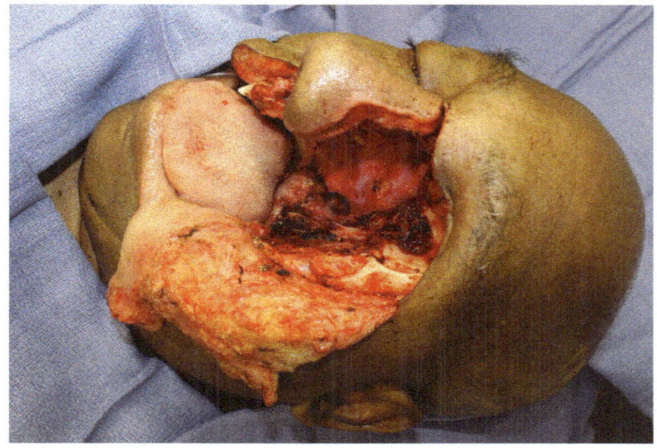

Fig. 12.17 View of the defect cav ty post-resection.

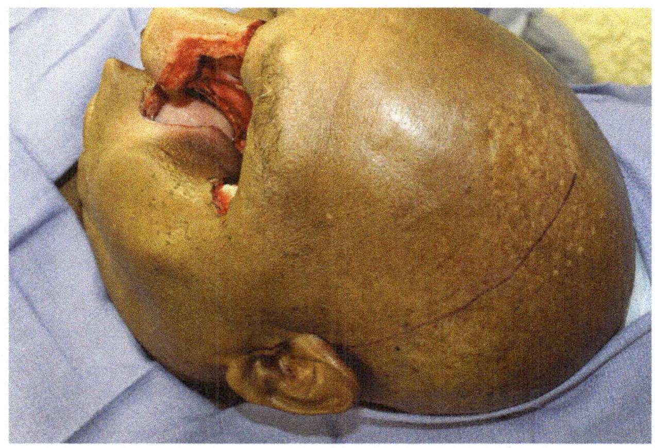

Fig. 12.18 View of the donor site prior to raising the temporalis flap to repair the cranial base defect.

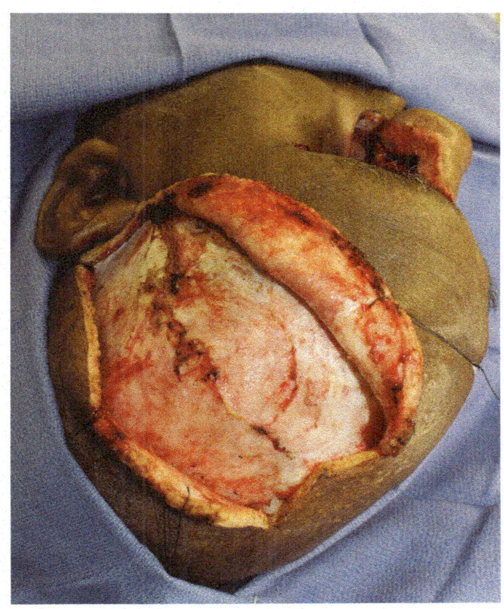

Fig. 12.19 Elevation of the scalp flaps revealing the temporalis muscle.

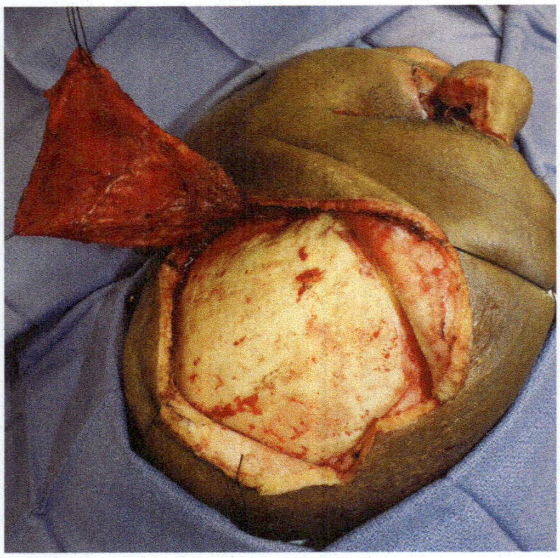

Fig. 12.20 Elevated temporalis muscle flap prior to transfer to the orbital cavity.

temporalis muscle flap to obliterate part of the defect and allow the patient to be later reconstructed with an obturator and orbital prosthesis (Figure 12.18).

The muscle was exposed in a wide fashion to allow for the harvest of the entire muscle (Figure 12.19). The muscle flap was elevated and the arc of rotation checked to be sure that it would transfer to the orbital and maxillectomy defect (Figures 12.20 to 12.22).

The flap was inset and the patient had an uneventful recovery with completion of the radiation therapy (Figures 12.23 and 12.24).

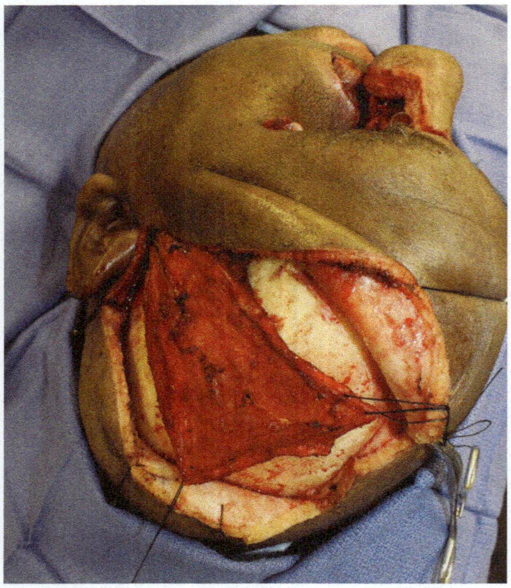

Fig. 12.21 View of the temporalis muscle flap prior to transfer. Note the position of the sutures at each corner; these sutures will aid in the transfer.

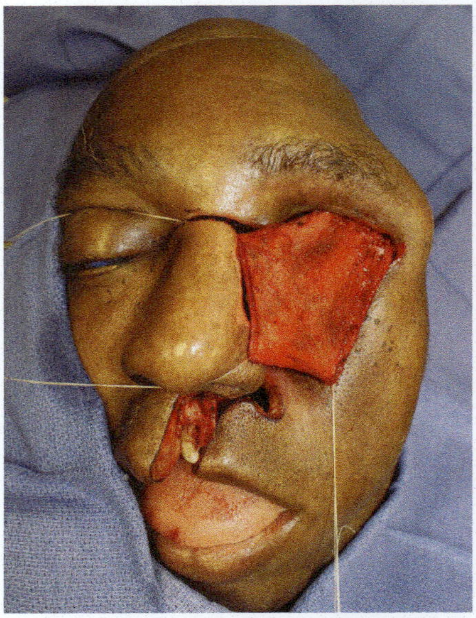

Fig. 12.22 Transfer of the flap into the orbital cavity to repair the skull base defect.

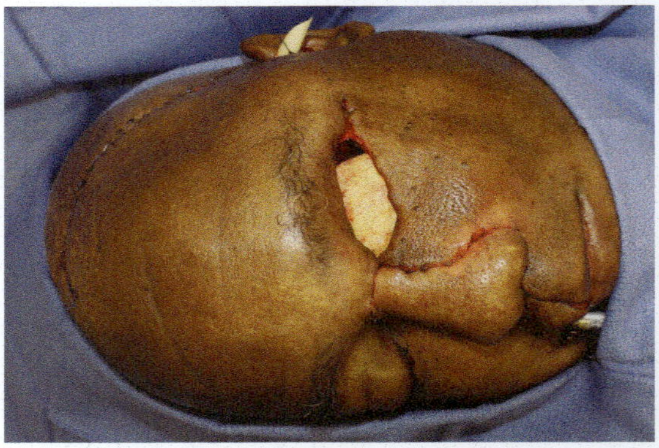

Fig. 12.23 Flap has been inset and packing was placed to keep the flap into position.

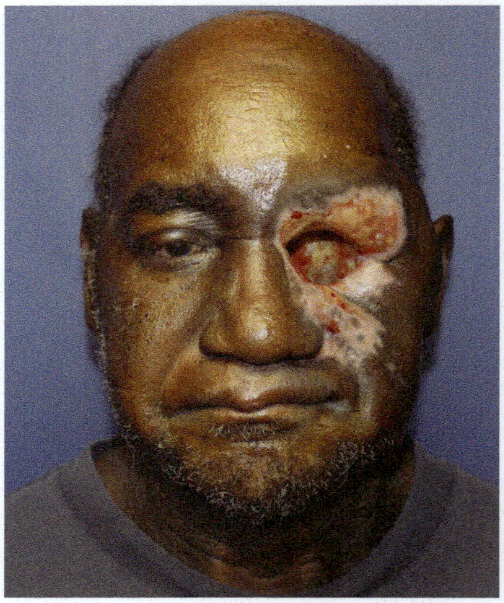

Fig. 12.24 Late view of the appearance of the defect after completion of radiation therapy.

References

1. Edwards SP, Feinberg SE. The temporalis muscle flap in contemporary oral and maxillofacial surgery. *Oral Maxillofacial Surg Clin N Am* 2003; 15:513–535.
2. Mathes SJ, Nahai F. Classification of the vascular anatomy of muscles: experimental and clinical correlation. *Plast Reconstr Surg* 1981; 67:177–187.
3. Nakajima H, Imanishi N, Minabe T. The arterial anatomy of the temporal region and the vascular basis of various temporal flaps. *Br J Plast Surg* 1995; 48:439–450.
4. Cheung LK. The vascular anatomy of the human temporalis muscle: implications for surgical splitting techniques. *Int J Oral Maxillofac Surg* 1996; 25:414–421.
5. Burggasser G, Happak W, Gruber H, Freilinger G. The temporalis: blood supply and innervation. *Plast Reconstr Surg* 2002; 109:1862–1869.

Chapter 13

Cervicofacial advancement flap

Introduction

The cheek is the widest skin expanse of the face and is an important cosmetic and functional unit that provides a platform for crucial midface structures while supporting the lips, nose, and lower eyelids.[1] Defects of the cheek region are therefore conspicuous and potentially difficult to reconstruct with minimal evidence of the surgical insult. The first author to describe the cervicofacial flap to tackle complex midface problems was Beare, who in 1969 described the use of this flap for the reconstruction of orbital exenteration defects.[2] The cervicofacial flap has also been referred to as the Mustarde flap, or as the cheek Mustarde flap since his publication of the use of the flap to reconstruct large defects in the periorbital region.[3] Since then the flap has been described in various forms including a cervicopectoral extension.[4–6]

Although frequently separated in the literature, and perhaps the lexicon, of reconstructive surgeons, cervicofacial and cervicothoracic (cervicopectoral) flaps represent different degrees of inferior extension for the same flap, allowing flexibility in defect management.[7]

The advantages of the cervicofacial flap are similar to other local regional flaps in the head and neck in that there is great color match and equal skin texture. The use of this flap enables placement of the scar in an ideal location where it is camouflaged. The use of the cervicofacial flap is made easier in older patients due to the likelihood of redundant tissues and rhytids, which enables the reconstructive surgeon to better hide the final scars.

The use of the cervicofacial or cervicopectoral flap has very few disadvantages. The potential downside of the flap is the increased risk to the branches of the facial nerve if the elevation of the flap is made deeper to the parotidomasseteric fascia. When reconstructing large defects, the superior tip of the flap may develop signs of venous congestion or ischemia and may eventually lead to the loss of that portion of the flap. Some authors have advocated raising the flap deep to the superficial musculoaponeurotic layer to minimize the potential for distal edge ischemia; this is especially recommended in smokers.[8]

Anatomy

The blood supply to this flap is a random pattern since it is elevated just below the subcutaneous layer. Multiple perforators to the skin arise from the deep facial artery, transverse facial artery, and superficial temporal artery.[9] These perforators are sacrificed as the dissection is carried in the subcutaneous layer. A modification of this flap includes the deep plane cervicofacial flap, which carries the dissection below the superficial musculoaponeurotic system (SMAS) in the face and deep to the platysma in the neck. With this design, the flap becomes a myofasciocutaneous flap with an axial blood supply. An anteriorly based flap derives it blood supply from the submental and perforating branches of the facial artery, while a posteriorly based flap receives its supply from perforators of the superficial temporal artery.[10–12] An extension of this flap includes a pectoral component, which as a fasciocutaneous flap receives its major supply from the first four internal mammary perforating vessels.[13] The venous drainage is mainly through paired vessels, emptying into the anterior and external jugular veins.

Local and Regional Flaps in Head & Neck Reconstruction: A Practical Approach, First Edition. Rui Fernandes.

Companion website: www.wiley.com/go/fernandes/flapsreconstruction

Flap harvest

- The head of the patient is rotated towards the contralateral side and the neck is extended to visualize the entire length of the neck.
- The chest is also prepped into the field.
- The anticipated defect is marked and a decision is made on where to base the flap, i.e., anterior or posterior.
- The superior aspect of the flap is extended towards the lateral canthus and slightly superior towards the anterior hairline. The marking is then extended along the pre-auricular region and extended posterior around the earlobe towards the hairline behind the ear and continues inferiorly towards the base of the neck along the anterior aspect of the trapezius muscle.
- If the defect is anticipated to be very large, the extension can be carried just above the nipple areolar complex.
- The patient is prepped and draped in the usual fashion and the resection is carried out.
- The elevation of the flap begins by making the incision along the previously marked flap outline.
- The flap is raised in the subcutaneous plane and extended towards the defect site. In the facial region, the flap is elevated superficial to the superficial musculoaponeurotic system (SMAS).
- As the dissection is carried out below the inferior border of the mandible, the dissection is transitioned below the platysma muscle.
- Flap elevation is stopped once adequate rotation of the flap is achieved to repair the defect with minimal tension.
- See Figures 13.1 to 13.6a, b.

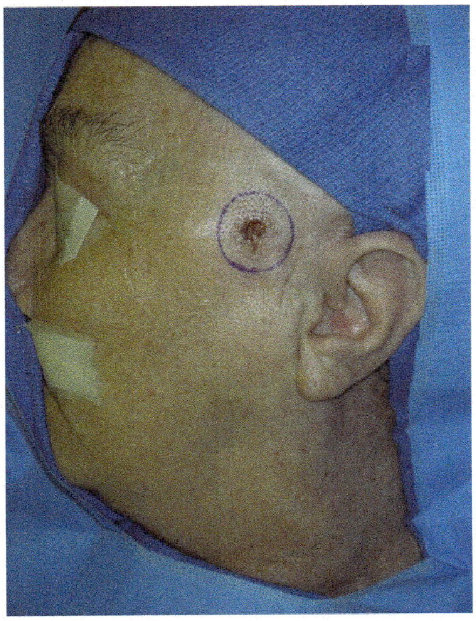

Fig. 13.1 Appearance of a left facial lesion with planned resection margins.

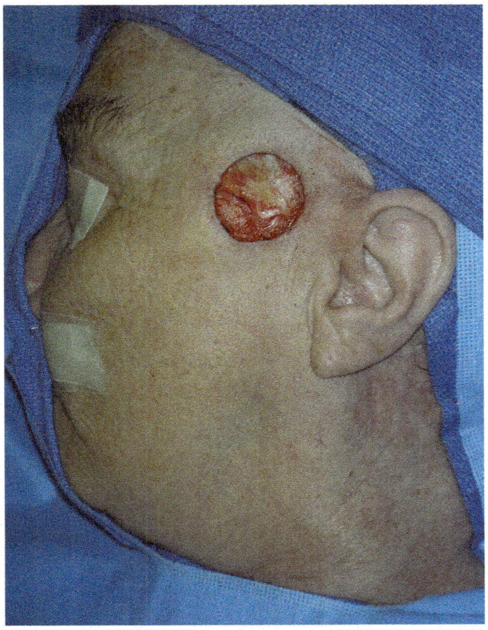

Fig. 13.2 Defect after excision of the lesion.

Extended cervicofacial (cervicopectoral/cervicothoracic) flap

- In cases where the defect is large or for complex defects of the cheek where there is a through-and-through defect, the reconstruction may be carried out using a combination of flaps such as a pedicle

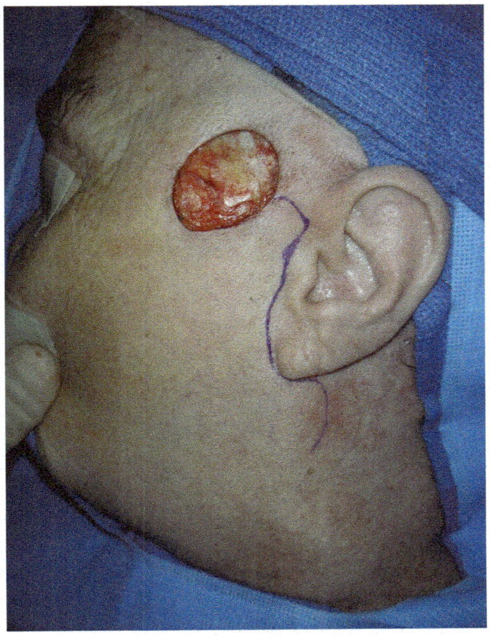

Fig. 13.3 Planning for the cervicofacial flap with incision in the preauricular region.

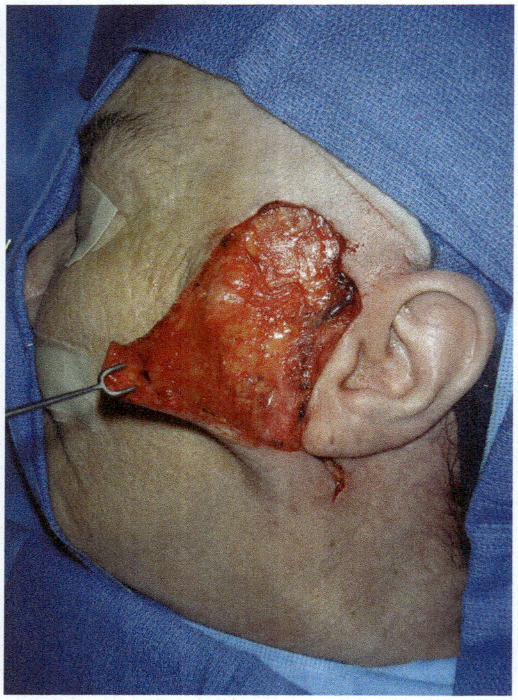

Fig. 13.4 Elevation of a facial flap prior to transfer.

pectoralis myocutaneous flap to repair the buccal defect and the extended cervicofacial (cervicopectoral) flap for the skin defect.

- A complex defect can also be reconstructed with a combination of a free flap and a cervicopectoral flap.

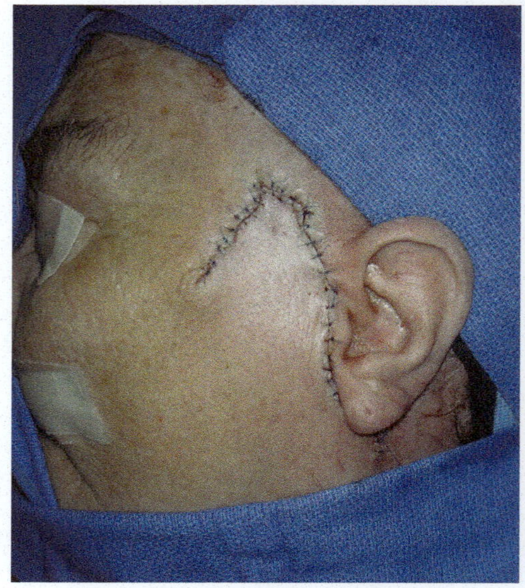

Fig. 13.6a Inset of the flap into the defect.

- In these cases, the elevation of the cervicopectoral flap is extended inferior to the clavicle and onto the pectoral muscle.
- The plane of dissection in this area should be suprafascial.
- Dissection towards the midline should be deliberate and cautious to avoid the perforators from the internal mammary artery, which serve to aid in the perfusion of the extended flap.

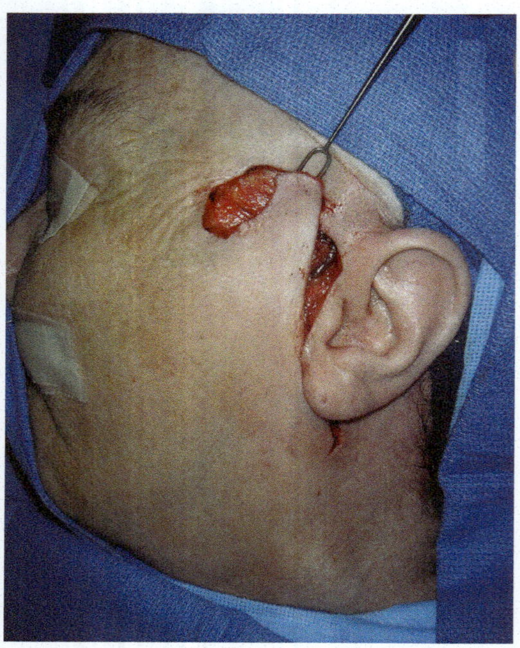

Fig. 13.5 Confirmation of the reach of the flap to repair the defect.

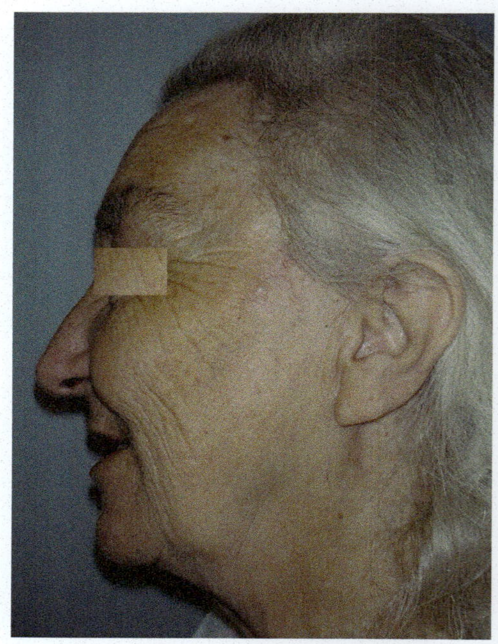

Fig. 13.6b Appearance after a few months post-surgery; note the well healed scar.

- The flap is advanced to the defect and checked to be sure that adequate tissue can be transferred to repair the defect.
- Often, there is enough redundant tissue that affords the surgeon the ability to contour the flap and place the incisions along the junctions of various subunits. Attention to this detail will render a more pleasing final cosmetic reconstruction.
- The donor site can often be closed primarily after wide undermining.
- If the donor site is unable to be closed primarily even after wide undermining, then a skin graft may be used to repair the remaining open area.

Case #1

A 66-year-old Caucasian male was referred for the management of a biopsy-proven melanoma of the medial cheek and infraorbital region (Figure 13.7). A plan was made for resection of the tumor in conjunction with a sentinel node dissection and immediate reconstruction of the defect with a cervicofacial rotation flap. The design of the flap was extended posterior to the ear and rotated inferiorly towards the low neck. The resection was performed with a resultant significant infraorbital/medial cheek defect (Figures 13.8 and 13.9). The flap was then elevated along the previously marked outline and raised in the supra SMAS plane (Figures 13.10 and 13.11). The flap was then rotated to the defect and inset without any tension (Figures 13.12 to 13.14). The final appearance of the patient was acceptable without any facial distortion (Figures 13.15 and 13.16).

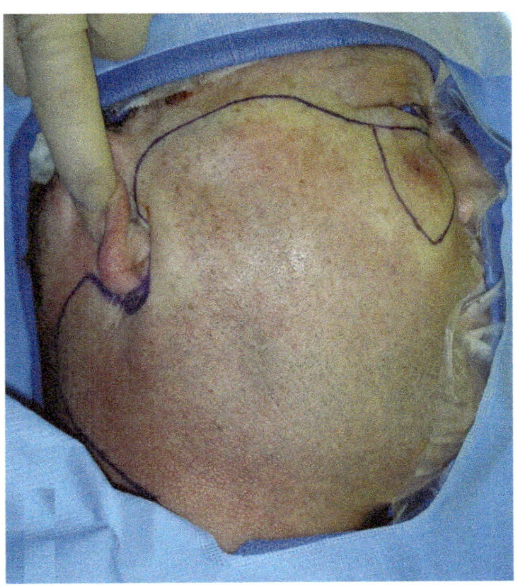

Fig. 13.7 Markings for excision of an infraorbital melanoma with immediate reconstruction of with a large cervicofacial flap.

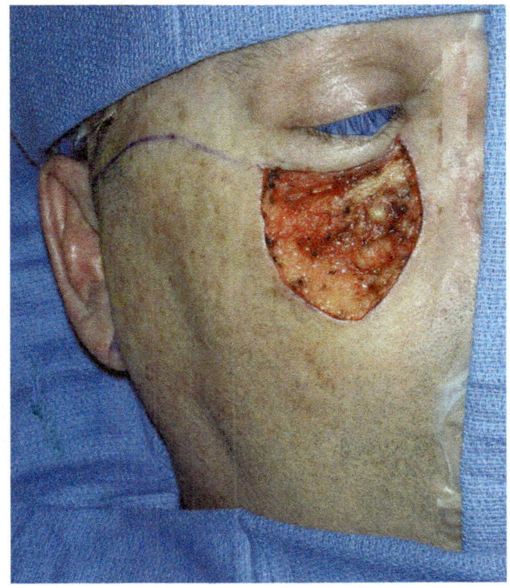

Fig. 13.8 Infraorbital defect after excision of the melanoma.

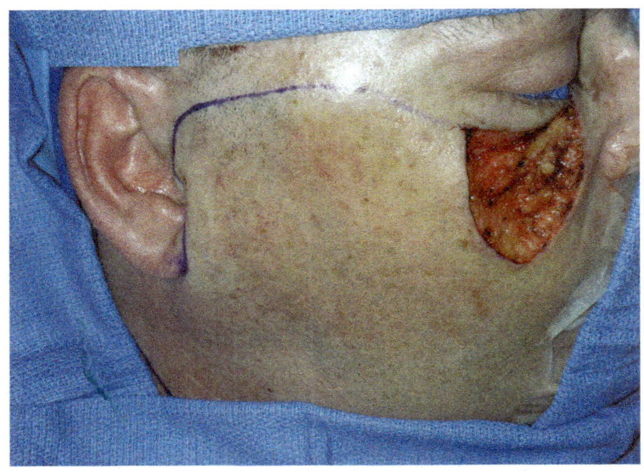

Fig. 13.9 Markings for the cervicofacial flap.

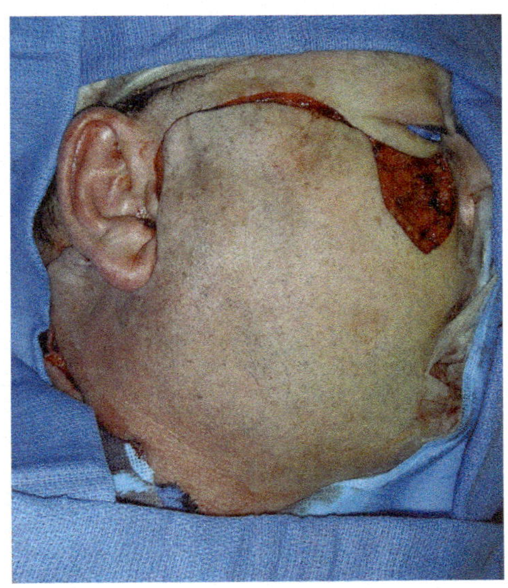

Fig. 13.10 Incision for the cervicofacial flap prior to transfer of the flap.

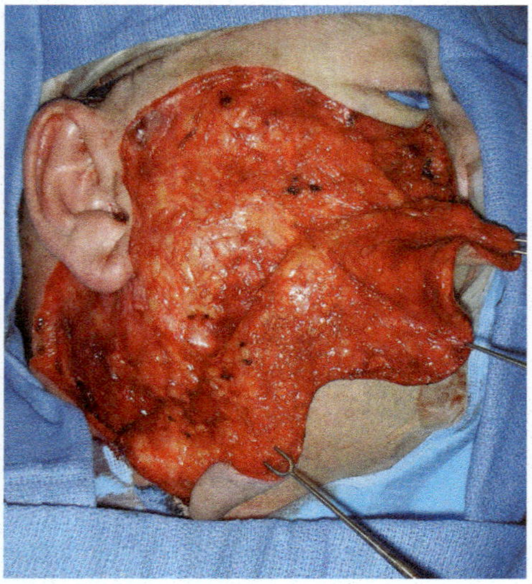

Fig. 13.11 Elevation of the cervicofacial flap.

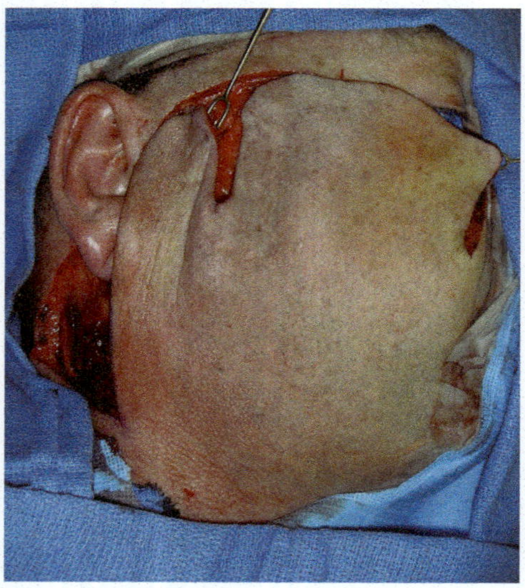

Fig. 13.12 Confirmation of the reach of the flap prior to inset.

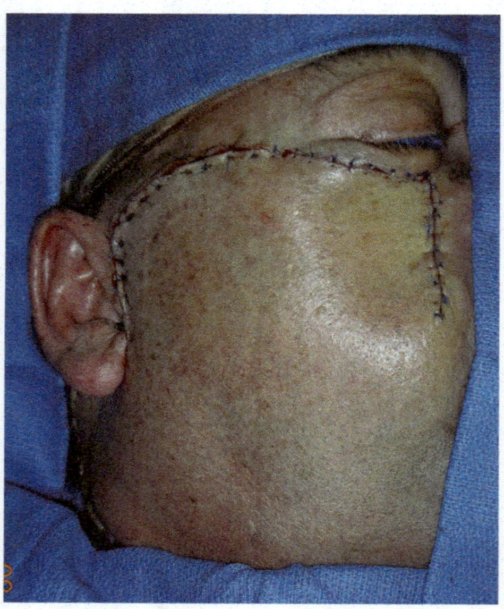

Fig. 13.13 Inset of the flap into the defect. Note the passive fit of the flap without distortion of the lower eyelid.

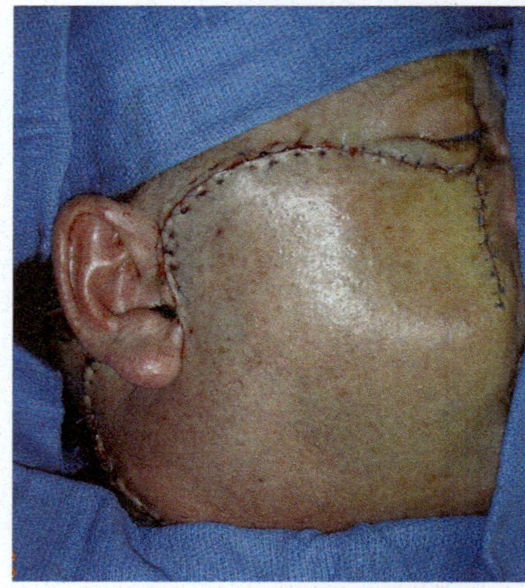

Fig. 13.14 Lateral facial appearance of the reconstruction.

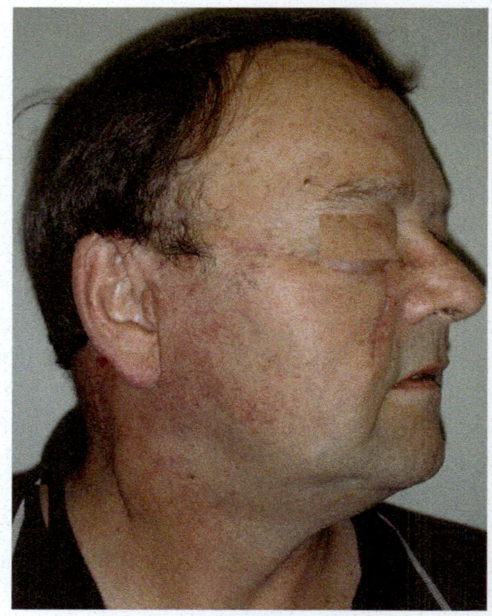

Fig. 13.15 Early postoperative appearance of the reconstruction. Note that the incision is well camouflaged.

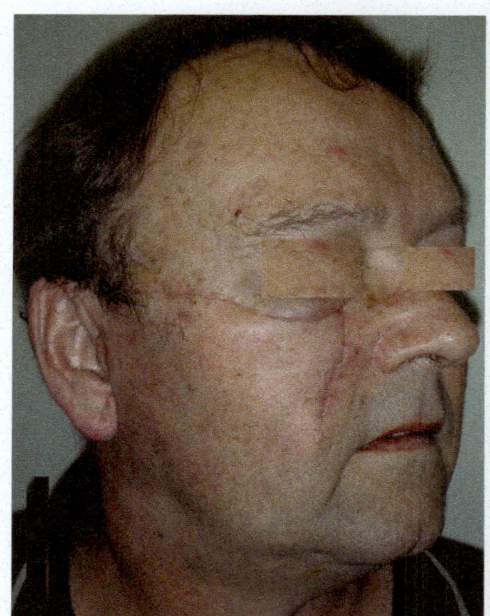

Fig. 13.16 Frontal view of the reconstruction.

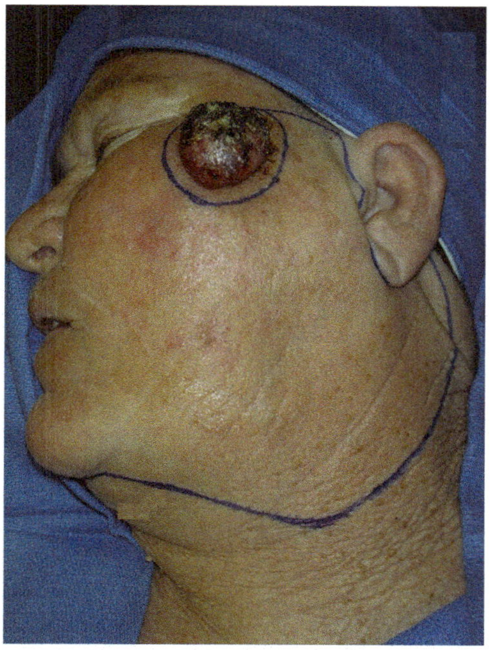

Fig. 13.17 Markings for the resection of a large facial carcinoma with planning for a cervicofacial flap.

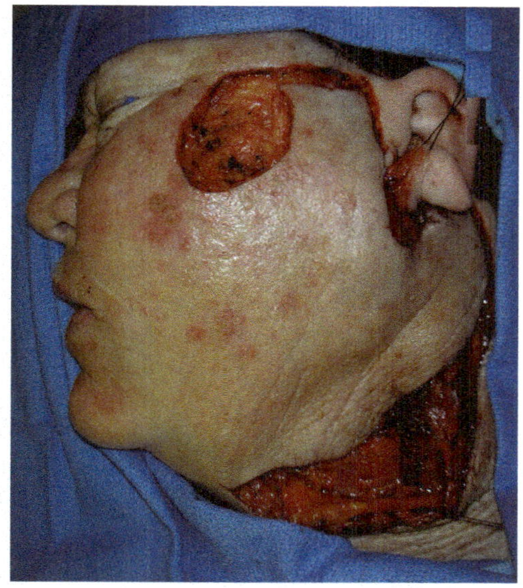

Fig. 13.18 View of the surgical defect and incision of the cervicofacial flap.

Case #2

A 67-year-old Caucasian female presented with a large, longstanding lesion of the left cheek region. She reported a recent increase in the size of the lesion as well as a palpable neck node. Workup revealed a squamous cell carcinoma with an enlarged level II node. A plan was formulated for a wide local excision of the lesion with simultaneous neck dissection and planned reconstruction of the defect with an anteriorly based cervicofacial rotational flap (Figure 13.17). The lesion was excised and the neck dissection was performed. The approach for the neck dissection was extended by elevating the cervicofacial flap (Figures 13.18 and 13.19). The flap was rotated to the defect and checked to be sure that it would allow for a tension-free repair of the defect without compromising the flap (Figure 13.20a). The flap was inset (Figure 13.20b). The late appearance of the patient was found to be acceptable with minimal evidence of the surgical resection and reconstruction (Figure 13.20c).

Case #3

A 55-year-old Caucasian male was referred for the management of a large, neglected skin malignancy with extension to the underlying parotid gland and invasion of the zygomatic arch and masseteric muscle (Figure 13.21). A plan was made for a radical resection and immediate reconstruction of the defect with a cervicopectoral flap due to multiple comorbidities which rendered the patient a poor candidate for microvascular reconstruction. The surgical markings for the resection as well as an extended cervicofacial/cervicopectoral flap were designed, stopping just superior to the nipple (Figure 13.22). A radical resection of the tumor was performed with sacrifice of the masseteric muscle, the parotid gland with facial nerve sacrifice, and resection of the zygomatic arch (Figure 13.23). The flap was then elevated with care taken not to injure the perforators from the internal mammary

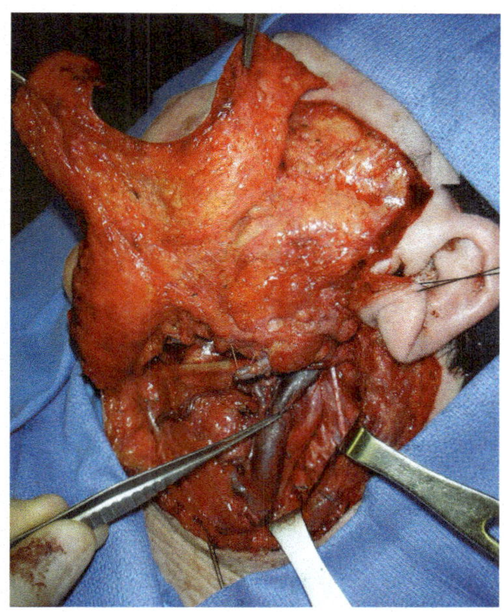

Fig. 13.19 View of the elevated flap revealing a selective neck dissection and a superficial parotidectomy performed at the same time.

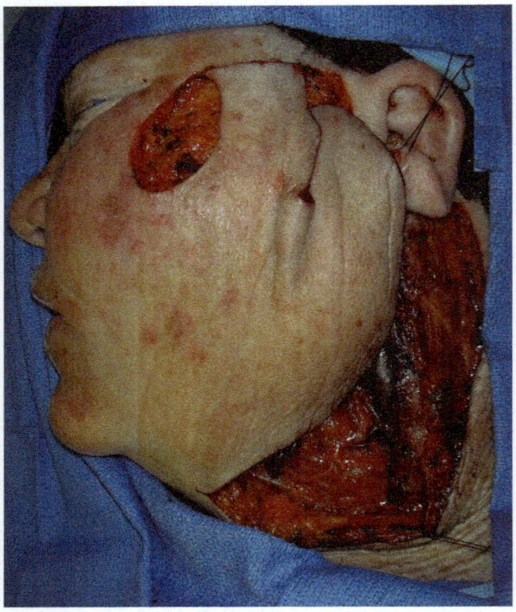

Fig. 13.20a Checking for the rotation of the flap into the defect.

artery accessing the flap between the first, second, and third intercostal spaces (Figure 13.24). The flap was then rotated to the defect to check the adequacy of reach, note the excess of tissue overlapping the defect (Figure 13.25). The flap was trimmed along the areas of excess taking care to place the incision along the junction of the esthetic zones (Figure 13.26). The final appearance of the patient was acceptable in terms of skin color and texture (Figure 13.27).

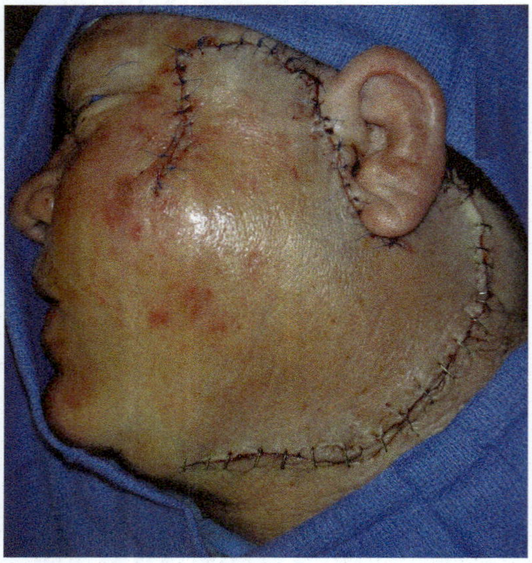

Fig. 13.20b Inset of the flap into the defect.

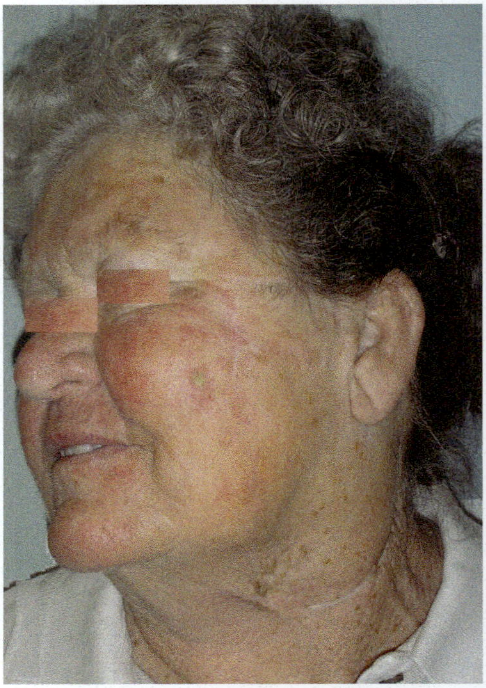

Fig. 13.20c Late appearance of the reconstructed defect. Note that the appearance of the scar is very subtle.

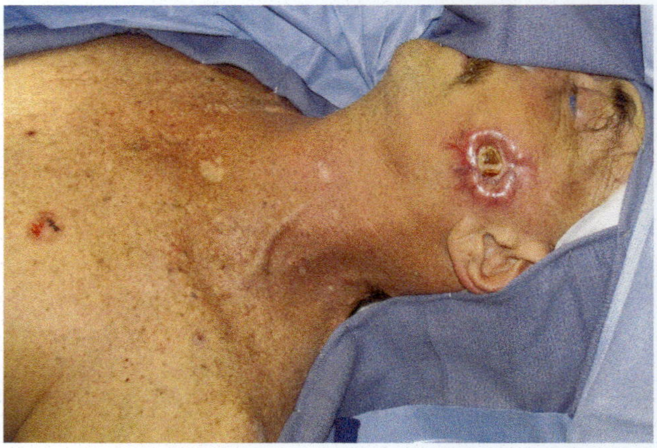

Fig. 13.21 View of a large facial tumor with deep extension to the parotid and masseteric muscle.

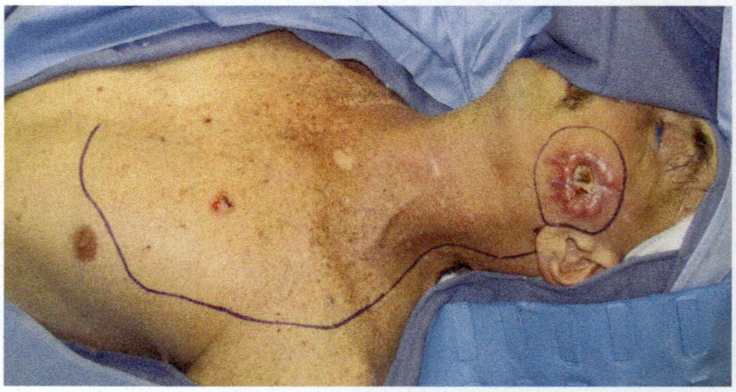

Fig. 13.22 Planning for the radical resection of the tumor with immediate reconstruction with a cervicopectoral flap.

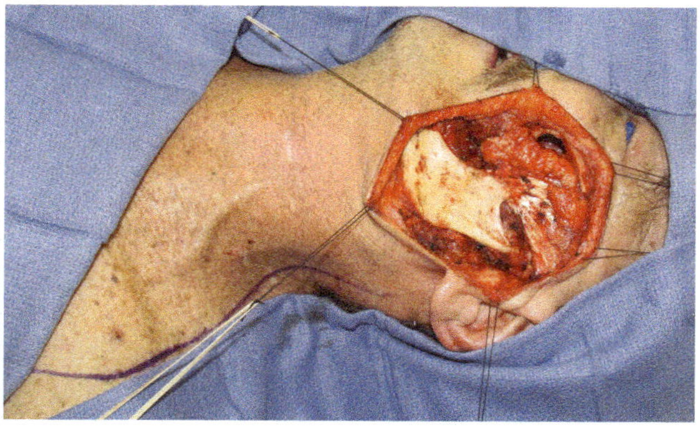

Fig. 13.23 Appearance of the radical resection with total parotidectomy and facial nerve sacrifice.

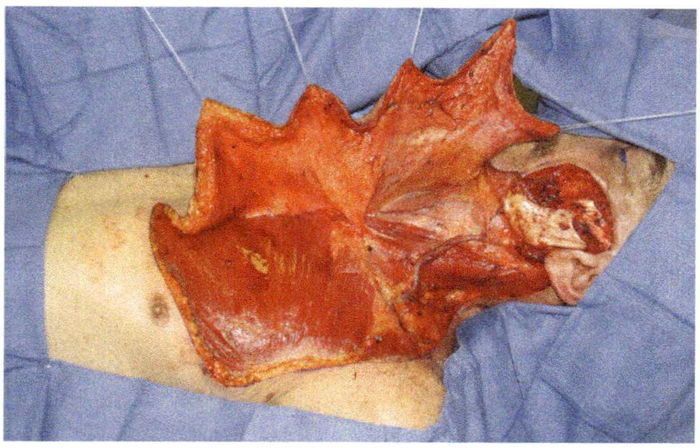

Fig. 13.24 View of the of the elevated cervicopectoral flap prior to transfer to the defect.

Case #4

A 79-year-old Caucasian male with a history of squamous cell carcinoma of the oropharynx previously treated with chemoradiation presented for management of a biopsy-proven recurrence. The tumor extended from the oropharyngeal region and the skull base towards the skin. The patient was also noted to have facial nerve paralysis at presentation and severe pain. A discussion was had with the patient for a palliative resection with a plan for immediate reconstruction with pedicled pectoralis major myocutaneous flap and a cervicopectoral flap (Figure 13.28). Once the resection was completed, the defect encompassed the entire buccal mucosa and the full thickness towards the skin and skull base (Figures 13.29 and 13.30). A cervicopectoral flap was elevated as previously described while preserving the skin paddle overlying the pectoralis major myocutaneous flap (Figures 13.31 and 13.32). The pectoralis flap was elevated and brought to the head and neck and used to repair the buccal defect and extended to fill the skull base defect (Figure 13.33).

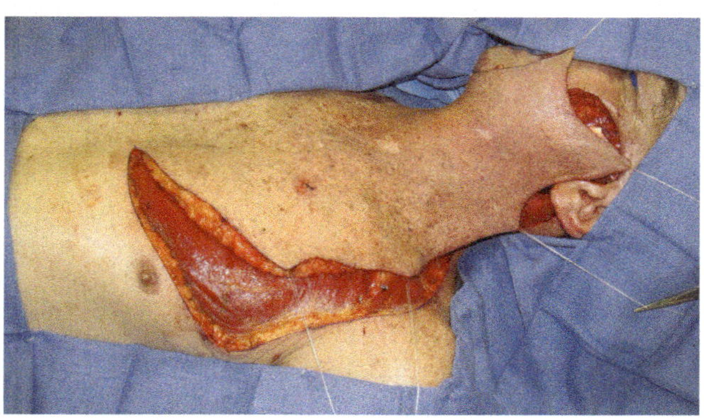

Fig. 13.25 Rotation of the flap into the defect to check for passive reach.

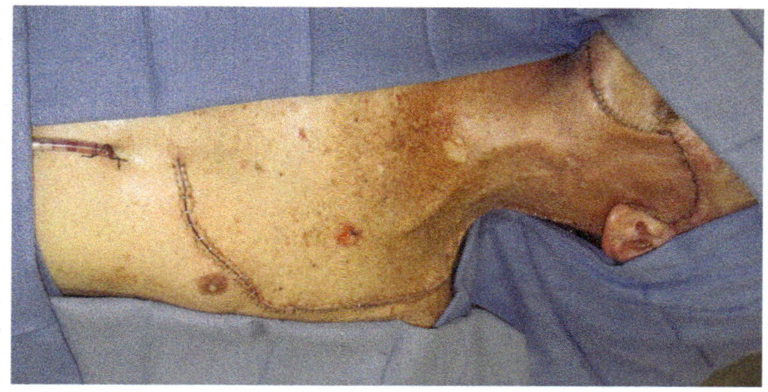

Fig. 13.26 Inset of the flap after trimming the flap and placing the incision lines along the labio mental crease.

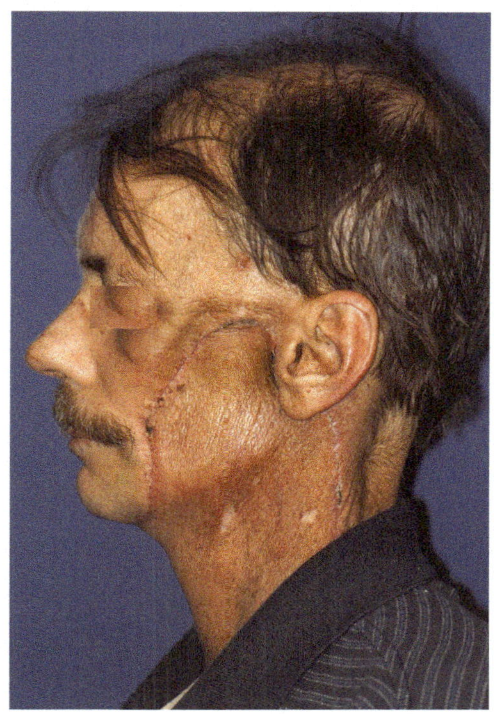

Fig. 13.27 Early postoperative appearance of the reconstructed defect; note the perfect skin color and texture match.

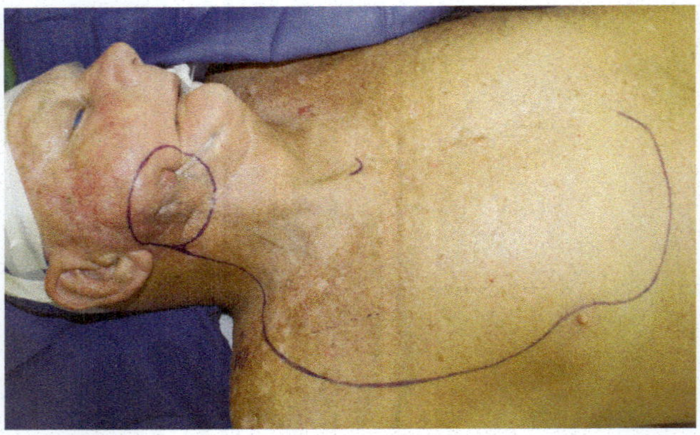

Fig. 13.28 Planning for a salvage surgery to resect a large recurrence post failed chemoradiotherapy. The markings are for a radical resection and a cervicopectoral flap.

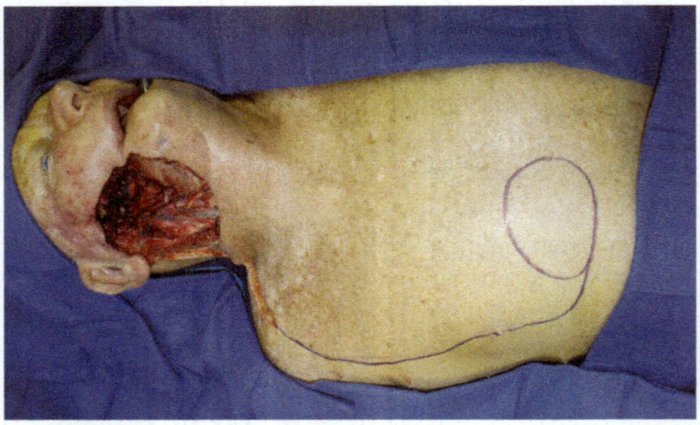

Fig. 13.29 View of the radical resection with exposed carotid vessels.

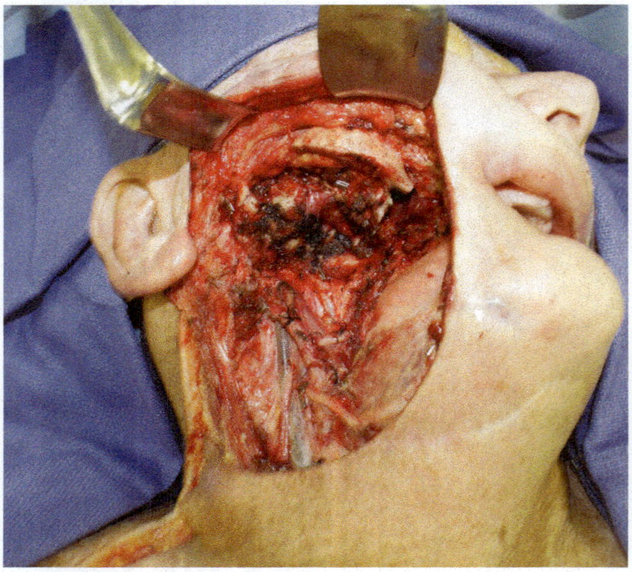

Fig. 13.30 View of the resection to the skull base.

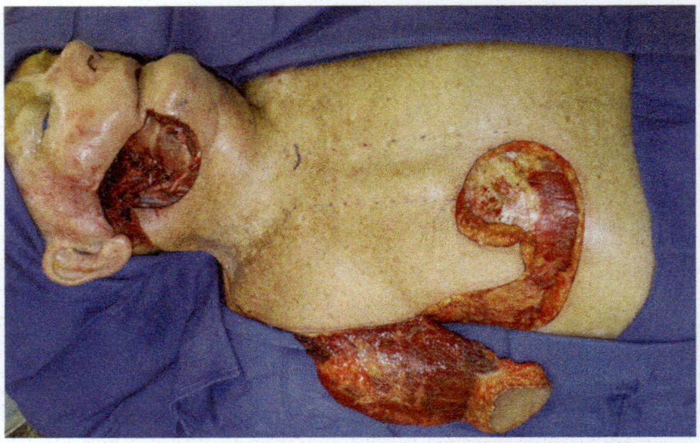

Fig. 13.31 Elevated pectoralis major flap and a cervicopectoral flap.

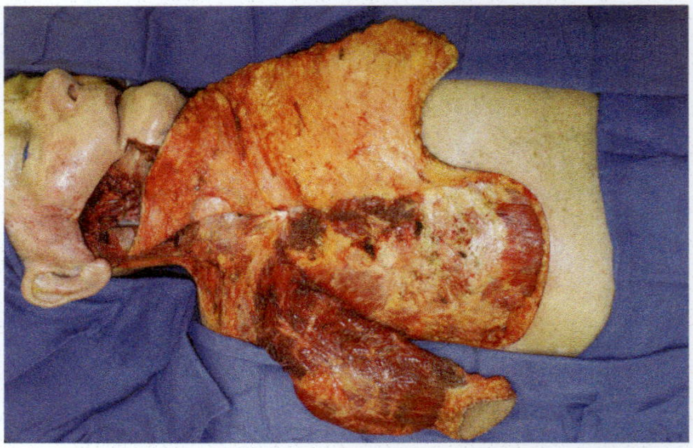

Fig. 13.32 Appearance of the elevated cervicopectoral flap and view of the pectoralis muscle flap.

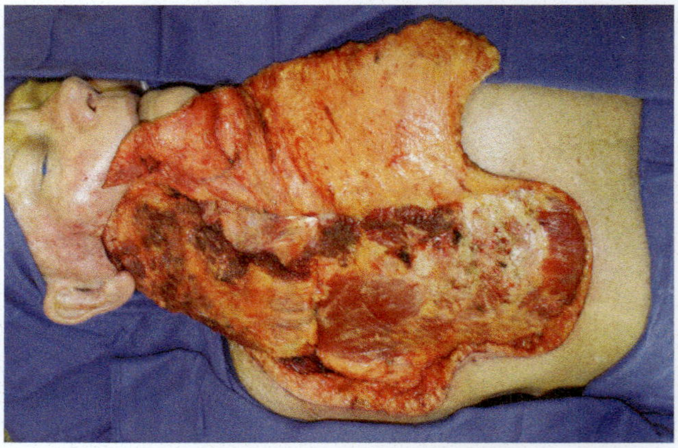

Fig. 13.33 Inset of the pectoralis major flap to repair the large skull base defect.

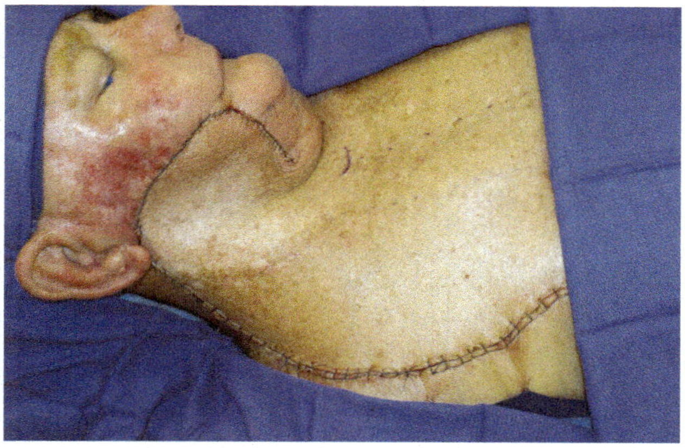

Fig. 13.34 Inset of the cervicopectoral flap to repair the facial skin defect.

The cervicopectoral flap was then rotated and inset to repair the large cheek defect (Figure 13.34). Early postoperative follow-up showed that the flap had an excellent take and great color match. The inferior site of the donor site was skin grafted (Figure 13.35). The frontal view of the patient as well as the intraoral view showed that the skin paddle for the pectoralis muscle had a good take and that there was adequate facial contour (Figures 13.36 and 13.37).

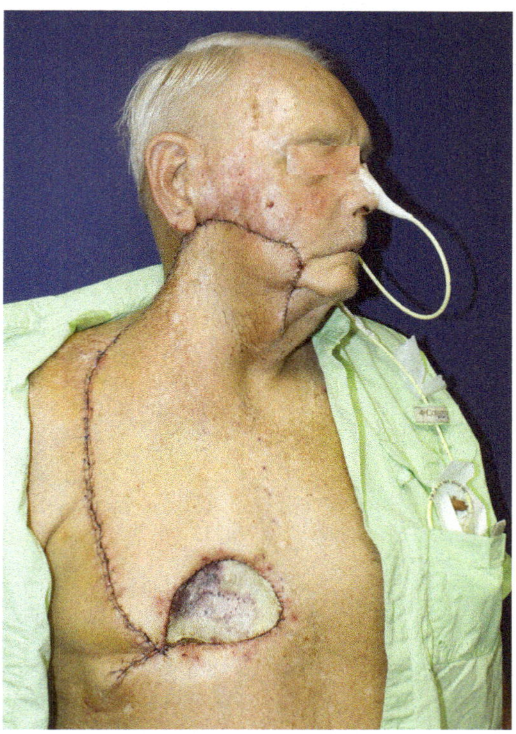

Fig. 13.35 View of the donor site with a skin graft in the lower chest.

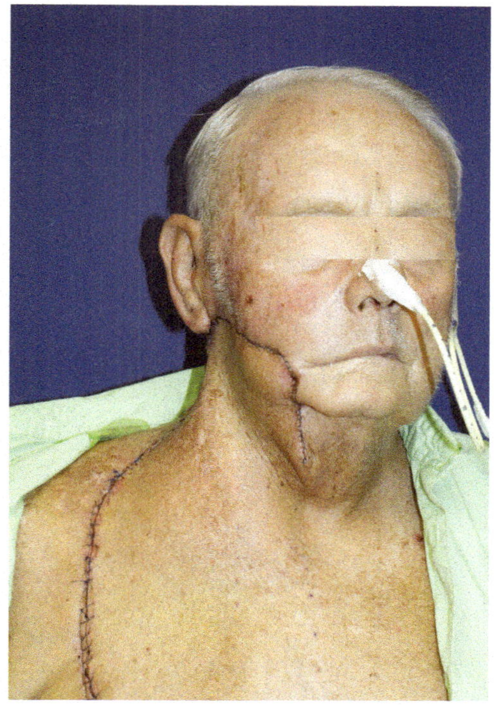

Fig. 13.36 Early postoperative appearance of the reconstruction.

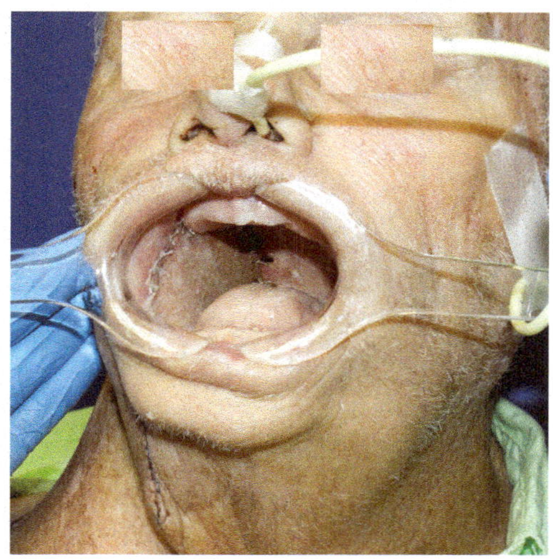

Fig. 13.37 Intraoral view of the pectoralis major reconstruction used not only for the skull base but also for the buccal mucosa defect.

References

1. Chandawarkar RY, Cervino AL. Subunits of the cheek: an algorithm for the reconstruction of partial thickness defects. *Br J Plast Surg* 2003; 56:135–139.
2. Beare RL. Flap repair following exenteration of the orbit. *Proc R Soc Med* 1969; 62 1087–1890.
3. Mustarde JC. The use of flaps in the orbital region. *Plast Reconstr Surg* 1970; 45:146–150.

4. Garrett WS, Giblin TR, Hoffman GW. Closure of skin defects of the face and neck by rotation and advancement of cervicopectoral flaps. *Plast Reconstr Surg* 1966; 38:342–346.
5. Becker DW. A cervicopectoral rotation flap for cheek coverage. *Plast Reconstr Surg* 1978; 61:868–870.
6. Shestak KC, Roth AG, Jones NF, Myers EN. The cervicopectoral rotation flap a valuable technique for facial reconstruction. *Br J Plast Surg* 1993; 46:375–377.
7. Moore BA, Wine T, Netterville J. Cervicofacial and cervicothoracic rotation flaps in head and neck reconstruction. *Head Neck* 2005; 27:1092–1101.
8. Becker FF, Langford FPJ. Deep plane cervicofacial flap for reconstruction of large cheek defects. *Arch Otolaryngol Head Neck Surg* 1996; 122:997–999.
9. Menick FJ. Discussion: simplifying cheek reconstruction: a review of over 400 cases. *Plast Reconstr Surg* 2012; 129:1300–1303.
10. Tan ST, Mackinnon CA. Deep plane cervicofacial flap: a useful and versatile technique in head and neck surgery. *Head Neck* 2006; 28:46–55.
11. Becker FF, Langford FP. Deep-plane cervicofacial flap for reconstruction of large cheek defects. *Arch Otolaryngol Head Neck Surg* 1996; 122:997–999.
12. Kroll SS, Reece GP, Robb G, Black J. Deep-plane cervicofacial rotation-advancement flap for reconstruction of large cheek defects. *Plast Reconstr Surg* 1994; 94:88–93.
13. Becker DW. A cervicopectoral rotation flap for cheek coverage. *Plast Reconstr Surg* 1978; 61:868–870.

Chapter 14
Submental island flap

Introduction

The submental island flap was first mentioned in the literature by Martin *et al.*, who described this new flap as a good option to reconstruct various defects in the head and neck[1]. Since this description, the submental island has struggled to gain a strong foothold as a reliable flap in the reconstruction of head and neck defects. Two likely reasons for the slow and reluctant acceptance of this flap into the everyday use by head neck reconstructive surgeons has been the difficult dissection of the flap along the submandibular gland area as well as concern for its use in patients with oral cavity cancers. The latter is due to the belief or fear of potentially transferring nodal disease to the reconstructed site. This concern has not been shown to be valid by the collective experience of most surgeons who routinely use the submental flap.

The submental island flap is a fantastic option for the reconstruction of defects in the head and neck extending from the oral cavity, oropharynx, hypopharynx, maxilla, as well as various sites in the face such as the parotid bed, chin, face, upper and lower lip, and in neck defects.

The main disadvantage of the submental island flap is the dissection of the pedicle near the takeoff of the facial artery and vein as the vessels travel through the submandibular gland. Dissection in this area can be very tedious and a potential site for problems, particularly of the veins leading to venous congestion of the flap.

Overall, this flap is a very reliable option for the reconstruction of small to fairly large defects in the head and neck while still providing the ability to primarily close the donor site. The location of the donor site scar is well hidden, particularly when the patient is standing upright.

Anatomy

The submental artery island flap is a type C fasciocutaneous flap with its dominant pedicle based on the submental artery, which arises approximately 5–6.5 cm from the origin of the facial artery.[1] The facial artery has a mean diameter of 2.7 mm at its origin form the external carotid artery. The submental artery emerges from the medial portion of the facial artery 5–7 mm inferior to the mandibular border, 3–5 cm anterior to the mandibular angle and with a mean diameter of 1.7 mm.[2] The submental artery arises deep to the submandibular gland and continues forward and medially across the mylohyoid muscle. As it continues its course, the artery gives branches to the submandibular gland, the platysma, digastric and mylohyoid muscles, small branches to the subplatysmal fatty layer, and 1–4 cutaneous perforators.[3] These perforators pierce the platysma and terminate in the subdermal plexus connected with the contralateral artery, allowing for skin perfusion of both the ipsilateral and contralateral neck.[4] This enables a flap to be raised from the mandibular left angle to the right angle with a width of 7–8 cm and a length of 15–18 cm, a territory of 45 ± 10.2 cm^2.[5] The submental artery terminates either deep to, superficial to, or within the anterior belly of the digastric and sends branches to the lower lip.[6] During flap harvest the ipsilateral anterior belly of the digastric is included, as the artery has been found to lie deep to the muscle in 70% of cases. The pedicle length ranges from 5 to 8 cm giving a significant arc of rotation extending from the medial canthus to the zygomatic arch. The venous drainage is via the submental vein, which has a mean diameter of 2.2 mm. It drains into the facial vein, which has a mean diameter of 2.5 mm. The caliber of the submental vessels, make this flap suitable for microvascular transfer. The sensory nerve supply to this region is via

Local and Regional Flaps in Head & Neck Reconstruction: A Practical Approach, First Edition. Rui Fernandes.

Companion website: www.wiley.com/go/fernandes/flapsreconstruction

the transverse cervical nerves. Motor innervation is via the cervical branch of the facial nerve. On dissection care must be taken to avoid injury to the marginal mandibular branch of the facial nerve as it can travel a mean of 12 mm away from the submental artery.

Flap harvest

- The first step in the harvest of the submental artery flap is the determination of the amount of skin that can be harvested while allowing for primary closure of the defect. This can be done with a pinch test. The skin inferior to the inferior border of the mandible is pinched to determine the greatest amount of skin which can be taken while allowing for advancement of the remaining neck skin to close to the skin at the inferior border of the mandible.
- Once the skin amount is determined, an elliptical skin island is marked out as needed. The amount of skin can extend laterally to the posterior border of the mandible or the mastoid area.
- If the flap is being raised in conjunction with a neck dissection, the ipsilateral posterior border of the skin island is extended to meet the neck dissection in an apron-type incision.
- A Doppler scan may be used to help determine the trajectory of the pedicle, but this is not necessary.
- Flap raising begins by making the superior skin incision on the distal part of the flap, i.e., on the side away from the pedicle.
- The incision is extended from the skin, the subcutaneous tissue, and to the fascia of the contralateral anterior belly of the digastric. Skin incision is also extended inferiorly towards the ipsilateral aspect of the pedicle.
- Dissection is extended to the midline over the mylohyoid muscle and the ipsilateral anterior digastric muscle.
- The attachment of the anterior digastric muscle is detached from the mandible and it is sectioned inferiorly at the intermediate tendon.
- At this point, dissection is carefully carried out towards the facial artery hugging the inferior border of the mandible where the submental vascular pedicle travels in a transverse horizontal fashion.
- As the dissection approaches the submandibular gland, a subplatysmal flap should be raised to facilitate the inspection and dissection of the pedicle. This portion of the dissection can also be carried out at the beginning of the flap harvest with a circumferential incision and elevation of the subplatysmal flap.
- Taking care to identify the facial vessels and the marginal mandibular branch of the facial nerve, the fascia is elevated superiorly to protect the nerve.
- Dissection in this region approaches the submandibular gland. At this point, dissection should be carried out with a bipolar electrocautery to minimize damage to the vascular pedicle.
- Larger vascular branches of the vascular pedicle should be clipped and divided.
- Once dissection of the pedicle is completed along the submandibular gland, the gland is often removed. At this point, the submental artery and vein are completely dissected to the takeoff at the facial vessels.

Transfer to the oral cavity

- Once the flap pedicle is completely dissected, the flap is ready to be transferred to the oral cavity if that is where the defect is located.
- Prior to the transfer of the pedicle, a tunnel from the neck to the oral cavity must be created.
- The usual transfer to the oral cavity is done by forming a tunnel along the mylohyoid muscle. This dissection can be done from the neck and the tunnel connected to the oral cavity via the resection defect.
- Care should be taken to insure that there is at least ample room to tolerate the pedicle size and so it is not compressed postoperatively as this can interfere with the venous outflow or perfusion.
- Once the tunnel is made, a large Kelly clamp is passed from the oral cavity to the neck. The skin edge of the flap is secured with the Kelly clamp and the flap is gently teased into the oral cavity. Once in the oral cavity, the contour and alignment is oriented for the most effective position and the pedicle in the neck is checked to insure that it is not twisted.
- The flap is then inset and the neck closed over a vacuum drain.
- See Figures 14.1 to 14.10.

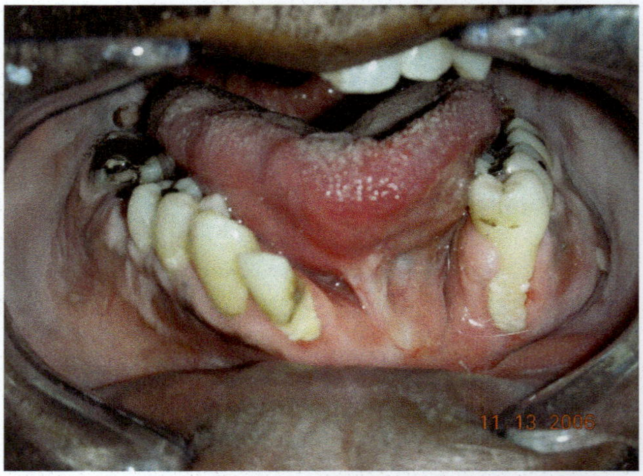

Fig. 14.1 Appearance of intraoral scaring in the anterior vestibule secondary to a gunshot injury.

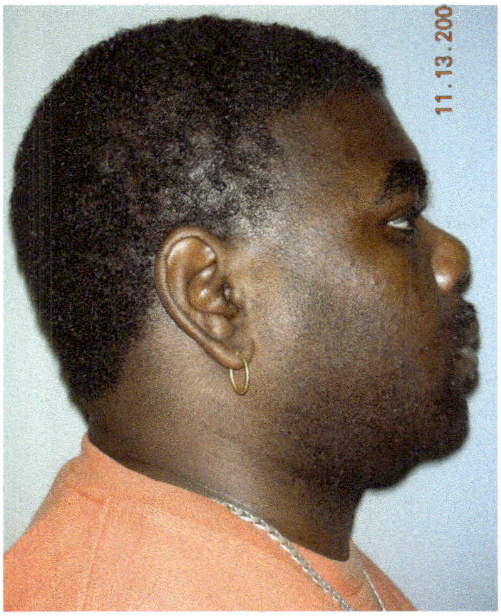

Fig. 14.2 Profile view of the patient prior to harvest of a submental island flap; note the redundancy of the submental tissue.

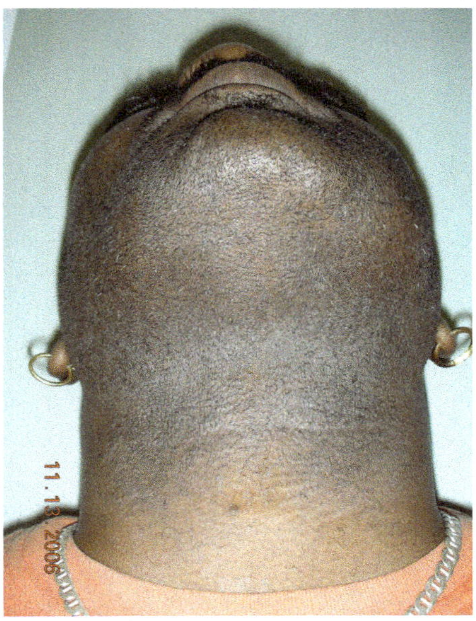

Fig. 14.3 Submental view, prior to flap harvest.

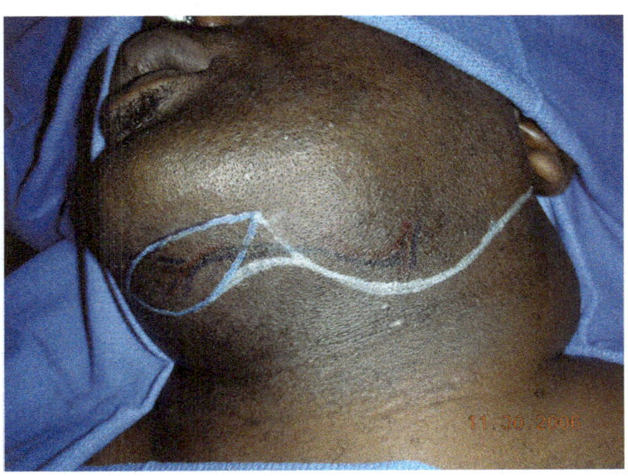

Fig. 14.4 Preoperative markings for the submental island flap to be used in the reconstruction of an intraoral defect.

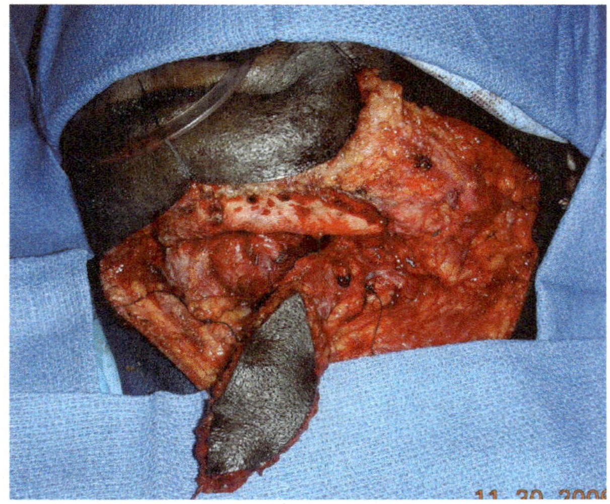

Fig. 14.5 Raised submental flap prior to transfer.

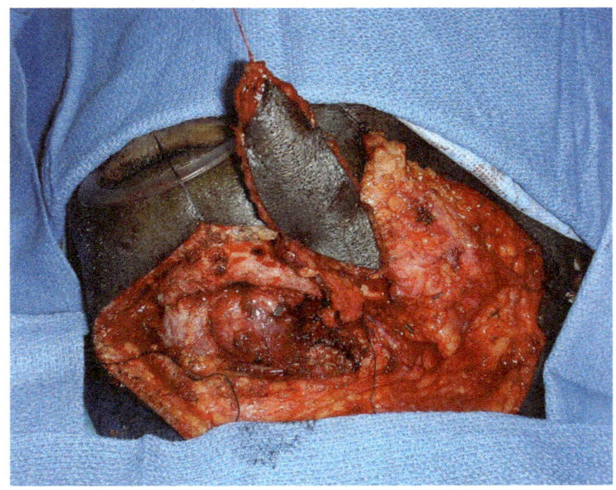

Fig. 14.6 Assessment of the rotation of the submental island flap.

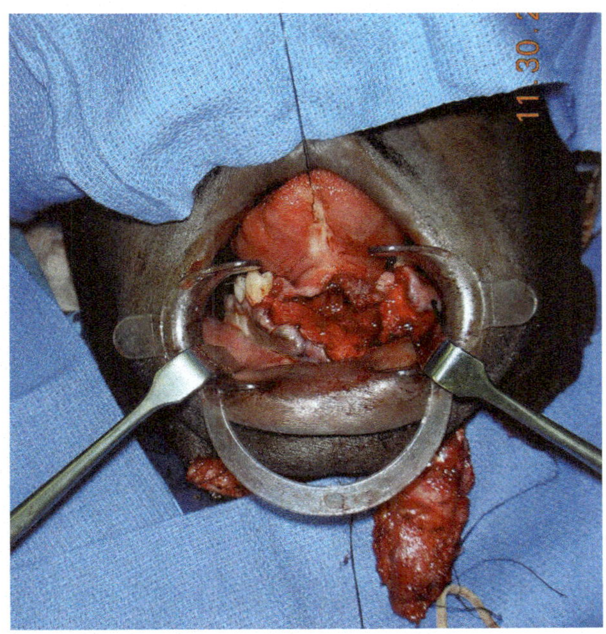

Fig. 14.7 Reestablishing the intraoral defect by releasing the scars.

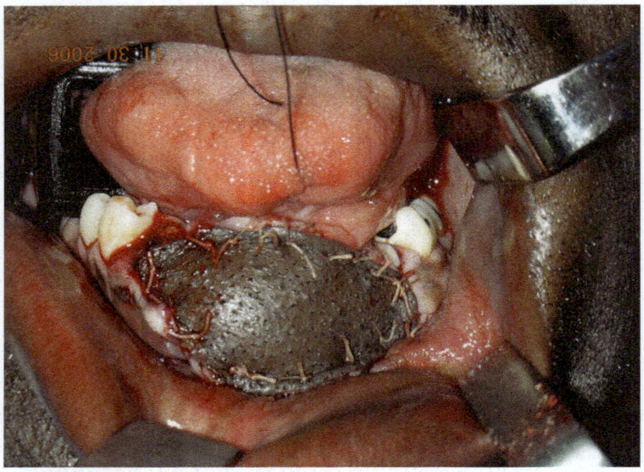

Fig. 14.8 Inset of the flap into the oral cavity defect.

Case #1

A 55-year-old male was referred to our service with a newly diagnosed squamous cell carcinoma of the tongue. Workup of the patient revealed a 2.5 cm lesion of the tongue and clinical as well as computer tomography of the neck did not show any enlarged nodes. The patient was staged as a T2N0M0, Stage II cancer of the posterior lateral tongue. A decision was made to perform a hemiglossectomy and a selective neck dissection. The reconstruction was going to be carried out with a submental island flap (Figure 14.11). The resection of the tongue was completed and the neck dissection was carried out simultaneous to the raising of the submental island flap. Care was taken to dissect and preserve the vascular pedicle while dissecting the submandibular gland with the rest of the neck dissection (Figure 14.12). The dissection of the pedicle allowed for a long reach of the flap which was confirmed by rotation of the pedicle along the arc Figures 14.13 and 14.14). A tunnel was then created in the floor of the mouth along the mylohyoid muscle and the flap was then transferred to the oral cavity and inset to repair the tongue defect (Figure 14.15).

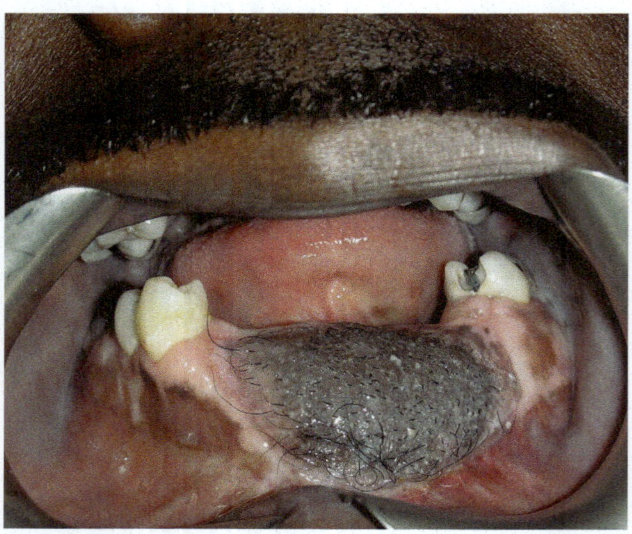

Fig. 14.9 Late appearance of the reconstructed defect with the submental island flap.

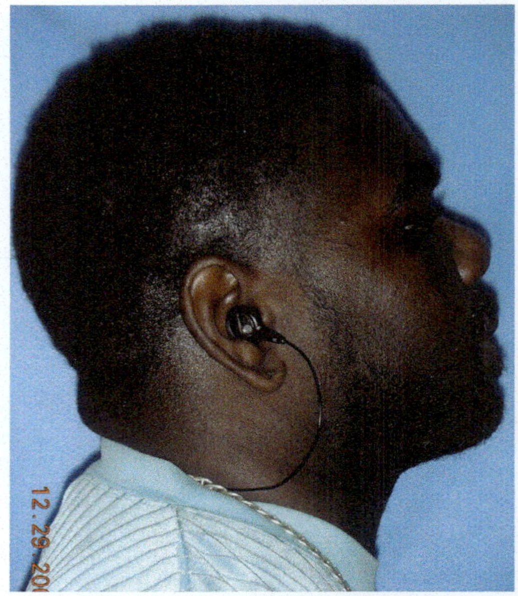

Fig. 14.10 Postoperative profile view of the patient. Note the more pleasing neck contour.

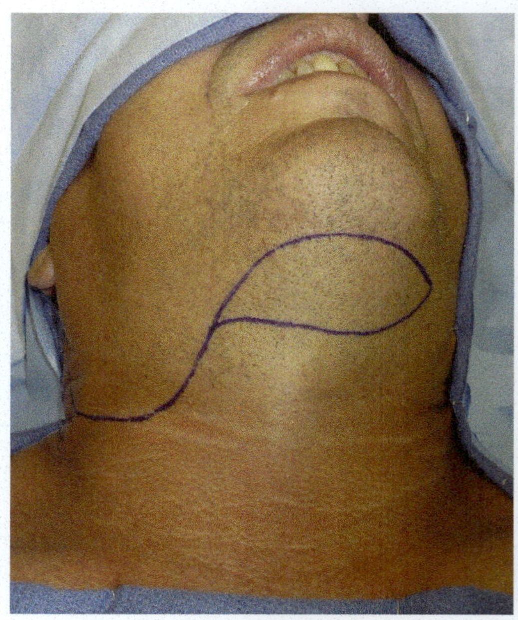

Fig. 14.11 Submental view of markings for a submental island flap.

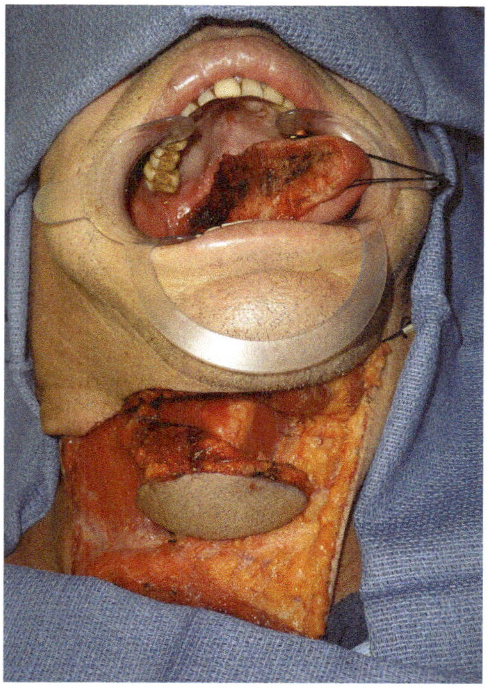

Fig. 14.12 View of the hemiglossectomy defect and a raised submental island flap prior to transfer into the oral cavity.

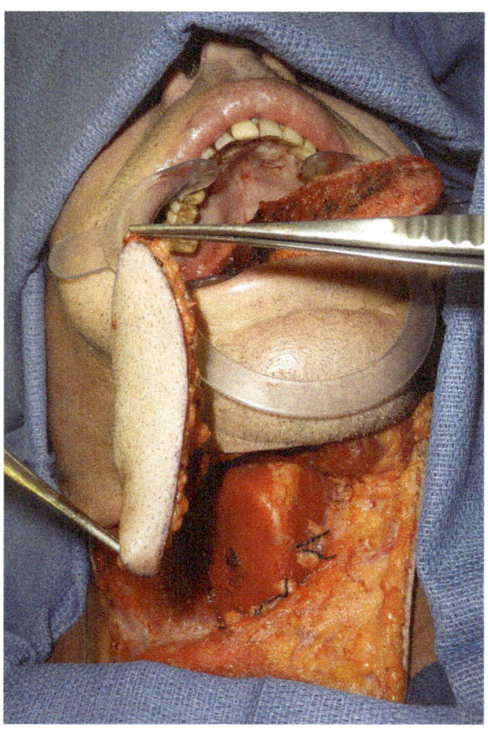

Fig. 14.13 Assessment of the arc of rotation of the submental island flap.

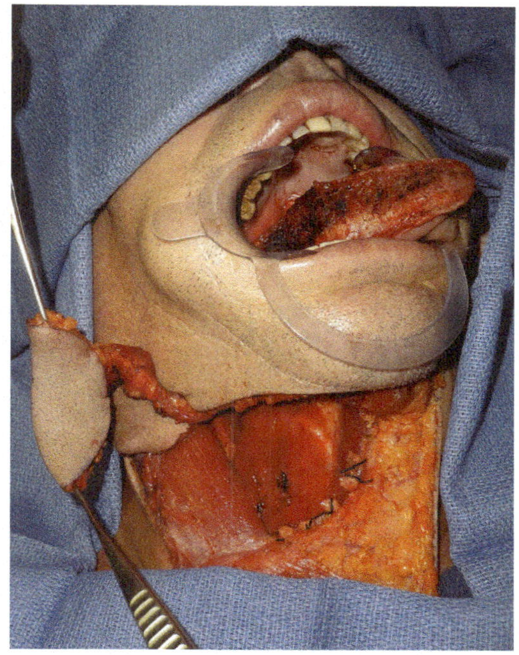

Fig. 14.14 Assessment of the arc of rotation of the submental island flap.

Case #2

A 75-year-old Caucasian female was referred for resection of a longstanding and neglected squamous cell carcinoma of the left temporal region. After evaluation and workup it was noted that the tumor had extended to the orbital contents and she was recently experiencing significant eye pain and changes in vision associated with

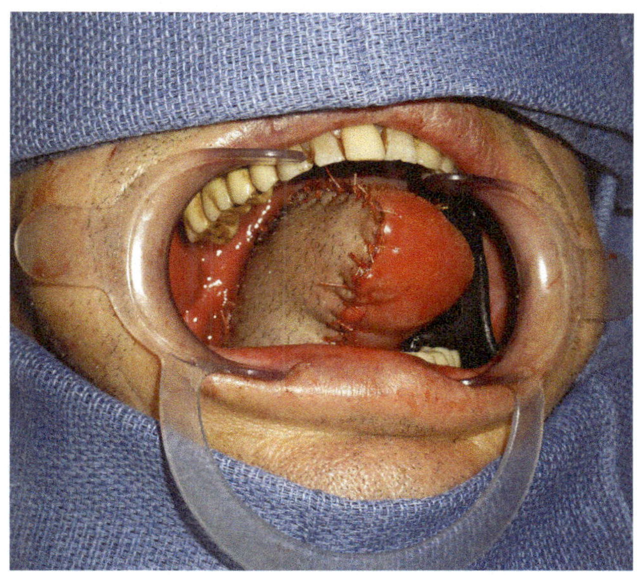

Fig. 14.15 View of the reconstructed hemiglossectomy defect with the submental island flap.

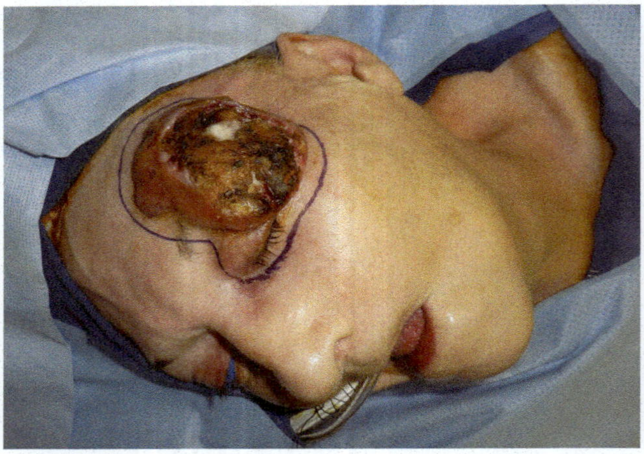

Fig. 14.16 View of a large facial carcinoma on an elderly female.

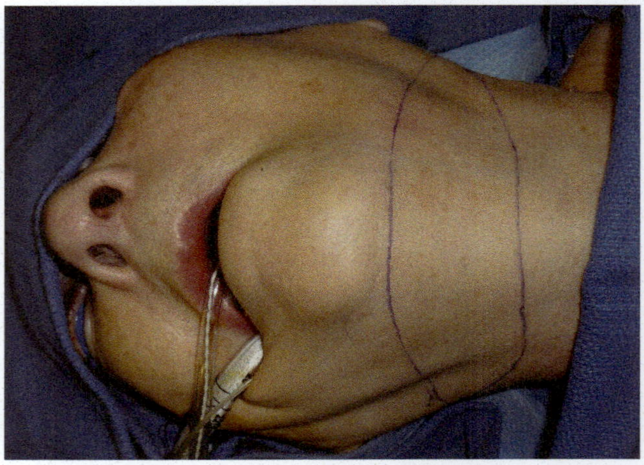

Fig. 14.18 Submental view of the planned submental island flap; note the large skin paddle design.

the left eye (Figure 14.16). She was presented at the multidisciplinary head and neck tumor board and a recommendation was made for resection of the tumor in conjunction with an orbital exenteration. The resection was executed without difficulties (Figure 14.17). A decision was made to reconstruct the defect with a cervicofacial flap and a submental island flap (Figure 14.18). The cervicofacial flap was elevated and rotated anteriorly to repair the periorbital defect thus creating a large preauricular defect, which would be reconstructed with the rotation of the submental island flap. The submental island flap was elevated and then rotated to the preauricular defect and inset (Figures 14.19 to 14.23). The final outcome was very acceptable as the tissues blended well with the surrounding area without any noticeable color or texture mismatch (Figures 14.24 to 14.26).

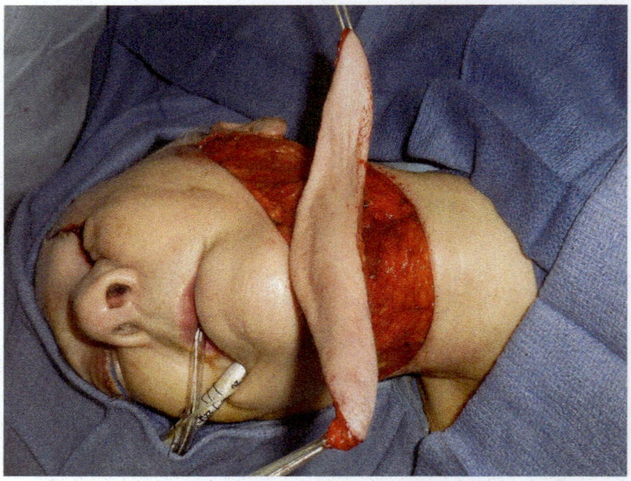

Fig. 14.19 View of the raised submental island flap prior to rotation and transfer.

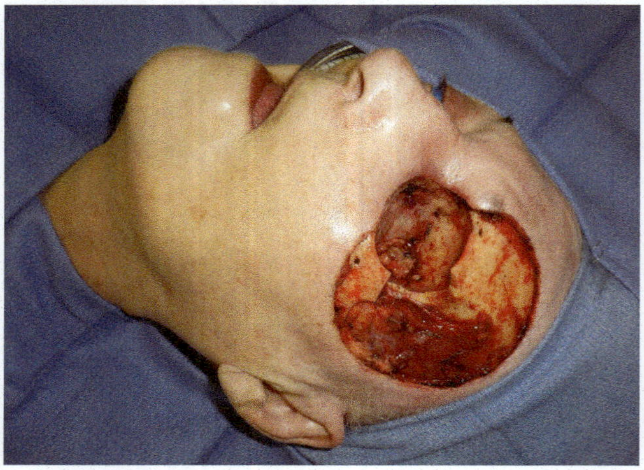

Fig. 14.17 Defect after radical resection of the tumor which included an orbital exenteration and lateral orbital bone resection.

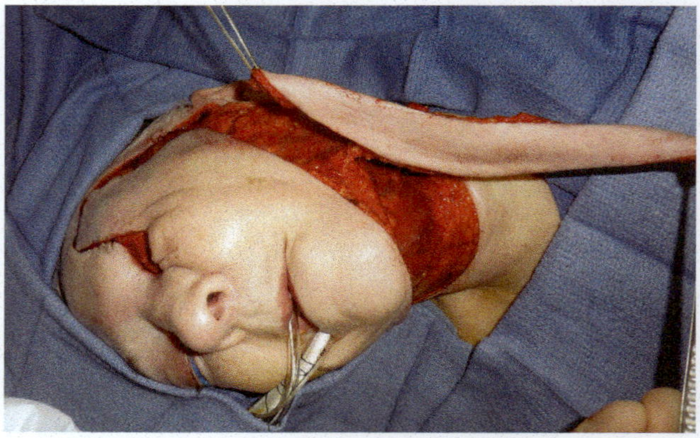

Fig. 14.20 Another view of the submental island flap prior to transfer to the defect.

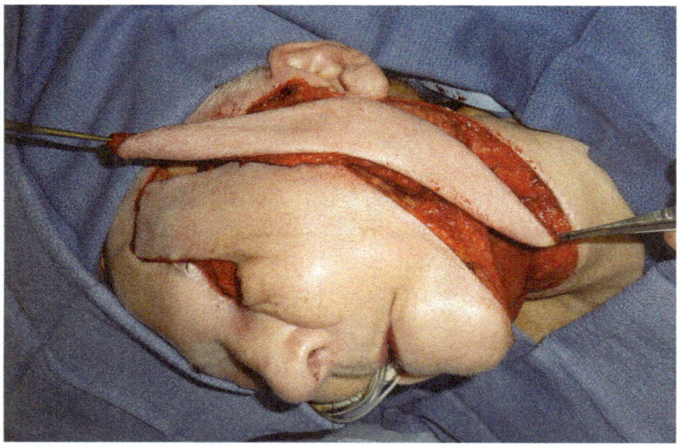

Fig. 14.21 Transfer of the submental island flap into the defect.

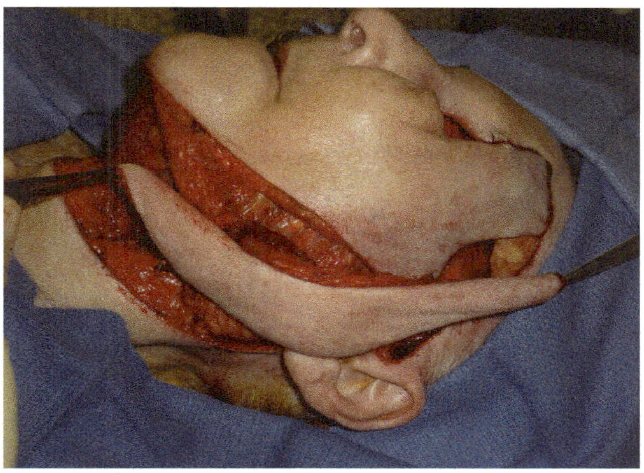

Fig. 14.22 Lateral view of the transferred flap.

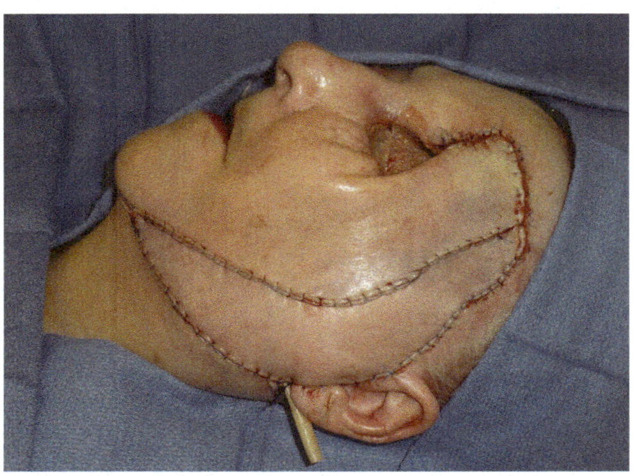

Fig. 14.23 Inset of the submental island flap along with the cervicofacial flap to repair the large facial defect.

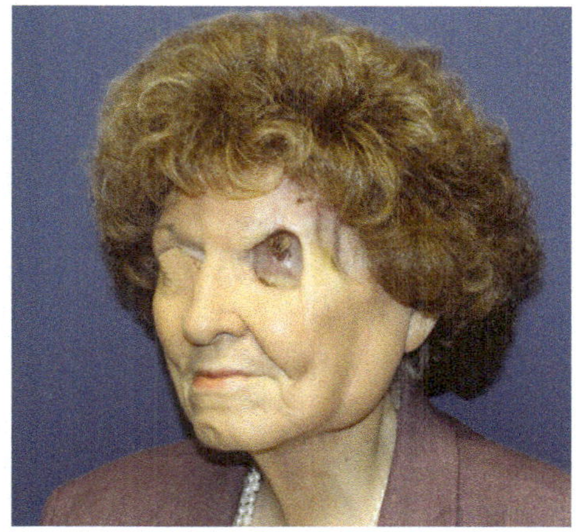

Fig. 14.24 View of the healed patient several weeks after reconstruction.

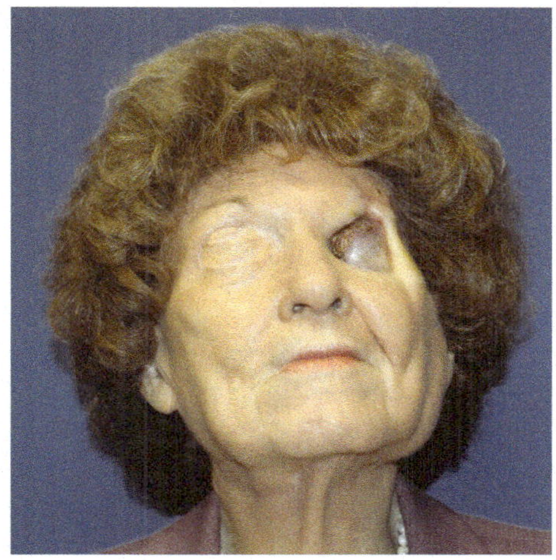

Fig. 14.25 Frontal view of the final reconstruction.

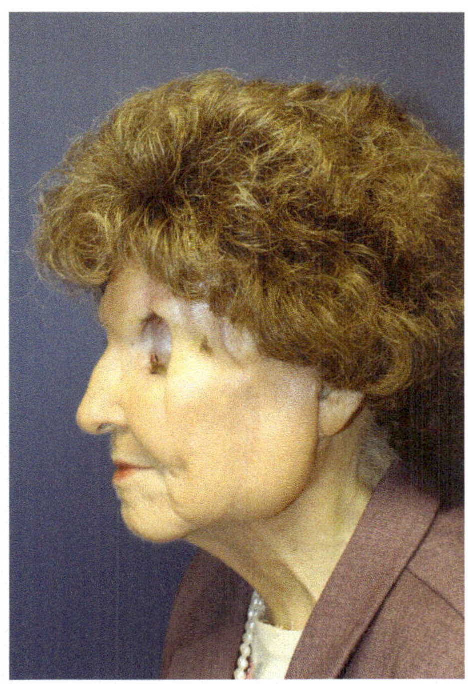

Fig. 14.26 Profile view of the reconstructed defect.

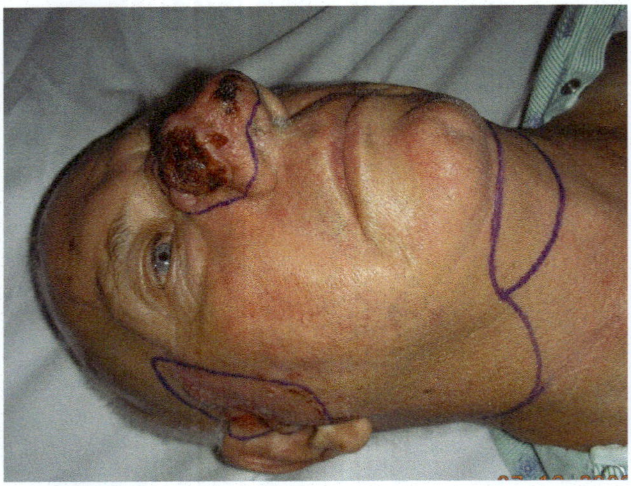

Fig. 14.27 View of the patient with the markings for a submental island flap prior to raising the flap.

Case #3

A 68-year-old male was referred to our service with advanced skin cancer in the preauricular region with extension to the underlying parotid tissue and another involving nearly the entire right nasal wall, Figure 14.27. A plan was made for resection of the preauricular lesion in conjunction with a parotidectomy and neck dissection with immediate reconstruction of the preauricular defect with a submental island flap (Figures 14.28 to 14.30). The flap was elevated, and rotated to confirm adequate reach without tension on the pedicle (Figure 14.31). The flap was inset, and several weeks later the patient had a

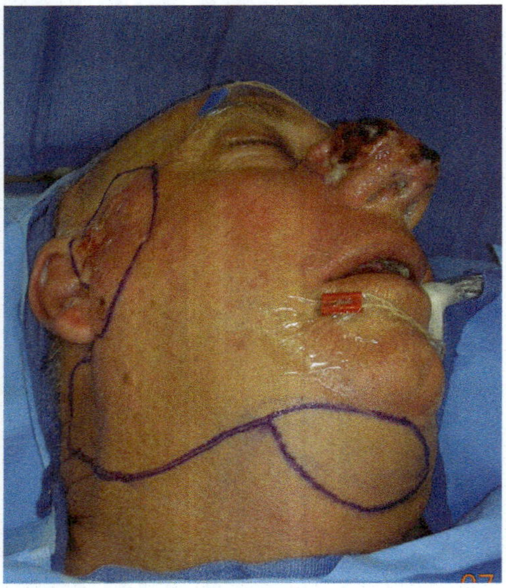

Fig. 14.28 Another view of the planned resection and submental flap.

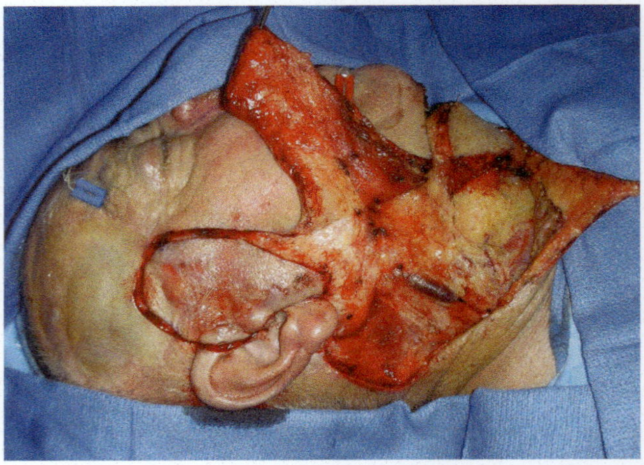

Fig. 14.29 Incision for the parotid resection including skin and submental island flap.

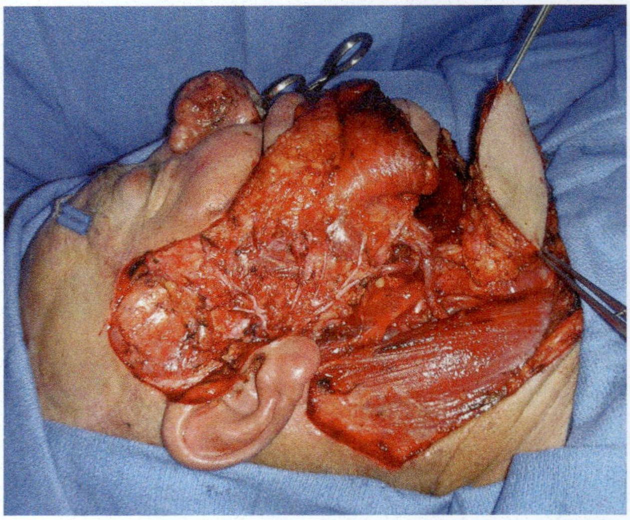

Fig. 14.30 View of the parotidectomy with a selective neck dissection and a submental island flap.

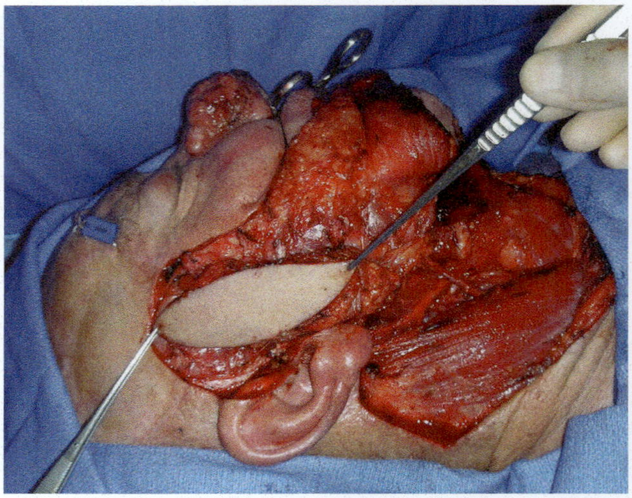

Fig. 14.31 Assessment of the reach of the flap into the parotidectomy defect.

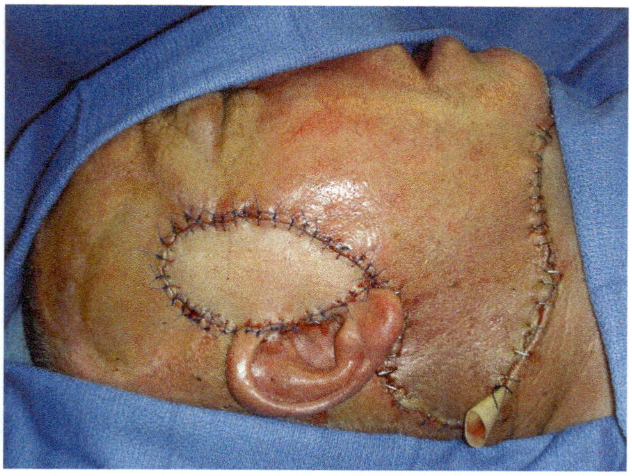

Fig. 14.32 Inset of the flap into the defect with repair of the donor site.

very acceptable appearance with good color and texture matches of the transplanted flap to the surrounding tissues (Figures 14.32 and 14.33).

Case #4

A 70-year-old male with advanced dementia and multiple other comorbidities was referred for surgical management of an advanced, neglected right facial squamous cell carcinoma which had progressed to encompass the midface, the upper lip, nose, and maxilla (Figure 14.34). A surgical plan was made for a radical resection that would include a wide resection of the facial skin extending into the upper lip, the nose, and a significant component of the cheek skin. Additionally, a maxillectomy would be performed. The markings for the skin flap and for an immediate reconstruction with a submental island flap was made (Figures 14.35 and 14.36). The resection was performed and several frozen section margins were confirmed to be negative (Figure 14.37). A submental island flap was raised, taking advantage of the thickness of the flap to reconstruct the facial defect (Figure 14.38). The maxillectomy was closed with the palatal flap that had been elevated off the maxilla prior to the maxillectomy. The submental island flap was tunneled under the bridge of skin and checked to see that the vessels were not kinked (Figure 14.39). The flap was then closed without any tension (Figure 14.40). Early postoperative appearance was very satisfactory (Figure 14.41).

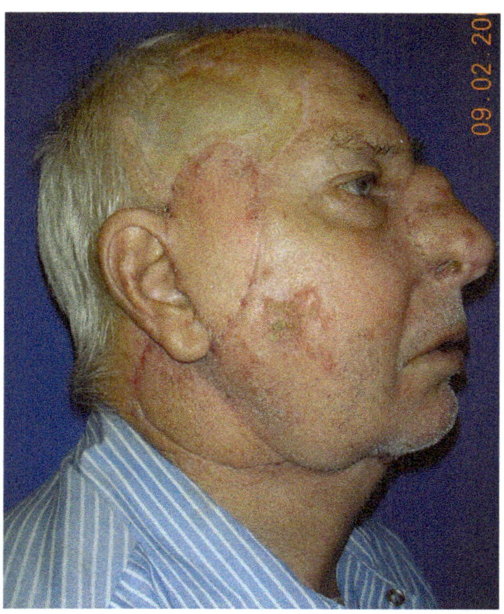

Fig. 14.33 Profile view of the reconstructed parotid bed and donor site.

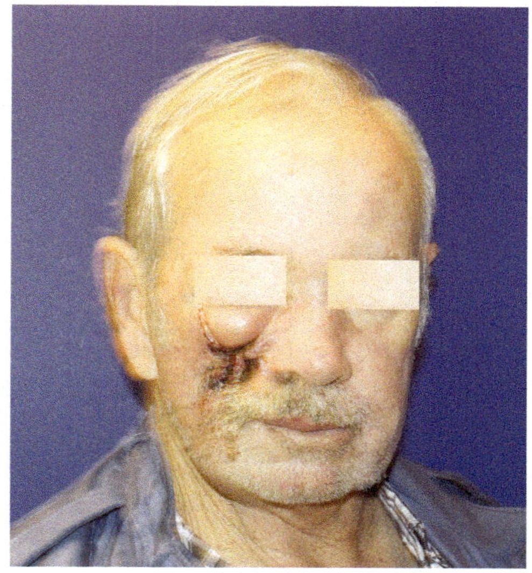

Fig. 14.34 Frontal view of a patient with a large neglected facial squamous cell carcinoma.

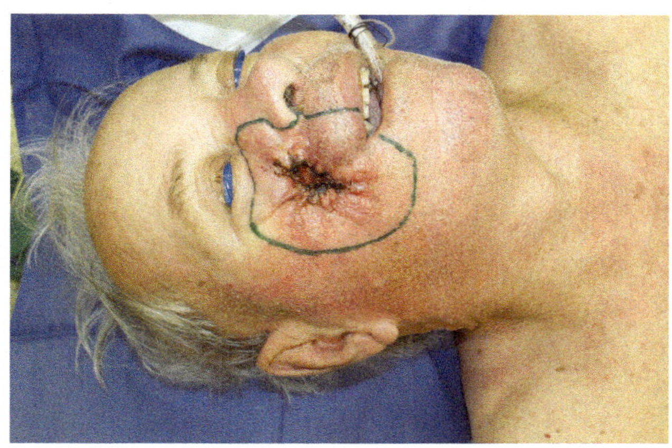

Fig. 14.35 Markings for a large composite facial resection with concurrent maxillectomy.

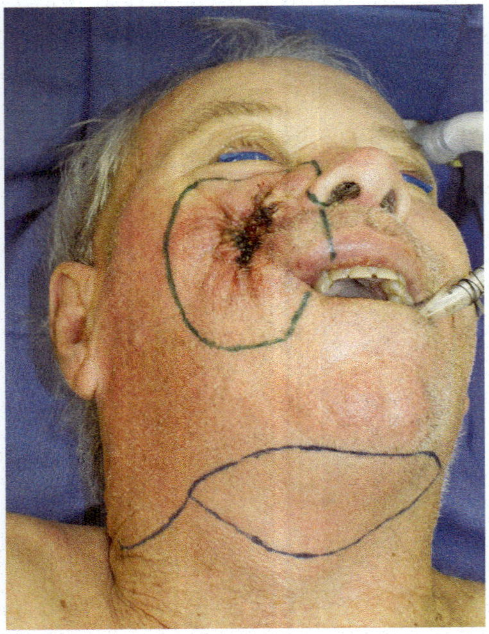

Fig. 14.36 Planning for a large skin paddle prior to raising a submental island flap.

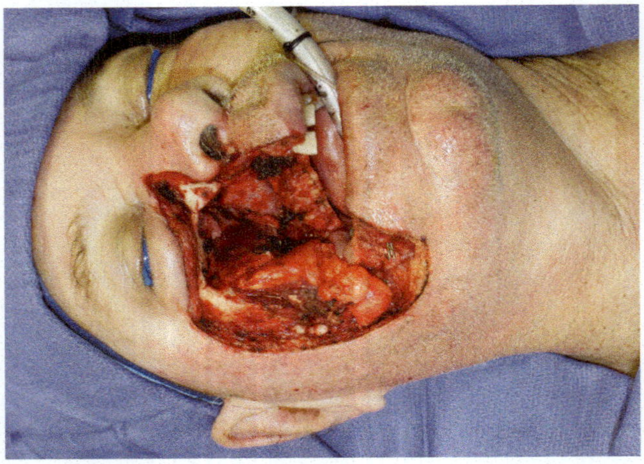

Fig. 14.37 View of the resected tumor bed revealing a large facial skin defect.

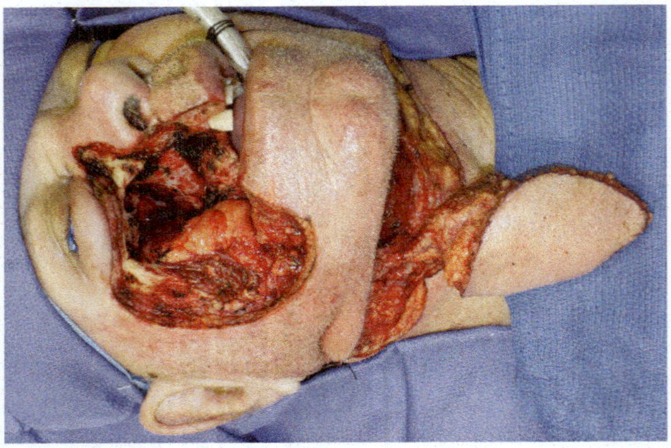

Fig. 14.38 The submental island flap has been raised and is ready for transfer.

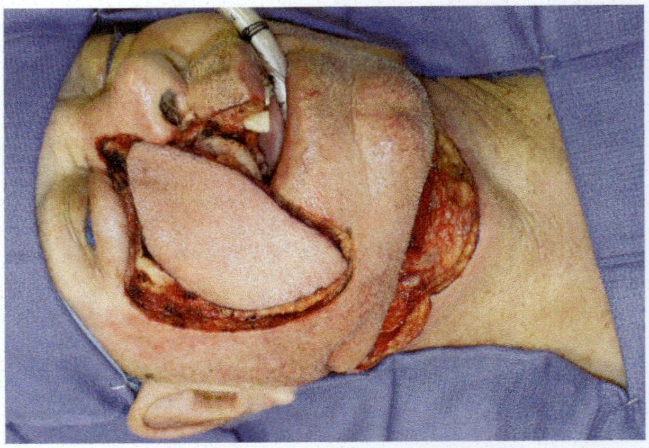

Fig. 14.39 Transfer of the flap into the defect prior to inset.

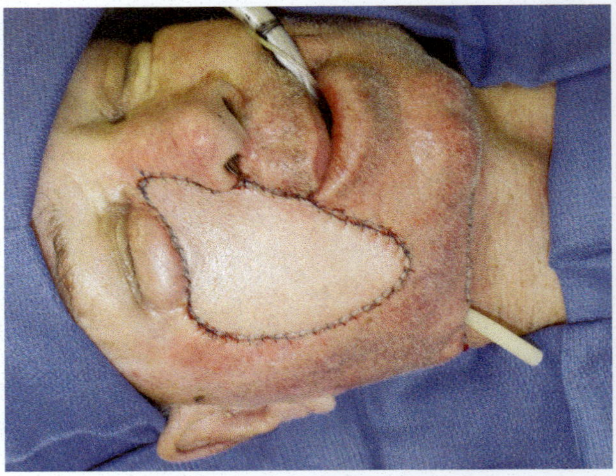

Fig. 14.40 Facial appearance after inset of the flap and repair of the donor site.

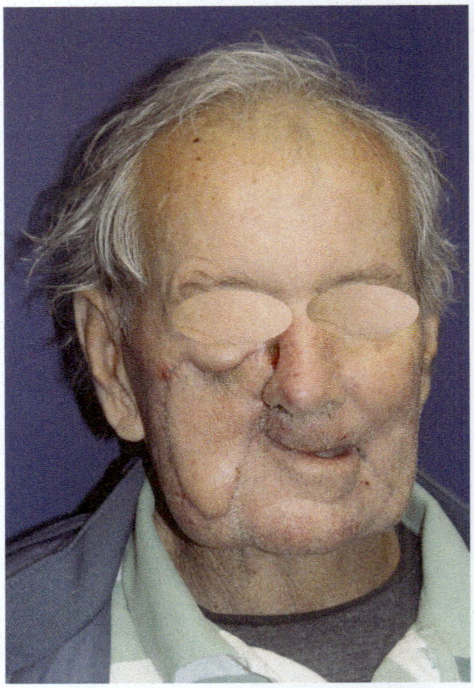

Fig. 14.41 Postoperative view of the patient several weeks after the reconstruction.

References

1. Martin D, Pascal JF, Baudet J, Mondie JM et al. The submental island flap: a new donor site. Anatomy and clinical applications as a free or pedicled flap. *Plast Reconstr Surg* 1993; 92:867–873.
2. Magden O, Edizer M, Tayfur V, Atabey A. Anatomic study of the vasculature of the submental artery flap. *Plast Reconstr Surg* 2004; 114:1719–1723.
3. Multinu A, Ferrari S, Bianchi B. The submental island flap in head and neck reconstruction. *Int J Oral Maxillofac Surg* 2007; 36:716–720.
4. Parmer PS, Goldstein DP. The submental island flap in head and neck reconstruction. *Curr Opin Otolaryngol Head Neck Surg* 2009; 17:263–266.
5. Tang M, Ding M, Almutairi K, Morris SF. Three dimensional angiography of the submental artery perforator flap. *J Plast Reconstr Aesthet Surg* 2011; 64:608–613.
6. Curran AJ, Neligan P, Gullane PJ. Submental artery island flap. *Laryngoscope* 1997; 107:1545–1549.

Chapter 15
Pectoralis major myocutaneous flap

Introduction

The first description of the pectoralis major flap for head and neck reconstruction was by Ayrian in 1978. The following year he published his work in the *Journal of Plastic and Reconstructive Surgery.*[1]

Since the description of this flap, its use quickly became widespread and within a short time it held the position as the flap of choice in head and neck reconstruction. The pectoralis muscle flap held its position as the workhorse flap in the reconstruction of defects in the head and neck for many years until the introduction of the radial forearm free flap.

The pectoralis flap has, however, not been relegated to the history books. It remains as one of the main flaps for salvage reconstruction secondary to the loss of microvascular flaps as well as in those patients in whom microvascular flaps is either contraindicated or cautioned due to existing comorbidities that diminish their ability to tolerate an extended operating time.

Advantages

The location of the donor site as it relates to the head and neck makes this flap a great option for reconstructing defects in this region. The harvest of the flap can be carried out with the patient in a supine position, i.e., in the same position as the ablative head and neck operation. The potential for a two-team approach is also available, although the surgical field would be slightly crowded.

One of the greatest advantages of the pectoralis major myocutaneous flap is the quality and quantity of tissue that can be harvested. The pectoralis major muscle enables the closure of a multitude of defects in the head and neck but its robust quantity allows for the coverage of the reconstruction plates used in mandibular surgery, therefore decreasing the likelihood of plate exposure through the skin or the mucosa. At the same time, the muscle coverage in the neck provides additional protection of the great vessels. This fact is of importance in patients who have had a radical neck or a type I or II modified radical neck dissection. The coverage of the vessels becomes even more significant in those patients needing adjuvant radiation therapy or those who have already received radiotherapy and may be faced with delayed wound healing.

Disadvantages

The main disadvantage is that the pectoralis major flap is a pedicle flap and therefore its use in reconstruction of head and neck defects is limited to sites within the arc of rotation of the flap. Equally, some of the reasons that make this flap a good option for reconstruction will also be potential downsides in certain cases. When the defect site demands a thin and pliable flap, this may not be the most ideal flap.

The tunneling of the flap in the neck to reach the defect creates a bulge over the clavicle and in the neck. This bulge has greater prominence in those patients in whom the sternocleidomastoid muscle is retained. The bulge of the muscle will eventually diminish as the muscle is not innervated and therefore will atrophy with time.

In cases where the flap is used as a myocutaneous flap with the skin island used to reconstruct a skin defect in the head and neck, there is often a very distinct color mismatch. In males there may also be a significant amount of hair growth on the skin component of the flap that may become bothersome to patients depending on the site of the reconstruction. This is often relieved, however, in patients receiving postoperative radiation therapy to the site. The radiation will affect the hair cells and

Local and Regional Flaps in Head & Neck Reconstruction: A Practical Approach, First Edition. Rui Fernandes.

Companion website: www.wiley.com/go/fernandes/flapsreconstruction

therefore the affected sites will no longer have any hair growth.

Anatomy

An anatomical understanding of the pectoralis muscle and its vasculature is of paramount importance to the surgeon. The muscle originates along the medial aspect of the clavicle, manubrium, sternum, and the cartilages of ribs 2 to 6. The fibers of the pectoralis major muscle form a large triangular muscle which travels obliquely to insert on the greater tubercle of the humerus. The pectoralis muscle functions by providing adduction and internal rotation of the arm.

The pectoralis muscle is a type V muscle according to the Mathis and Nahai classification.[2] This means that the muscle has one dominant pedicle and several segmental pedicles. The main arterial supply to the pectoralis muscle is the thoracoacromial artery which is a branch of the second portion of the axillary artery. The pectoralis muscle also receives perfusion from the lateral thoracic artery to supply the lateral aspect of the muscle. Perforating branches from the internal mammary artery supply the medial aspect of the muscle and continue to perfuse the overlying skin.

The venous drainage to the muscle and the region is by the accompanying venae commitantes, which drain in the axillary vein. On the superior aspect of the muscle, along the deltopectoral groove, the cephalic vein is encountered as it drains the upper extremity on its way to drain into the axillary vein.

The motor innervation to the muscle comes from the medial and lateral pectoral nerves. The lateral pectoral nerve, a branch from the brachial plexus, innervates the majority of the medial and sternal aspect of the muscle while the medial pectoral nerve (also a branch from the brachial plexus) innervates the lateral aspect of the pectoralis major and the pectoralis minor muscle.

Flap harvest

The flap is harvested with the patient in a supine position. Upon completion of the preparation of the recipient site, the size of the needed skin paddle is measured. The other important information needed is the location of the defect.

- Using either a suture string or the string from the lap towel, one end is positioned over the clavicle on the ipsilateral side of the defect and pivoted lying in a passive form along the neck and into the farthest point of the defect.
- The string is then rotated caudally to the chest and the inferiormost reach is marked. This location will be the most inferior point of the skin paddle. The location of the majority of the potential skin paddle must be positioned over the underlying pectoralis muscle.
- The skin paddle is designed according to the needs of the defect and the outside perimeter of the skin island is shaped into a fusiform shape to aid in later closure of the defect.
- A point near the junction of the arm to the chest and another at the superior-lateral point of the flap are marked and a curvilinear line is marked. The curvilinear design allows for the potential use of a deltopectoral flap in the remote chance that the pectoralis muscle flap fails.
- The initial incision is made on the lateral aspect of the skin paddle and along the curvilinear line.
- The incision along the skin paddle should be made outward to insure that the base of the skin paddle is wider than the skin paddle itself.
- Once the position of the skin paddle is confirmed as being located over the muscle bed, the curvilinear extension is elevated in the suprafascial plane towards the lateral border of the muscle.
- The remainder of the skin island is completed and the skin edge is then sutured to the pectoralis fascia to prevent shearing of the skin paddle from the underlying muscle.
- Starting laterally, the lateral edge of the pectoralis muscle is elevated in the plane between the pectoralis major and minor. This is a relatively avascular plane. The inferior edge of the flap is released from its origin along the lower ribs. Perforating vessels should be clipped and hemostasis insured.
- The medial attachment of the pectoralis muscle is released beginning inferiorly in a cephalad direction. The medial release should be lateral to the row of the internal mammary perforators, especially the second and third perforators that are saved in case a bailout with the deltopectoral flap is needed.
- Once the flap is released medially, the lateral and medial pectoral nerves are divided and the thoracoacromial pedicle is identified and preserved.
- The lateral attachment of the pectoralis muscle to the humerus is then released by placing a hemostat between the muscle and sequentially segmenting the muscle. While performing the lateral release of the muscle care should be taken not to injure the cephalic vein superiorly or the lateral arterial branch to the muscle.
- The next aspect is the creation of the tunnel to transfer the flap into the neck and into the defect site. The usual circumstance is that a neck incision would have already been made to carryout the resection. A subplatysmal flap elevation is extended to the

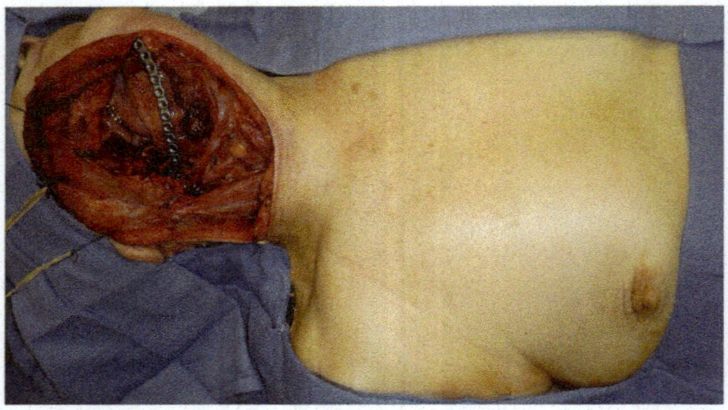

Fig. 15.1 View of an oral defect in a patient who has undergone a composite resection and a neck dissection.

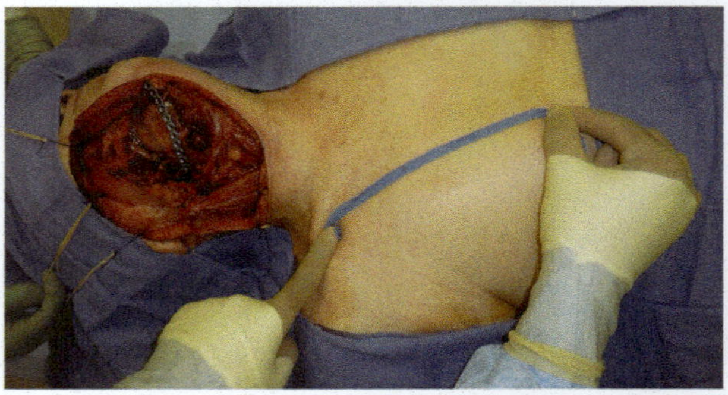

Fig. 15.3 The measurement is then transferred to the chest wall prior to design of the skin paddle as well as to ensure that the skin paddle is located over the pectoralis muscle.

clavicle. Inferiorly from the pectoralis aspect, the skin is elevated suprafascially in a cephalad direction towards the clavicle until it communicates with the neck.

- The dimension of the tunnel should be sufficient to accommodate the flap transfer without impingement and constriction of the perfusion.
- The flap is transferred to the neck taking care to not cause undue shearing of the skin paddle during transfer.
- Once in the defect, the flap can be inset depending on the particular site to be reconstructed. In cases where the flap is being used for mandibular soft tissue reconstruction, the flap is brought into the mouth medial to the reconstruction plate and the muscle is wrapped over the bar to diminish the chance of plate exposure.
- The chest is closed in layers with care to not alter the position of the breast in females and nipple in males. Draining of the donor bed is recommended.

Figures 15.1 to Figure 15.11 illustrate the steps of harvesting the flap described here.

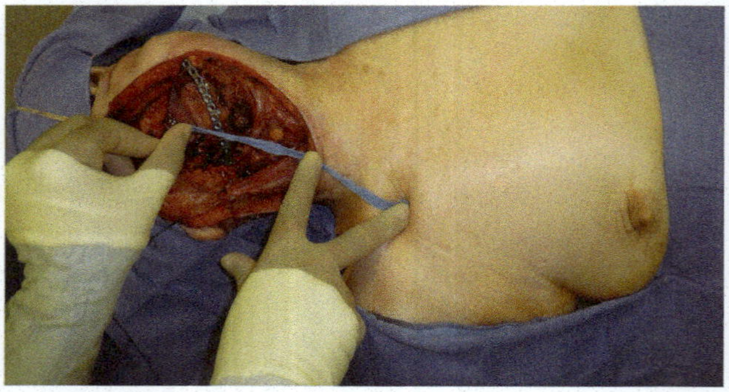

Fig. 15.2 Measurement for the pectoralis major flap begins by assessing the distance from the clavicle, the pivot point, to the defect.

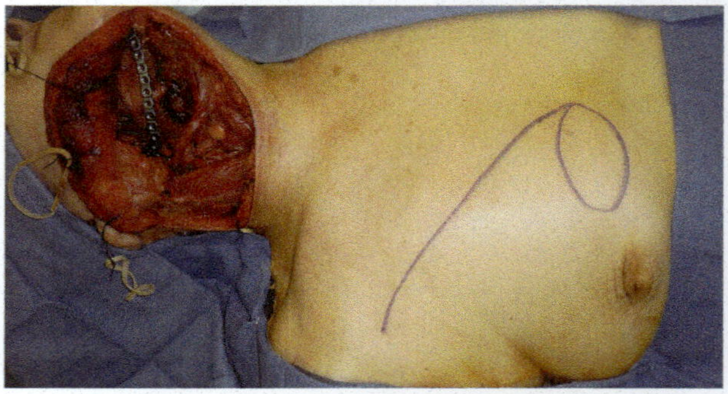

Fig. 15.4 Design of the skin paddle and a curvilinear releasing incision towards the shoulder.

Special circumstances

Harvesting in female patients

When harvesting a pectoralis muscle flap on a female patient with medium to large breast tissues, the location and design of the skin flap has to be taken into consideration. In cases where the esthetics is not of

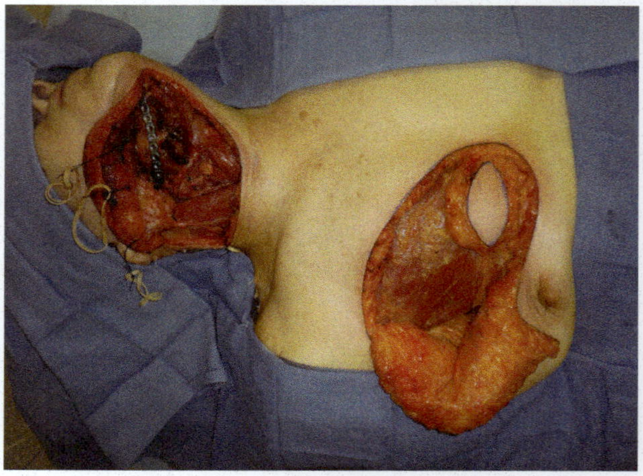

Fig. 15.5 Elevated skin flap away from the pectoralis muscle and skin paddle.

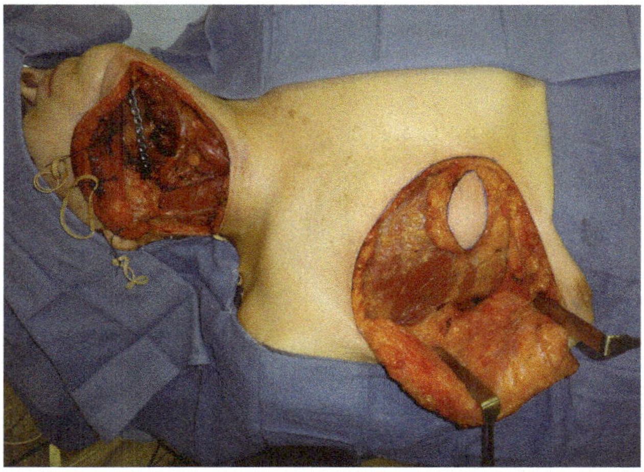

Fig. 15.6 The dissection and reflection of the skin flap is continued until the lateral border of the pectoralis muscle is well visualized.

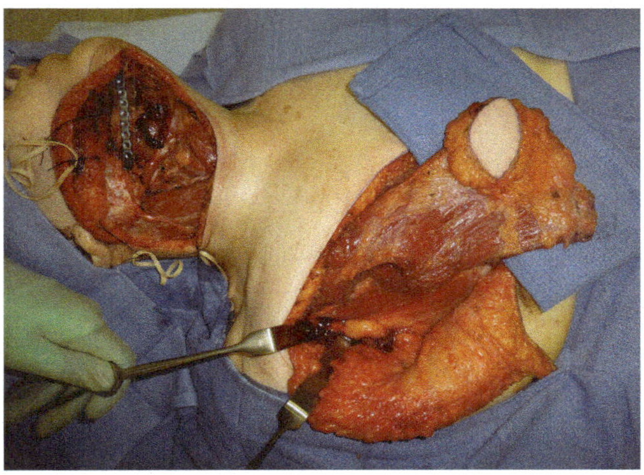

Fig. 15.7 The flap is elevated and its insertion along the humerus bone.

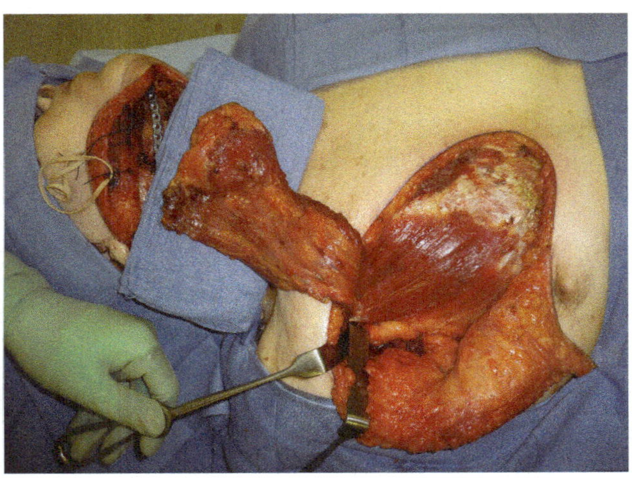

Fig. 15.8 The pectoralis muscle reflected to reveal the vascular pedicle and the underlying pectoralis minor.

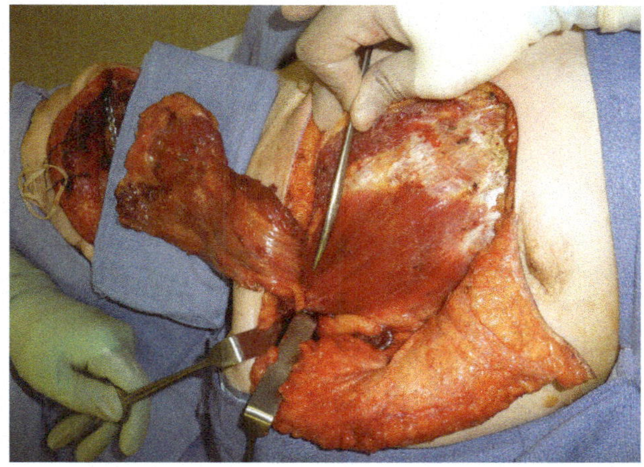

Fig. 15.9 The surgical instrument is pointing towards the vascular pedicle on the undersurface of the flap.

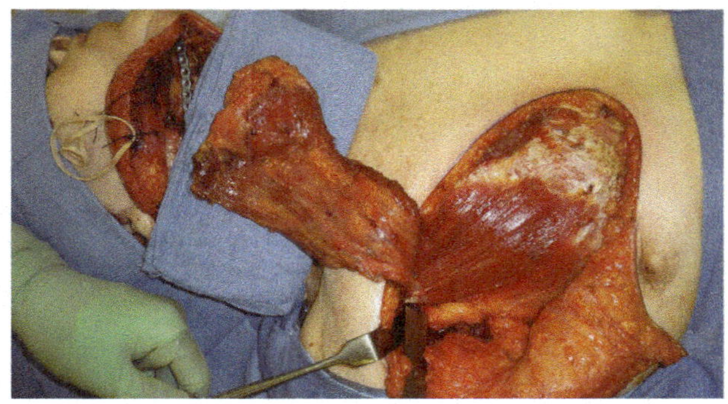

Fig. 15.10 The insertion of the muscle has been completely severed to improve the arc of rotation.

concern, the conventional design of the flap can be done as previously described. If esthetics is of concern, the incision can be brought caudally from the distal clavicular region and lateral to the breast. Once the incision is in the inframammary fold, it is extended medially and into the shape of the desired skin island. The harvest of the flap is

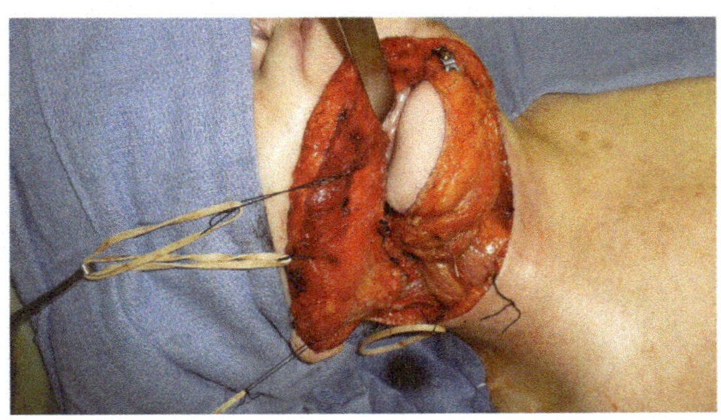

Fig. 15.11 The myocutaneous flap has been transferred to the defect in the subcutaneous tunnel.

otherwise similar to conventional harvest with care not to shear the skin paddle from the underlying muscle. This concept is especially important in cases where there is a large amount of subcutaneous fat.

Patients with breast implants

In patients who may have had a previous breast enhancement procedure and still retain the implant in place, it is imperative to discuss with the patient that the implant will likely be lost and the implication of this fact on the final esthetics of the donor side compared to the unaffected side. In some selected cases, one may still retain the implant or re-implant the patient at the completion of the flap harvest. In these rare cases, attention must be taken to have a meticulous closure to minimize the potential for extrusion of the implant. It is critical to remember that in these situations, the flap will most likely compose a muscle only flap.

Complications

The most dreaded complication of the pectoralis major myocutaneous flap is the loss of the flap. This unfortunate event is often a consequence of a technical mistake in either the harvesting of the flap or on the inset. When harvesting the flap, care must be taken to avoid the sharing forces on the skin paddle from the underlying muscle. Placement of significant forces will cause disruption of the perforating vessels to the overlying skin and potentially lead to the loss of the skin paddle. Another reason for the eventual loss of the skin paddle due to a technical mistake during harvest is the undermining of the skin leading to a larger skin island over a small base of fat connecting to the muscle. In these cases, the lateral edges of the unsupported skin may not be perfused and could potentially become ischemic later.

Technical mistakes can also be made at the time of the inset, which can lead to the loss of the flap. In this scenario, the most common culprit is closure of the flap under significant tension. In cases where there is tension on closure, the shoulder roll should be taken out allowing the shoulder to drop, and at the same time the neck should be flexed to further diminish the distance from the donor site and the reach of the flap. Once this is done, the tension should be relieved and the closure performed in a safer manner.

Complications can also occur at the donor site. The most commonly seen complications in this region are: formation of a hematoma, dehiscence of the wound closure, loss of alignment of the breast as it relates to the contralateral breast, ischemia of the skin, and the formation of a seroma.

The donor site should always be drained at the time of wound closure. The placement of a drain will not prevent the development of a hematoma but it may diminish the likelihood of its formation. In cases where there is seroma formation, the seroma can be aspirated in the office setting after prepping the skin. A large gauge needle is used to penetrate the skin and the aspirate is suctioned using a 60 cm^3 syringe. The needle is kept in place and the procedure is repeated until all of the seroma is aspirated. A pressure dressing is then placed around the chest to prevent reformation of the seroma. In cases where the seroma recurs after several episodes of aspiration, the patient is brought back to the operating room and the area is explored. A common finding is that of a pseudocapsule lining of the cavity. The capsule is removed and a sclerosing agent, such as tetracycline powder, or sutures are used to prevent the reformation of the cavity.

Case #1

A 58-year-old male was referred for salvage surgery after failure of previous neck dissection and radiation therapy for a high-grade mucoepidermoid carcinoma. He was noted to have a large left neck recurrence that was adherent to the thyroid gland and extending to the overlying skin. The area of the skin involved was marked out with plans for the incorporation of the neck dissection and thyroidectomy Figure 15.12. A salvage neck dissection was performed in conjunction with the thyroidectomy (Figures 15.13 and 15.14). A template was used to determine the optimal size of the skin portion of the flap to be harvested and transferred to the defect. This was then drawn on the donor site after the arc of rotation was confirmed (Figure 15.15). The myocutaneous flap was then elevated

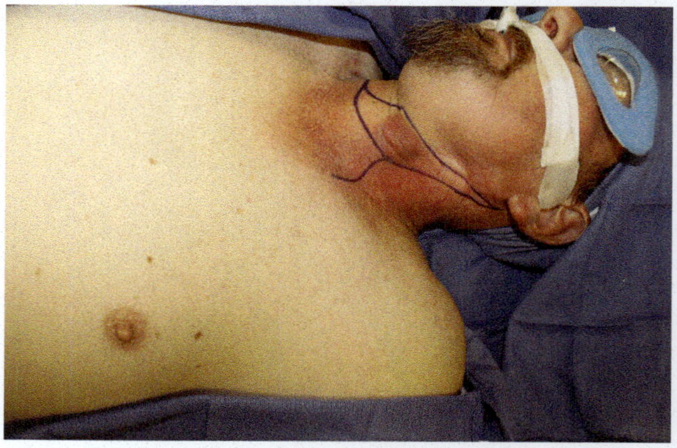

Fig. 15.12 View of a patient for a salvage surgery after failed surgery, and chemoradiotherapy. Note the area of cervical recurrence and the damaged skin from the radiation.

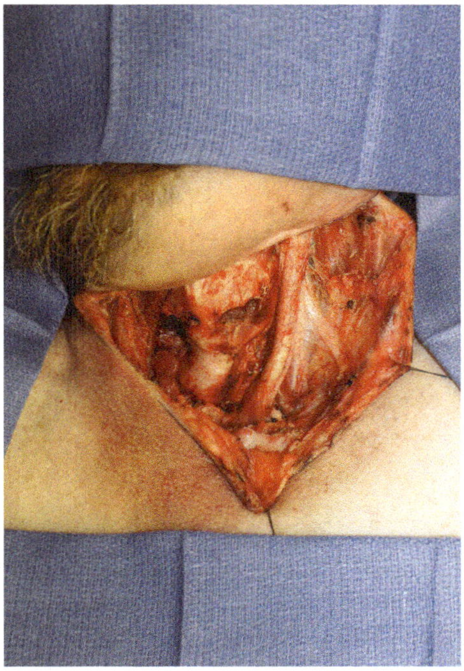

Fig. 15.13 View of the neck after an extended radical neck dissection with exposed carotid vessels and large missing skin.

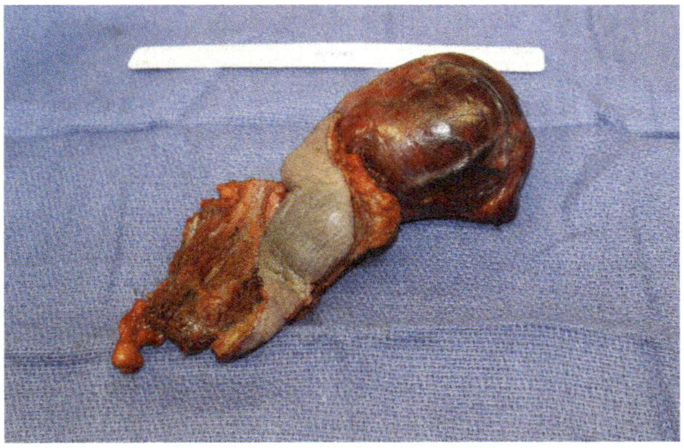

Fig. 15.14 View of the resection along with a hemithyroid lobectomy.

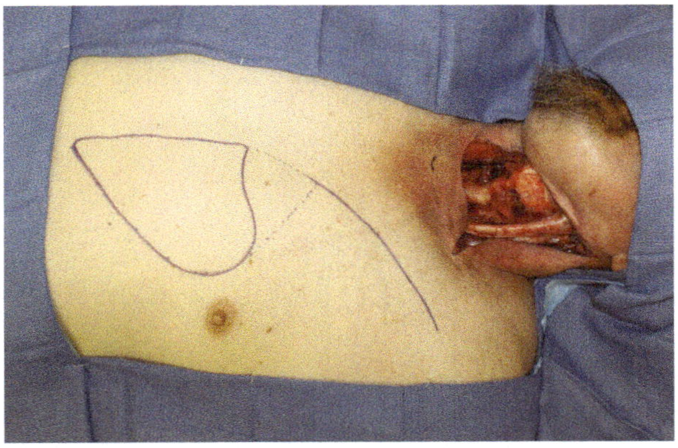

Fig. 15.15 Design for a large skin paddle over the pectoralis major muscle.

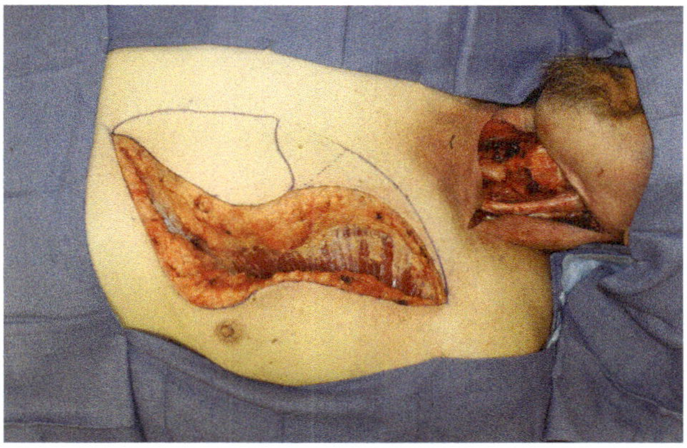

Fig. 15.16 Elevation of the lateral chest skin flap exposing the underlying pectoralis muscle.

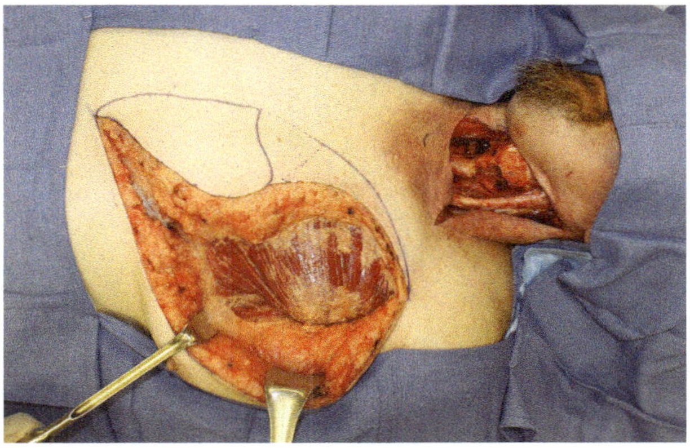

Fig. 15.17 Exposure of the lateral aspect of the pectoralis muscle.

as previously described (Figures 15.16 to 15.20). Once the flap was elevated, a tunnel was created in the subcutaneous plane to the defect in the neck (Figure 15.21) and then inset (Figure 15.22). The final appearance of the patient is seen in Figure 15.23.

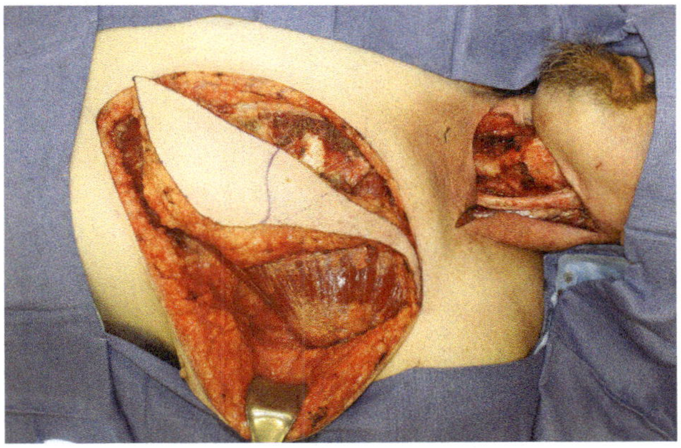

Fig. 15.18 Completed exposure of the pectoralis myocutaneous flap.

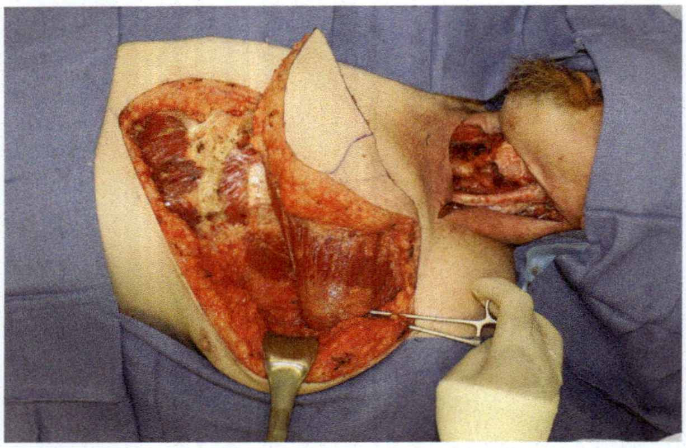

Fig. 15.19 Preparation for the disinsertion of the muscle from the humerus attachment; note the position of the hemostat.

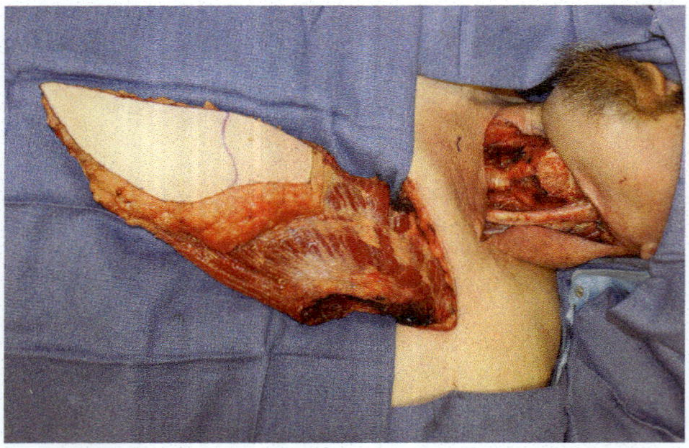

Fig. 15.20 Completion of the disinsertion; the flap is ready for transfer.

Case #2

A 33-year-old female was referred after failed radiotherapy and surgery for a retromolar trigone squamous cell carcinoma. She presented with a large recurrence in the primary site and extension to the neck. The surgical plan

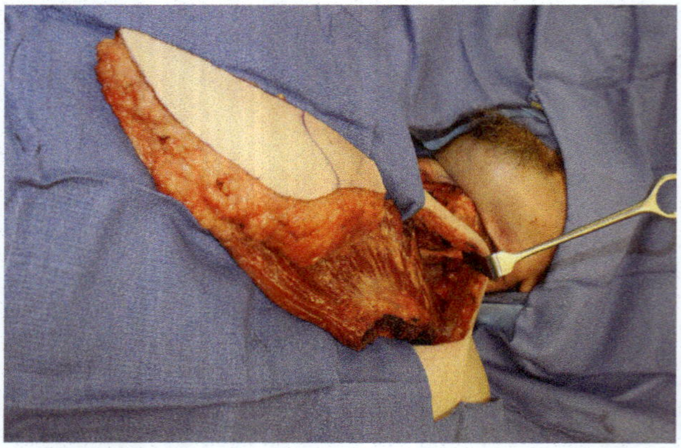

Fig. 15.21 Development of a subcutaneous tunnel for the flap transfer to the neck.

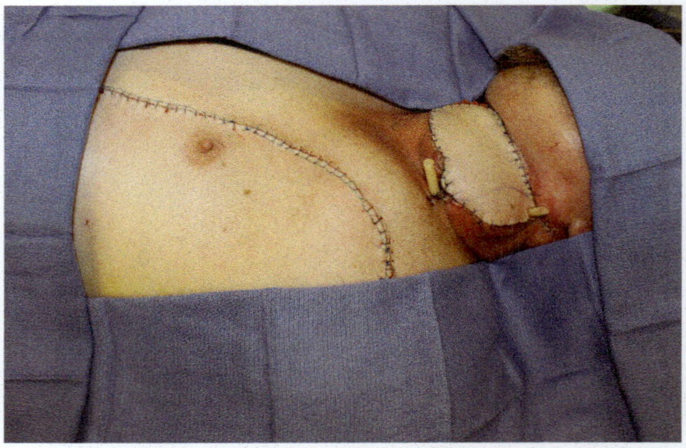

Fig. 15.22 Inset of the flap in the neck.

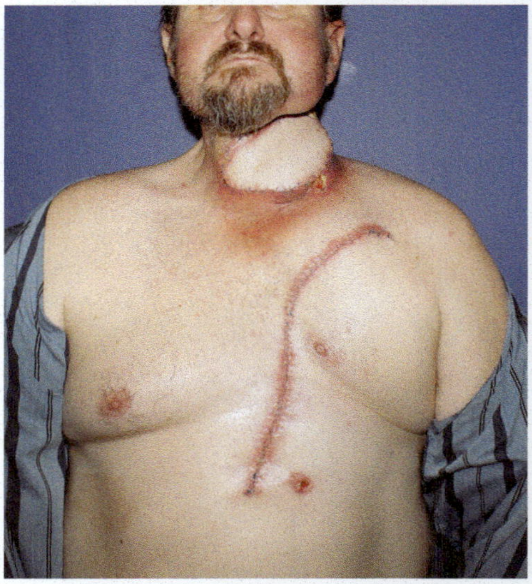

Fig. 15.23 Postoperative view of the healed flap and view of the chest donor site. Note the altered position of the nipple areolar complex due to the large size of the harvested skin paddle.

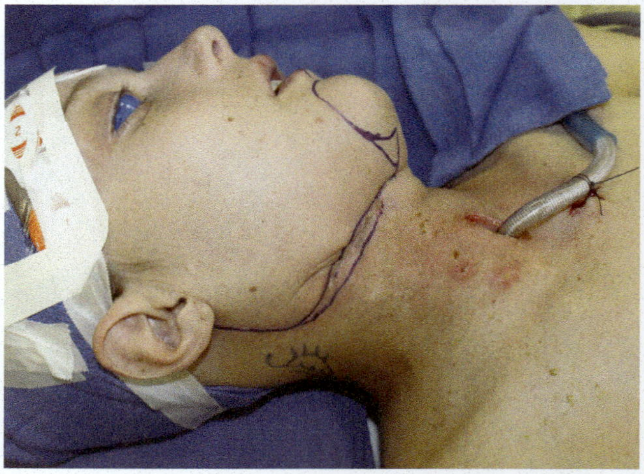

Fig. 15.24 Appearance of the patient prior to salvage resection for an oropharyngeal recurrence after triple therapy.

involved resection of the neck skin and approach to the tumor via a lip split approach and mandibulotomy (Figure 15.24). The tumor was resected with a radical clearance of the pharynx and external carotid artery (Figure 15.25). The plan for the flap was transferred to the chest in

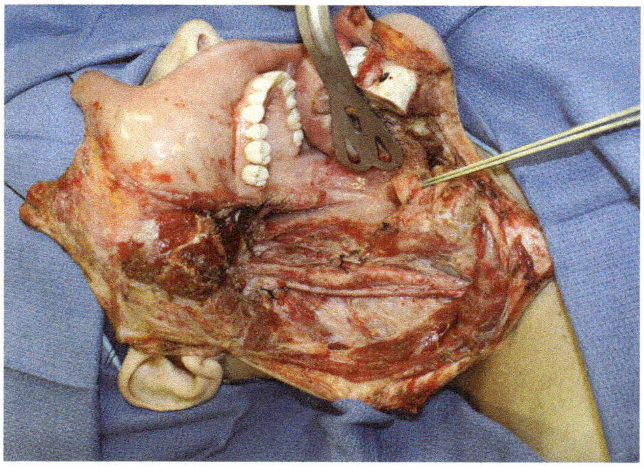

Fig. 15.25 Appearance of the completed resection; the resultant defect is large and complex.

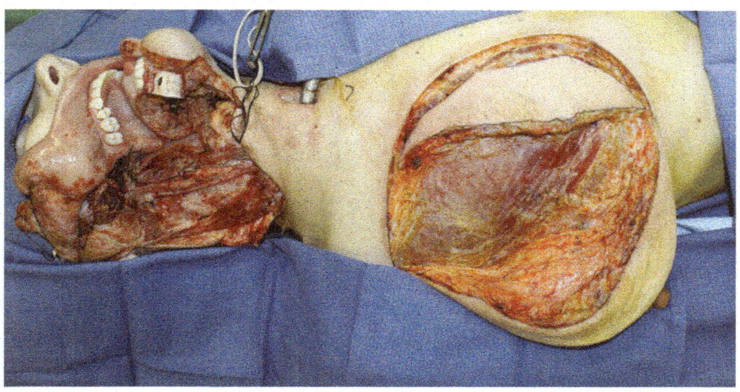

Fig. 15.26 Elevation of the myocutaneous pectoralis major flap. Note that the breast has been elevated off the muscle and positioned laterally.

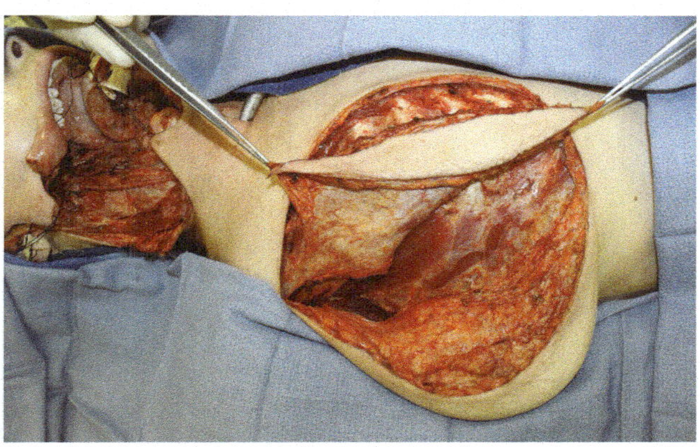

Fig. 15.27 Elevation of a large fusiform skin paddle prior to transfer.

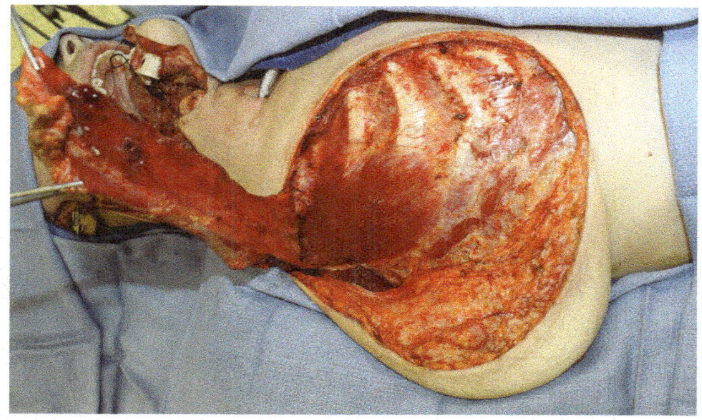

Fig. 15.28 Assessment for the adequacy of the reach of the flap to the defect.

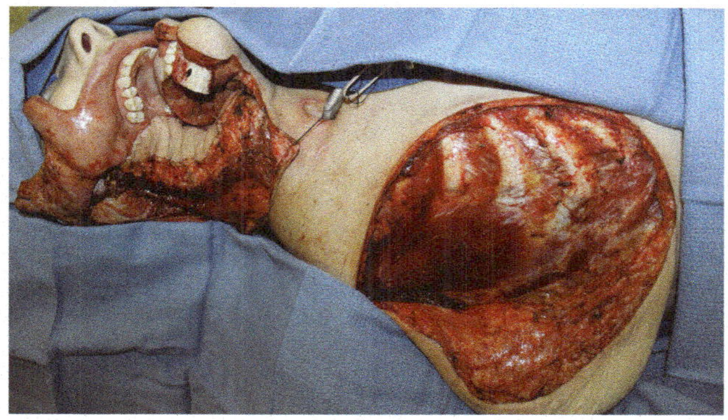

Fig. 15.29 Inset of the flap prior to the closure of the donor site and neck.

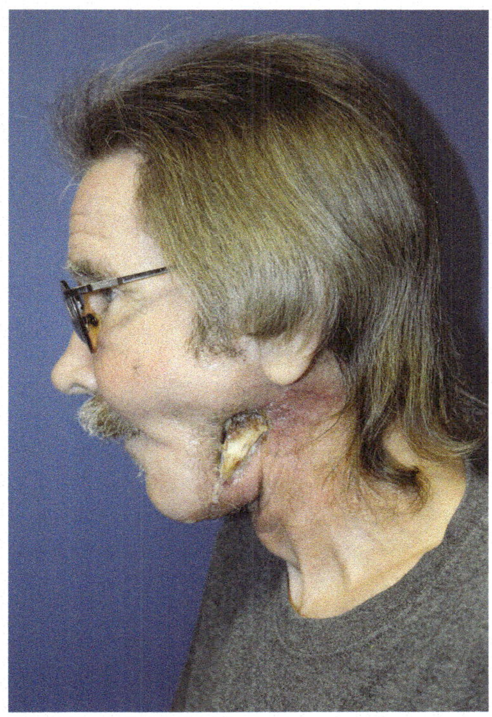

Fig. 15.30 View of a patient with a large exposure of the mandible secondary to ORN.

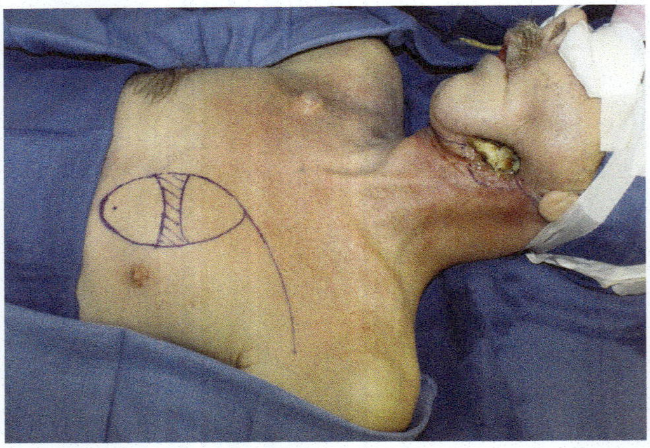

Fig. 15.31 Design of a large skin paddle with planning for de-epithelializing the middle portion to repair both intraoral and extraoral defects.

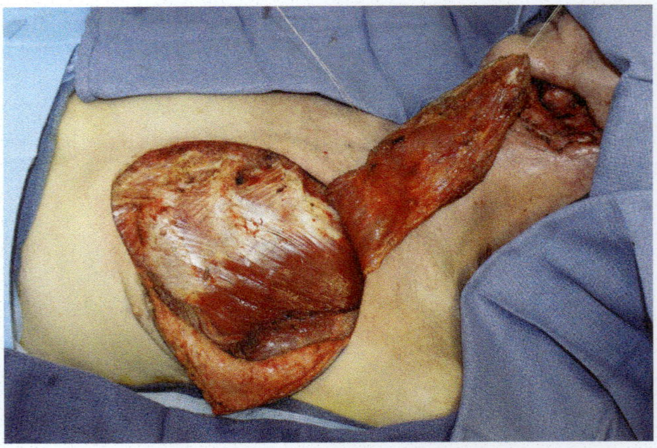

Fig. 15.33 Assessment of the arc of rotation and reach of the flap.

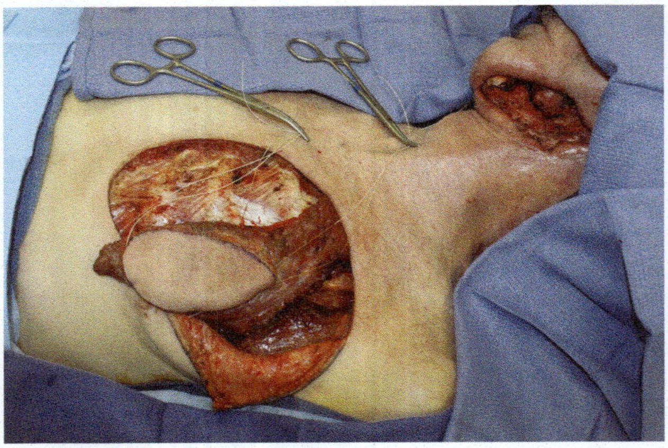

Fig. 15.32 Completion of the elevation of the flap prior to transfer to the neck.

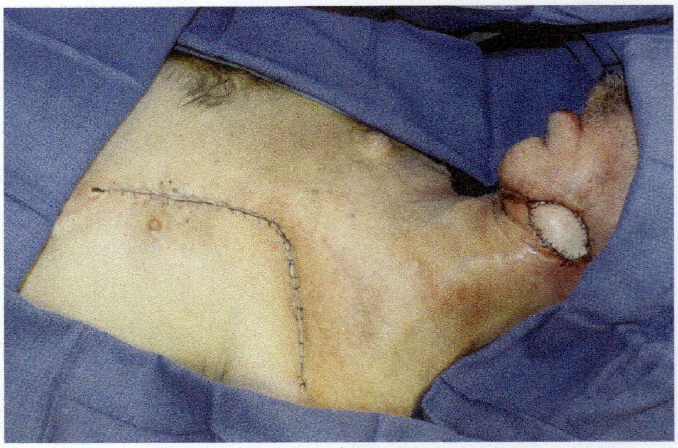

Fig. 15.34 Inset of the flap repairing both the oral and neck defects.

a curvilinear skin paddle design and a broad muscle harvest to cover the exposed great vessels in the neck (Figure 15.26). A myocutaneous flap was harvested and then transferred to the neck in a subcutaneous tunnel and inset to the defect site (Figures 15.27 to 15.29). The donor site was closed by advancing the chest with minimal distortion to the chest wall.

Case #3

A 54-year-old male with Buerger's disease, a history of squamous cell carcinoma, and previous treatment with surgery and radiation therapy was referred due to a recent development of osteoradionecrosis with exposed bone in the neck (Figure 15.30). The patient was taken to the operating room where the mandible was resected to bleeding bone and the proposed skin paddle was marked on the chest with the anticipation of de-epithelializing the middle section of the skin paddle to allow for the creation of a double paddle flap with skin closure intraorally and skin closure of the skin defect of the neck (Figure 15.31). The flap was elevated, a subplatysmal flap was created to the defect in the neck, and the flap was then transferred to the site, and the bridge de-epithelialized and inset into the defect (Figures 15.32 to 15.34).

References

1. Ariyan S. The pectoralis major myocutaneous flap. A versatile flap for reconstruction in the head and neck. *Plast Reconstr Surg* 1979; 63(1):73–81.
2. Mathes SJ, Nahai F. Classification of the vascular anatomy of muscles: experimental and clinical correlation. *Plast Reconstr Surg* 1981; 67(2):177–178.

Chapter 16
Latissimus dorsi myocutaneous flap

Introduction

The latissimus dorsi flap was first described by Tansini in 1896.[1,2] The latissimus dorsi myocutaneous flap is one of the most commonly used free flaps in microvascular reconstructive surgery. It's used primarily for the repair of breasts and extremity defects. The use of this flap in the head and neck is also commonplace as a microvascular transfer, especially in cases where a large volume of muscle or skin is needed. The scalp is probably the most common site in the head and neck region where the latissimus dorsi flap is utilized. Although most surgeons think of the utility of this flap as a free flap only, it can also have significant utility to the head and neck surgeon as a pedicled flap. The first description of its use as a pedicled flap in head and neck reconstruction was by Quillen *et al.* in 1978.[3] Typically the use of the pedicled latissimus dorsi flap for the reconstruction of head and neck defects are for those selected cases where the neck is vessel depleted and the pectoralis major muscle has already been used before or is somehow compromised.

The latissimus flap can reach a number of areas in the head and neck when used as a pedicle flap. The flap can be used for defect located as high as orbital exenteration defects, temporal bone defects, as well as for pharyngeal reconstruction as in cases of laryngo-pharyngectomy resections.

The main concern for this flap is the potential for venous congestion and loss of the skin paddle. This result is often due to compression or kinking of the vascular pedicle in the axilla or as it travels in the tunnel to reach the defect.

Although the use of the latissimus dorsi muscle as a pedicle flap for head and neck may not be the first or second option for most reconstructive surgeons, it should be considered as a "bailout" option to the surgeon and for the very difficult cases stated earlier.

Anatomy

The latissimus dorsi muscle is a broad fan-shaped muscle with its origin from the lower six thoracic vertebrae as well as the fascia from the iliac crest and the lower four ribs. The muscle inserts into the medial aspect of the humerus.

The vascular supply to the latissimus muscle is from the thoracodorsal artery and vein. The thoracodorsal artery is a branch of the subscapular artery and the same is true for the vein.

The action of the latissimus flap is to aid in the adduction and inward rotation of the arm.

Flap harvest

The flap can be harvested with the patient in the prone position, supine position or most commonly, the lateral decubitus position.

Once the patient is intubated on the operating room table, the patient is placed in a lateral decubitus position and secured with the aid of a bean bag and straps. The position of the bean bag should allow for exposure of the spine and inferiorly to the iliac crest. A gel roll should be placed under the contralateral axilla in order to minimize pressure to the brachial plexus. The ipsilateral arm should be prepped and included placed in the operating field. The patient should be secured to the operating table with at least two straps. The area to be prepped should include the head and neck extending inferiorly to the ipsilateral anterior chest and back up to the spine. Inferiorly, the prep should end at the iliac crest. The bed is rotated towards the donor side so the patient is in a more horizontal position to allow for the ablative portion of the surgery. Once the resection is completed, the patient is then once again rotated to the opposite side, this time to

Local and Regional Flaps in Head & Neck Reconstruction: A Practical Approach, First Edition. Rui Fernandes.

Companion website: www.wiley.com/go/fernandes/flapsreconstruction

allow for the harvest of the flap. The prepped arm can be positioned away from the operative field by the assistant and manipulated as needed during the harvest and transfer of the flap.

- The anterior edge of the latissimus dorsi muscle is palpated and marked from the axilla extending caudally towards the insertion along the iliac crest.
- The desired shape of the skin paddle is marked. Care should be taken to place the skin paddle well over the underlying muscle.
- The skin incision is made along the anterior marked edge of the skin paddle and extended both towards the axilla superiorly and towards the iliac crest inferiorly.
- The incision is extended to the fascia over the latissimus. A suprafascial dissection is then extended in the same way as the skin incision. The dissection is completed when the whole length of the anterior border of the latissimus muscle is well delineated.
- At this point, the location of the skin paddle over the muscle is confirmed and, once deemed to be in the correct location, the remainder of the skin paddle is incised and extended to the fascia of the latissimus.
- The skin paddle is sutured to the muscle fascia to prevent shearing of the skin from the muscle during the remainder of the flap elevation as well as during the muscle transfer.
- The anterior edge of the latissimus muscle is elevated and the plane between the latissimus muscle and the serratus anterior muscle is dissected.
- The plane under the latissimus muscle should be relatively avascular. The dissection towards the axilla should be done carefully to identify the thoracodorsal artery and its accompanying venae commitantes. The insertion of the vascular pedicle is approximately 12 cm inferior from the muscle insertion to the humerus.
- The inferior portion of the flap (inferior to the skin paddle in cases of a musculocutaneous flap) at the desired muscle length is separated and dissection is extended in a cephalad direction and medially along the vertebral column.
- Once the desired muscle length is harvested along the medial aspect of the skin island, the dissection is then devoted to the vascular pedicle.
- The thoracodorsal vessels are dissected towards the subscapular vessels. Care is taken to identify and protect the long thoracic nerve.
- Once the vessels are dissected, the muscle is divided superior to the insertion of the vascular pedicle in the undersurface of the muscle.
- With the flap mobilized, the vascular pedicle should be checked to avoid any twisting or kinking.

Creation of the tunnel

- The tunnel in the neck should be made in the subplatysma plane. Care should be taken not injure the external jugular vein when developing the neck tunnel. The dissection is continued until the clavicle is reached and extended above the clavicle.
- Once the tunnel reaches the clavicle, attention is then turned to the development of the axillary tunnel.
- Using the incision from the flap harvest, dissection is extended in the axilla towards the lateral aspect of the pectoralis major muscle. Once the pectoralis major muscle is identified, the pectoralis minor is identified under the pectoralis major. A tunnel can be developed either above or below the pectoralis major muscle. If the tunnel is above the muscle it will result in a slight loss of the pedicle length as it travels to the neck.
- If the tunnel is developed between the pectoralis muscles, the path to the neck will have to be developed by making a skin incision below the clavicle and incision of the pectoralis muscle insertion along the clavicle to allow for the flap transfer. The tunnel should be wide enough to accommodate the flap without constriction.

Transfer of the flap to the neck

- The flap is ready to transfer to the recipient site in the head and neck once the tunnel is completed.
- A large clamp is introduced from the subclavicular incision and advanced in the tunnel towards the axilla. Using large retractors, the axillary tunnel is elevated and the inferior portion of the flap is turned towards the clamp and the muscle is clamped.
- The flap is mobilized to the neck by a combination of pulling from the neck and pushing from the axilla with care to not shear the skin paddle.
- Once the flap is transferred to the neck in the subplatysma tunnel, the path of the thoracodorsal pedicle is once again checked to make sure it is not stretched or kinked.

Closure of the donor site

- The donor site is evaluated to make sure it is hemostatic. The small bleeding points are cauterized.
- A closed system drain (usually a 19 Jackson Pratt drain) is inserted and the incision is closed in layers. The drain is left in place for at least a week or until a time when there is consistently less than 20 cm^3 output in a 24-hour period.

Figures 16.1 to 16.11 depict the raising of the flap and the creation of the tunnel with transfer to the neck.

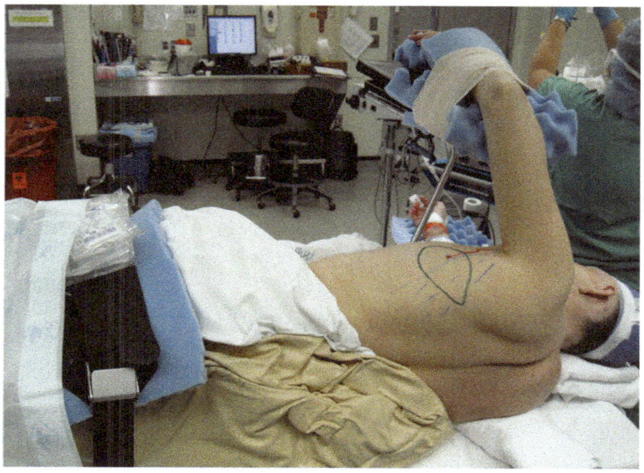

Fig. 16.1 Positioning of the patient in a lateral decubitous position for harvest of the latissimus dorsi flap.

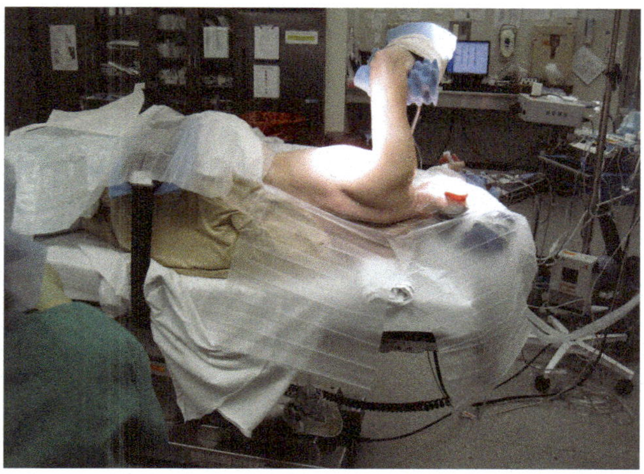

Fig. 16.2 Rotating the bed allows for resection of the primary while at the same time access to the latissimus dorsi without the need for re-prepping.

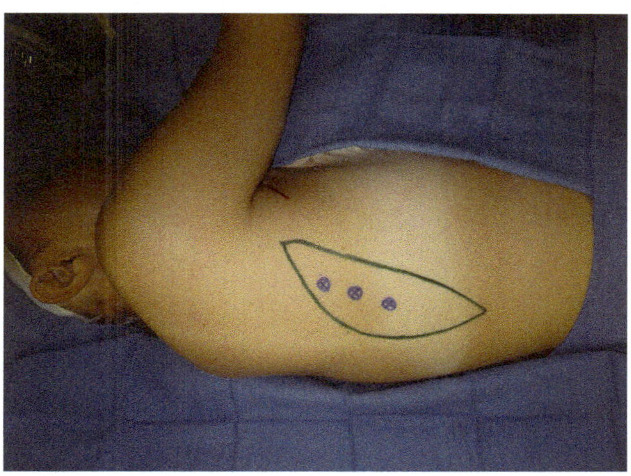

Fig. 16.3 Markings for the skin paddle directly overlying the anterior edge of the muscle.

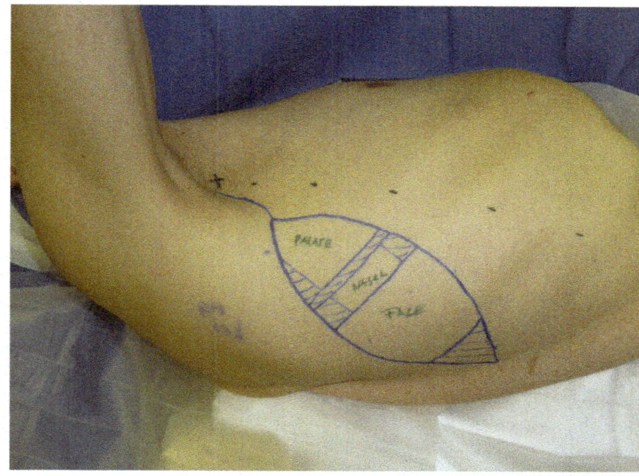

Fig. 16.4 View of the skin paddle design positioned at a different angle than in Figure 16.3.

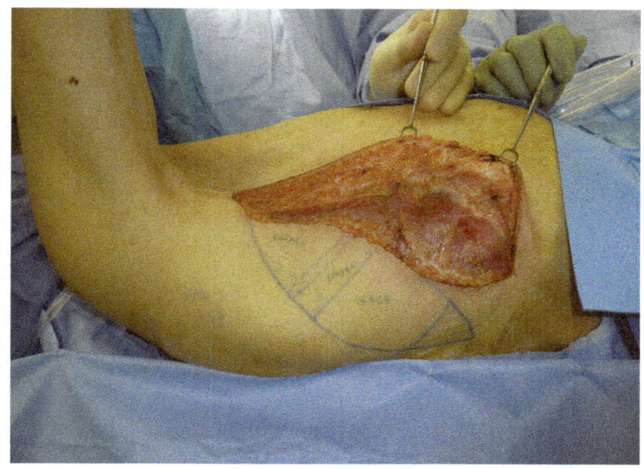

Fig. 16.5 Elevation of a skin flap revealing the latissimus dorsi muscle until the anterior border of the muscle was fully visualized.

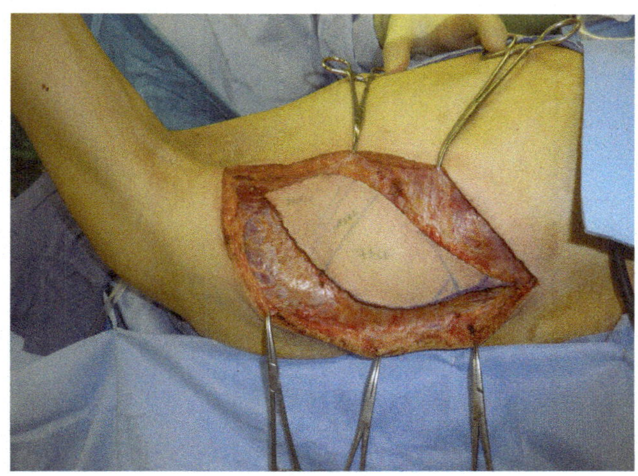

Fig. 16.6 Circumferential elevation of the surrounding skin away from the skin paddle exposing the underlying muscle.

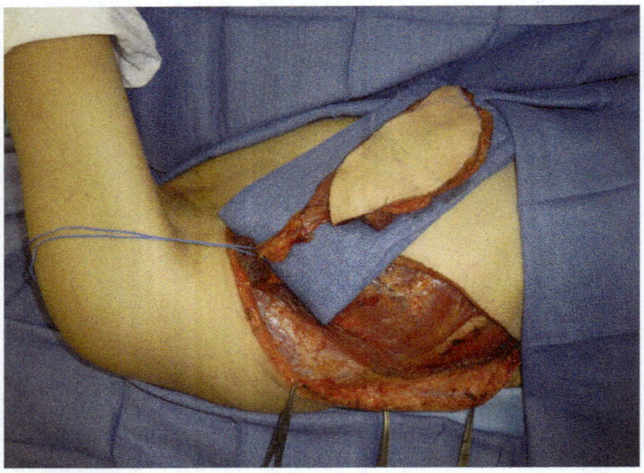

Fig. 16.7 Completed elevation of the flap prior to transfer.

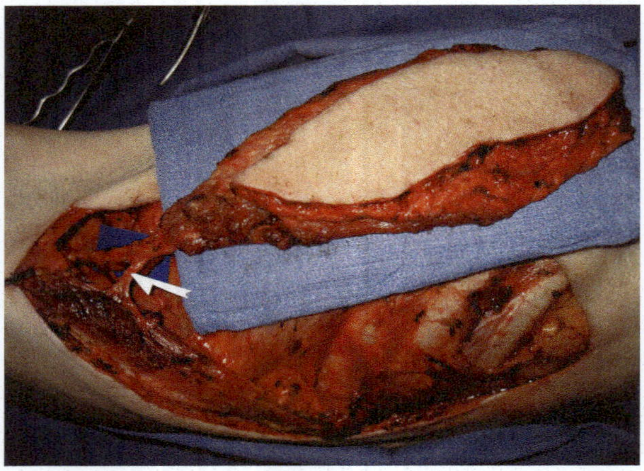

Fig. 16.8 Close-up view of the vascular pedicle of the flap.

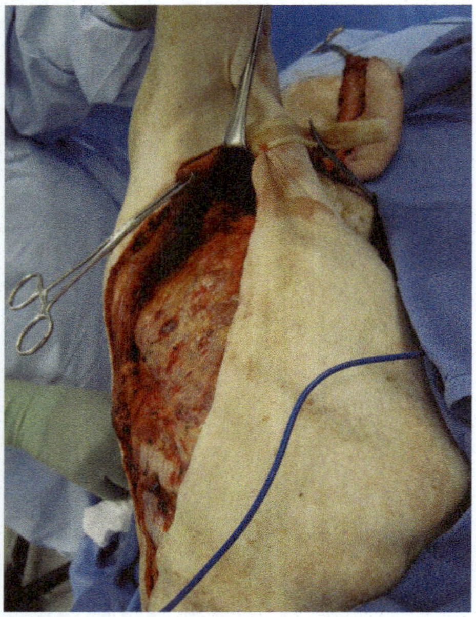

Fig. 16.9 Development of a tunnel for the transfer of the flap into the neck region.

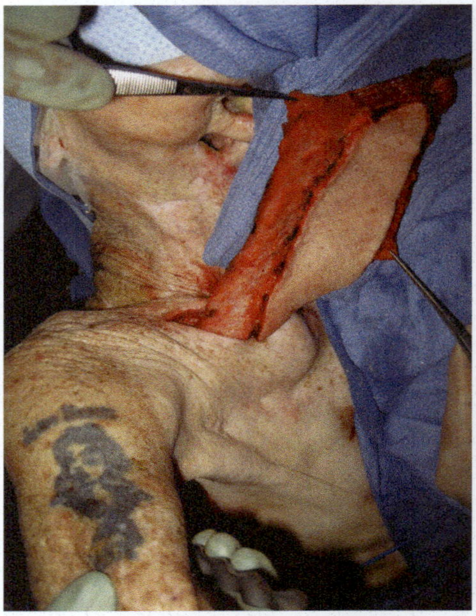

Fig. 16.10 Transfer of the flap along the flap and into the neck.

Complications

The potential complications associated with the latissimus dorsi flap can be separated into those affecting either the flap itself or the donor site. Regarding the donor site, the most commonly encountered postoperative complication is the formation of a seroma. The best way to avoid the formation of a seroma is to keep the drain in place until the output is negligible. In cases where there is persistent drain, the use of a chest corset can also be

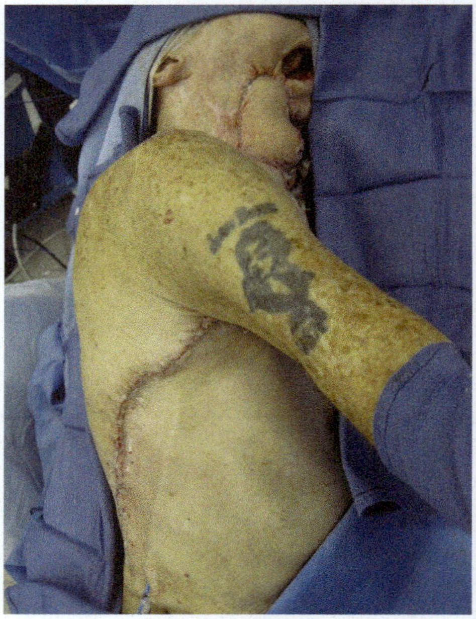

Fig. 16.11 Closure of the donor site.

used to propagate the adhesion of the skin to the underlying muscle. A hematoma can also form at the donor site. If this happens, the management is the same as with any other site, i.e., evacuation if warranted or expectant observation and wait for resolution.

Complications of the flap can be manifested most commonly secondary to either kinking of the pedicle or compression of the pedicle in its transition from the tunnel to the neck. The best way to deal with these two issues is to not have them at all. It is imperative to develop a wide tunnel for the transfer of the flap but also to account for the eventual postoperative swelling which can lead to compression of the pedicle and venous congestion. The transfer of the flap can lead to kinking or twisting of the pedicle. This problem can be increased when the circumflex scapular artery is divided to improve the rotation. The division of the artery allows for a better rotation and further reach of the flap but it creates the potential for twisting. The potential for twisting can be minimized by using methylene blue to cover one of the surfaces of the pedicle so a possible twist is more apparent.

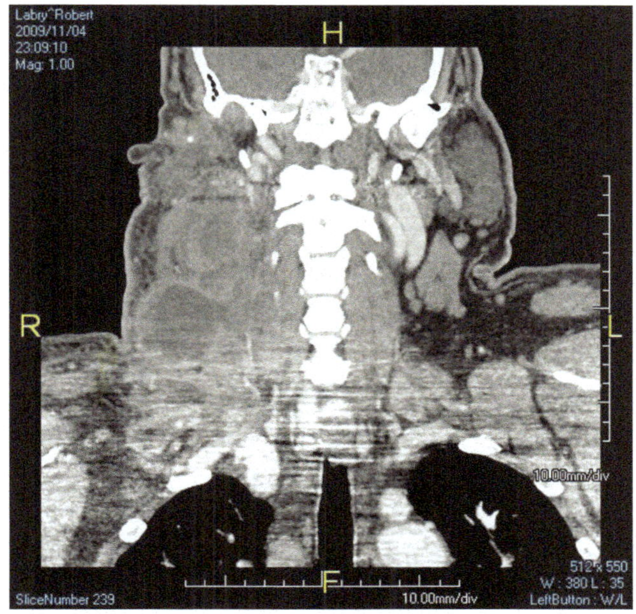

Fig. 16.13 Coronal view of the neck showing the multiple nodal disease.

Case# 1

The patient is a 67-year-old with a history of melanoma of the temporal region treated with surgical resection and postoperative chemotherapy. He failed treatment and presented with a large neck mass suspicious for recurrence. Computer tomography of the neck revealed a large conglomerate of matted nodes extending from the superior aspect to the supraclavicular region (Figures 16.12 and 16.13). Clinical examination revealed a large ulcerated mass of the posterior neck region (Figure 16.14). The treatment plan included resection of the neck mass and immediate reconstruction of the defect with a pedicled latissimus dorsi flap (Figure 16.15). An extended radical neck dissection was performed with resulting exposure of the carotid vessels and the neuromuscular contents of the neck (Figure 16.16). The resected specimen is shown in Figure 16.17. A pedicled musculocutaneous latissimus

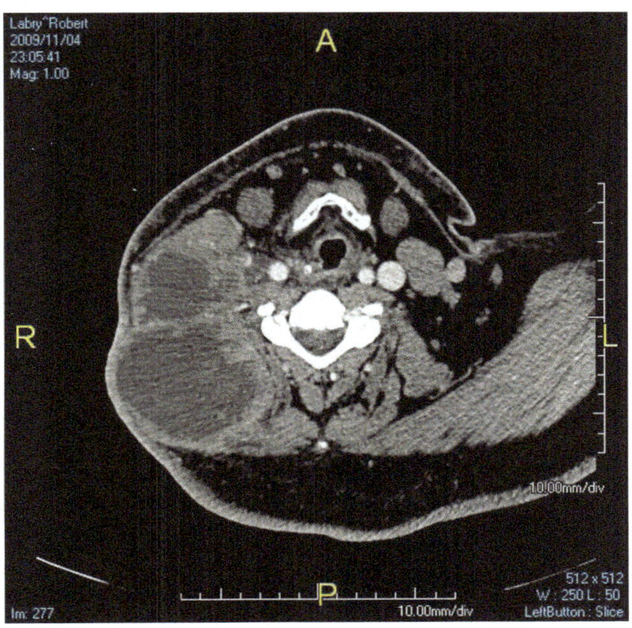

Fig. 16.12 CT scan of neck depicting multiple large nodal disease.

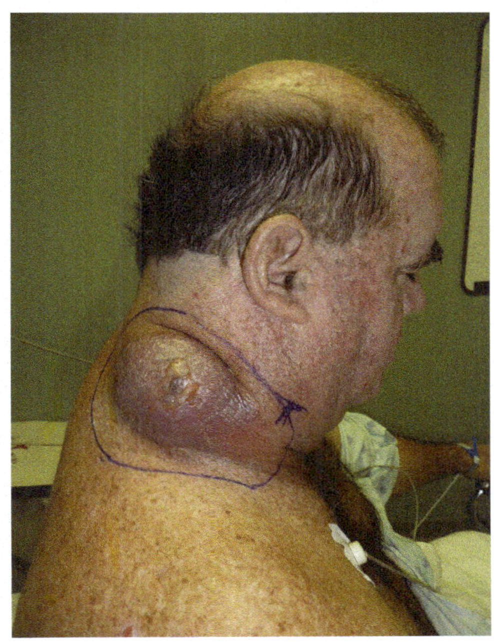

Fig. 16.14 View of the patient prior to resection; view of the planned resection.

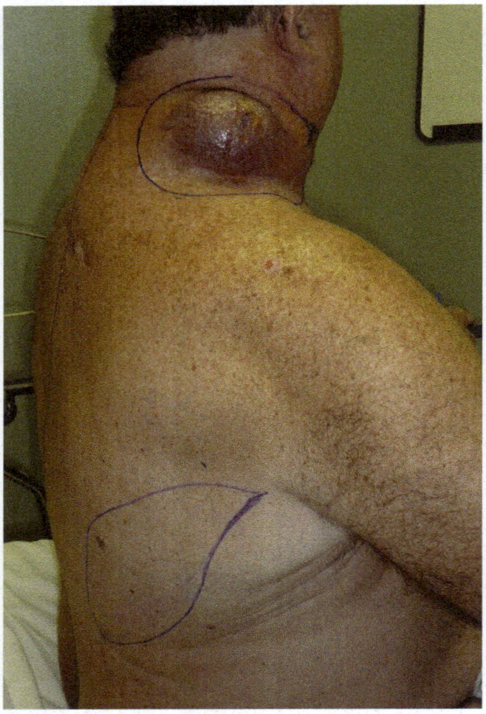

Fig. 16.15 View of both the planned resection and the latissimus donor site.

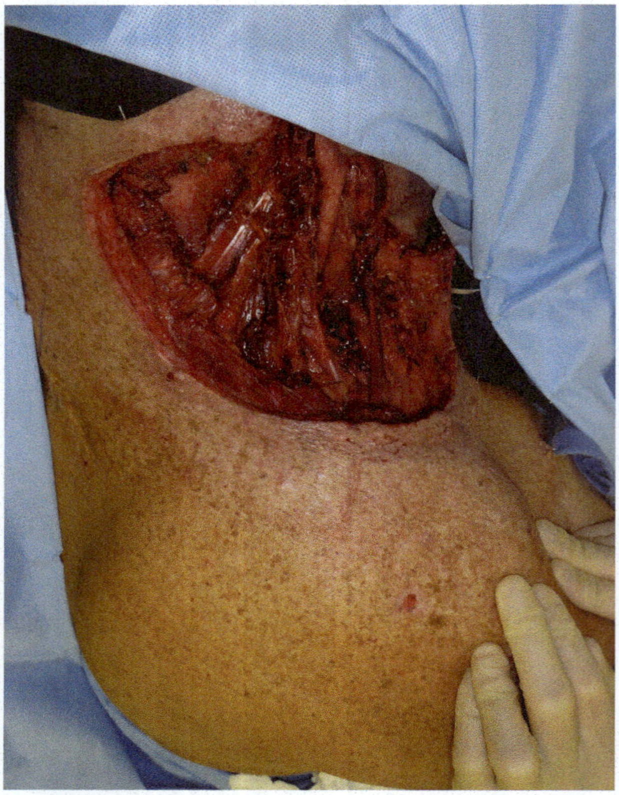

Fig. 16.16 Appearance of the resection with exposure of the great vessels and a large skin paddle defect.

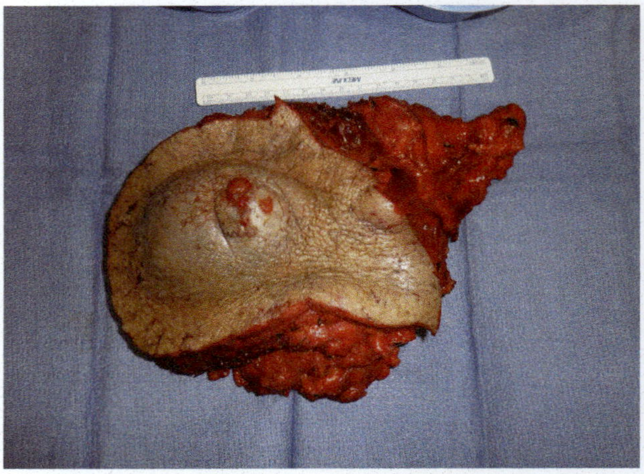

Fig. 16.17 Resected specimen.

dorsi flap was elevated and transferred to cover the defect site (Figure 16.18). The patient healed well from the surgery and the reconstruction. A small dehiscence developed at the superior portion of the reconstruction that eventually healed by secondary intention. The donor site healed without any obvious deficit (Figures 16.19 and 16.20).

Case #2

A 69-year-old male with history of renal transplantation and immunosuppression was referred for evaluation and treatment of facial squamous cell carcinoma.

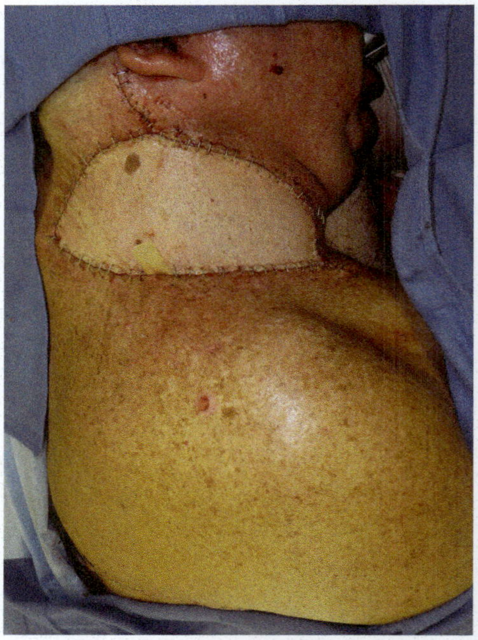

Fig. 16.18 Appearance of the latissimus dorsi myocutaneous flap reconstruction of the cervical defect.

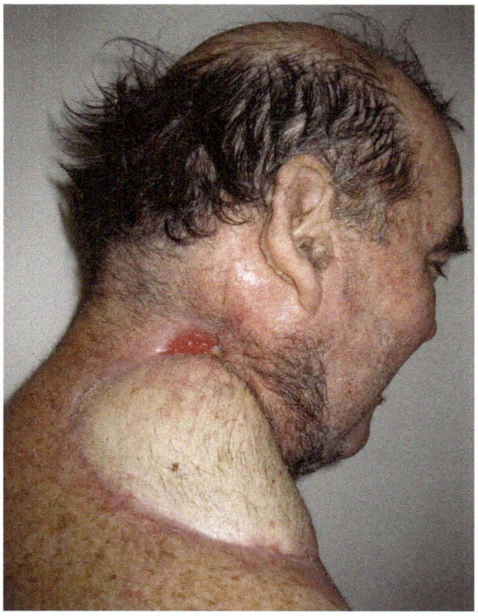

Fig. 16.19 Early postoperative healing with only a minor dehiscence in the superior portion.

The patient had an extensive history of excision of squamous cell carcinomas of the head and neck region and most recently had failed radiation therapy to the left facial region for a large multicentric squamous cell carcinoma. He presented with recurrent squamous cell carcinoma encompassing nearly the entire left face with gross tumor extension to the left orbit. He was also complaining of difficulty with vision from the left eye. He was presented to

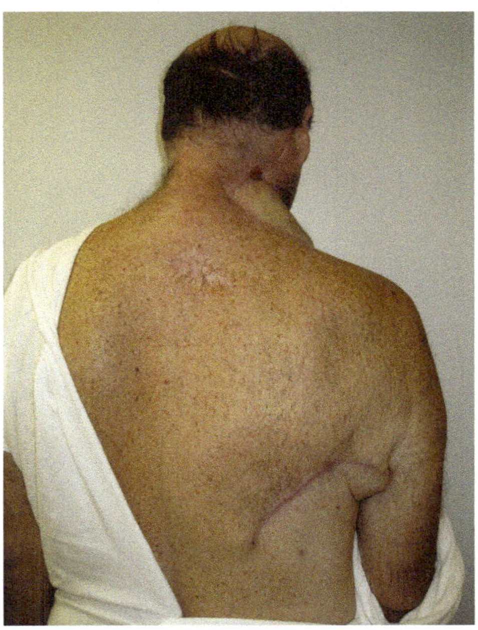

Fig. 16.20 Appearance of the healed donor site.

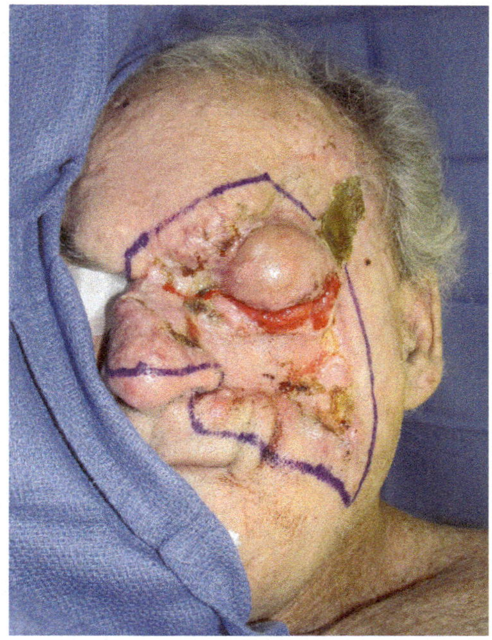

Fig. 16.21 View of the facial malignancy with a planned resection area.

the head and neck tumor board and a recommendation was made for a radical resection of the left facial tumor along with orbital exenteration and immediate reconstruction with a pedicled latissimus dorsi flap (Figures 16.21 and 16.22). The resection was completed and clearance was confirmed with the aid of numerous frozen section margins (Figures 16.23 and 16.24).

A pedicled latissimus dorsi myocutaneous flap was elevated and a long pedicle was dissected to the subscapular artery (Figure 16.25). A tunnel was created under the pectoralis major and over the pectoralis minor muscle. A small incision was made in the supraclavicular area of the neck and the flap was transferred to the neck ensuring that the pedicle was not kinked or compressed along its path in the tunnel (Figure 16.26). The flap was inset into the donor site. A small area of exposed muscle along the nasal dorsum was grafted with a full thickness

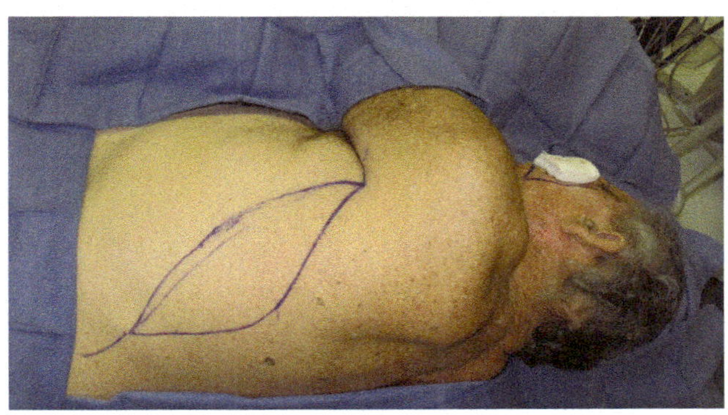

Fig. 16.22 Positioning of the patient for the harvest of the latissimus dorsi flap.

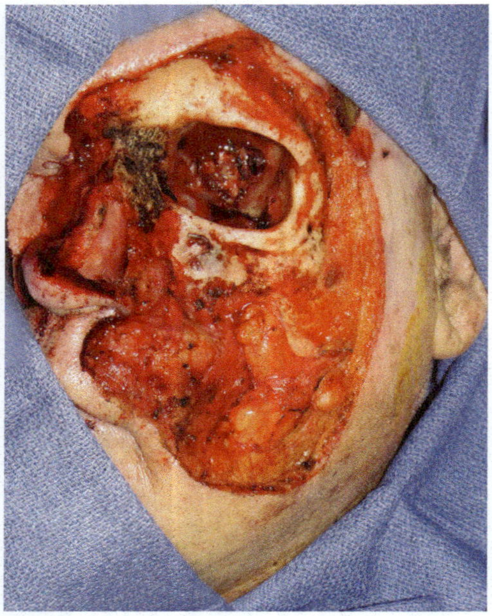

Fig. 16.23 View of the large defect which includes an orbital exenteration.

skin graft (Figure 16.27). The patient healed well from the reconstruction and has been disease-free for nearly 3 years since the surgery (Figures 16.28 and 16.29).

Case #3

A 78-year-old female with a prolonged history of basal cell carcinoma of the lower cervical region with extension

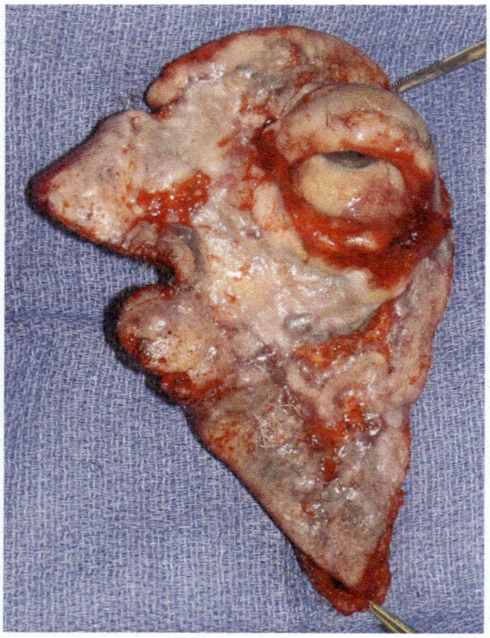

Fig. 16.24 View of the resected specimen

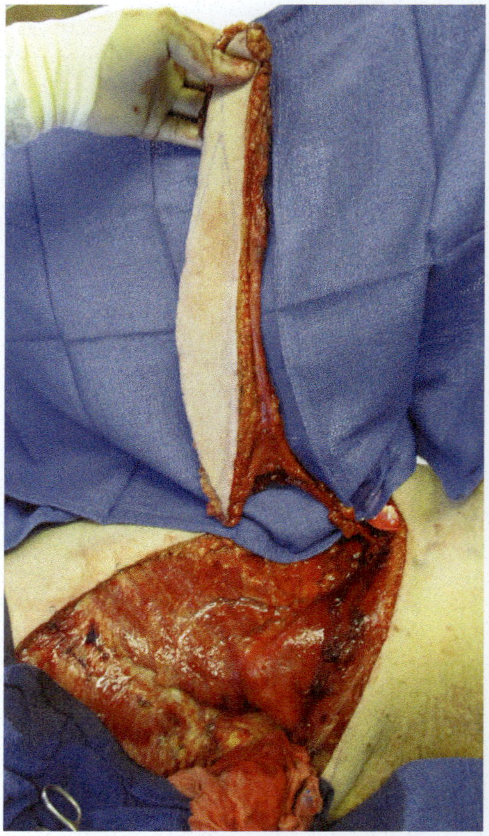

Fig. 16.25 Elevated latissimus dorsi flap prior to its transfer into the neck.

and invasion of the clavicle and sternal bone was referred after failed radiation therapy. She underwent an extensive resection of the lesion by the cardiothoracic surgical team. The resection included the clavicular as well as sternal bone (Figure 16.30).

Given her overall fragile state, she was deemed best suited for a shortened operation and therefore a decision

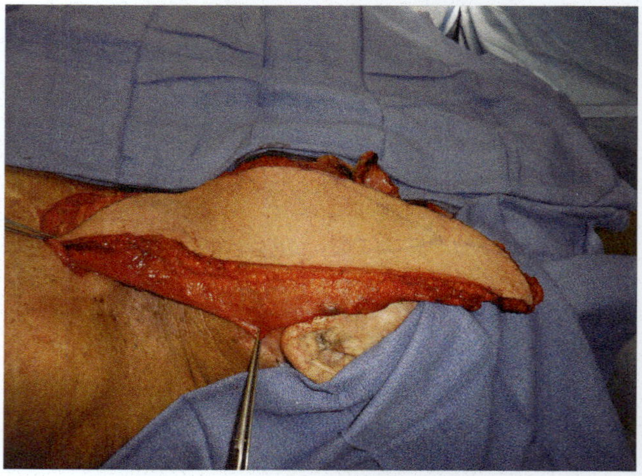

Fig. 16.26 Transfer of the flap into the neck; note the reach of the flap.

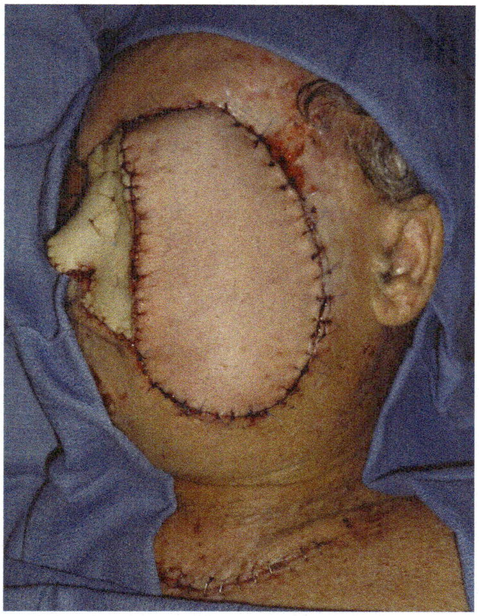

Fig. 16.27 Final appearance of the inset of the flap with a small portion of a full-thickness skin graft over the latissimus muscle portion over the nose.

was made to reconstruct her defect with a pedicled latissimus dorsi myocutaneous flap. The flap was elevated with the patient in the supine position. A broad quantity of muscle was harvested to obliterate the extensive defect. The flap was then transferred to the upper chest via a tunnel created between the pectoralis muscles (Figures 16.31 and 16.32). Once the flap was transferred, the position of the pedicle was checked to confirm proper alignment without kinking, the muscle was tucked into

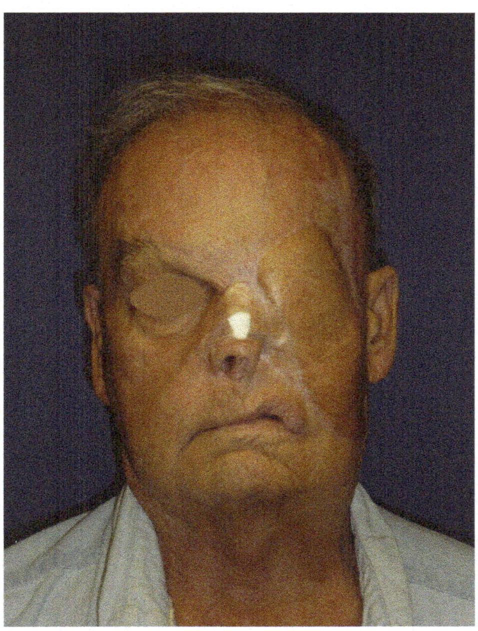

Fig. 16.28 Frontal view of the healed patient.

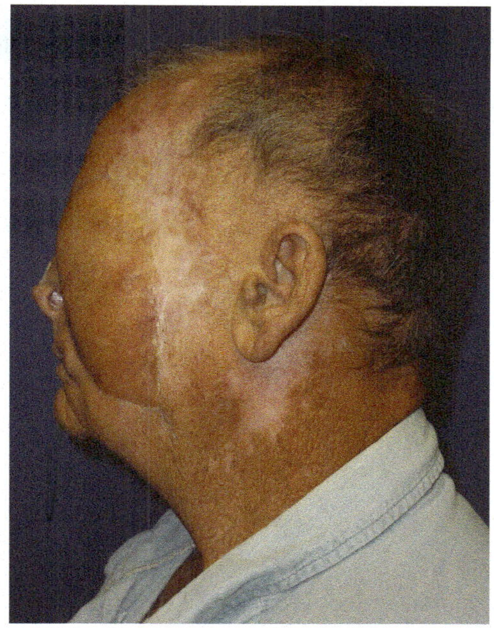

Fig. 16.29 Profile view of the patient after healing of the reconstruction.

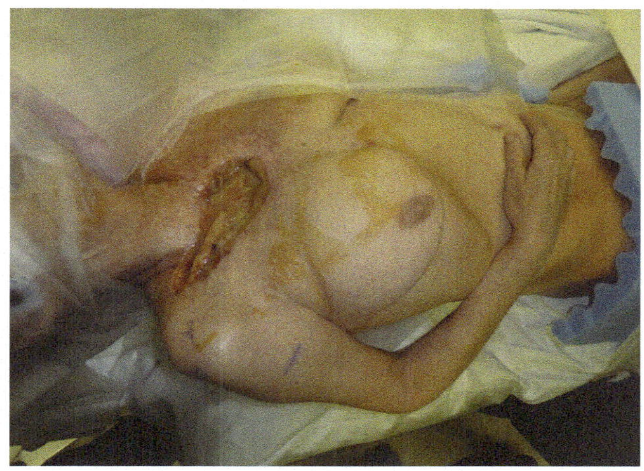

Fig. 16.30 View of a patient with a large defect in the upper chest region.

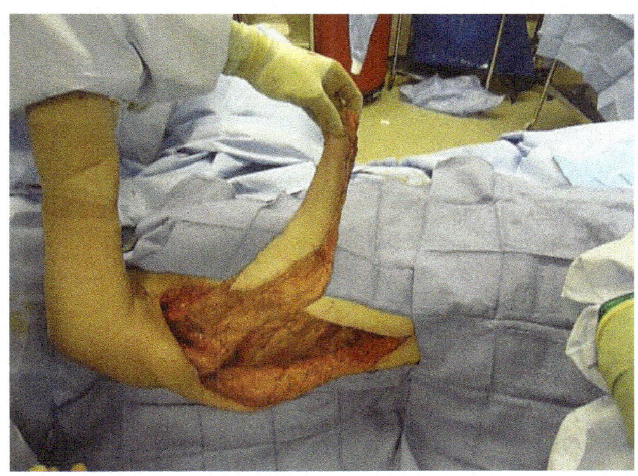

Fig. 16.31 Elevated flap prior to transfer.

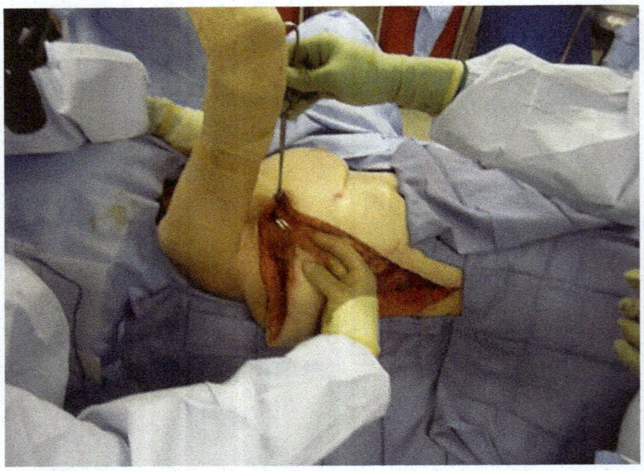

Fig. 16.32 Transfer of the flap into the chest defect.

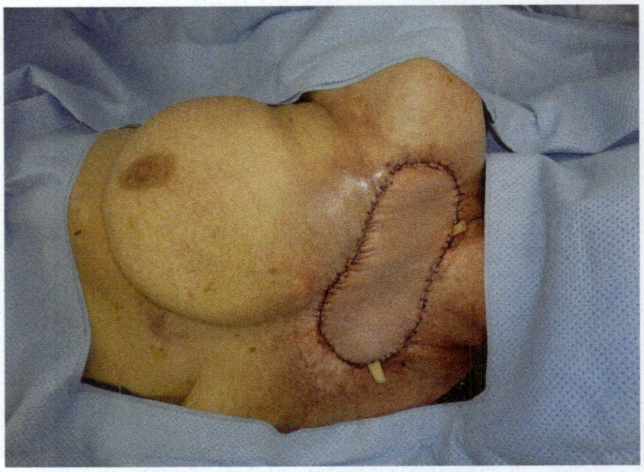

Fig. 16.33 View of the transferred flap after inset.

the defect area, and the skin was inset using interrupted sutures (Figure 16.33).

References

1. Tansini I. Spora il mio nuovo processo di amputazione della mammaella per cancre. *Riforma Med (Palermo, Napoli)* 1896; 12:3.
2. Maxwell GP. Iginio Tansini and the origin of the latissimus dorsi musculocutaneous flap *Plast Reconst Surg* 1980; 65(5):686–692.
3. Quillen CG, Shearin JC Jr, Georgiade NG. Use of the latissimus dorsi myocutaneous island flap for reconstruction in the head and neck area: case report. *Plast Reconstr Surg* 1978; 62(1):113–117.

Chapter 17
Sternocleidomastoid flap

Introduction

Owens described the sternocleidomastoid (SCM) flap in 1955 utilizing the entire length of skin overlying the muscle.[1] Later, the flap design was modified by Ariyan to include only the lower third of the skin.[2] Since its description, the flap has had a diminished role in the reconstruction of head and neck defects. Although numerous authors have published variations of the use of the SCM flap and espouse the advantages of the flap, it has always retained the role of a seldom-used flap for head and neck reconstruction.[3,4] The diminished role of the SCM in reconstruction of head and neck defects stems from two main reasons. The first is that its use as a myocutaneous flap continues to be viewed as unreliable due to the common loss of the skin component of the flap. Second is the fact that the most common head and neck defects are a result of ablation of malignancies and therefore there is often an accompanying neck dissection, which may result in the compromise of the flap. In cases where a neck dissection has already been done, the blood supply to the SCM is often compromised. The site where this may occur is the blood supply entering the muscle as either the superior or middle third. The occipital vessels are often ligated in the dissection of level IIb nodes. As most head and neck defects are located in the upper third of the neck or within the oral cavity, using the SCM as a superiorly based flap is no longer a possibility.

The SCM receives its blood supply from several blood vessels and is commonly divided into thirds, the superior, middle, and inferior third. This segmental blood supply enables the flap to be used in three possible ways: superiorly based, inferiorly based, or as a perforator based on the middle third.[5] The limitations of the SCM flap are similar to any other pedicled flap, i.e., the arc of rotation and the ability to reach the location of the defect. The use of the flap as a superiorly based flap allows for the reconstruction of various defects in the head and neck as well as the oral cavity. The inferiorly based flap can be used to repair defects around the inferior aspect of the mandible, and the upper, central, and lower neck region. The SCM may be of particular use in reconstructing pharyngeal fistulas.

Anatomy

The sternocleidomastoid is a paired muscle in the anterior neck, enclosed by the superficial cervical fascia, directly beneath the platysma. The external jugular vein and the great auricular nerve cross the surface of the muscle vertically. The muscle has a medial sternal head that originates from the upper part of the anterior surface of the manubrium sterni and a clavicular head that arises from the superior and anterior surface of the medial third of the clavicle. As the muscle ascends obliquely beyond the supraclavicular fossa, the two heads fuse together and insert into the lateral surface of the mastoid process and the superior nuchal line of the occipital bone. It is classified as a type II pattern of vascular circulation.[6] The dominant blood supply to the muscle is from branches of the occipital artery. These branches form a rich anastomosis within the muscle that can supply its entire length with the exception of the inferior 3–5 cm.[7] The middle third of the muscle receives its blood supply from branches of the superior thyroid artery and external carotid artery.[8] The vascular supply from the upper and middle third of the muscle can maintain viability of the entire muscle and overlying skin. The lower third of the muscle has shown the most variability in its vascular supply with branches arising from the thyrocervical trunk, suprascapular artery, and the transverse cervical artery. The venous drainage is through the accompanying occipital vein, posterior auricular vein,

Local and Regional Flaps in Head & Neck Reconstruction: A Practical Approach, First Edition. Rui Fernandes.

Companion website: www.wiley.com/go/fernandes/flapsreconstruction

external jugular vein, and branches from the internal jugular vein. The motor innervation to the muscle is via a branch of the spinal accessory nerve as it courses to the trapezius.

Flap harvest

- The flap is raised with the patient in a supine position with the donor side exposed and the head rotated to the contralateral side.
- A shoulder roll should be placed to help elevate the base of the neck and therefore provide better exposure for harvest.
- The SCM should be easily visualized and or palpated; this is easier in thin patients and those with long necks.
- The markings for the flap should be made by outlining the muscle from the mastoid region as it travels in a diagonal path to the insertion in the clavicle and sternum.
- If the flap is to be raised as myocutaneous flap, the skin paddle should be outlined with care to center it over the belly of the muscle.
- Regardless of whether the flap is to be raised as an inferiorly based or superiorly based flap, the surgeon should determine the arc of rotation and confer the reach of the flap, particularly if it is a myocutaneous flap. This will ensure that the skin component will reach the defect in a safe manner without tension.
- Once the skin paddle is designed, the next step is to incorporate the rest of the incision with that of the skin paddle.

Superiorly based flap

- The incision for the harvest of the flap is often done in conjunction with that of the neck dissection, this is often a low apron incision which begins behind the sternocleidomastoid area, extends inferiorly along a neck crease, and transverses the neck to the contralateral side.
- Using either electrocautery with a Colorado tip or a 15 blade, the skin is incised down to and through the platysma.
- A subplatysma flap is then raised to the inferior border of the mandible. This should allow for visualization of the SCM along the neck from its origin to the superior aspect of the skin paddle.
- The area inferior to the skin flap is equally raised in the subplatysmal plane as was done superiorly.
- The skin paddle is sutured to the overlying fascia of the sternocleidomastoid muscle. This maneuver minimizes sharing of the skin flap and potential compromise of the skin paddle.
- The muscle is dissected inferiorly to identify the insertion of the muscle at the sternal and clavicular areas. The muscle is then elevated from the respective attachments.
- At this time, along the inferior third of the muscle, the vascular pedicle from the transverse cervical vessels should be identified, ligated, and divided.
- Dissection of the muscle is then carried out in a superior fashion towards the middle portion of the muscle. The pedicle from the superior thyroid artery to the muscle should be identified, ligated, and divided in this area.
- The division of the superior thyroid arterial contribution to the muscle gives an improved arc of rotation of the flap and therefore the likelihood that it will reach a superior defect without tension.
- The last part of the dissection is towards the upper third portion of the muscle.
- In this region, two main structures should be kept in mind: one is the occipital vessels that will be the main blood supply to the superiorly based flap and the other is the spinal accessory muscle.
- The spinal accessory muscle will be identified along the superior portion of the muscle as it travels diagonally from the skull base towards the muscle from medial to lateral.
- At this point, rotation of the flap is carried out to check if the flap will reach the defect.
- If the flap reaches the defect without tension then the inset can begin; otherwise, careful dissection on the posterior superior aspect of the muscle should be carried out, as this is most often the area of restriction.

Inferiorly based flap

- The inferiorly based flap is raised in a similar way to the superiorly based flap with the exception that the branches from the thyrocervical trunk maintain the blood supply to the muscle.
- The main difference when raising the inferiorly based flap will be the dissection and preservation of the spinal accessory nerve in the upper portion of the muscle.

Closure of the donor site

- The donor site is evaluated to make sure it is hemostatic. The small bleeding points are cauterized.
- A closed system drain (usually a 19 Jackson Pratt drain) is put in place and the incision closed in layers. The drain is in left in place for at least a week or until there is consistently less than a 20 cm^3 output in 24 hours.

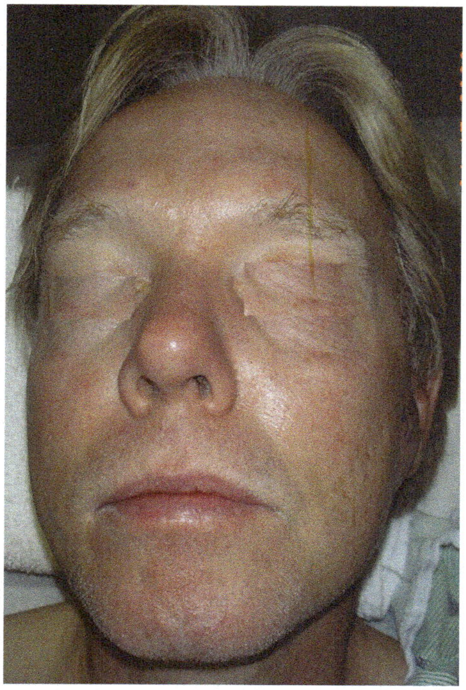

Fig. 17.1 View of a patient with a parotid adenoid cystic carcinoma.

Case #1

A 48-year-old Caucasian male was referred for the management of a biopsy-proven adenoid cystic carcinoma of the left parotid region. At the time of presentation, he was noted to have facial nerve deficit on the ipsilateral side (Figure 17.1). After presentation at the multidisciplinary head and neck tumor board, a decision was made for a total parotidectomy with facial nerve sacrifice and immediate reconstruction with a graft from the greater auricular nerve (Figures 17.2 and 17.3). The resultant facial depression was addressed with a sternocleidomastoid flap. The flap was elevated as a superiorly based flap and the arc of rotation was checked to ensure that there would be minimal tension at the inset of the flap (Figures 17.4 to 17.6). The flap was then inset and the

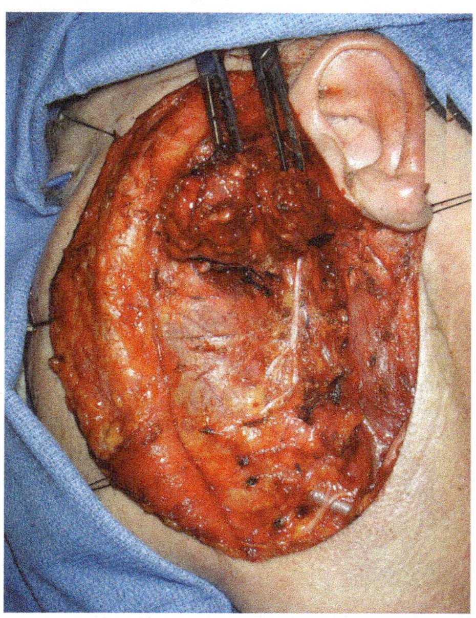

Fig. 17.2 Parotidectomy with visualization of the portion of the facial nerve.

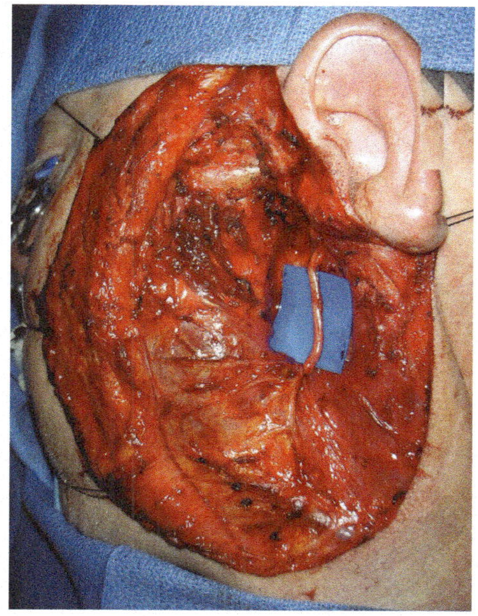

Fig. 17.3 View of a nerve graft in the surgical bed.

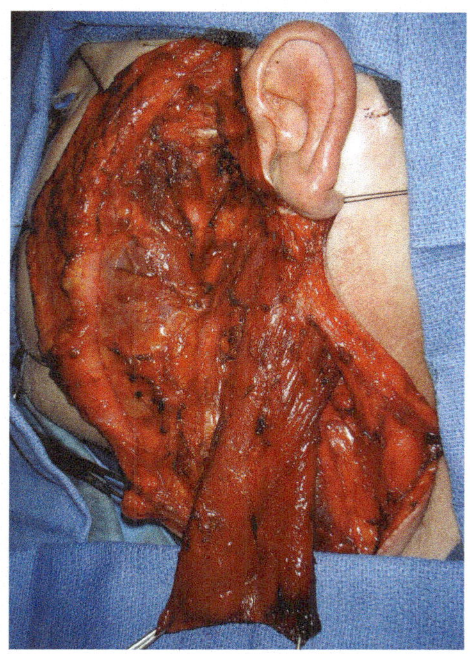

Fig. 17.4 Elevation of the sternocleidomastoid muscle flap based on the superior occipital vessels.

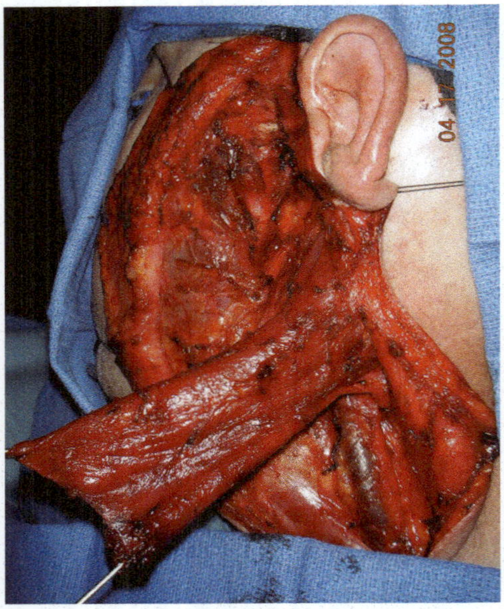

Fig. 17.5 Arc of rotation of the flap to assess the reach.

defect was closed (Figure 17.7). The final facial appearance of the patient was acceptable with minimal depression noted at the resected side (Figure 17.8a and b).

Case #2

A 63-year-old Caucasian male was referred for the management of a recurrent right facial squamous cell carcinoma. The patient had a remote history of renal transplantation and numerous head and neck skin squamous cell carcinomas. He had undergone several extensive

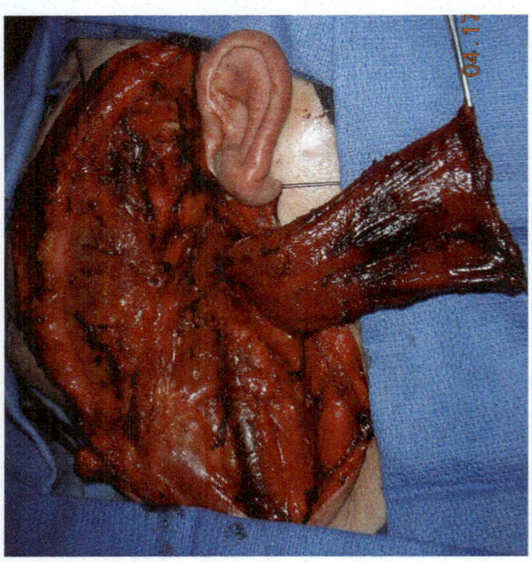

Fig. 17.6 Exposure of the undersurface of the sternocleidomastoid flap prior to transfer.

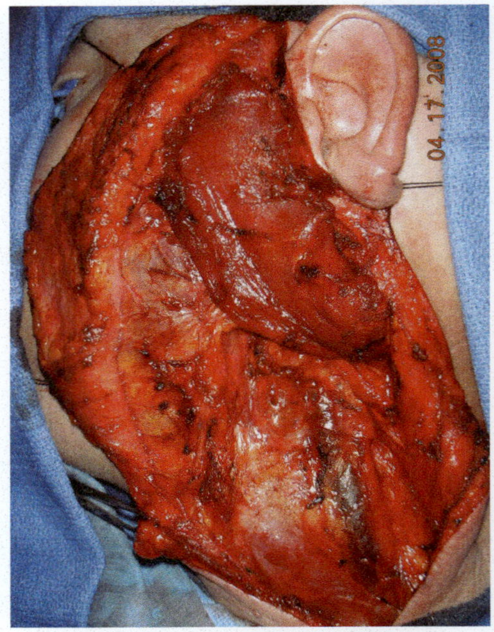

Fig. 17.7 Inset of the sternocleidomastoid flap into the defect site.

resections in the past with various reconstructive techniques and adjuvant radiation therapy to the sites. He was recently noted to have a rapidly enlarging tumor on the right preauricular region with loss of function of the facial nerve on the ipsilateral side (Figure 17.9). He was presented at the multidisciplinary tumor board and a recommendation was given for a radical resection with

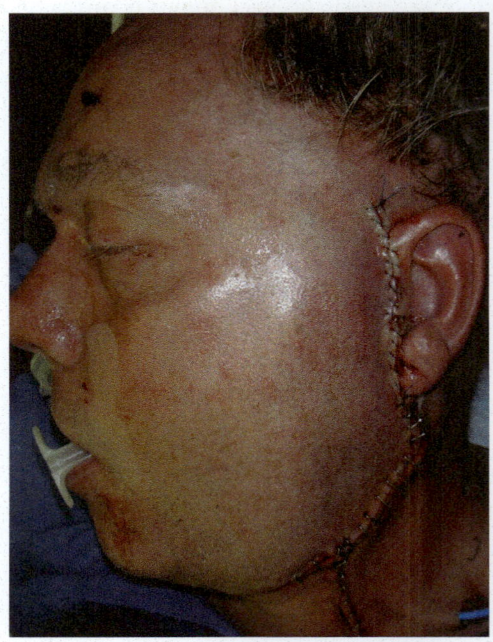

Fig. 17.8a Immediate view of the surgical reconstruction demonstrating the normal facial architecture.

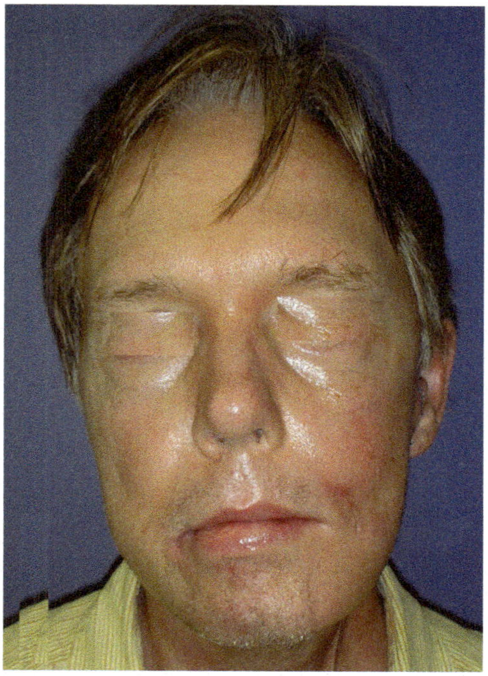

Fig. 17.8b Postoperative facial appearance demonstrating the normal facial contour.

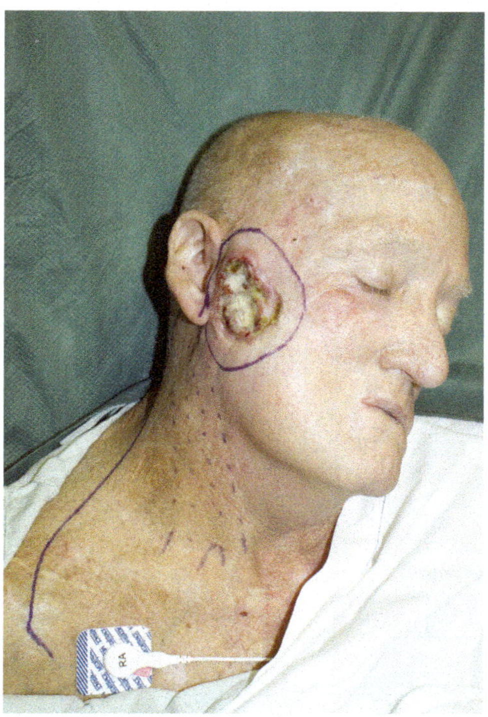

Fig. 17.9 View of a patient with a large, right facial recurrent carcinoma. Markings denote the planned radical resection and a cervicopectoral flap.

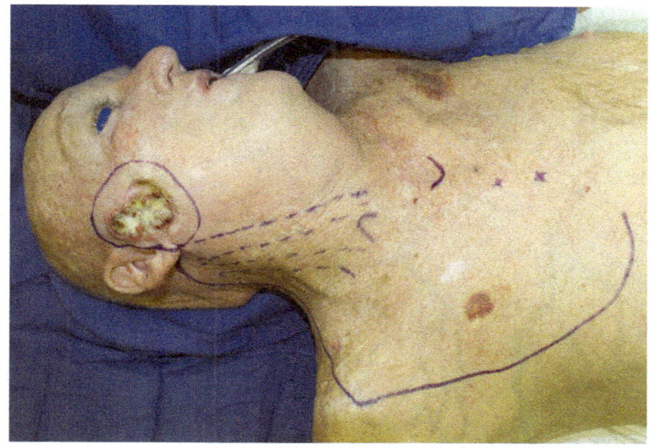

Fig. 17.10 Surgical plan demonstrating the outline of the sternocleidomastoid muscle prior to surgery.

sacrifice of the facial nerve and resection of the zygomatic arch due to tumor extension evident on the computer tomography examination. The reconstructive plan was to carry out a superiorly based SCM flap to cover the mandible and resection bed and to rotate a cervicofacial flap to repair the skin defect (Figure 17.10). The resection was carried out as planned (Figure 17.11). A cervicofacial flap was then elevated and extended inferior to the clavicular region and exposing the entire length of the SCM flap (Figure 17.12). The SCM flap was then raised by first disinserting the two heads of the muscle from the clavicle and sternum (Figure 17.13). The flap was then elevated in a superior fashion and the superior thyroid vessels ligated during the dissection (Figure 17.14). The rotation of the flap was then checked to confirm that it would be adequate to obliterate the defect without tension (Figure 17.15). The flap was then inset and the cervicofacial flap was rotated to repair the skin defect (Figures 17.16 and 17.17). The facial appearance a few days after surgery was acceptable with a proper contour of the right face and good color and perfusion to the entire cervicofacial flap (Figure 17.18).

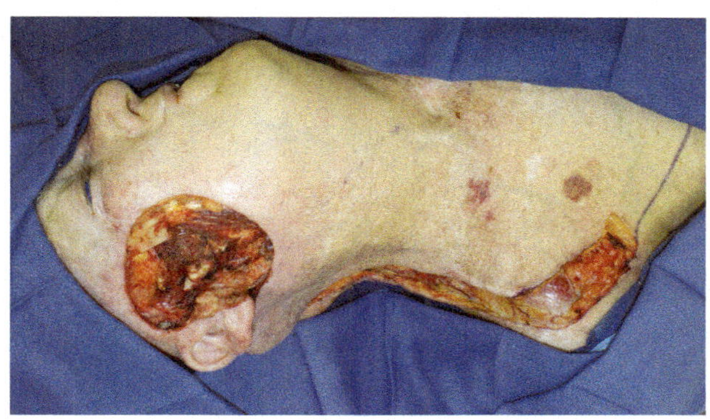

Fig. 17.11 View of the resection bed and incision for the elevation of the cervicopectoral flap.

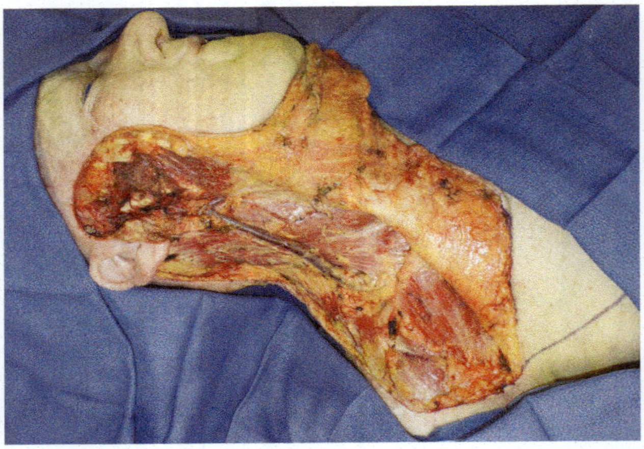

Fig. 17.12 The cervicopectoral flap is reflected anteriorly giving view of the sternocleidomastoid muscle.

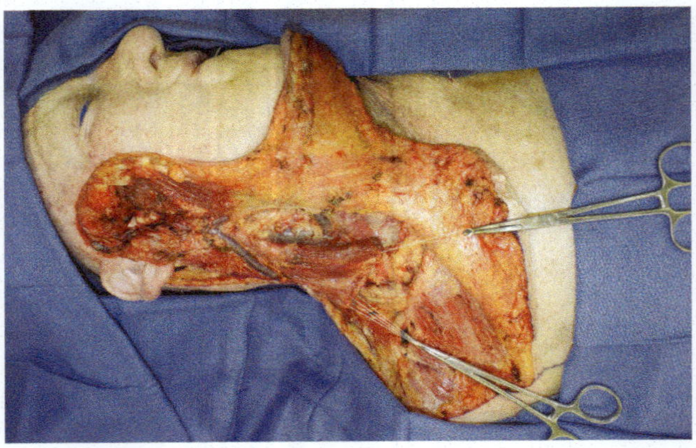

Fig. 17.13 Complete exposure and elevation of the sternocleidomastoid flap prior to rotation.

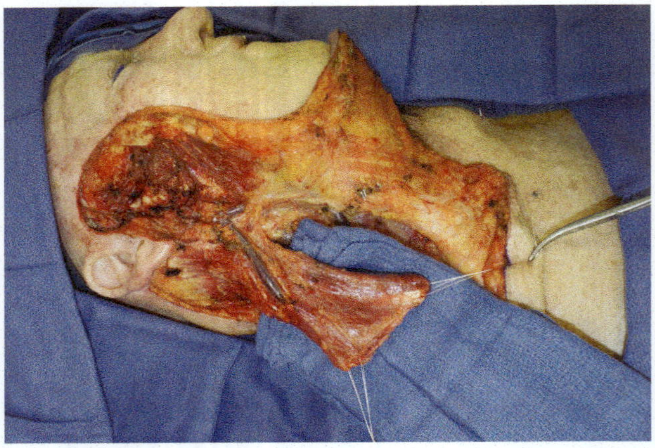

Fig. 17.14 View of the elevated flap.

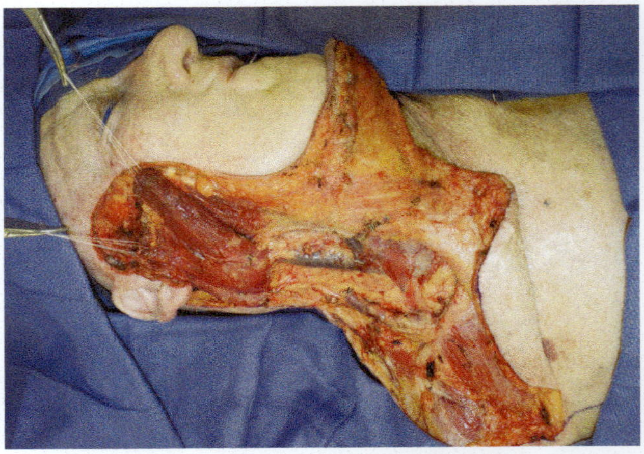

Fig. 17.15 Rotation of the sternocleidomastoid flap into the parotid defect.

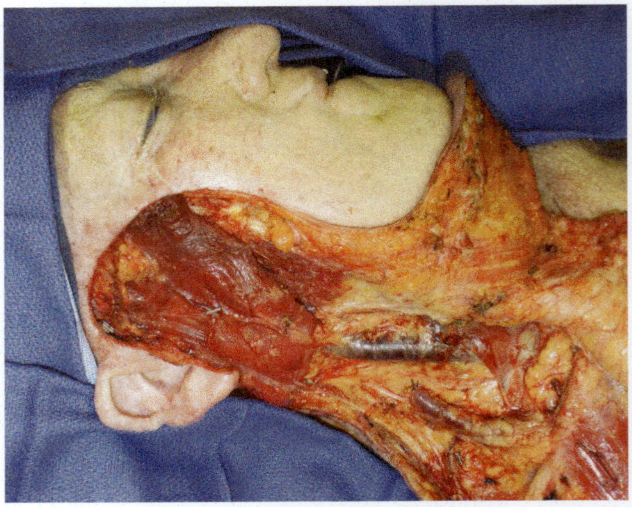

Fig. 17.16 View of the inset of the flap.

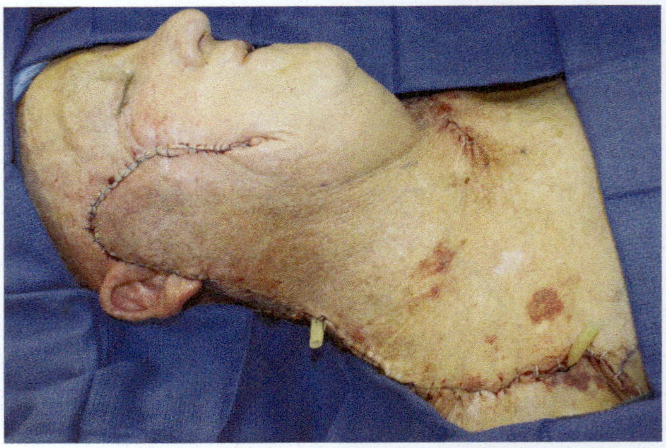

Fig. 17.17 Closure of the surgical defect with a cervicopectoral flap.

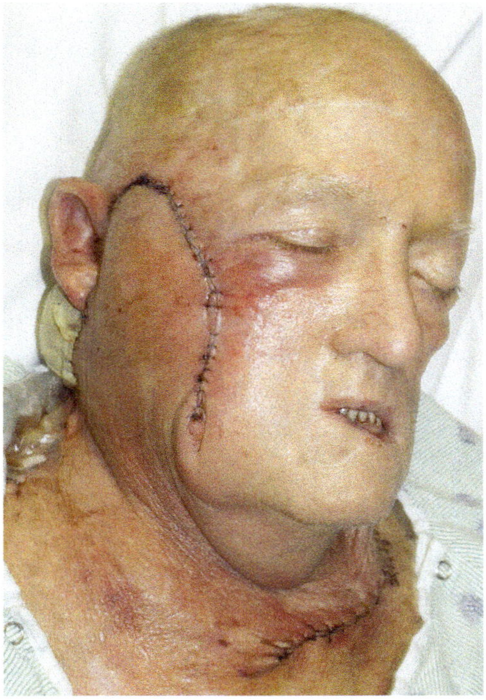

Fig. 17.18 Early postoperative view of the reconstruction.

References

1. Owens NA. Compound neck pedicle designed for the repair of massive facial defects: development and application. *Plast Reconstr Surg* 1955; 15:369–389.
2. Ariyan S. One-stage reconstruction for defects of the mouth using a sternocleidomastoid myocutaneous flap. *Plast Reconstr Surg* 1979; 63:618–620.
3. Conley J, Gullane PJ. The sternocleidomastoid muscle flap. *Head Neck Surg* 1980; 2:308–311.
4. Hill HL, Brown RG. The sternocleidomastoid flap to restore facial contour in mandibular reconstruction. *Br J Plast Surg* 1978; 31:143–146.
5. Avery CM. The sternocleidomastoid perforator flap: short communication. *Br J Oral Maxillofac Surg* 2011; 49:573–575.
6. Mathes SJ, Nahai F. Classification of the vascular anatomy of muscles: experimental and clinical correlation. *Plast Reconstr Surg* 1981; 67:177–178.
7. Marx RE, McDonald DK. The sternocleidomastoid muscle as a muscular or myocutaneous flap for oral and facial reconstruction. *J Oral Maxillofac Surg* 1985; 43:155.
8. Kierner AC, Aigner M, Zelenka I, Riedl G, Burian M. The blood supply of the sternocleidomastoid muscle and its clinical implications. *Arch Surg* 1999; 134:144.

Chapter 18
Trapezius flap

Many reports of the trapezius myocutaneous flap have centered on a single form of the flap. However, three distinct myocutaneous segments—the superior, the lateral island, and the extended island flaps—can be harvested from the trapezius muscle and its overlying skin.[1] In 1972, Conley described the superior trapezius flap, based on the paraspinous perforating branches of the posterior intercostal vessels.[2] Panje and Demergasso described the lateral island trapezius flap, based on the transverse cervical vessels.[3,4] Mathes and Nahai described the vertical trapezius myocutanous flap in 1979.[5] Baek *et al.* described the lower island flap, based on the transverse cervical vessels, in 1980.[6]

The role of the trapezius flap in reconstruction of defects of the head and neck remains relegated to salvage cases or those selected patients with significant morbidities who otherwise cannot withstand extended operations. One of the main reasons why this flap continues to lack popularity is due to the positioning of the patient to raise the flap as well as the potential for vascular compromise to the skin island. Given the location of defects in the head and neck, the use of the trapezius flap requires repositioning the patient from a supine position to a prone position to harvest and then repositioning the patient for the inset of the flap. The need for multiple repositioning can sometimes be avoided when the preparation of the defect and raising of the flap can be carried out with the patient in the lateral decubitus position.

The trapezius flap can be used to reconstruct numerous defects in the head and neck region ranging from defects in the oral cavity, resurfacing of various sites in the neck, and coverage of mandibular and temporal defects.

Anatomy

The trapezius muscle is a triangular muscle that covers the back of the neck and shoulder region and extends inferiorly in the back. It arises from the medial third of the superior nuchal line of the occipital bone, the external occipital protuberance, the ligamentum nuchae, the spine of the seventh cervical vertebra, the spines of all the thoracic vertebrae, and the corresponding supraspinous ligament. The upper part of the trapezius passes obliquely downward, laterally and forward to the lateral third of the clavicle. The middle part passes transversely to the medial edge of the acromion and the upper border of the spine of the scapula. The lower part passes obliquely upward and laterally to terminate in the tubercle at the medial end of the spine of the scapula.[7] The actions of the trapezius muscle can be divided based on the region, the upper region elevates the shoulder, the middle retracts the scapula and aids in the abduction of the upper extremity, and the lower portion aids in the depression of the scapula.

The blood supply to the trapezius flap had been a source of confusion in the literature for many years. Netterville and his colleagues are credited with clarifying the blood supply to the flap in their publication of a cadaveric study published in 1991.[8] The skin overlying the trapezius muscle receives its blood supply from four sources: the transverse cervical artery, the dorsal scapular artery, the intercostal perforators lying just off the midline, and the branches from the occipital artery.

The blood supply to the trapezius muscle and overlying skin is primarily from the superficial and deep descending branches of the transverse cervical artery,

Local and Regional Flaps in Head & Neck Reconstruction: A Practical Approach, First Edition. Rui Fernandes.

Companion website: www.wiley.com/go/fernandes/flapsreconstruction

as well as the occipital artery. The superficial descending branch arises directly from the thyrocervical trunk in 75–80% of cases and is known as the transverse cervical artery.[9] The dorsal scapular artery arises from the subclavian artery in 75% of cases; however, in 25% of cases, it arises from the transverse cervical artery, and in these cases, the vessel is named the deep descending branch of the transverse cervical artery, and the junction of the two descending branches is the cervicodorsal trunk. The transverse cervical artery enters the trapezius muscle at the base of the neck and descends vertically along the deep surface of the trapezius. The dorsal scapular artery runs under the levator muscle before it divides, giving a major branch and a descending branch. The major branch exits between the rhomboid major and minor to gain access in the deep surface of the trapezius to supply its lower trapezius. The descending branch continues under the rhomboid major muscle and does not supply the trapezius.

The neural supply to the trapezius muscle comes from the spinal accessory nerve.

Flap harvest

- The flap is raised with the patient in either the prone position or in the lateral decubitus position.
- When the flap is to be raised with the patient in the lateral decubitus position, using a beanbag helps to facilitate the positioning as well as securing the patient.
- The skin paddle component of the flap is positioned by measuring the location of the defect from the pivot point in the shoulder.
- Once the measurement from the pivot point to the defect is measured, the information is then transferred to the trapezius. The marking for the skin island should overlie the trapezius muscle.
- The incision is begun on the lateral aspect of the skin flap and carried down to the fascia of the trapezius muscle.
- The positioning of the skin island is checked to be sure that it is placed over the muscle. The preference is that the entire skin island is placed directly over the muscle; if this is not possible, the skin paddle is usually not extended further than 15 cm below the inferior tip of the scapula.
- Once the positioning of the skin island is confirmed, the incision is extended superiorly towards the base of the neck.
- The skin flap is elevated laterally until enough exposure is performed to enable elevation of the myocutaneous trapezius flap.
- The medial skin is then elevated medially towards the spine with the inferior aspect around the previously marked skin island.
- The skin paddle is then sutured to the fascia of the muscle to minimize shearing of the skin island from the underlying muscle.
- Incising the muscle around the skin paddle just superficial to the latissimus muscle enables the beginning of flap elevation.
- The incision of the trapezius muscle is begun inferiorly and extended superiorly taking care to identify the medial paraspinal perforators.
- Once the dissection reaches the rhomboid major muscle, care should be taken to identify the dominant branch of the dorsal scapular artery as it emerges between the rhomboid major and minor muscles.
- The descending branch of the dorsal scapular artery and accompanying veins should be ligated while protecting the dominant branch to the trapezius.
- The arc of rotation of the flap should be checked to see if there is adequate reach of the flap to reconstruct the defect.
- If further reach is needed, the rhomboid minor may be divided on either side of the pedicle. This maneuver will increase the laxity of the muscle and improve the rotation and reach of the flap.
- A subcutaneous tunnel is dissected to accommodate the passive transfer of the flap into the head and neck region.
- Alternatively, a release incision can be extended towards the base of the neck to accommodate the flap.

Closure of the donor site

- The donor site is evaluated to make sure it is hemostatic. The small bleeding points are cauterized.
- A closed system drain (usually a 19 Jackson drain) is put in place and the incision is closed in layers. The drain is in left in place for at least a week or until there is a consistently less than a 20 cm^3 output in a 24-hour period.
- See Figures 18.1 to 18.7.

Case #1

A 74-year-old Caucasian female with a long history of osteoradionecrosis was referred for resection and coverage of a large oral cutaneous fistula. Due to her numerous comorbidities, she was not a candidate for microvascular surgery and previous attempts at repairing the defect had used other possible pedicled flaps. A decision was made to use the trapezius flap to repair the defect (Figure 18.8). The incision was marked to extend from the back and to connect to previous incisions in the base of the neck (Figures 18.9 and 18.10). The flap was elevated by raising the skin flap surrounding the skin paddle and confirming the location of the paddle relative to the muscle (Figure 18.11). The flap was elevated as already

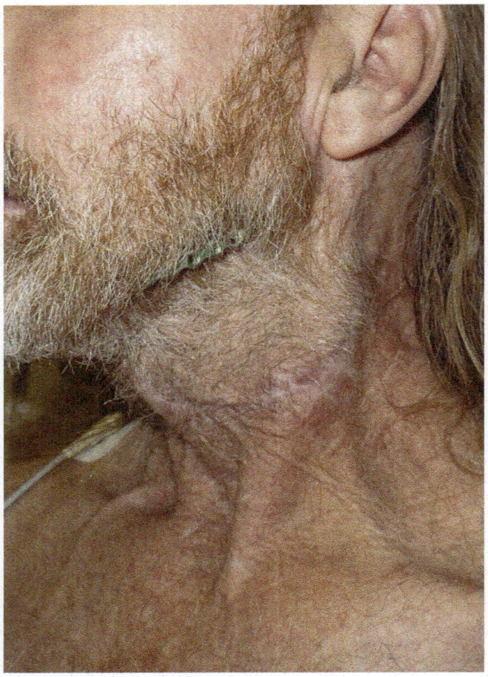

Fig. 18.1 View of a patient with exposed mandibular reconstruction plate in a previously radiated and operated bed.

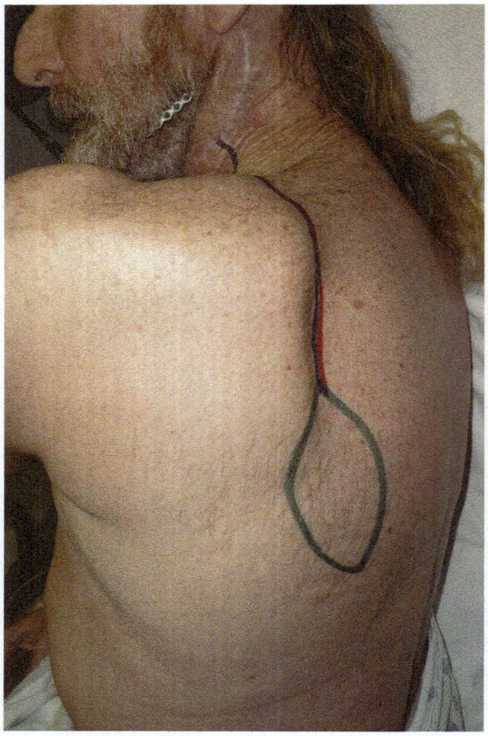

Fig. 18.2 Markings for an extended vertical trapezius flap.

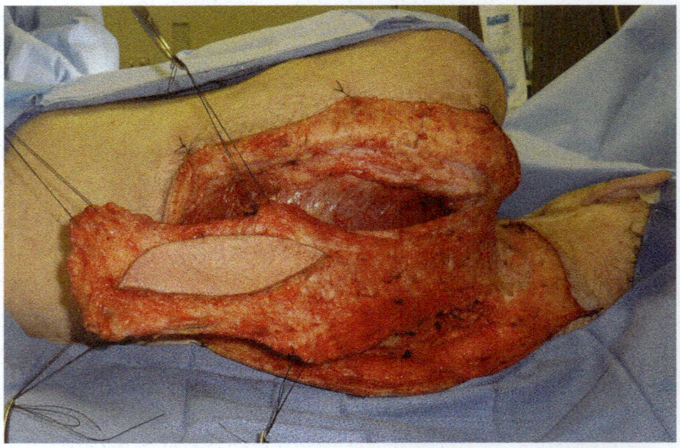

Fig. 18.3 The trapezius flap has been elevated and sutures placed in different points to better expose the flap prior to transfer.

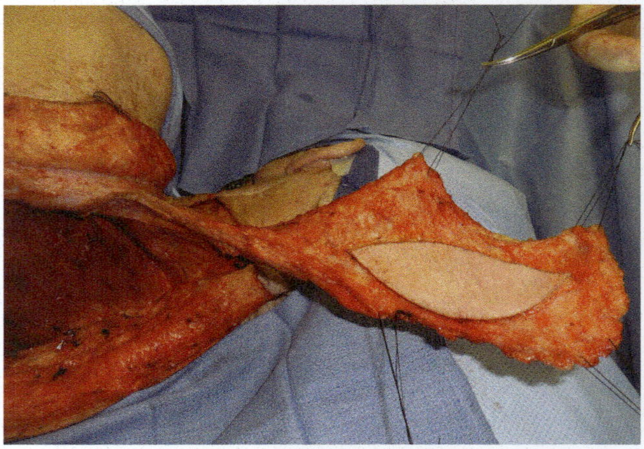

Fig. 18.4 Assessment of the arc of rotation and reach of the flap to the defect.

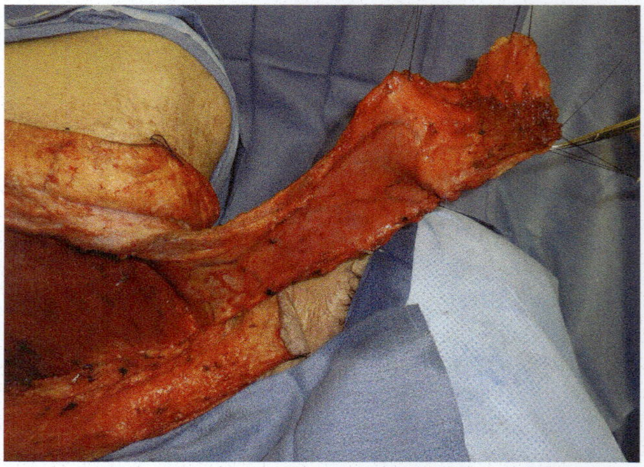

Fig. 18.5 View of the vascular pedicle on the undersurface of the trapezius flap.

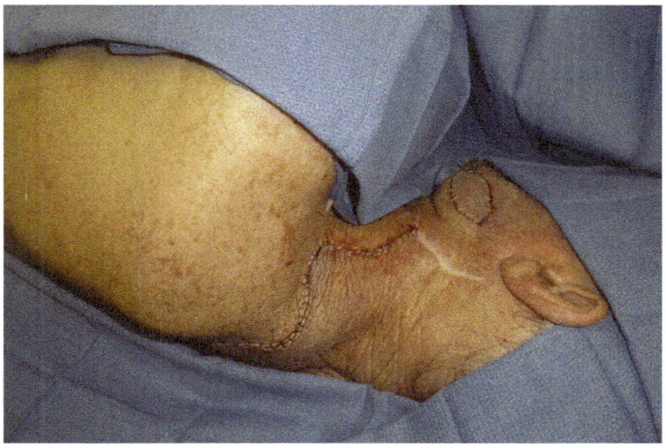

Fig. 18.6 Inset of the flap and closure of the donor site.

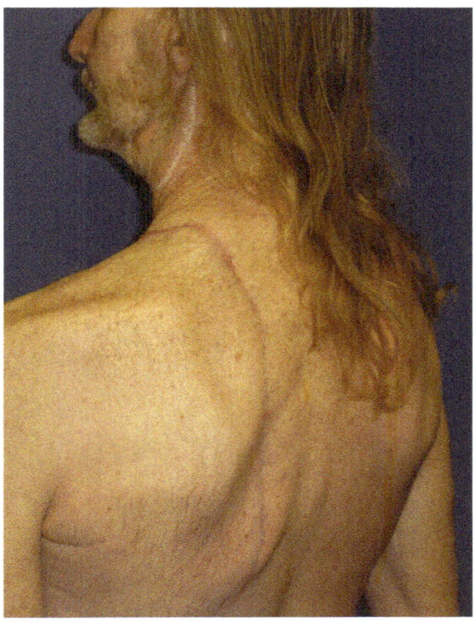

Fig. 18.7 Late postoperative view of the donor site and recipient site.

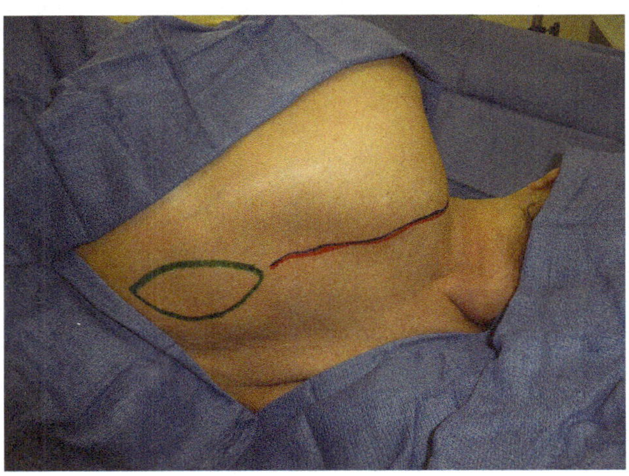

Fig. 18.8 View of a patient in a lateral decubitous position with markings for a trapezius flap.

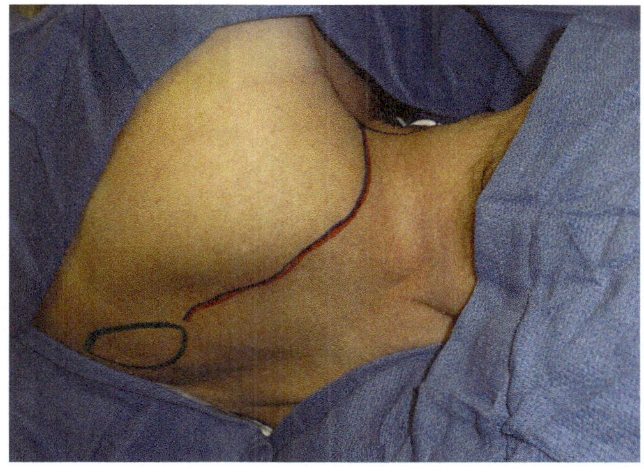

Fig. 18.9 Another view of the markings for the flap with extension of the incision towards the neck.

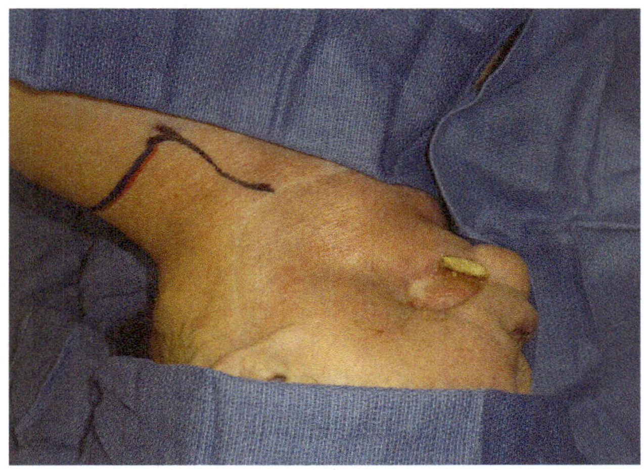

Fig. 18.10 View of the exposed mandible in a patient with ORN and a large oral cutaneous fistula.

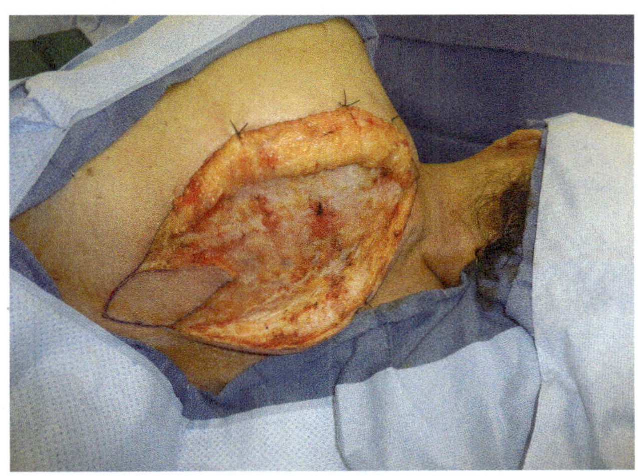

Fig. 18.11 Reflection of the skin flaps exposing the trapezius flap with location of the skin paddle at the inferior extent.

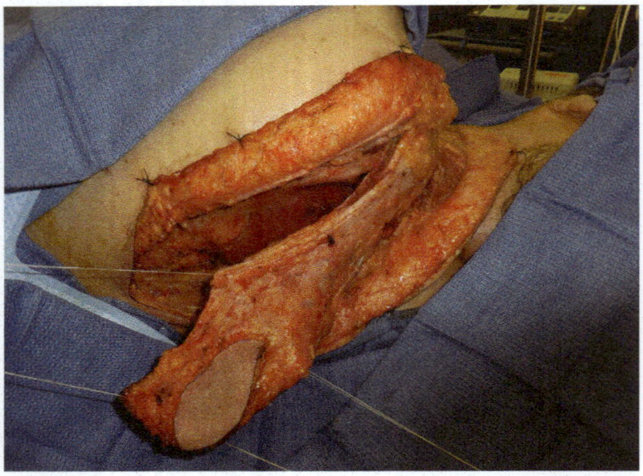

Fig. 18.12 View of the elevated flap prior to rotation and transfer to the defect site.

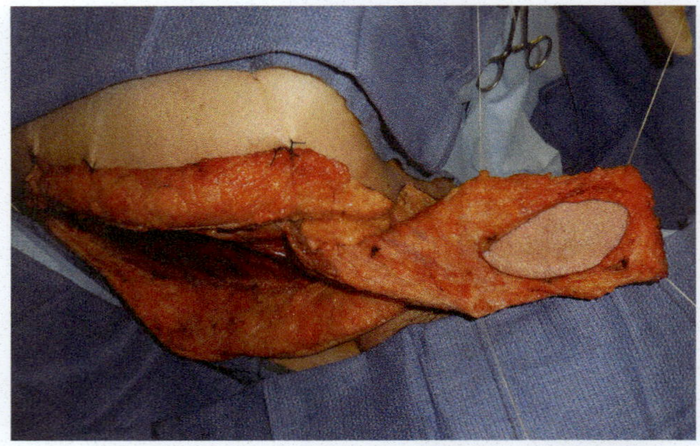

Fig. 18.14 Rotation of the flap to expose the skin paddle prior to inset.

described and the location of the dorsal scapular vessels were confirmed and protected. The arc of rotation of the flap was then assessed (Figures 18.12 and 18.13). After the necrotic mandibular bone was resected, the flap was transferred to the defect and the oral cavity, and the skin defects were also repaired (Figures 18.14 and 18.15).

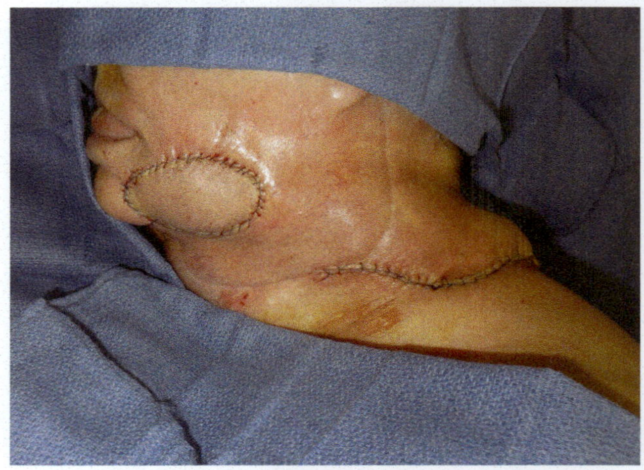

Fig. 18.15 Inset of the flap and closure of the donor site.

Case #2

A 60-year-old Caucasian female was referred for the management of a recalcitrant scalp wound. She had a history of meningioma, which had been treated with multiple surgical resections and radiation therapy. She had failed those therapeutic modalities and was now left with a persistent scalp wound composed of missing and unstable skin as well as necrotic bone with underlying exposed dura (Figure 18.16). After discussion at the tumor board, a

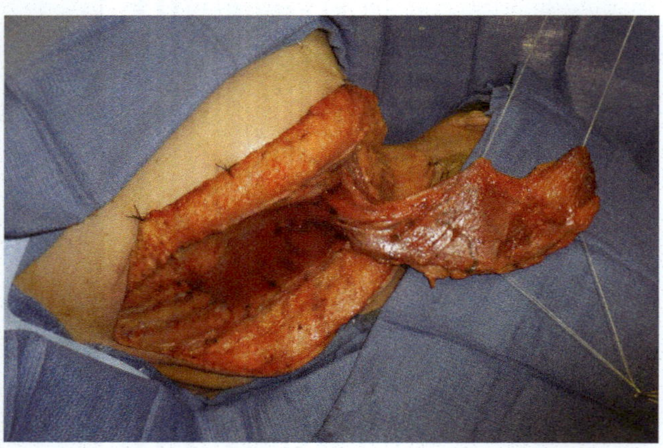

Fig. 18.13 Assessment of the arc of rotation and reach of the flap to the defect site.

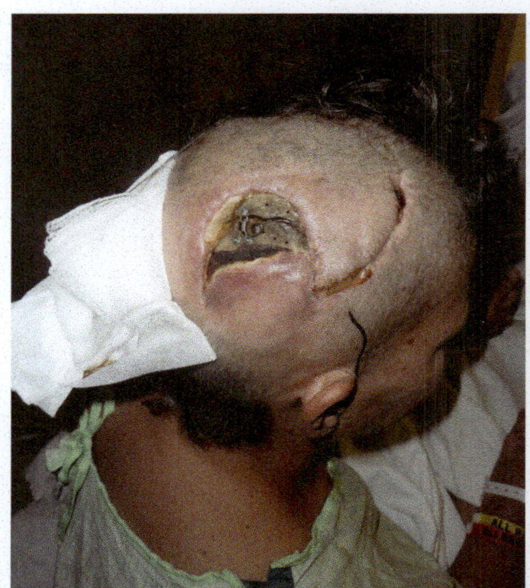

Fig. 18.16 View of a patient with refractory skull and scalp lesion following radiotherapy and multiple failed surgical interventions.

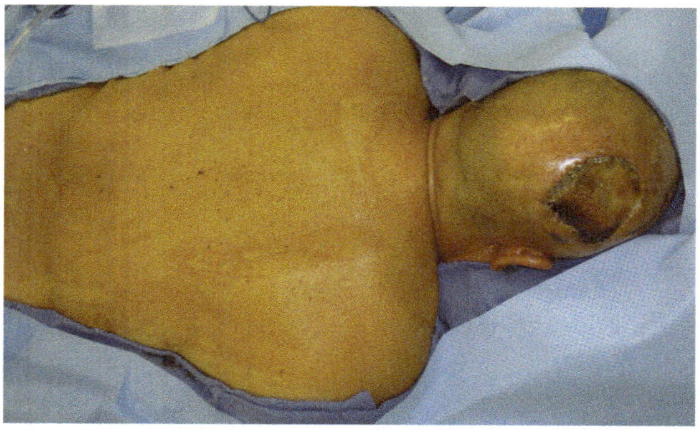

Fig. 18.17 Patient is placed in a prone position for the harvest of an extended vertical trapezius flap to repair the defect.

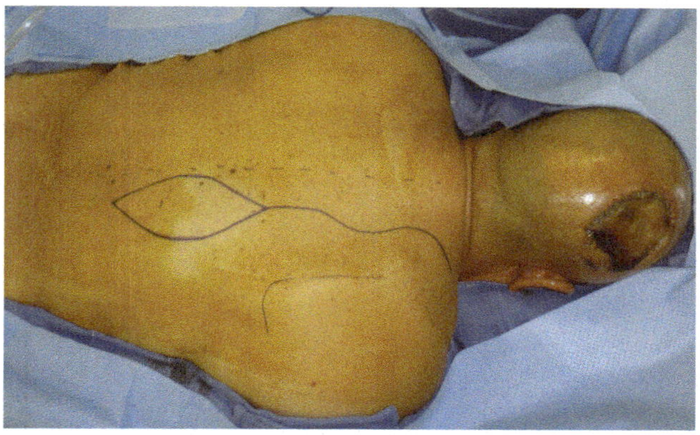

Fig. 18.18 Markings for the flap with placement of a skin paddle.

decision was made to offer the patient a palliative repair of the wound to allow her to return home. The patient was taken to the operating room and placed in a prone position not only to expose the scalp wound but also to allow for the eventual harvest of an extended trapezius flap (Figure 18.17). The markings for the musculocutaneous flap were made after measuring the location of the

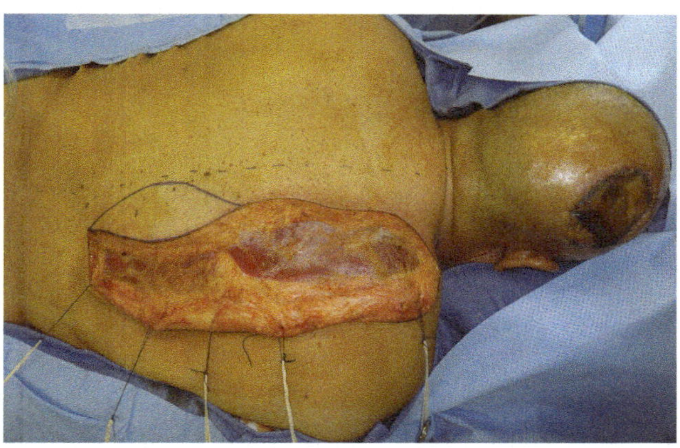

Fig. 18.19 Exposure of the trapezius muscle with confirmation of the placement of the skin paddle over the muscle.

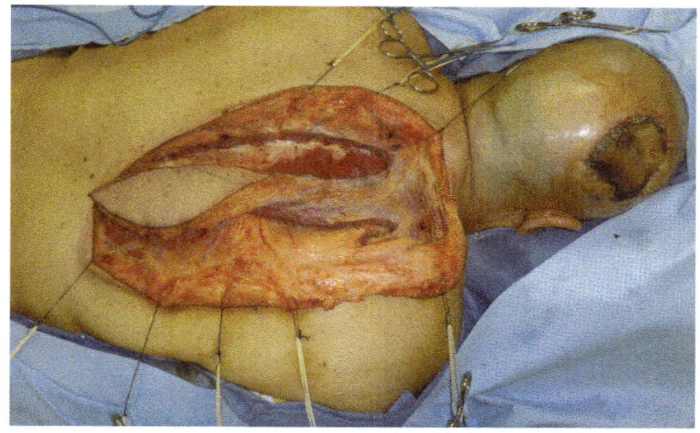

Fig. 18.20 Final exposure of the flap prior to rotation and transfer.

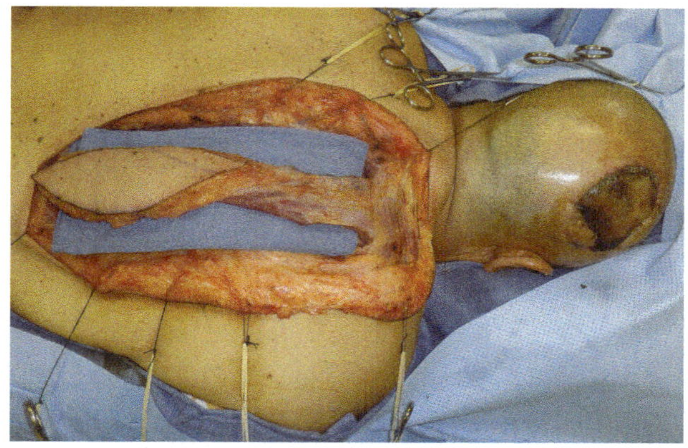

Fig. 18.21 Another view of the raised flap prior to transfer.

defect from the pivot point and transferring the information to the back (Figure 18.18). The flap was then elevated as described earlier by first raising the skin flaps and assuring that the skin paddle was located over the trapezius muscle (Figure 18.19). The medial component of the flap was dissected and the flap elevated towards the base of the neck and the dorsal scapular artery (Figures 18.20 and 18.21). The flap was then rotated and inset into the defect after the wound bed had been prepared (Figure 18.22).

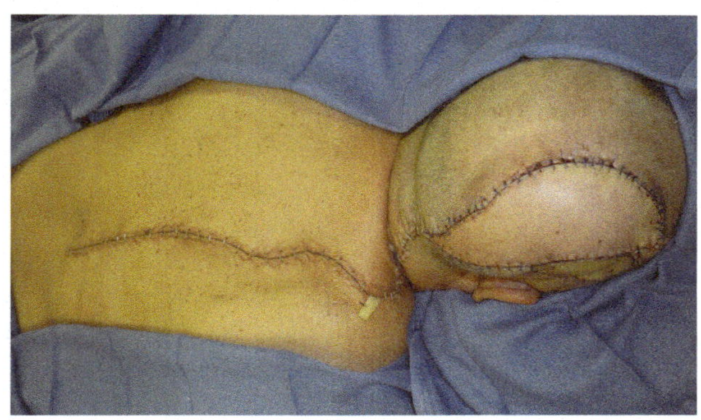

Fig. 18.22 Transferred flap and primary closure of the donor site.

References

1. Netterville JL, Panje WR, Maves MD. The trapezius myocutaneous flap dependability and limitations. *Arch Otolaryngol Head Neck Surg* 1987; 113:271–281.
2. Conley J. Use of composite flaps containing bone for major repairs in the head and neck. *Plast Reconstr Surg* 1972; 49:522–526.
3. Panje WR. The island (lateral) trapezius flap. Presented at the Third International Symposium of Plastic and Reconstructive Surgery; New Orleans, LA; April 29–May 4, 1978.
4. Demergasso F. The lateral trapezius flap. Presented at the Third International Symposium of Plastic and Reconstructive Surgery; New Orleans, LA; April 29–May 4, 1978.
5. Mathes SJ, Nahai F. *Clinical Atlas of Muscle and Musculocutaneous Flaps*. St. Louis, MO: Mosby. 1979. p. 396.
6. Baek S, Biller HF, Krespi YP, et al. The lower trapezius island myocutaneous flap. *Ann Plast Surg* 1980; 5:108–114.
7. Krespi YP, Oppenheimer RW, Flanzer JM. The rhombo-trapezius myocutaneous and osteocutaneous flaps. *Arch Otolaryngol Head Neck Surg* 1988; 114:734–738.
8. Netterville JL, Wood DE. The lower trapezius flap vascular anatomy and surgical technique. *Arch Otolaryngol Head Neck Surg* 1991; 117:73–76.
9. Chen WL, Deng YF, Peng JS, et al. Extended vertical lower trapezius island myocutaneous flap for reconstruction of cranio-maxillofacial defects. *Int J Oral Maxillofac Surg* 2007; 36:165–170.

Chapter 19
The supraclavicular artery island flap

The supraclavicular island flap has only recently gained popularity as a definitive option in head and neck reconstruction. The beginnings of this flap date back to Kazanjian and Converse when they described the acromial flap or "in Charretera".[1] Since this description, there has been a significant improvement in the understanding of the regional anatomy, which has led to a more predictable and robust flap. The step towards better understanding of the supraclavicular flap began with the publication of Lamberty and Cormack[2] where they described the vascular anatomy of the flap and demonstrated its reliability. The supraclavicular flap continued to exist in the surgical background without gaining a foothold in the reconstructive options of most surgeons. Pallua and his colleagues are credited with the first description of the flap as a "supraclavicular artery island flap"[3] and with a modification which eventually helped the establishment of this flap as a true contender in head and neck reconstruction. Since this description, there have been several publications in the literature describing the reliability of the flap in several options for reconstructing head and neck defects as well as in the anterior chest region.

The supraclavicular flap has several advantageous properties which has rendered it a preferred flap for the reconstruction of the lower face and neck for many reconstructive surgeons. One of the main advantages is that it is a thin and pliable flap. This property allows it to be used in situations where there is a need for resurfacing of the face or neck without the added bulk encountered in myocutaneous flaps. An additional advantage is that it also provides a very similar color match to the defect area and has a similar texture. The pliability of the flap allows it to be tubed when needed for pharyngeal reconstruction as well as for the reconstruction of stomal defects in cases where there is a soft tissue defect above or below the stoma following ablation of stomal recurrences. The supraclavicular flap is an easy flap to harvest. In the hands of experienced surgeons, the average time to raise the flap is less than one hour.[4,5] Additionally, the supraclavicular flap remains a viable reconstructive option even in patients who have undergone a previous neck dissection.[6] The use of this flap in the multiply operated and often vessel-depleted neck makes it a very attractive option for these challenging cases.

The supraclavicular island flap has relatively few disadvantages. The main one is that the quantity of tissue available for transfer is restricted to what can be harvested while still allowing for primary closure. Another disadvantage related to the tissue available for harvest is the length of the flap. The ideal is to not travel beyond the insertion of the deltoid muscle as this will begin to render the tip of flap more dependent on random perfusion and thus susceptible to ischemia and necrosis.

Anatomy

The main blood supply to the flap is the supraclavicular artery which is a branch from the transverse cervical artery. The artery can be found in a triangle formed by the sternocleidomastoid muscle, the external jugular vein, and the clavicle. The artery exits 3.0 – 0.7 cm above the clavicle at a distance of 8.2 ± 1.7 cm from the sternoclavicular joint and approximately 2.1 ± 0.9 cm dorsal to the sternocleidomastoid muscle.[7] The mean diameter of the artery is 1.5 mm.

The venous drainage to the flap consists of two veins. One runs along the artery as a venae commitantes and eventually drains into the transverse cervical artery, while the other is a branch of the external jugular vein and drains into the subclavian vein.

The skin area that can be harvested with this flap ranges from 10–16 cm wide to 22–30 cm long. The distal end of this flap can extend to the midportion of the

Local and Regional Flaps in Head & Neck Reconstruction: A Practical Approach, First Edition. Rui Fernandes.

Companion website: www.wiley.com/go/fernandes/flapsreconstruction

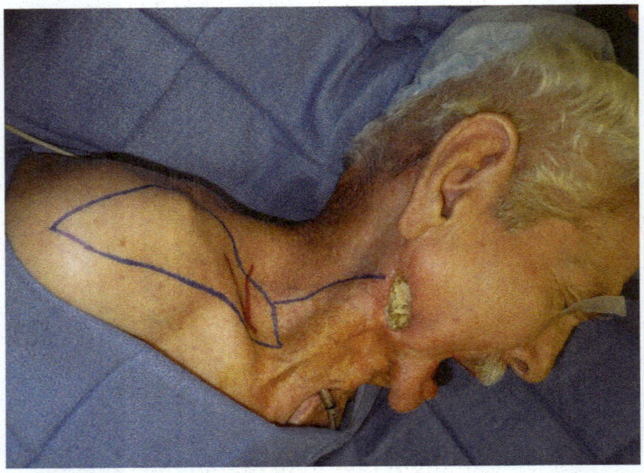

Fig. 19.1 View of exposed mandible with ORN in a previously operated and radiated patient.

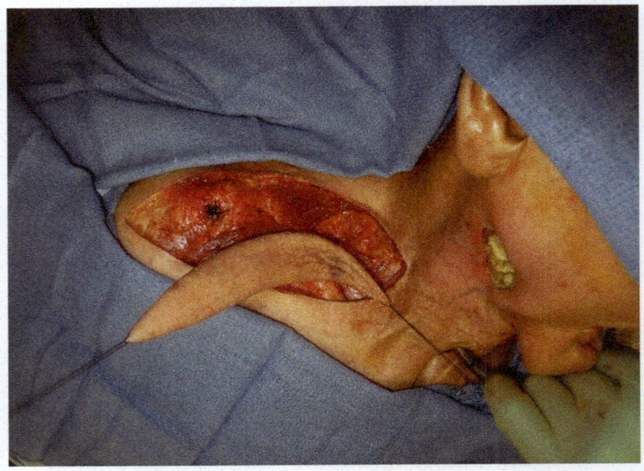

Fig. 19.3 Elevation of the supraclavicular flap.

deltoid with a slight anterior placement. The design of the skin flap is usually fusiform.

Flap harvest

The flap harvest is depicted in Figures 19.1 to 19.10.

The patient is positioned in a lateral decubitous position or supine with a roll under the ipsilateral shoulder. The defect area is measured and the shape of the defect is noted and transferred to the ipsilateral shoulder directly overlying the angiosome of the flap. Using a handheld Doppler, the main pedicle is identified and traced both laterally as well as medially towards the transverse cervical artery and the thyrocervical trunk.

- The elevation of the flap begins from the distal to the medial direction.
- An incision is made at the distal tip of the flap and deepened to the fascia overlying the deltoid muscle.
- A subfascial dissection is elevated in a medial approach towards the mid-third of the clavicle.
- At this region, some deltoid perforators to the skin may be encountered. These perforators can be divided with bipolar cautery.
- Completion of the skin incision is performed circumferentially along the skin island. Care should be taken not to extend the incision deeper than the subcutaneous tissue so the vascular pedicle is not injured.
- The vascular pedicle may be seen coursing through the skin island if transilluminated.
- Dissection is continued in a medial direction in a combination of blunt and bipolar dissection.
- Once the vascular pedicle is identified, a large dominant vein and a smaller venae commitante may be seen; if the second vein from the external jugular vein

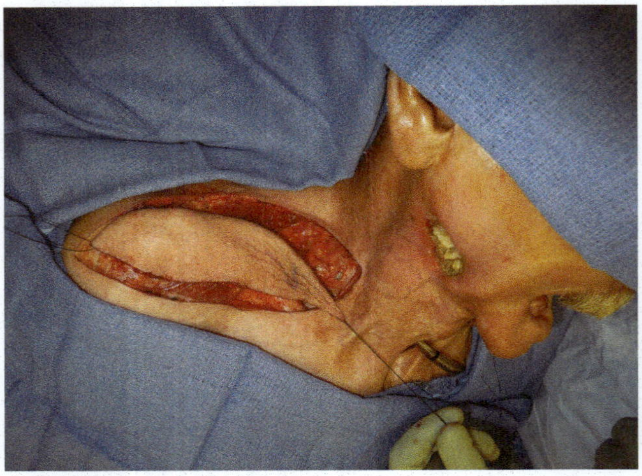

Fig. 19.2 Elevation of a supraclavicular flap prior to transfer.

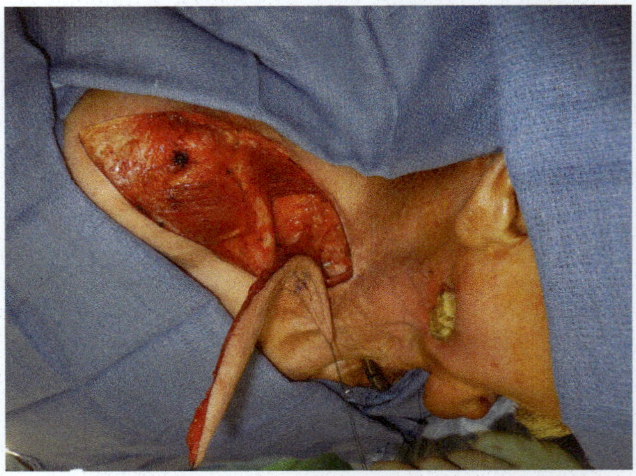

Fig. 19.4 Exposure of the vascular pedicle of the supraclavicular flap.

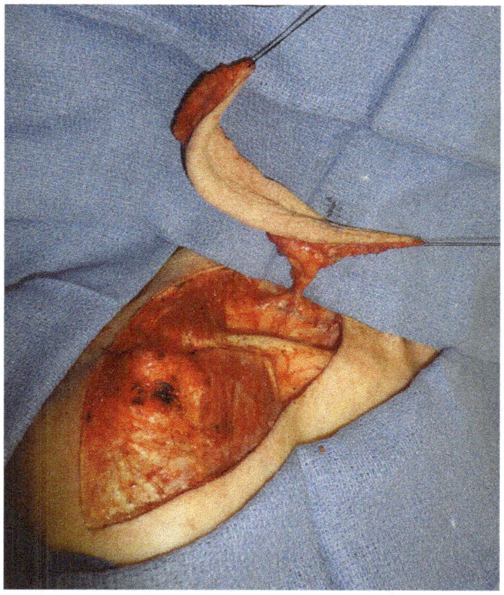

Fig. 19.5 Dissected vascular pedicle demonstrating good length of the pedicle.

is limiting the arc of rotation, a decision to sacrifice it can be made after placing an Auckland clamp on it and waiting several minutes to see if venous congestion develops on the skin flap.

- As the dissection proceeds medially and posteriorly, a small artery and vein may also be encountered; this is often the dorsal scapular artery and again, if it is limiting the arc of rotation, it too can be ligated and divided.
- Once the flap is elevated and there is sufficient pedicle dissection, adequate tension-free rotation of the flap to the defect should be checked. If the flap is able to reach the desired defect without any impediment, then dissection is complete. If there is tension or need for further reach, an attempt can be made at further freeing any restriction to the rotation and advancement of the flap along the base of the pedicle.

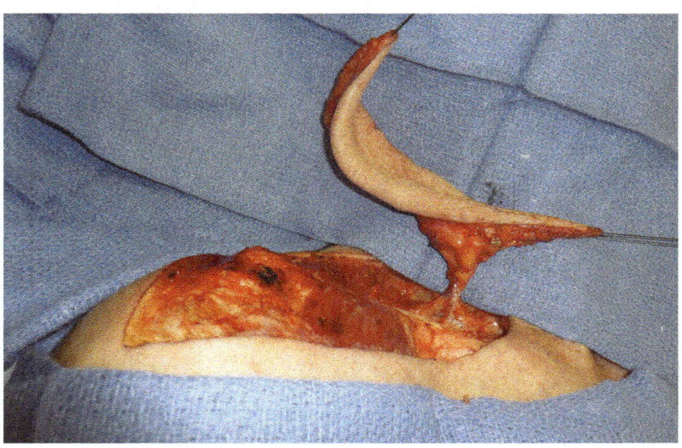

Fig. 19.6 Another view of the vascular pedicle to the supraclavicular flap.

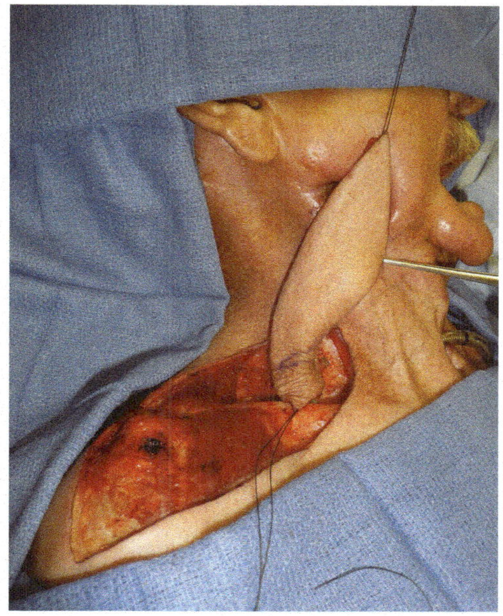

Fig. 19.7 Assessment of the rotation of the flap towards the defect.

- The transfer of the flap to the defect side can be made by a releasing skin incision along the bridge of skin between the donor site and the defect site or, if chosen, the flap can be tunneled to the recipient site.
- In cases where a tunneled flap is chosen, particular careful needs to be taken when de-epithelializing the skin so the entire flap is not compromised. Equally important is the adequate development of a wide unrestricting tunnel. If the tunnel is too narrow, it can cause compression of the flap and potentially lead to flap loss.
- The closure of the donor site can nearly always be done primarily. Only in rare circumstances will there be a need for skin grafting.

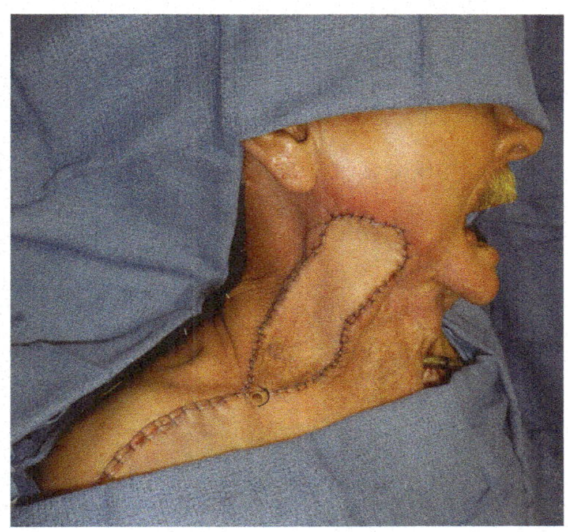

Fig. 19.8 Inset of the flap, repairing the skin defect and providing coverage for the mandible.

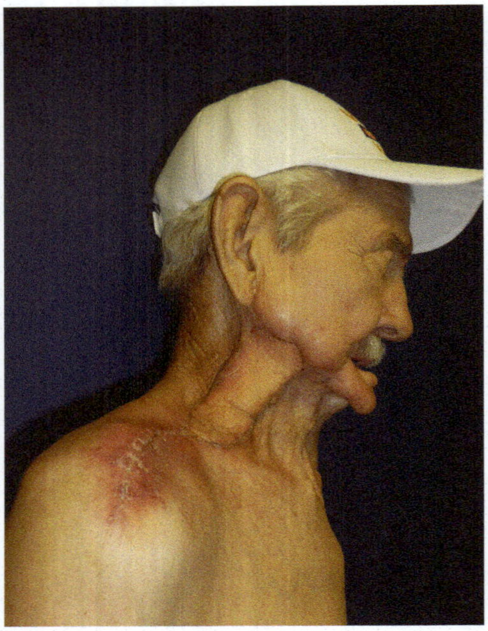

Fig. 19.9 Early postoperative view of the reconstruction.

- Prior to closing the defect, the tissues anteriorly as well as posteriorly should be widely undermined. The undermining should frequently reassessthe advancement of the two skin edges to enable closure without significant tension.
- The inset of the flap is carried out as dictated by the defect site.

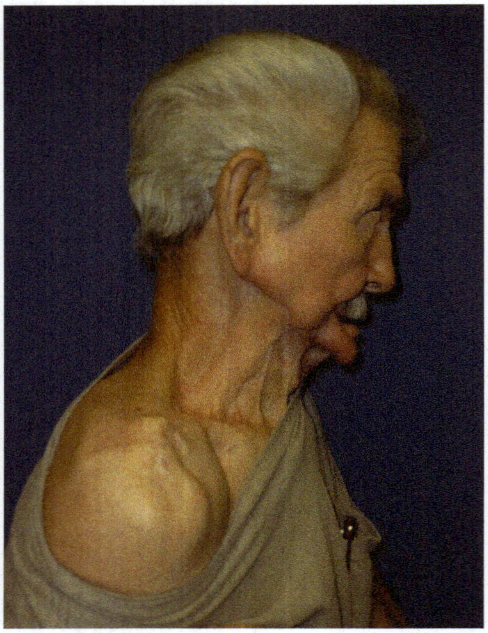

Fig. 19.10 Late postoperative view of the reconstruction; note the excellent color match.

Special circumstances

One of the best properties of the supraclavicular artery island flap is not only the color and texture but the thickness of the flap. This makes it an ideal flap in circumstances where a large volume of thin, pliable tissue is needed for resurfacing of the neck or face, particularly in burn contracture patients. Given that the maximum width that can be harvested from the donor site and that still allows closure is 16 cm, in cases where a greater volume of tissue is needed, consideration should be given to pre-expansion of the tissue.

The supraclavicular tissue is expanded until the desired amount of tissue is obtained. Once the expansion is complete, the patient is taken back to the operating room for the definitive reconstruction. The pseudocapsule on the undersurface of the expanded tissue is removed and the remainder of the flap harvest is executed as previously described.

Advantages

The advantages of the supraclavicular artery island flap are several. The color and texture of the skin is very similar to the surrounding area which makes it a great option for reconstructing regional defects of the head and neck. Additionally, the lack of hair on this region also renders it a good option to reconstruct non-hair bearing regions of the head and neck. The supraclavicular island flap also has the added advantage of ease of harvest, usually taking less than one hour to elevate the flap. Also, the donor site can be easily concealed with everyday clothing. These facts and the reliability of the flap, render the supraclavicular artery island flap one of the key options for the reconstruction of defects on the neck and lower face.

Disadvantages

The main disadvantage of this flap is in fact one of its advantages, that is, it is a thin flap. Often when reconstructing oncologic defects in the head and neck region, additional tissue bulk is desired to restore the defect site. Given that this is a fasciocutaneous flap, it does not allow for a true re-establishing of the lost bulk. Also, the limited quantity of tissue available for transfer without pre-expansion can be a disadvantage in certain situations.

Complications

The most feared complication of this or any other flap is the partial or full loss of the skin paddle. Bearing in mind that this is a regional axial pattern flap, the distal portion of the skin island is most at risk for ischemia and loss. In cases where the viability of the flap is in question, the surgeon may choose to trim the distal portion until viable bleeding tissue is encountered.

In patients previously treated with radiation therapy for their head and neck malignancies, the donor site may pose some additional problems. The most commonly encountered complication in this scenario is dehiscence of the donor site. The dehiscence can be treated with wet to dry dressing in most instances but in rare cases, the exposure of the clavicle warrants a speedier resolution to the problem. In the radiated patient, leaving an exposed bone in order to attempt secondary healing can lead to the eventual development of osteoradionecrosis of the clavicle. Taking this potential complication into account, the exposure should be addressed in a timely fashion in the operating room with debridement and primary closure.

Finally, patients need to be aware of the potential for a widened scar at the donor site. The risk for widening of the scar is often related to the tension at closing. When closure of the donor site is achieved without tension, there is a minimal risk of scar widening, while tension at closure increases the risk.

Case #1

A 65-year-old Caucasian man presented for reconstruction of a large oropharyngo-cutaneous fistula involving the left neck (Figure 19.11). He had a history of squamous cell carcinoma of the left tonsil region, which had been treated initially with radiation therapy to a total of 72 Gray. Following completion of his radiation therapy he underwent a staged modified radical neck dissection for persistent enlarged left cervical nodes. He later developed osteoradionecrosis (ORN) of the left mandible which warranted exploration and debridement through a transcervical approach. Since that intervention, he stated that the defect continued to enlarge and several attempts were made at closure with local tissue flaps but they were not successful. A discussion was undertaken with the patient regarding the complexity of the defect and the potential use of a free tissue transfer. Given the overall medical condition of the patient, it was decided that a supraclavicular flap would be a potential alternative to reconstruct the defect. A decision to use the supraclavicular flap, folded with one skin paddle on the pharyngeal side and the remainder of the flap replacing the missing cervical skin tissues.

The markings for the skin flaps were made on the ipsilateral side of the defect in the preoperative holding and again confirmed intraoperatively with the use of a handheld Doppler (Figures 19.12 and 19.13). The flap was then raised circumferentially, beginning at the distal aspect of the deltoid and moving medially towards the vascular pedicle and the defect site (Figures 19.14 and 19.15). The flap was dissected to the takeoff of the transverse cervical artery (Figure 19.16) and adequate, tension-free rotation to the defect was ensured (Figure 19.17). A small area of the skin paddle was de-epithelialized and the flap was inset into the defect, folded so part of the skin paddle repaired the pharyngeal defect and the rest replaced the missing skin on the neck. The donor site was closed primarily (Figure 19.18).

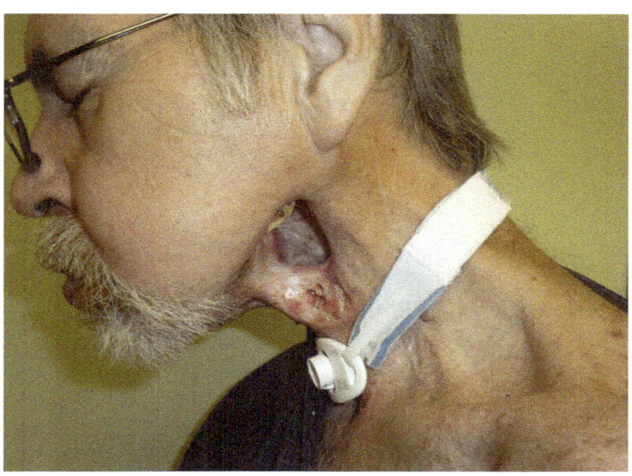

Fig. 19.11 View of a large, complex pharyngeal cutaneous defect in a patient post-chemoradiation.

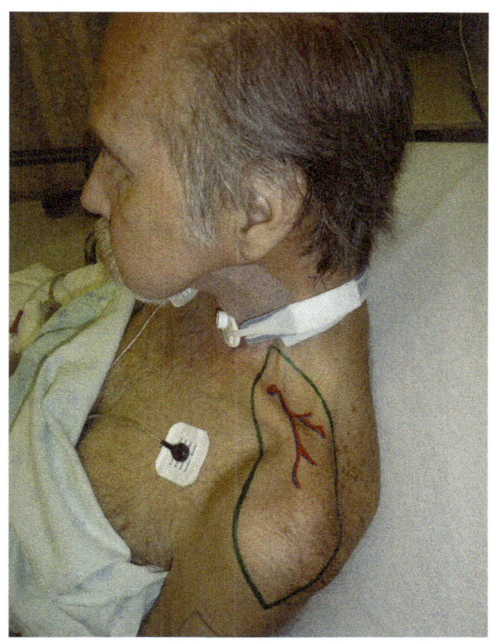

Fig. 19.12 Markings for a large supraclavicular flap to be used in repairing the defect.

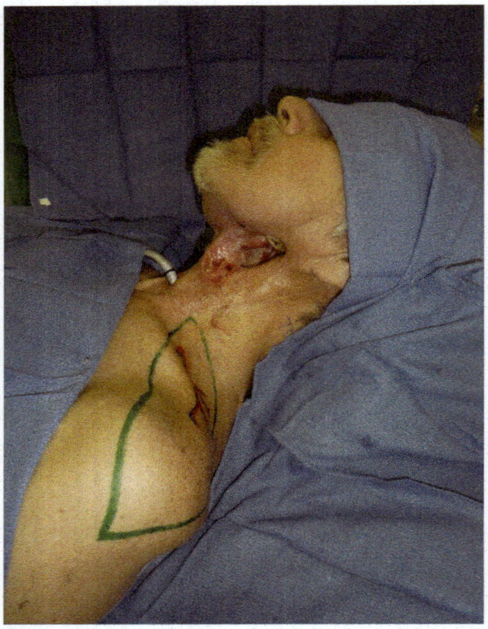

Fig. 19.13 Intraoperative view of the surgical field with the planned flap.

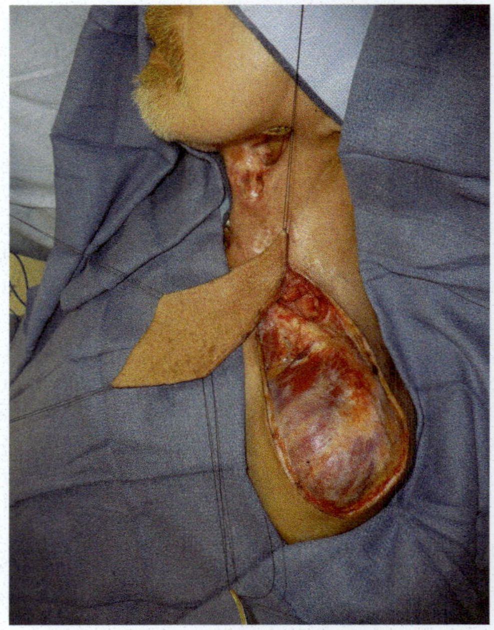

Fig. 19.15 Rotation of the flap with exposure of the left shoulder donor site.

Case #2

A 25-year-old African American male presented for consultation regarding relapsing massive cervicofacial keloids (Figure 19.19). He had a history of multiple attempts at resection of the keloids at another institution including low-dose radiation all of which had failed. Inspection of his face, neck, and anterior and posterior torso revealed numerous keloids with very limited area for harvesting a potential flap.

Given the concern for the formation of additional keloids at the donor sites, the use of a thin free flap or skin graft was abandoned. A discussion was then undertaken with the patient about the potential use of

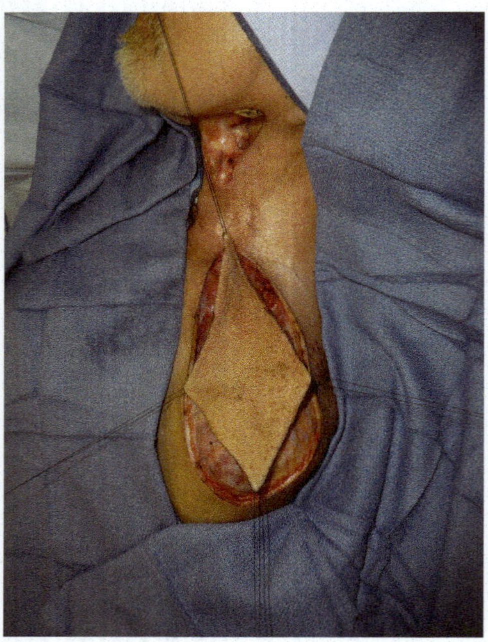

Fig. 19.14 Elevation of the supraclavicular flap.

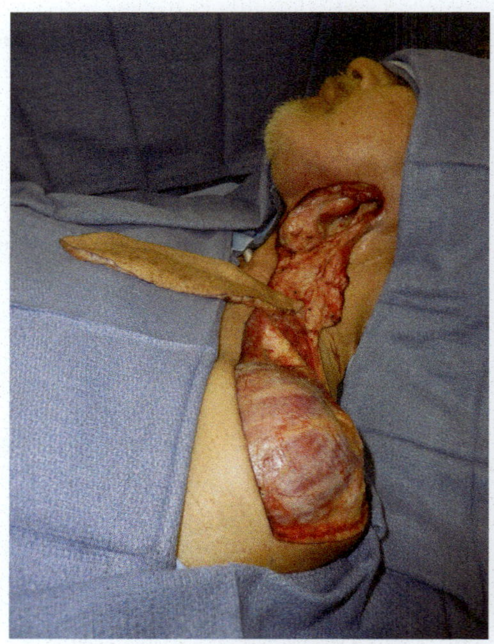

Fig. 19.16 Exposure of the recipient flap with the flap prior to inset.

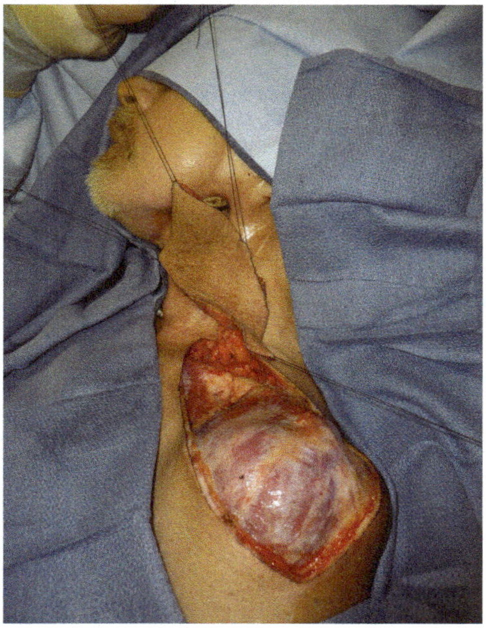

Fig. 19.17 Assessment of the passive rotation of the flap into the defect.

a supraclavicular artery island flap. This decision was made after inspection of both shoulder regions and noting that although he had some keloids in the area, there still existed the potential for raising two flaps to close the defect. Equally importantly, the donor site could be closed primarily and both the donor and recipient site

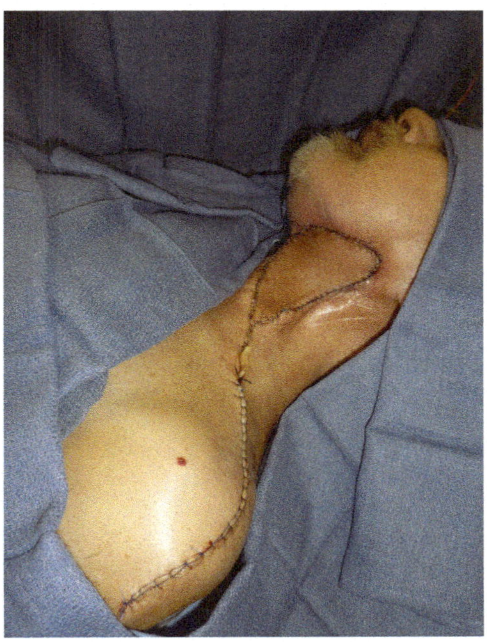

Fig. 19.18 Inset of the flap into the defect as a folded flap with portion of the skin flap repairing the pharyngeal defect and the remaining as a cutaneous coverage.

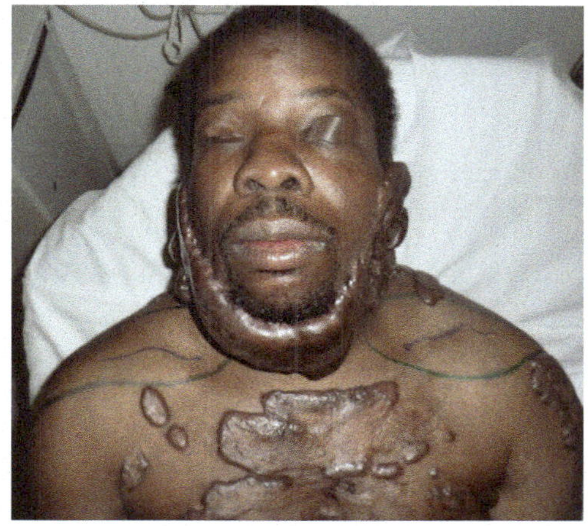

Fig. 19.19 View of a patient with multiple large keloid lesions which have been refractory to surgical and radiation therapy.

could be radiated on postoperative day one as per standard protocol in treating the recalcitrant keloids.

Markings for the bilateral supraclavicular artery island flap were made with care to avoid the existing keloids in the region (Figures 19.20 and 19.21). The flaps were elevated after the excision of the keloids and preparation of the recipient bed. The right supraclavicular flap was tunneled to the defect site while the left was rotated to the defect site (Figures 19.22 to 19.26). A late postoperative

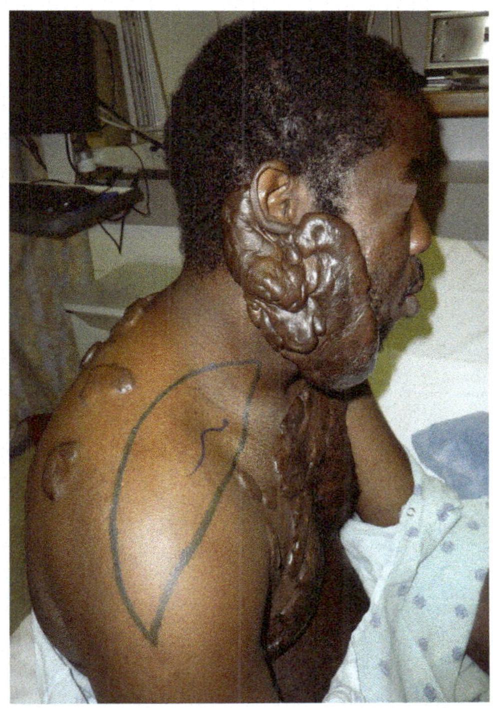

Fig. 19.20 Planning for a supraclavicular flap prior to excision of the extensive facial keloids.

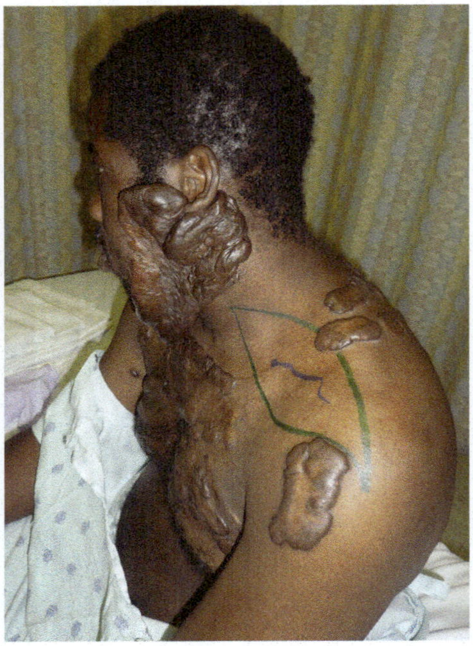

Fig. 19.21 View of the contralateral shoulder with planning for the supraclavicular flap.

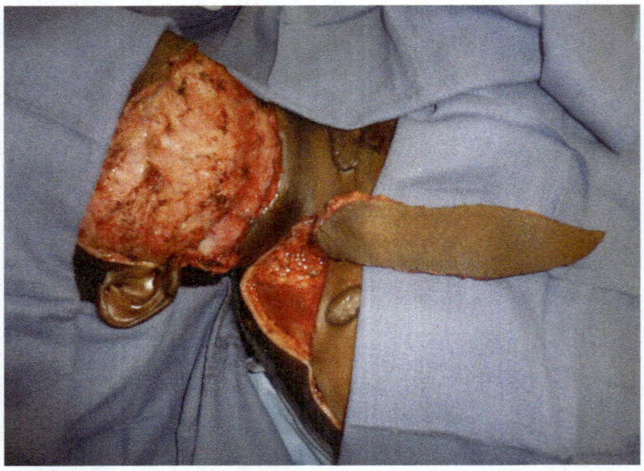

Fig. 19.22 View of the facial skin defect and elevated supraclavicular flap prior to transfer.

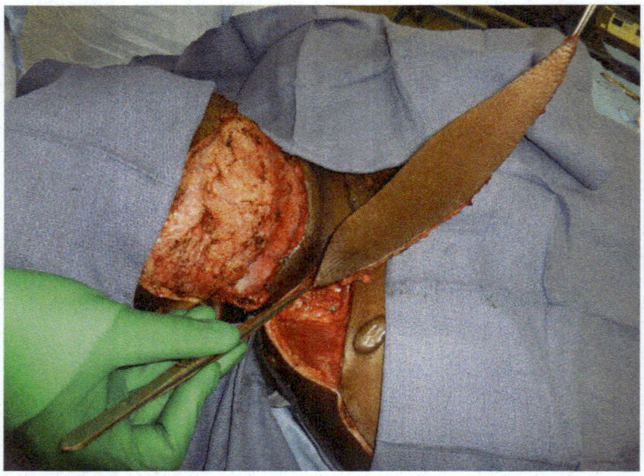

Fig. 19.23 Assessment of the arc of rotation of the right supraclavicular flap prior to inset.

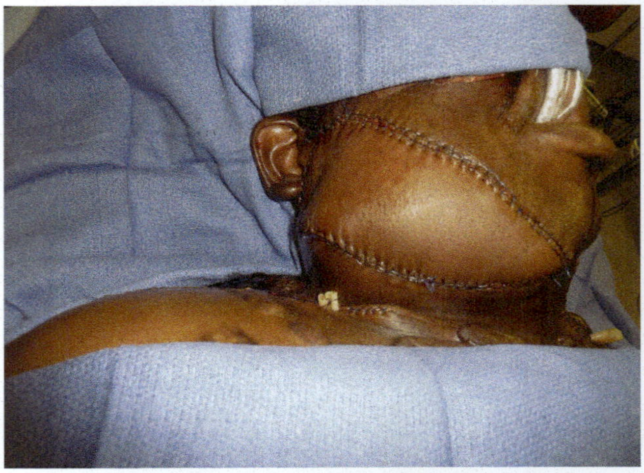

Fig. 19.24 Inset of the right supraclavicular flap into the facial defect.

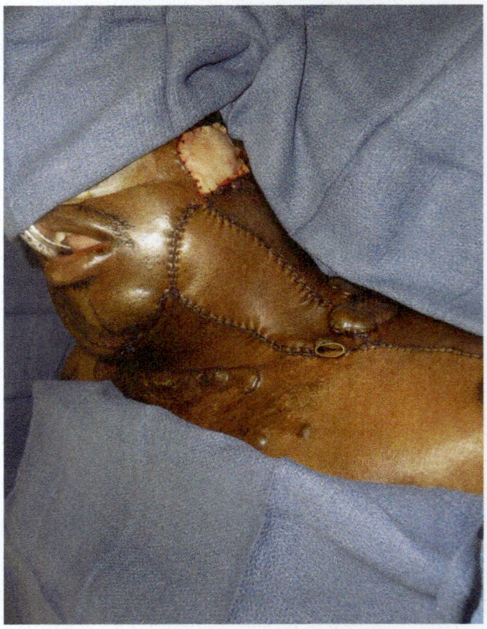

Fig. 19.25 Inset of the left supraclavicular flap into the facial defect.

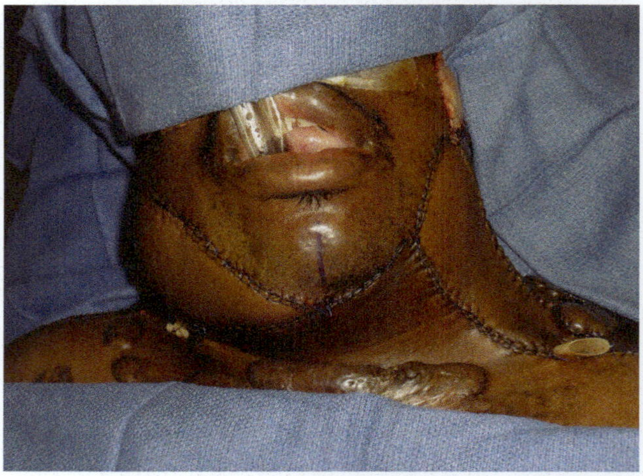

Fig. 19.26 Frontal view of the reconstructed facial defects after removal of the keloids.

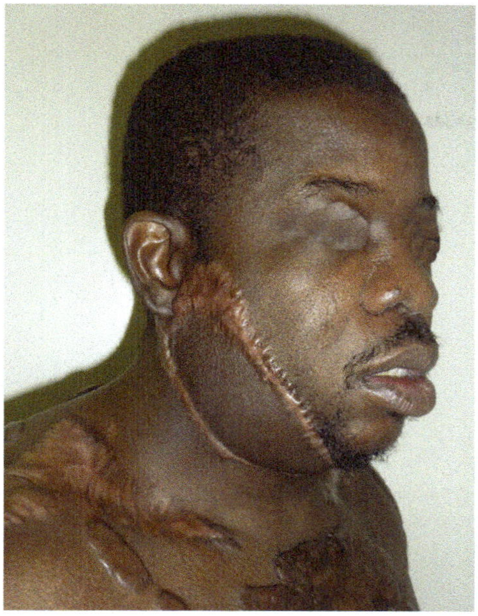

Fig. 19.27 Late view of the reconstructed facial defect with the good color match from the supraclavicular flap.

view of the patient with the keloids removed and the reconstructions in place, show a marked improvement in facial appearance (Figures 19.27 and 19.28).

Case #3

A 75-year-old Caucasian male was referred for the management of a recurrent floor of mouth squamous cell car-

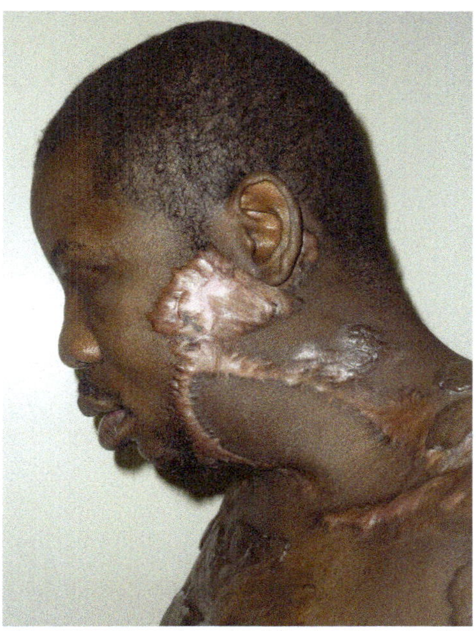

Fig. 19.28 View of the left facial reconstruction with the supraclavicular flap.

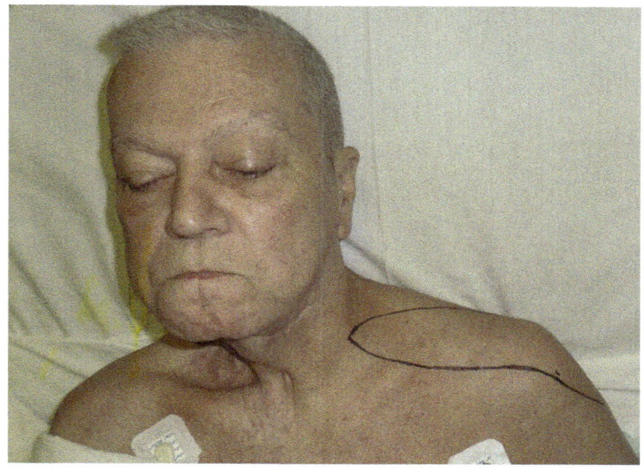

Fig. 19.29 Planning for a supraclavicular flap reconstruction in a patient with a recurrence of an anterior floor of mouth carcinoma after previous resection and radiation therapy.

cinoma (SCCA). He had a history of previous surgical resection for a floor of mouth SCCA treated with a wide local excision, a right radical neck dissection, and selective left neck dissection followed by postoperative adjuvant radiotherapy. At presentation, he was noted to have a small floor of mouth recurrence abutting the mandible but without evidence of invasion. Given his previous treatment and current morbidities, a decision was made to use the supraclavicular island flap to reconstruct the planned defect from a wide local excision with a marginal mandibulectomy. The patient's appearance at the time of surgery is shown in Figure 19.29. The resection was carried out via a midline lip split approach (through the previous incision, note the exposed left shoulder with the marked flap in Figure 19.30).

The flap was harvested in a standard manner as shown in Figure 19.31 and then rotated to the defect to confirm passive reach (Figure 19.32). The flap was then inset into

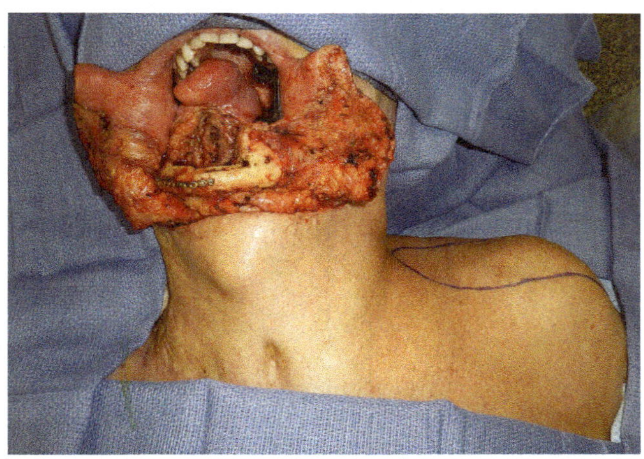

Fig. 19.30 View of the completed resection of the floor of mouth recurrence.

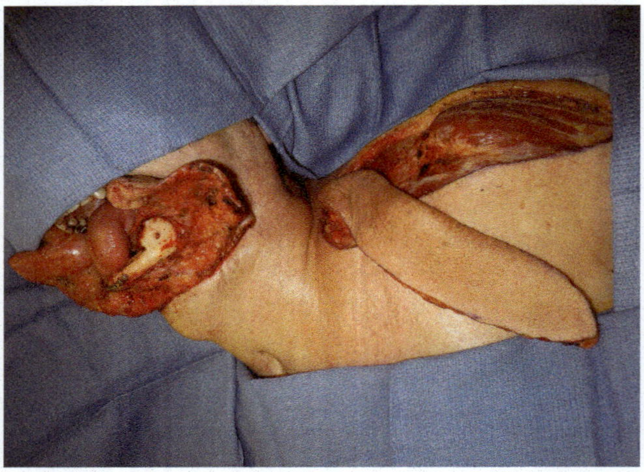

Fig. 19.31 Elevated supraclavicular flap prior to transfer into the oral cavity.

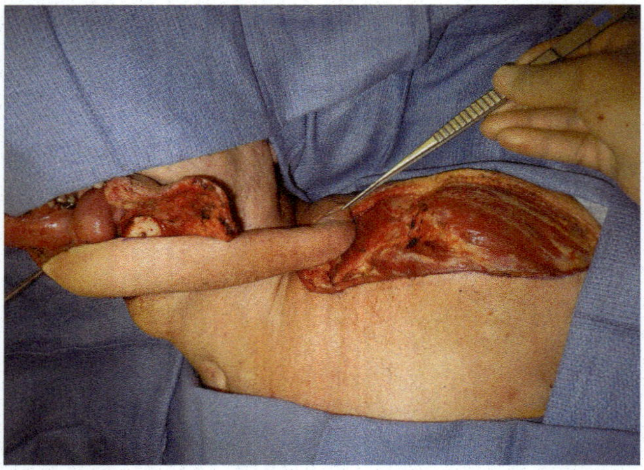

Fig. 19.32 Assessment of the arc of rotation of the flap to confirm passive reach into the oral defect.

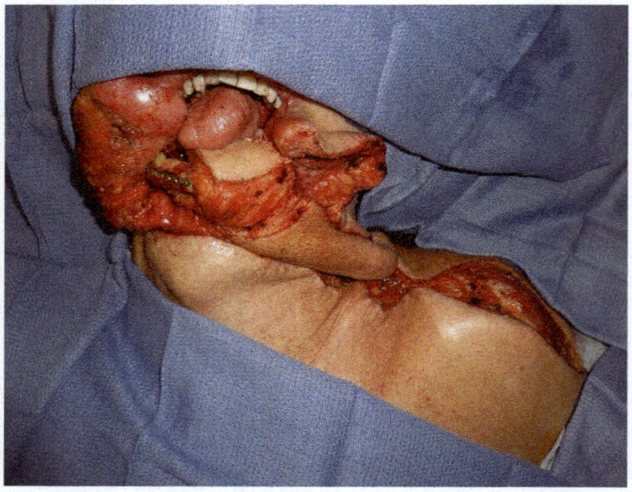

Fig. 19.33 Inset of the flap with de-epithelialized segment prior to replacement and closure of the facial flaps.

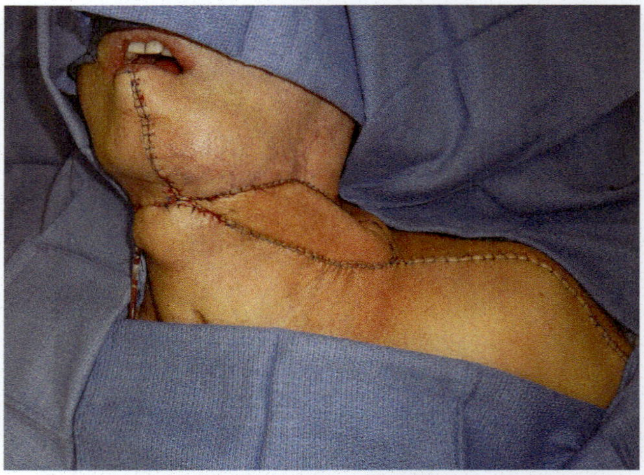

Fig. 19.34 View of the immediate closure with portion of the supraclavicular flap in the neck.

the defect and the buried skin area of the flap was de-epithelialized as shown in Figure 19.33.

The lip split was closed as well as the neck and donor site (Figure 19.34). The early postoperative view of the patient is shown in Figure 19.35.

Case #4

This very pleasant 85-year-old female presented nearly 3 years after resection of a large anterior floor of mouth SCCA. She had undergone a surgical resection that

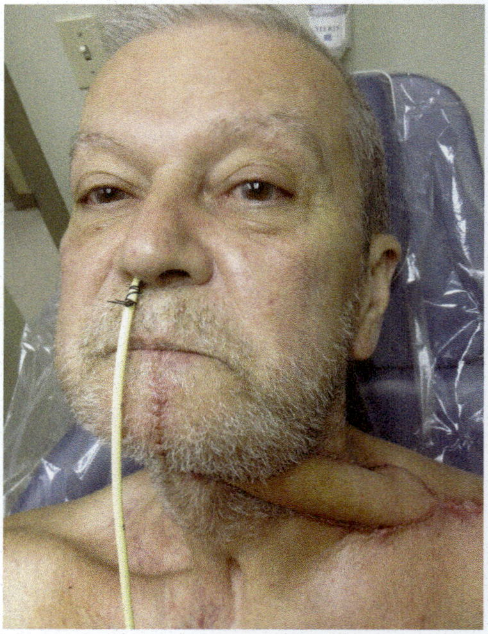

Fig. 19.35 Early postoperative view of the patient with good view of the external flap portion.

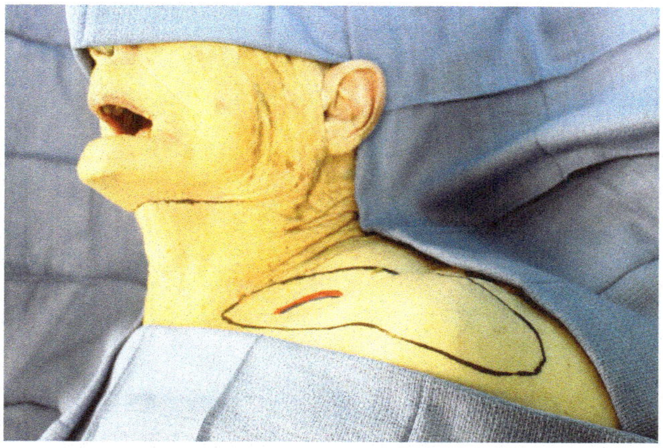

Fig. 19.36 View of a patient with planning for a supraclavicular flap to repair an oral defect.

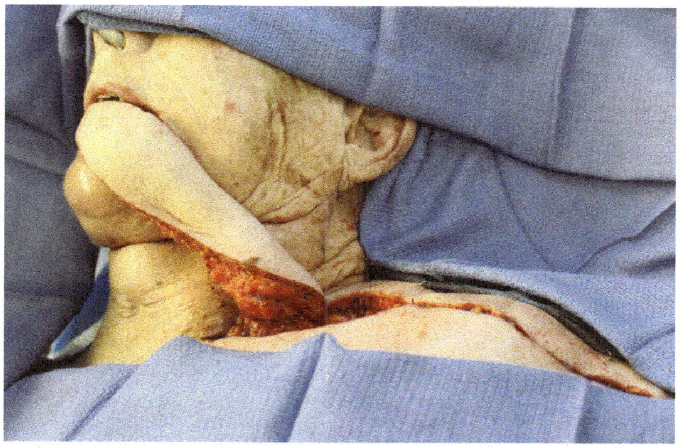

Fig. 19.38 Assessment of the reach of the flap towards the oral cavity.

included segmental mandibulectomy, floor of mouth resection, and bilateral selective neck dissection. At the time of her surgical intervention, it was her's and the her family's wishes that the least invasive surgical therapy be performed due to concerns about her tolerating the procedure, her age, and her life expectancy. Given these concerns, she was reconstructed with local tissue rearrangement and a mandibular reconstruction bar. Three years later, she had recovered well from her cancer treatment but was not pleased with her lip projection, difficulty speaking, and inability to use a denture (Figure 19.36).

A plan was devised to use a supraclavicular island flap and simultaneous repair of the anterior mandibular defect with a non-vascularized iliac crest bone graft that would be covered by the vascularized flap (Figure 19.37). A very nice and thick (due to a larger than normal subcutaneous adipose tissue) flap was harvested and rotated to the planned defect area, ensuring that there would be adequate reach and no tension on closure (Figures 19.37 and 19.38). The portion of the flap that would be tunneled in the neck was de-epithelialized (Figure 19.39). The flap was then inset along with the bone reconstruction of the mandible (Figure 19.40). The patient had an uneventful postoperative healing and was extremely pleased with her reconstruction (Figures 19.41 and 19.42).

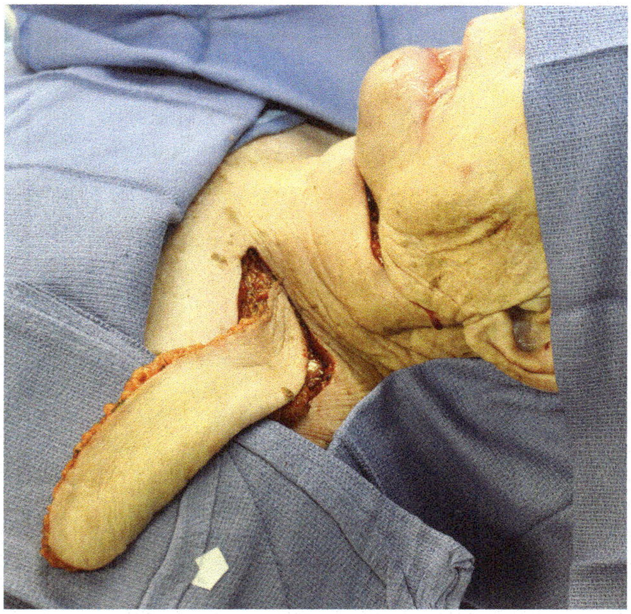

Fig. 19.37 View of the elevated supraclavicular flap prior to transfer.

Case #5

This patient is a 59-year-old Caucasian male with a history of tonsil carcinoma. The patient was referred for salvage surgery after failed chemoradiation therapy. He

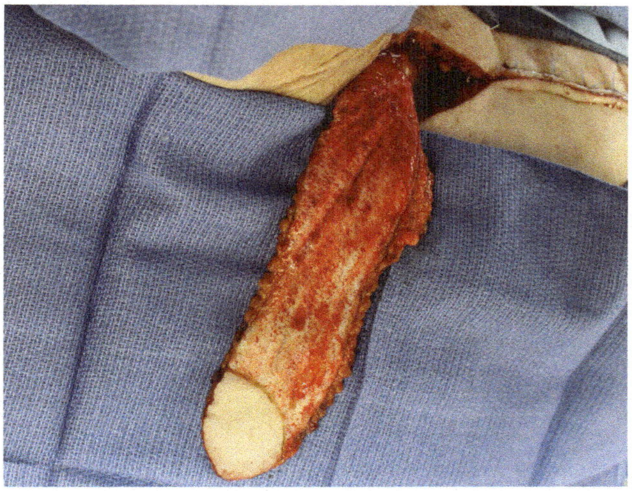

Fig. 19.39 View of the de-epithelialized flap with the skin paddle for the oral cavity repair.

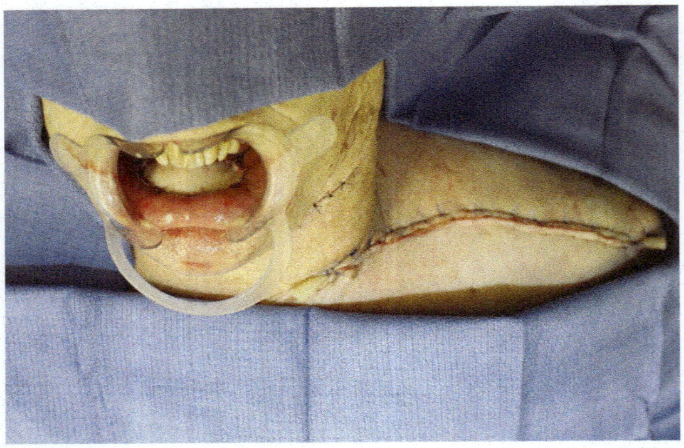

Fig. 19.40 View of the inset of the flap in the oral cavity and closure of the donor site.

presented with a large nodal disease to the neck, which encroached his external carotid artery and other neck vessels, as well as recurrent disease at the primary site. He was treated with a wide excision of the primary and a radical resection of the cervical nodes including sacrifice of the external carotid artery and its branches as well as the jugular venous systems (Figure 19.43). Given the vessel-depleted neck and the presence of the supraclavicular vessels, a decision was made to use the supraclavicular island flap to reconstruct his defect. The planned flap was marked on the ipsilateral neck as seen in Figure 19.44. The flap was elevated and the vascular pedicle was dissected and isolated (Figure 19.45 and 19.46). The flap was then rotated to the defect and the area to be submerged was

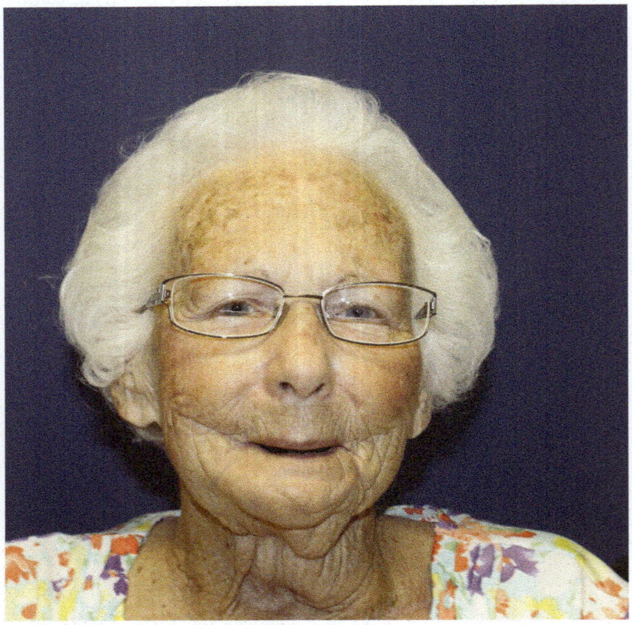

Fig. 19.41 Late postoperative facial appearance.

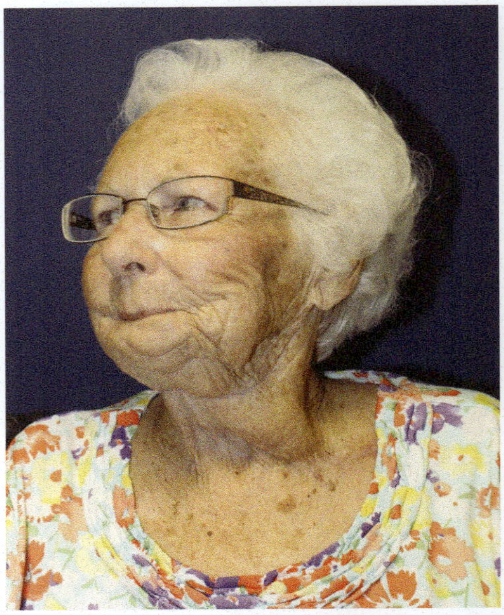

Fig. 19.42 View of the neck which shows that the bulk of the flap is not very large and therefore not conspicuous.

de-epithelialized (Figure 19.47). The inset was then completed and the neck and donor site closed (Figure 19.48). The view of the patient on early postoperative follow up with a good flap contour of the oropharynx is shown in Figure 19.49.

Case #6

This pleasant 83-year-old Caucasian female had undergone a total laryngopharyngectomy and immediate

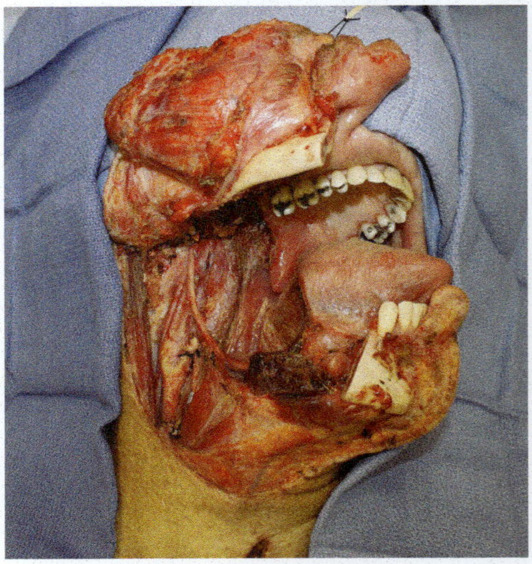

Fig. 19.43 View of a salvage surgery for an oropharyngeal recurrence after failed chemoradiation.

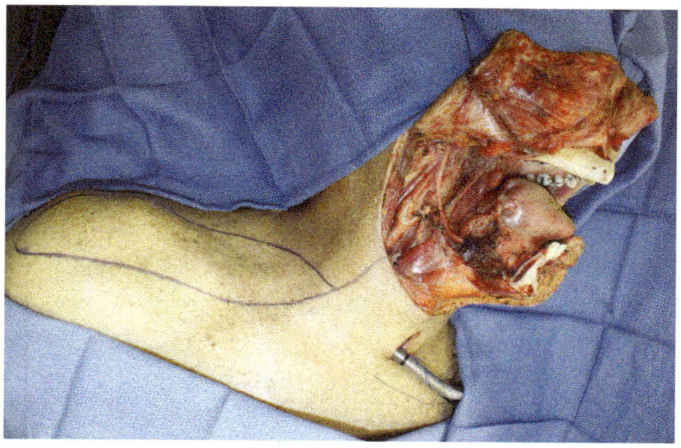

Fig. 19.44 Planning for a supraclavicular flap to be used in the repair of the pharyngeal defect.

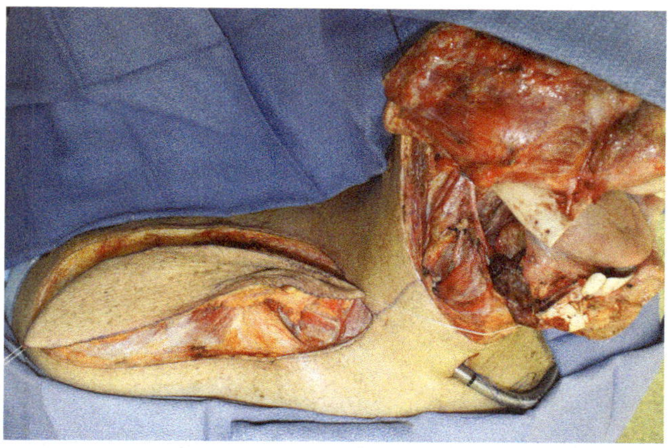

Fig. 19.45 Elevation of the flap prior to transfer.

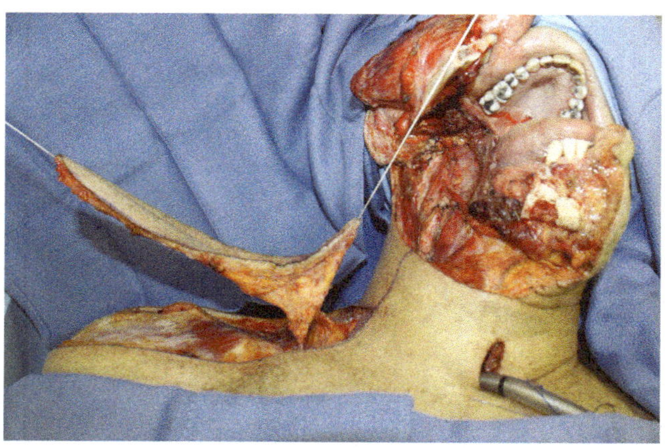

Fig. 19.46 View of the elevated flap with dissected pedicle prior to transfer.

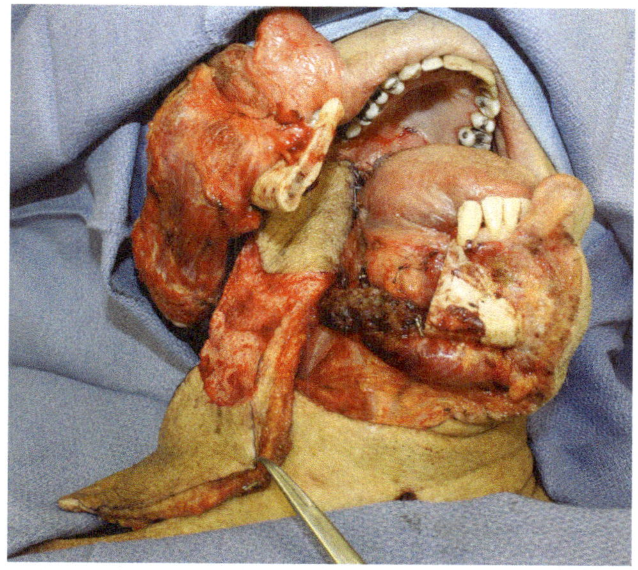

Fig. 19.47 Transfer of the flap with de-epithelialized segment.

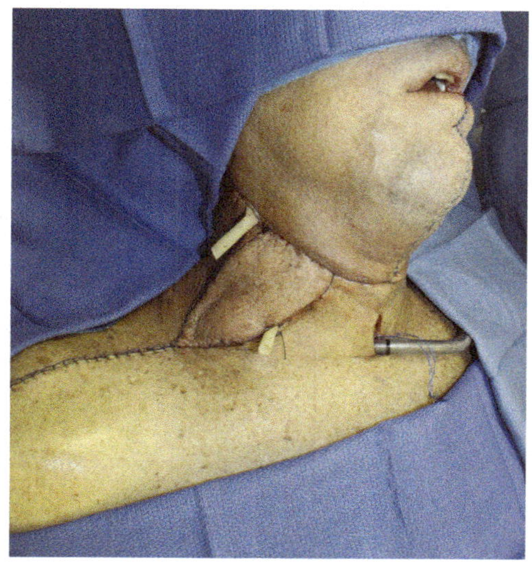

Fig. 19.48 View of the closure of the defect and donor site.

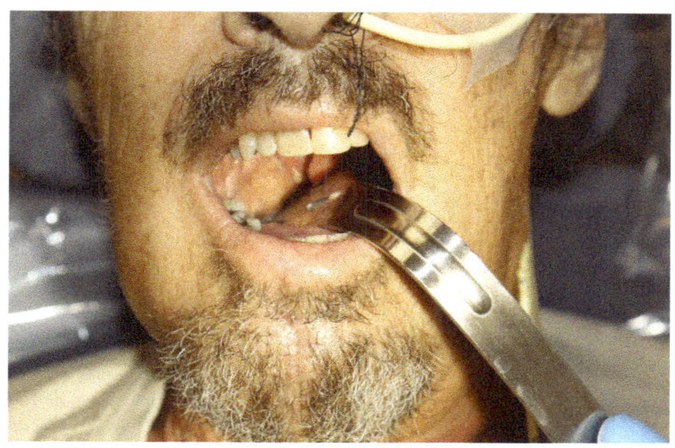

Fig. 19.49 Intraoral view of the reconstructed pharynx.

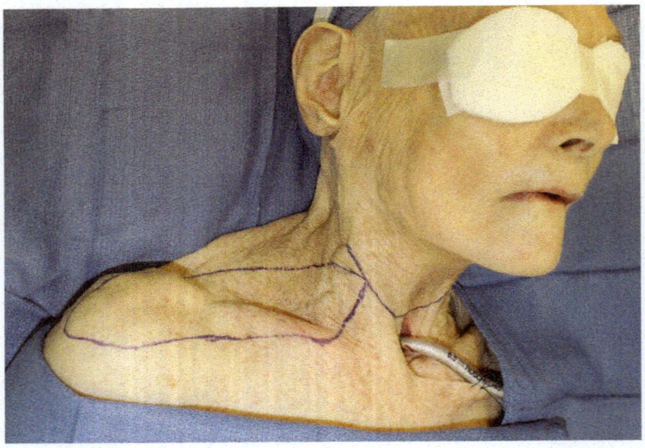

Fig. 19.50 View of the markings for a supraclavicular flap in a patient with pharyngeal stricture.

reconstruction of her pharyngeal defect with a tubed radial forearm free flap. She then received postoperative radiation therapy which she tolerated well. She had an uneventful course and was doing well for nearly 1 year before she began to experience difficulty swallowing. She had a number of dilations, to which she responded well for a few weeks before relapsing. A decision was made to perform an interpositional graft to increase her cervical pharyngeal/esophageal diameter in an attempt to return her to taking food by mouth. She was brought to the operating room where the flap was planned and designed as seen in Figure 19.50. The cervical stricture was opened and the stricture relieved resulting in an anterior pharyngeal defect (Figure 19.51). The flap was then rotated to the defect site, and then the right wall of the defect was repaired (Figures 19.52 and 19.53). The amount of

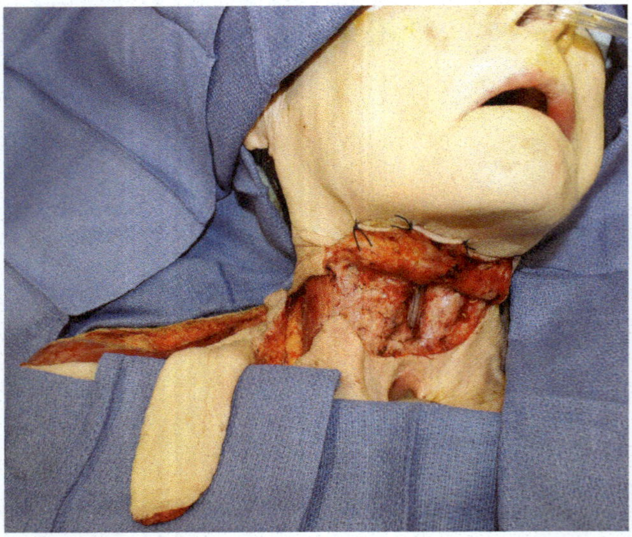

Fig. 19.51 View of the raised pharyngeal flap and opening of the anterior pharyngeal wall.

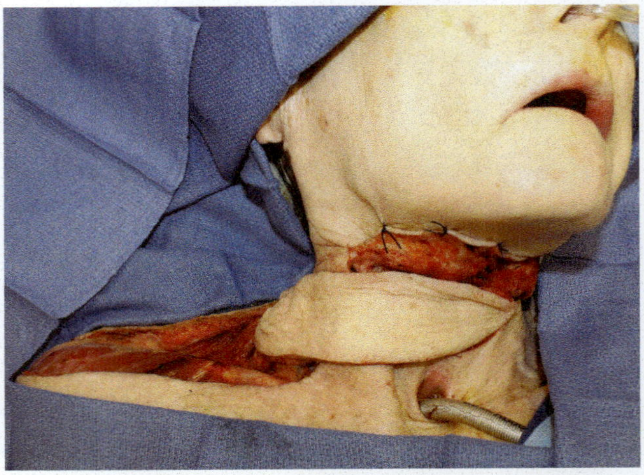

Fig. 19.52 Assessment of the arc of rotation of the flap prior to repair of the pharyngeal stricture.

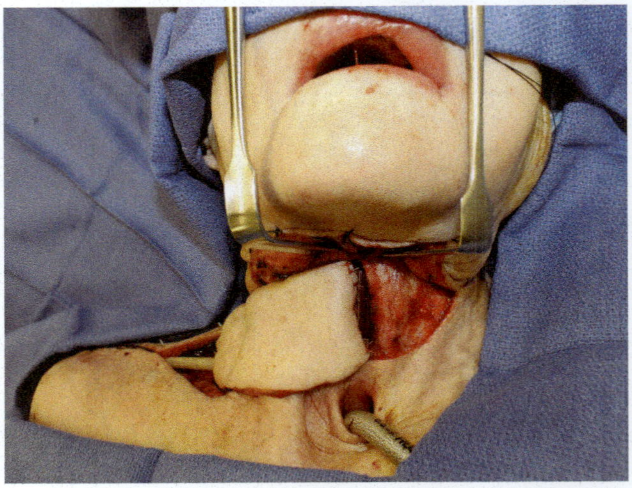

Fig. 19.53 Inset of the flap into the pharyngeal wall to create a new anterior wall.

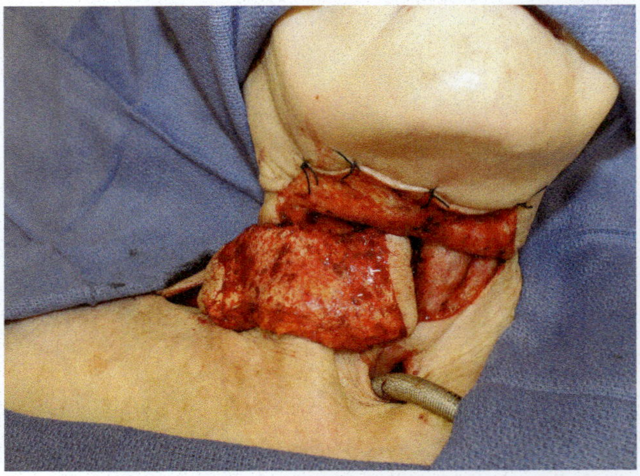

Fig. 19.54 De-epithelialized segment of the flap which will be covered by the neck flap.

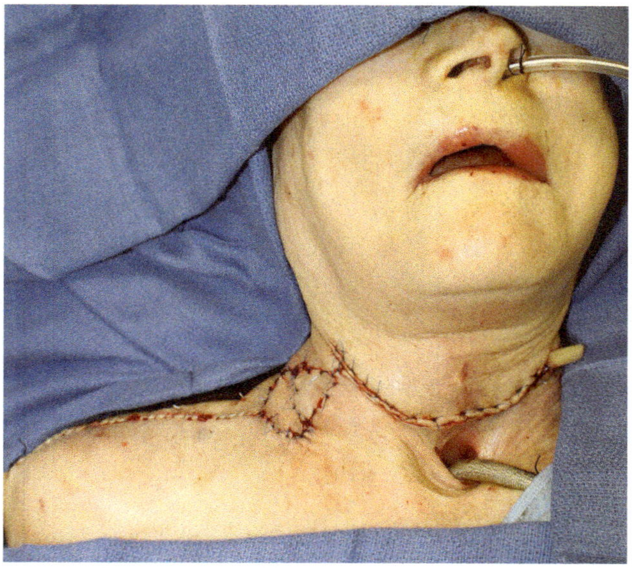

Fig. 19.55 View of the repair at the end of surgery.

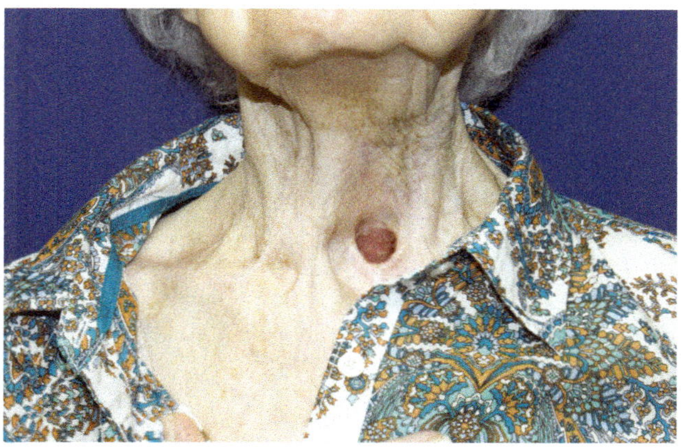

Fig. 19.56 Late view of the patient with restoration of oral intake.

skin needed to repair the anterior defect was measured and the remaining skin was de-epithelialized (Figure 19.54). The edge of the skin of the flap was then advanced to the left pharyngeal wall and inset. The neck and donor site was then closed in a standard manner (Figure 19.55). She tolerated the short procedure well and with the support of speech therapy, she was able to resume per oral intake of foods (Figure 19.56).

References

1. Kazanjian VH, Converse JM. *The Surgical Treatment of Facial Injuries*. Baltimore: Williams & Wilkins, 1949.
2. Lamberty BGH, Cormack GC. Misconceptions regarding the cervico-humeral flap. *Br J Plast Surg* 1983; 36:60–63.
3. Pallua N, Machens HG, Rennekampff O, Becker M, Berger A. The fasciocutaneous supraclavicular artery island flap for releasing postburn mentosternal contractures. *Plast Reconstr Surg* 1997; 99:1878–1884.
4. Levy JM, Eko FN, St. Hilaire H, Friedlander PL, Melgar MA, Chiu ES. Posterolateral skull base reconstruction using the supraclavicular artery island flap. *J Craniofac Surg* 2011; 22:1751–1754.
5. Alves HR, Ishida LC, Ishida LH, Besteiro JM, Gemperli R, Ferreira MC. A Clinical experience of the supraclavicular flap used to reconstruct head and neck defects in late-stage cancer patients. *J Plast Reconstr Aesth Surg* 2012; 65(10):1350–1356.
6. Su T, Pirgousis P, Fernandes R. Versatility of the supraclavicular island flap in head and neck reconstruction of vessel depleted and difficult necks. *J Oral Maxillofac Surg* 2013; 71(3):622–627.
7. Pallua N, Noah EM. The tunneled supraclavicular island flap: an optimized technique for head and neck reconstruction. *Plast Reconstr Surg* 2000; 105:842–851.

Chapter 20
The internal mammary perforator flap

Introduction

The internal mammary perforator (IMAP) flap is a relatively new flap for the reconstruction of head and neck defects. It was first described by Kalender and colleagues for the reconstruction of breast defect.[1] Subsequently, the flap was described as an island flap for the treatment of chest wall radionecrosis.[2] One of the first descriptions of the IMAP in the repair of head and neck defects was by Yu for the repair of a tracheostoma reconstruction.[3] Later, Neligan described the IMAP in a case where the flap was used to resurface a large neck defect.[4]

Since the first description of the IMAP, several publications have further clarified the vascular distribution to the flap and the extent of perfusion from the arterial perforators to the anterior chest wall.[5,6] This improved understanding has made the use of the IMAP predictable and reliable for the reconstruction of various head neck defects.

The IMAP flap has several advantages for the reconstruction of head neck defects. This flap is often used in cases of previously radiated necks with unstable skin and in patients with laryngectomies who have developed pharyngocutaneous fistulas. In these cases, the primary goal is the closure of the fistula. The guiding principle in these reconstructions is to repair the fistula while minimizing obstruction to the stoma.

The IMAP serves as a good flap option because it has the advantage of being distant from the previously radiated field, while also being a thin and pliable fasciocutaneous flap. Another obvious advantage of this flap is that it enables the repair of the fistula and the overlying skin while minimizing the need to enter the previously operated and radiated neck. This makes the reconstruction becomes more predictable and easier to execute. The location of the donor site is also favorable for most donors as it is easily concealed.

One of the disadvantage of this flap is that its use can be limited to the anterior neck and the arc of rotation.

The IMAP flap is an easy flap to harvest. When the reach will be adequate without the need for intramuscular perforator dissection, the flap may be raised rapidly with careful dissection along the medial aspect where the perforators emerge from the muscle.

Anatomy

The arterial supply to this flap is from the perforating branches of the internal thoracic artery (also known as the internal mammary artery). This is a paired artery arising from the subclavian artery near its origin, it travels downward approximately 1 cm lateral to the sternum and terminates as the superior epigastric and musculophrenic arteries. Cutaneous perforators arise from the internal thoracic artery in the first 5 to 6 intercostal spaces. They pierce through the intercostal muscles and medial fibers of the pectoralis major, travel in the subcutaneous tissue in a laterocaudal direction supplying the overlying skin.[7] In their course, the perforators are accompanied by their venae comitantes. The anterior cutaneous branch of the intercostal nerves can provide sensory innervation to the flap.[8] The perforators segmentally supply the skin of the anterior chest from the clavicle to below the submammary fold and from the midline to the anterior axillary line. From cadaveric studies, a reliable anatomy has been determined and the mean size of the skin area perfused by a single perforator is 13×7 cm, with the second perforator having the largest area of skin supplied measuring 16×9 cm.[9] This allows a flap harvest size ranging from 13×7 cm up to 20×13 cm when based on adjacent perforators. The mean diameter of the perforators is 1.3 ± 0.5 mm with the second perforator consistently having the largest diameter with a mean of 1.6 ± 0.5 mm.[10] Flaps

Local and Regional Flaps in Head & Neck Reconstruction: A Practical Approach, First Edition. Rui Fernandes.

Companion website: www.wiley.com/go/fernandes/flapsreconstruction

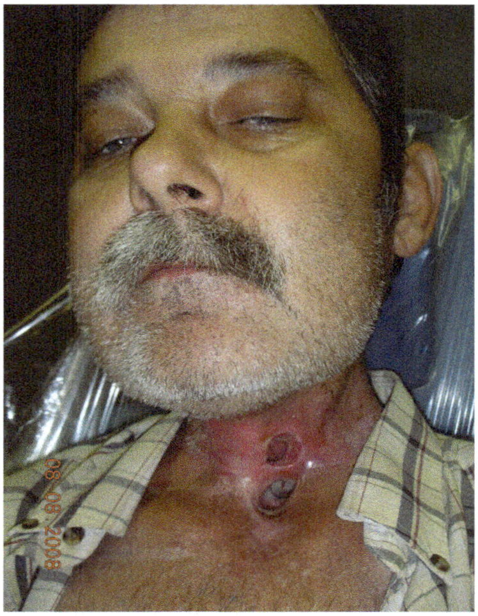

Fig. 20.1 View of a patient with multiple pharyngeal fistulae located suprastomal and within. The neck is clearly hostile, with evidence of previous surgeries and radiotherapy.

based on the first and second internal mammary artery perforators are routinely used for anterior neck reconstruction.

Flap harvest

Flap harvest is depicted in Figures 20.1 to 20.8.

- The patient is positioned in the supine position. Before making the flap design, a Doppler should be used to confirm the most prominent perforator and its intercostal location. Another option for confirming the

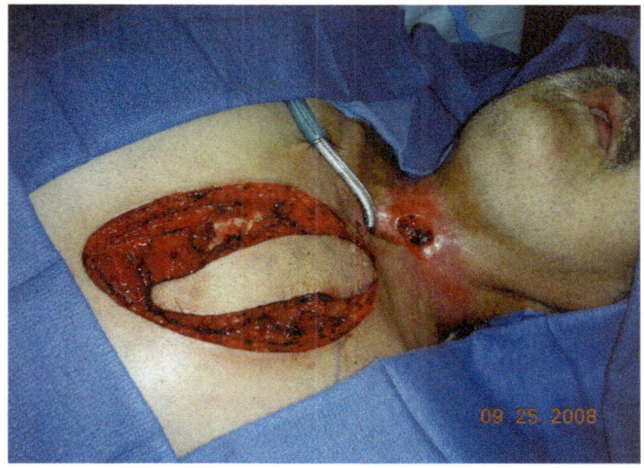

Fig. 20.3 Incised IMAP flap prior to elevation and rotation.

location and best caliber of the perforator is to use a color flow ultrasound to inspect the size of the perforator as well as the path it takes towards the skin.
- The location and size of the defect is inspected and measured. Using a cord from the lap sponge or any other measuring string, the pivot point is placed directly over the main perforator. The opposite end of the string is then placed at the distal end of the defect. Care should be made to insure that the string is passive and not tented as this would result in a deficiency of the length and a potential problem with the reach of the flap.
- The string is then rotated to the thorax and the distal end is marked. This point represents the most distal end of the flap. The markings are then transferred to the chest wall. The design of the flap may be placed in several positions, either horizontally, vertically, or obliquely. It is most important to insure that the width and length of the flap will be sufficient to cover the

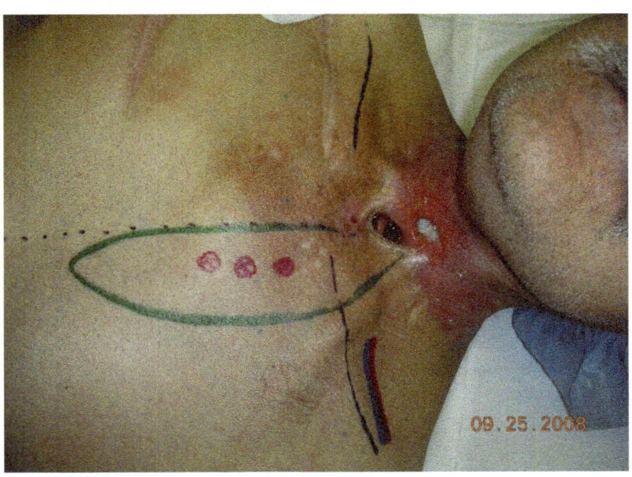

Fig. 20.2 Markings for an IMAP flap; flap is designed in a vertical orientation.

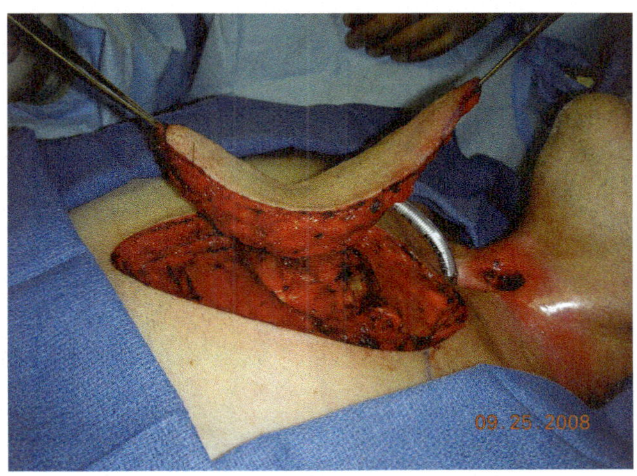

Fig. 20.4 Elevation of the IMAP flap prior to rotation and transfer.

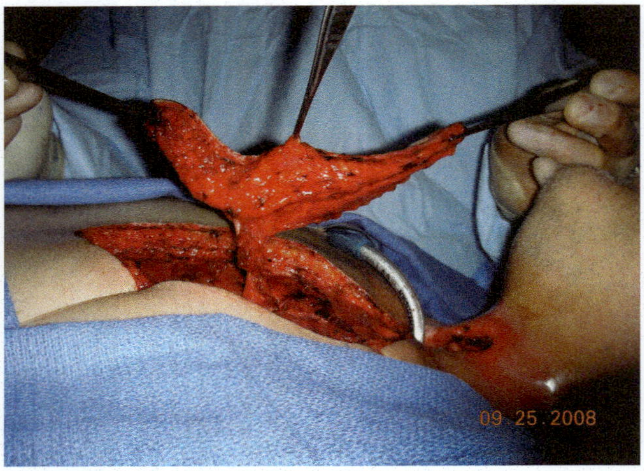

Fig. 20.5 View of the elevated flap with dissected pedicle.

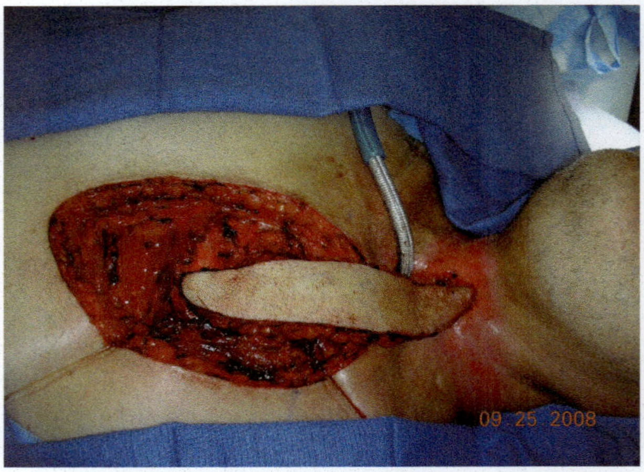

Fig. 20.7 Rotation of the flap toward the defect.

defect and that flap placement is such that it will be perfused by the perforator.

- The flap may be elevated from either the distal end and dissected toward the midline where the location of the perforators are expected or by beginning at the medial aspect, directly inferior to the expected location of the perforator flap.
- If the elevation is begun inferior to the perforator, the dissection is extended to the subfascial plane and then the direction is changed to a superior or cephalad direction towards the expected perforator. Once the dissection nears the perforator, attention should be taken to not injure it. At this time, the use of monopolar electrocautery should be limited and bipolar electrocautery should be used more liberally.
- Once the location and adequacy of the caliber of the perforator is confirmed, the design of the flap is once again confirmed and, if needed, a new design made so that the perforator is better placed.
- With the flap design confirmed and the perforator dissected, the remainder of the flap is elevated in a subfascial plane.
- At this point, the rotation and reach of the flap is tested. If the flap is able to reach the defect without any tension then no further dissection of the pedicle is needed.
- If there is tension on the flap in order for it to reach the defect site, intramuscular dissection of the perforator is performed towards the axial vessel, i.e., the internal mammary artery.
- Once the vessels are reached, the portion of the vessel inferior to the takeoff of the perforator is then mobilized, ligated, and divided.
- Dissection of the vascular pedicle is then carried out in a cephalad direction; the next site of obstruction will be the costal cartilage of the rib. If the flap is still unable to reach the desired location, then a portion of the rib is removed to further mobilize the flap.

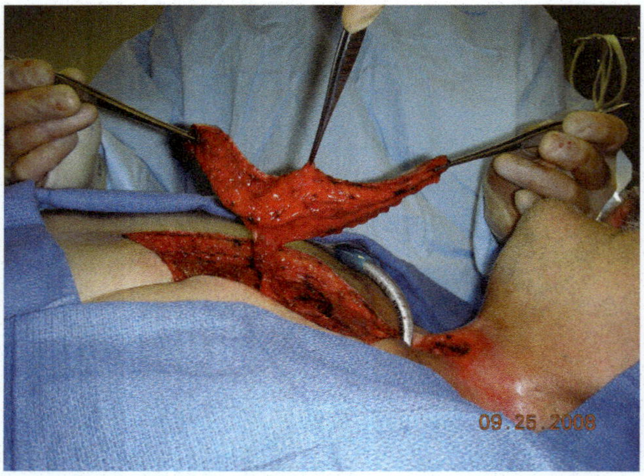

Fig. 20.6 Another view of the vascular pedicle going on to the undersurface of the flap.

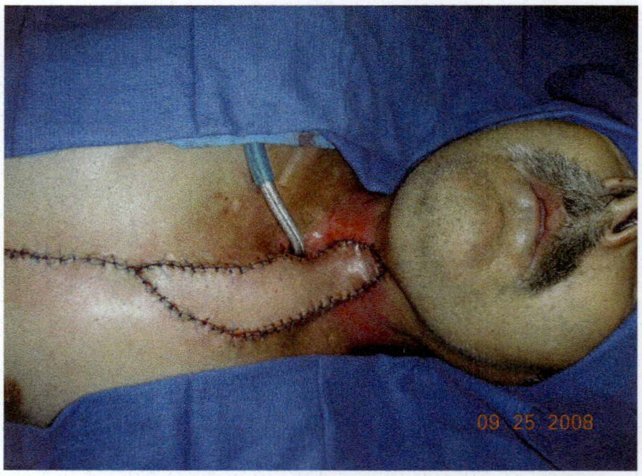

Fig. 20.8 Flap inset to repair the fistula. Note that it does not have a large bulk and thus it does not obliterate the stoma.

- The next decision to be made is the method of transfer for the flap into the defect. Usually there will be an intervening bridge of skin between the flap and the defect. The choices for transfer will be to either tunnel the flap or to make an incision on the skin between the donor site and the defect site to lay down the flap.
- If the choice is made to tunnel the flap, the area under the skin bridge will need to be de-epithelialized. This is easily achieved using sharp scissors to remove just the epithelium and leaving the dermis intact.
- If the transfer method chosen is the skin incision, then a skin flap is elevated to accommodate the width of the flap as it travels in its superior direction. The flap is then inset into the defect.
- The donor site is closed by undermining the skin and the area is closed primarily. Usually a drain is used in the donor site for a few days.

Special circumstances

The IMAP flap can be used in the situations where the chest is pristine. The circumstances where its use may be limited or challenged are those where a previous incision has been made in the ipsilateral anterior chest. The history as well as a thorough physical exam are needed to assess the amount of skin that can be raised and, more importantly, if the perforators to the overlying skin remain intact and patent. In cases where a previous pectoralis major flap was elevated, there is still a small possibility that the perforators to the skin remain intact and, depending on the incision used for the pectoralis flap, a potential for a vertical flap design may be possible.

Advantages

The advantages of the IMAP in head and neck reconstruction are the location of the donor scar, which can be easily hidden. The thickness of the flap is also an advantage in situations when there has been a previous laryngectomy. In these cases, one should always be cognizant of the possibility of partial occlusion of the stoma by the use of a bulky flap. The IMAP takes advantage of the fact that it is a perforator flap and therefore the muscle is not used, thus allowing for the transfer of the skin, subcutaneous fat, and fascia only. Another advantage of this flap is that it allows minimal dissection of the neck. This fact is only relevant when the patient has received radiation.

Disadvantages

The main disadvantage of the IMAP flap is its use in female patients. The placement of the incision in the chest of females carries a higher risk for the formation of keloids. The transfer of the flap and the repair of the donor site can also result in a displacement and distortion of the breast. These two facts must be kept in mind and communicated to the patients. The reality is that in most patients when the need to use the IMAP is being contemplated, the issue of cosmesis is often less important, and the disadvantages described are only relative.

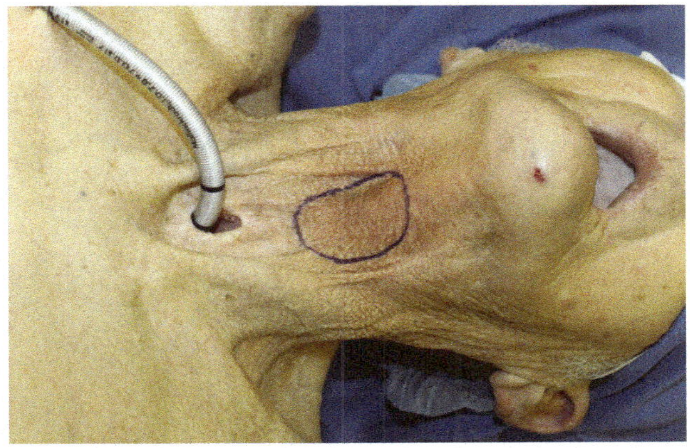

Fig. 20.9 View of a patient with a suprastomal recurrence.

Case #1

The patient is a 68-year-old male with a history of a salvaged total laryngectomy after failed radiotherapy. He was noted on routine follow-up to have a suprastomal recurrence and he was referred for a salvaged surgery for this (Figure 20.9). A suprastomal resection was performed leaving a pharyngeal defect and a cutaneous defect as seen in Figures 20.10 and 20.11. The pharyngeal

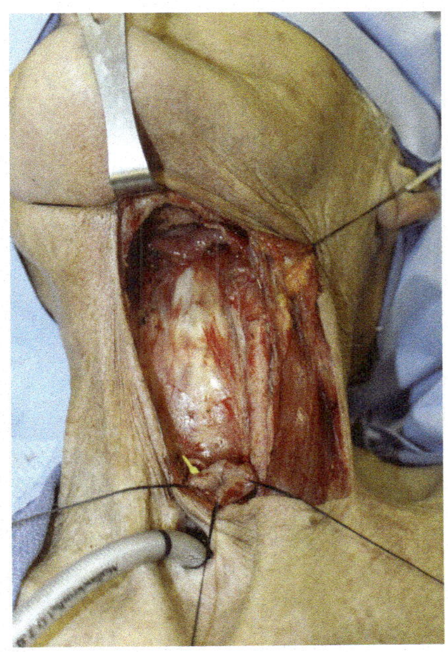

Fig. 20.10 Defect after salvage surgery depicting the superior extent of defect.

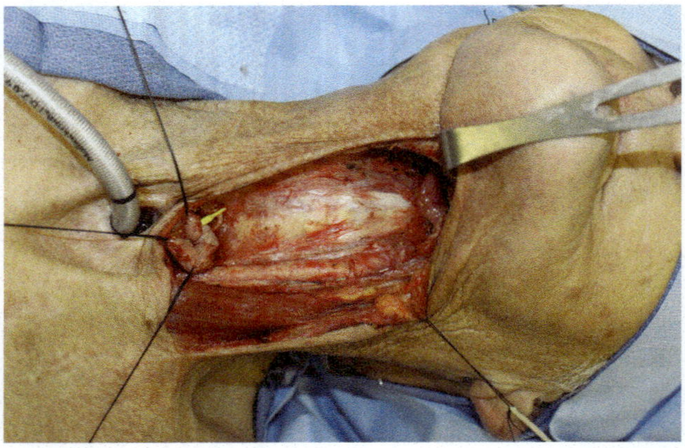

Fig. 20.11 View of the inferior defect.

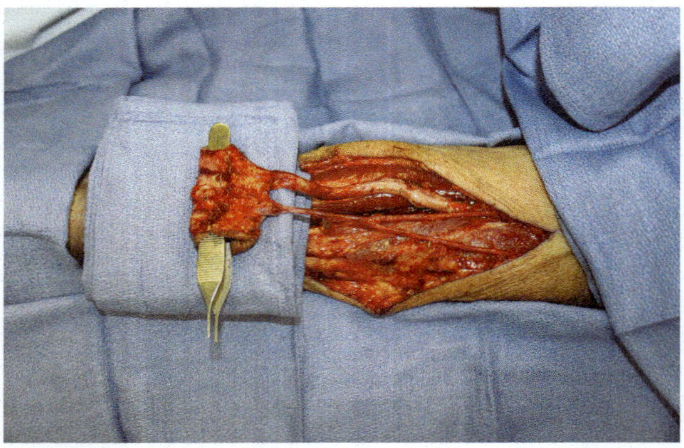

Fig. 20.12 View of a tubed radial forearm flap to be used for the pharyngeal reconstruction.

defect was reconstructed with a tubed radial forearm flap (Figures 20.12 and 20.13). Once the pharyngeal defect was completed, a horizontally oriented IMAP flap was elevated (Figure 20.14). The flap was elevated based on two arterial perforators (Figure 20.15). The arc of rotation was checked and deemed appropriate to repair the skin defect without tension (Figures 20.16 and 20.17). The patient seen a few months postoperative with a healed IMAP flap and nearly inconspicuous donor site is shown in Figure 20.18.

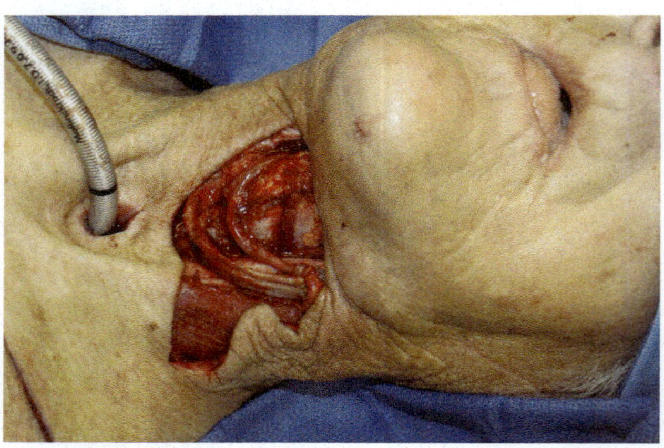

Fig. 20.13 Completion of the inset of the pharyngeal reconstruction with the radial forearm flap.

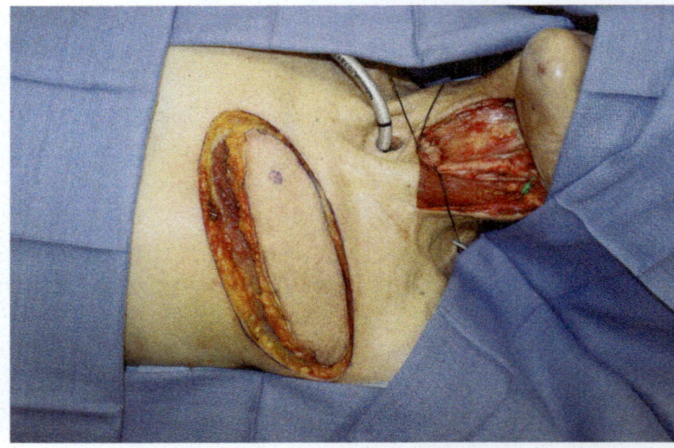

Fig. 20.14 Markings for the IMAP flap prior to elevation.

Case #2

This 70-year-old African American man was referred for repair of a pharyngocutaneous fistula which he developed after having to salvage a total laryngectomy and neck dissection secondary to failed organ preservation radiation therapy (Figure 20.19). A plan was made to repair the fistula with a combination of a turn-in flap and coverage with a non-radiated, thin, IMAP flap (Figures 20.22 to 20.22). Once the turn-in flap was done for the first layer closure, a horizontally designed IMAP flap was elevated based on the 3rd intercostal perforator originating from the internal mammary artery (Figures 20.23 to 20.26). The dissected intermuscular perforator was of good caliber and length, which allowed for an easy rotation of the flap into the defect site (Figure 20.27). The

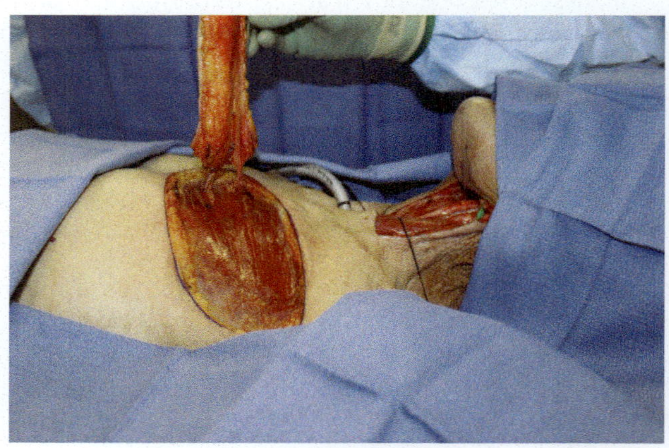

Fig. 20.15 Elevated IMAP flap based on two IMAP perforators.

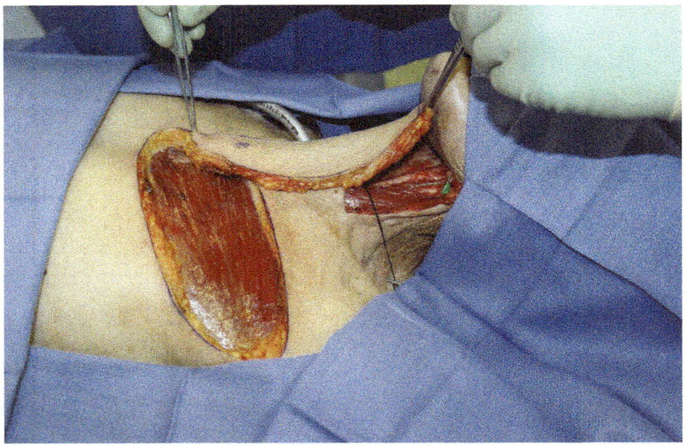

Fig. 20.16 Rotation of the flap to reach the neck defect.

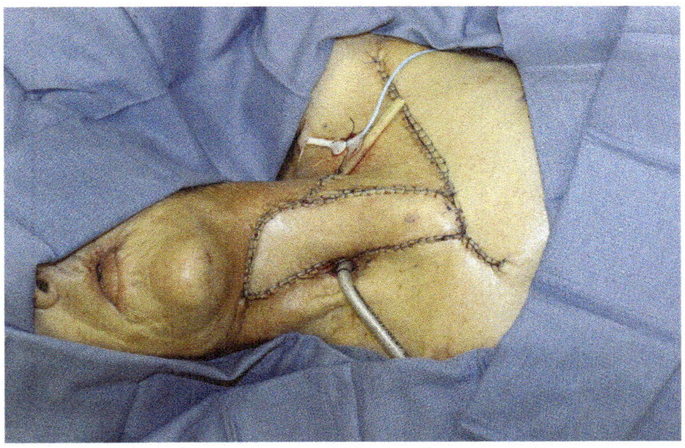

Fig. 20.17 Inset of the flap and immediate primary repair of the donor site.

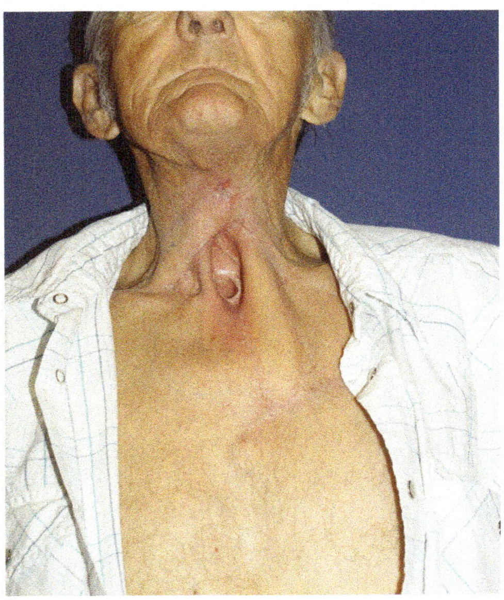

Fig. 20.18 Late appearance of the donor site and neck.

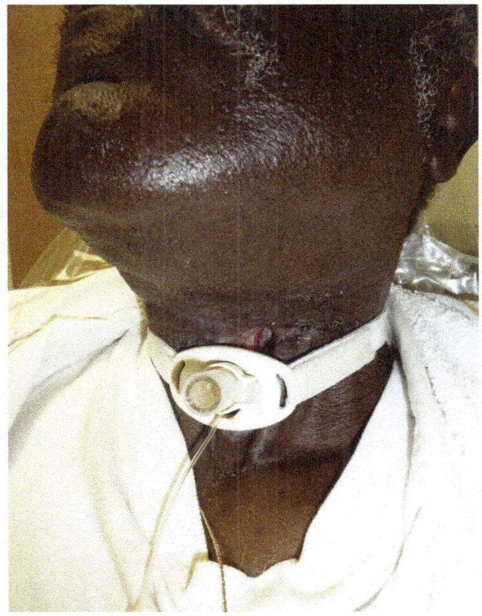

Fig. 20.19 View of a patient with a suprastomal pharyngeal fistula.

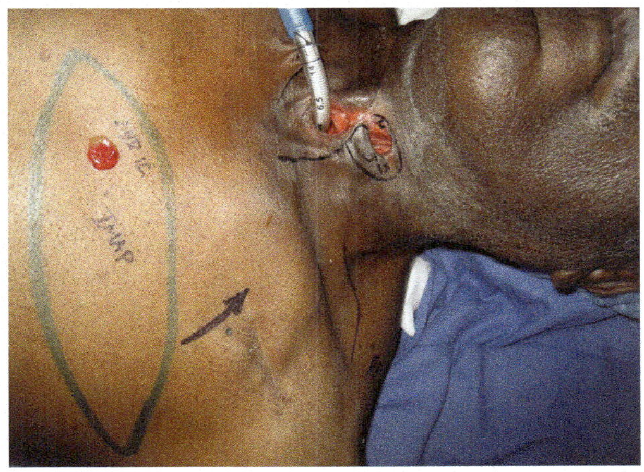

Fig. 20.20 Markings for a horizontal IMAP flap and turn-in flap at the fistula site.

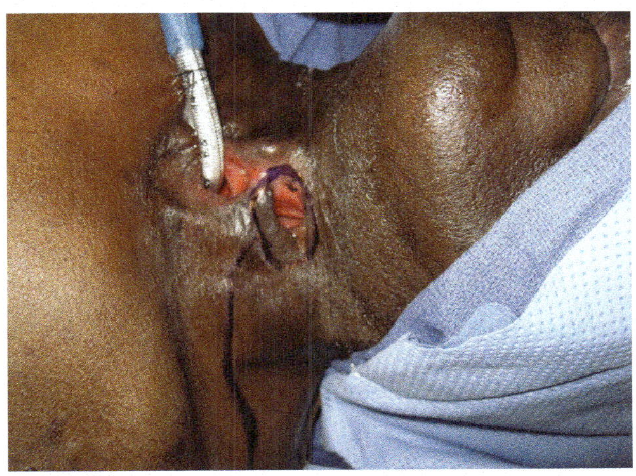

Fig. 20.21 Close-up view of the marking for the turn in flap.

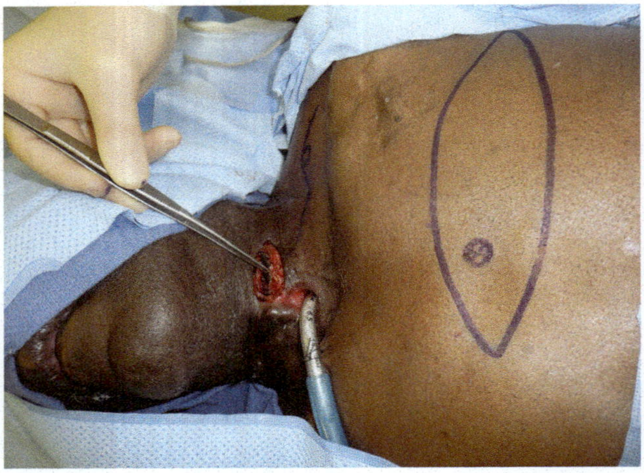

Fig. 20.22 Elevation of perifistula tissue for the first layer closure.

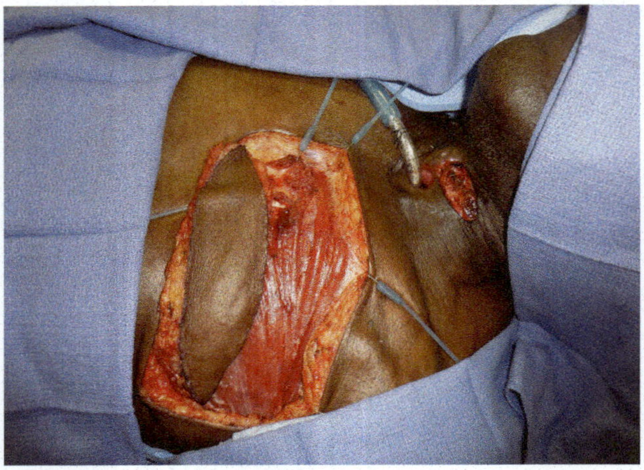

Fig. 20.23 Incision for the IMAP flap prior to elevation.

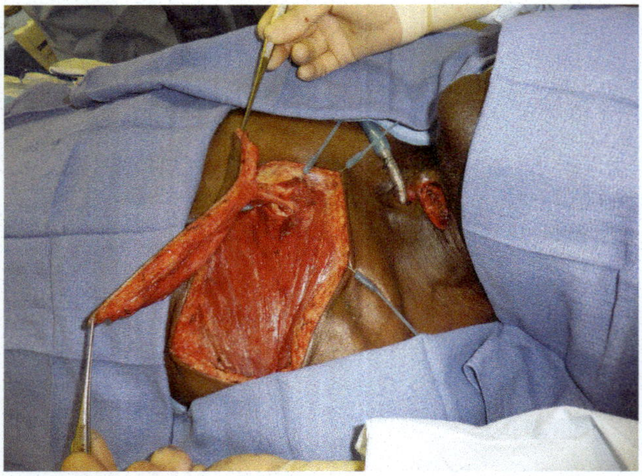

Fig. 20.24 Superior view of the pedicle after elevation of the IMAP flap.

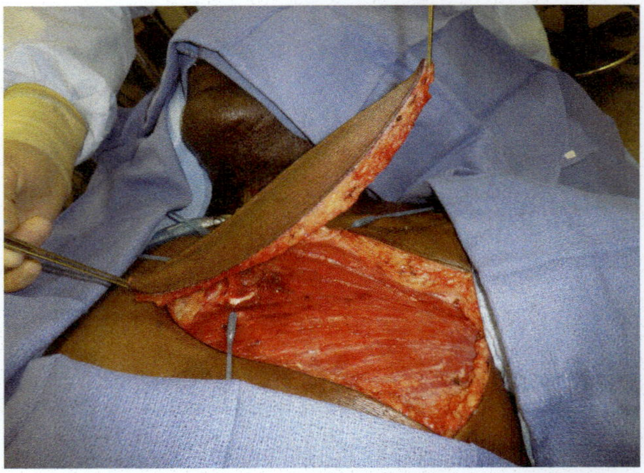

Fig. 20.25 Inferior view of the dissected pedicle between the pectoralis major muscle fibers.

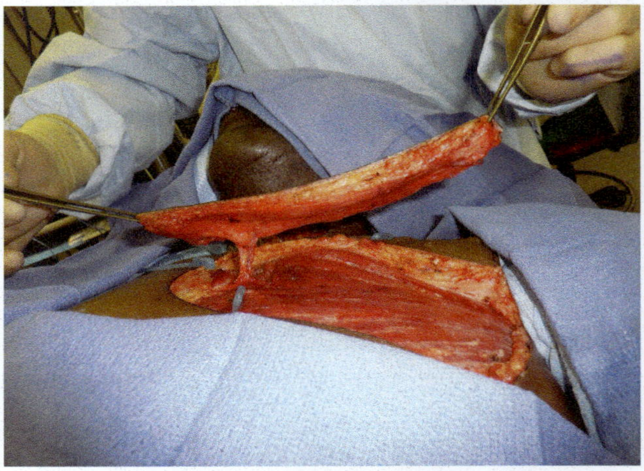

Fig. 20.26 View of the IMAP pedicle revealing good pedicle length.

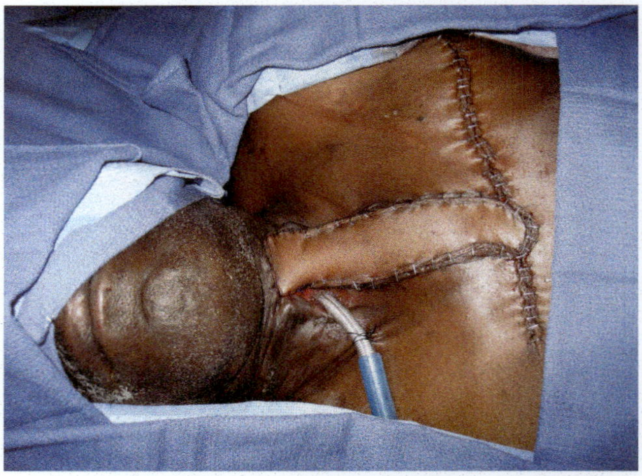

Fig. 20.27 View of the inset of the flap with primary repair of the donor site.

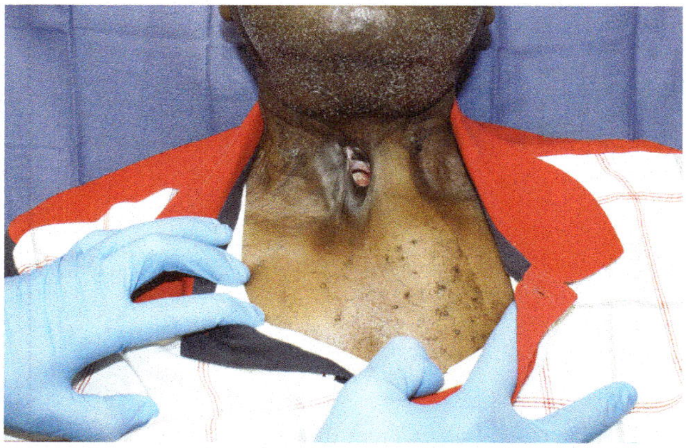

Fig. 20.28 Late postoperative view of the reconstructed pharynx.

patient did very well from his reconstruction and had a resolution of the fistula with minimal morbidity from the donor site (Figure 20.28).

References

1. Kalender V, Aydm H, Karabulut AB, et al. Breast reconstruction with the internal mammary artery pedicled fasciocutaneous island flap: description of a new flap. *Plast Reconstr Surg* 2000; 106:1494–1498.
2. Karabulut AB, Kalender V. Internal mammary artery pedicled island flap for the treatment of chest wall radionecrosis. *Plast Reconstr Surg* 2001; 108:583–584.
3. Yu P, Roblin P, Chevray P. Internal mammary artery perforator (IMAP) flap for tracheostoma reconstruction. *Head Neck* 2006; 28:723–729.
4. Neligan PC, Gullane PJ, Vesely M, et al. The internal mammary artery perforator flap: new variation on an old theme. *Plast Reconstr Surg* 2007; 119:891–893.
5. Vesely MJ, Murray DJ, Novak CB, et al. The internal mammary artery perforator flap: an anatomical study and a case report. *Ann Plast Surg* 2007; 58:156–161.
6. Rosson GD, Holton LH, Silverman RP, et al. Internal mammary perforators: a cadaver study. *J Reconstr Microsurg* 2005; 21: 239–242.
7. Vesely MJ, Murray DJ, Novak CB, Gullane PJ, Neligan PC. The internal mammary artery perforator flap an anatomical study and case report. *Ann Plast Surg* 2007; 58:156–161.
8. Gillis JA, Prasad V, Morris SF. Three-dimensional analysis of the internal mammary artery perforator flap. *Plast Reconstr Surg* 2011; 128:419e–426e.
9. Schmidt M, Aszmann OC, Beck H, Frey M. The anatomic basis of the internal mammary artery perforator flap: a cadaver study. *J Plast Reconstr Aesth Surg* 2010; 63:191–196.
10. Schellekens PP, Paes EC, Hage JJ, van der Wal MB, Bleys RL, Kon M. Anatomy of the vascular pedicle of the internal mammary artery (IMAP) flap as applied for head and neck reconstruction. *J Plast Reconstr Aesth Surg* 2011; 64:53–57.

Chapter 21

Ear reconstruction

Introduction

The ear plays an important role in facial appearance. Its prominence is not as high compared with the nose but when it is missing, over-projected, or deficient in some capacity, the eyes will be drawn to the defect. Perhaps even more important is the role this deficiency plays on the psyche of the patient.

The reconstruction of auricular defects range from the simple to the complex. The complexity is often associated with the size and composition of the defect. In some cases, a simple skin graft will enable the reconstruction of small to moderate defects. In other instances, the reconstruction will demand a more sophisticated approach due to the complexity of the defect.

Defects affecting the auricle can be broadly divided to traumatic (including burns), oncologic, or congenital (Figures 21.1a,b and 21.2). In rare circumstances defects secondary to infection can lead to the loss of cartilage and therefore deformation of the ear.

This chapter will describe the anatomical features of the external ear and the relevance to reconstruction. Various classifications of auricular defects will be reviewed and finally, the reconstructive options will be discussed. The reconstruction of the microtic ear will not be discussed much as that is not typically encountered in a head and neck surgical practice. Surgeons involved in microtia repair tend to be most commonly, pediatric craniofacial surgeons.

When the defect is encountered secondary to oncological trauma, a thorough understanding of the histology, size of the tumor, and nodal status becomes very important when reconstructive options are being contemplated. The need for adjuvant therapy needs to be determined. For patients who will need to receive adjuvant radiation therapy, undertaking a long multistage reconstruction may not be the most desirable option. Equally, the reconstructive surgeon also has to consider this when reconstructing secondary defects.

Anatomy

External ear anatomy (pinna)

The ear plays a prominent role in our facial esthetics. The anatomy of the external ear is complex due to the intricacies of the convexities and concavities formed by the skin drape over the cartilaginous structure.

In simple terms, one can divide the ear into large areas: helix and antihelix, the tragus, the concha, and the lobule.

The external ring of the auricle is the cartilaginous helix, anterior and parallel to it lays the Y-shaped antihelix. This cartilaginous concave area at the superior aspect of the auricle between the helix and antihelix is referred to as the scapha. The concave space immediately anterior to the antihelix is the cymba. Between the scapha and the cymba exists a small depression between two convexities (crura); this space is the triangular fossa.

The anterior aspect of the ear at the junction with the cheek is the crus of the helix and inferior to it is the tragus. The external auditory meatus is found in this area and is contiguous with the cavum.

The inferior portion of the auricle is formed by the lobule. The lobule is composed of fat and fibrous tissues and lacks any cartilage (Figure 21.3).

The position of the ear in a cranial caudal and anterior posterior aspect is important, as the spectator can perceive small differences with the contralateral ear. The average head-to-ear angle is 31.1 degrees and for the scapha-to-concha angle it is 106.7 degrees.[1]

Local and Regional Flaps in Head & Neck Reconstruction: A Practical Approach, First Edition. Rui Fernandes.

Companion website: www.wiley.com/go/fernandes/flapsreconstruction

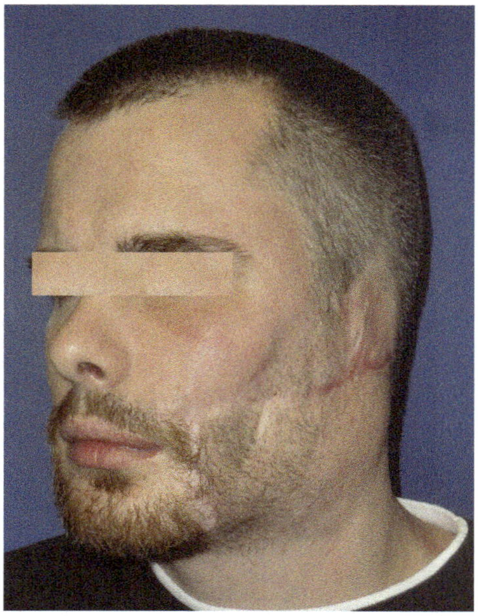

Fig. 21.1a View of a patient after traumatic loss of the ear due to an automobile accident.

The arterial supply to the ear comes from several vessels. Anteriorly, branches from the superficial temporal artery supply the ear; posteriorly the supply comes from the posterior auricular artery and the occipital artery. The venous drainage comes from the veins accompanying the named arteries.

The external ear receives innervation from the auriculotemporal nerve (anterior superior one-third), the greater auricular nerve (anterior and posterior lower two-

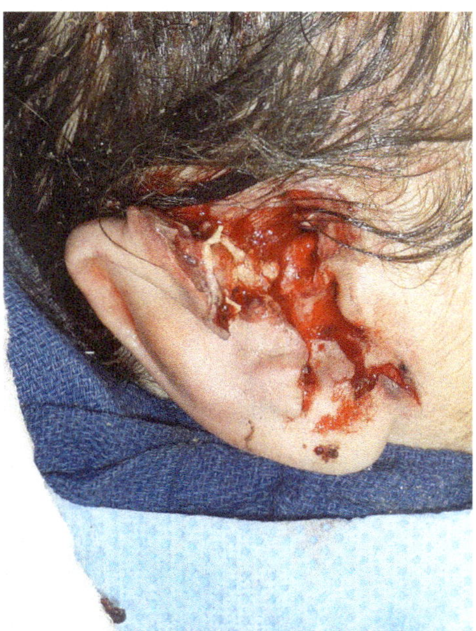

Fig. 21.1b Near amputation of the ear secondary to trauma; only inferior pedicle remains.

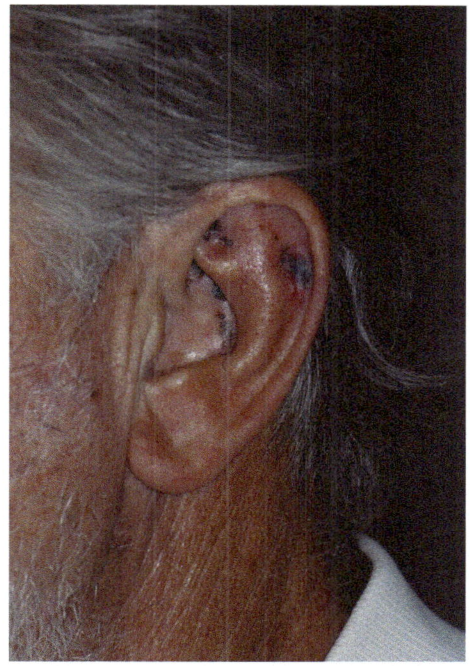

Fig. 21.2 View of multiple sites of melanoma in the left auricle.

thirds), the lesser occipital nerve (posterior superior one-third), and the auricular branch of the vagus, Arnold's nerve (external auditory canal floor and concha).

Defect classification

Reconstructive options can be categorized by either the characteristics or location of the ear defect (e.g., partial

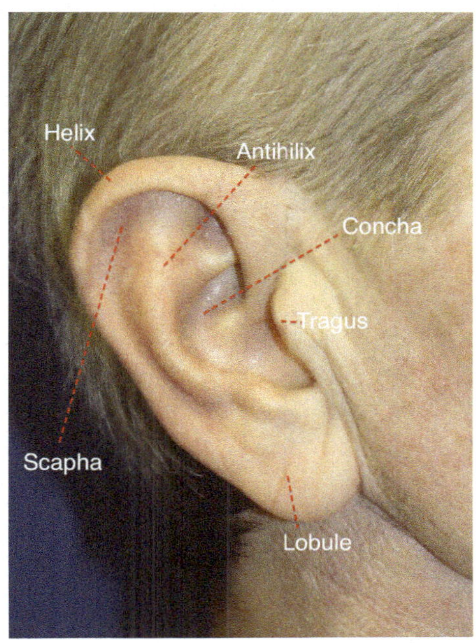

Fig. 21.3 Markings for various subsites of the ear.

or full-thickness, or upper, middle, or lower third of the auricle) or the type of surgical technique employed.[2] The description of the acquired defects as auricular thirds is commonly used and allows the surgeon a quick visual understanding of the location of the defect as well as its potential complexity.

Reconstructive options

The most common defect encountered is a partial helical defect. The helix is the most prominent portion of the ear and is therefore more susceptible to trauma as well as ultraviolet rays, which lead to the development of skin malignancies.

The following section will illustrate various reconstructive options when faced with acquired defects secondary to trauma or primary defects after resection of malignancies affecting the ear.

The cases will demonstrate some reconstructive options for the repair of these varied defects.

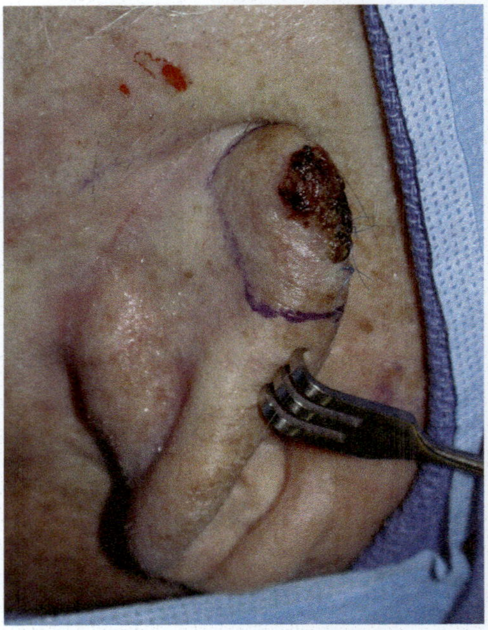

Fig. 21.5 Posterior view of the helical lesion.

Upper third

Case #1

A 78-year-old Caucasian male was referred for evaluation and treatment of a biopsy-proven squamous cell carcinoma of the upper helix (Figures 21.4 and 21.5). The area was marked for excision and was then resected (Figure 21.6). The defect was then evaluated for immediate reconstruction. The helix was undermined and a Burrow's triangle was removed in order to advance the helix to obtain primary closure (Figure 21.7).

Case #2

An 85-year-old male presented with a small helix lesion which was later diagnosed as a squamous cell carcinoma

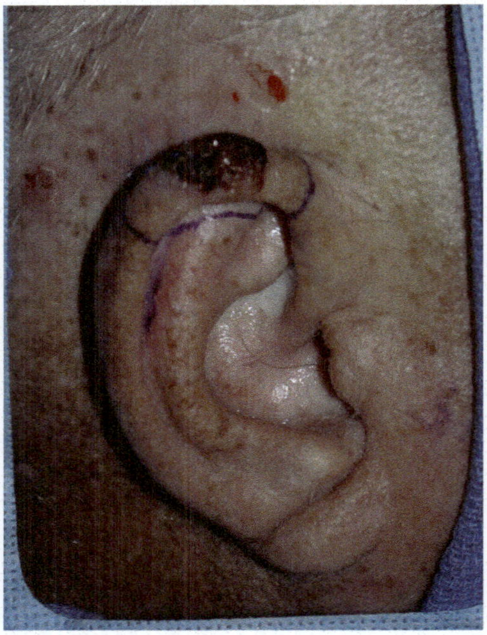

Fig. 21.4 Initial marking for the resection of a malignant lesion in the helix.

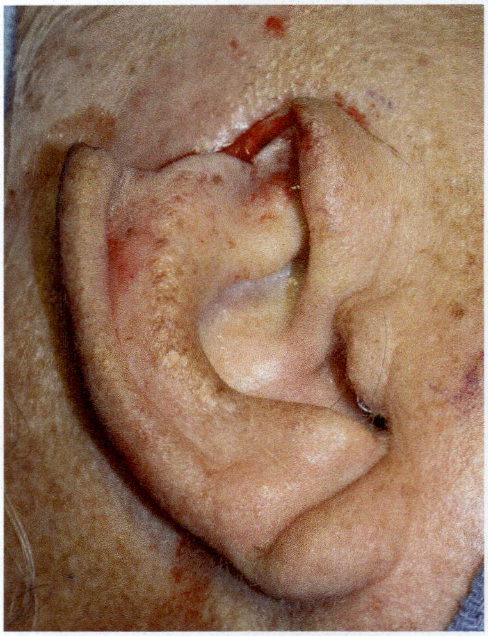

Fig. 21.6 Aspect of the defect after resection of the lesion.

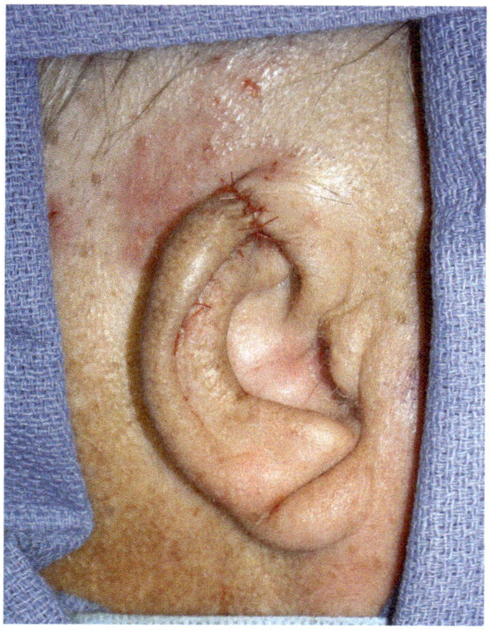

Fig. 21.7 Initial repair after undermining and advancement of the helix to obtain primary closure.

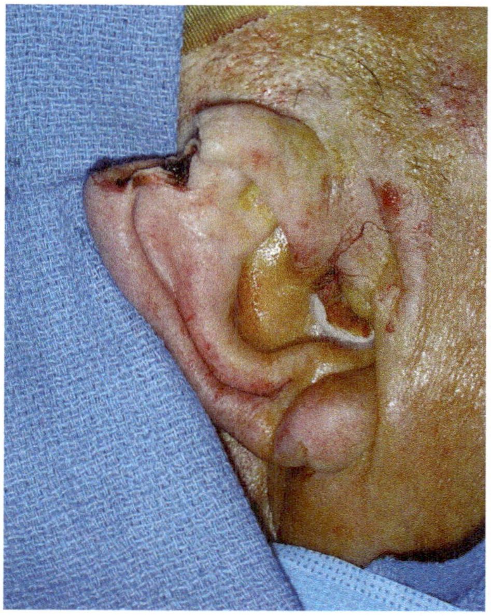

Fig. 21.9 View of the defect after resection of the lesion.

(Figure 21.8). The area was excised as a triangle or pie shape so as to allow for the primary closure of the defect without significant external defect (Figure 21.9). Once the area was excised, the defect was able to be closed primarily (Figure 21.10).

Case #3

A young man was involved in a motor vehicle accident and suffered loss of the upper and middle external ear. The avulsed ear was de-epithelialized and buried in a pocket in the posterior superior area (Figure 21.11). The patient was later brought back to the operating room where the ear was elevated and skin grafted onto the posterior and superior aspect of the reattached ear

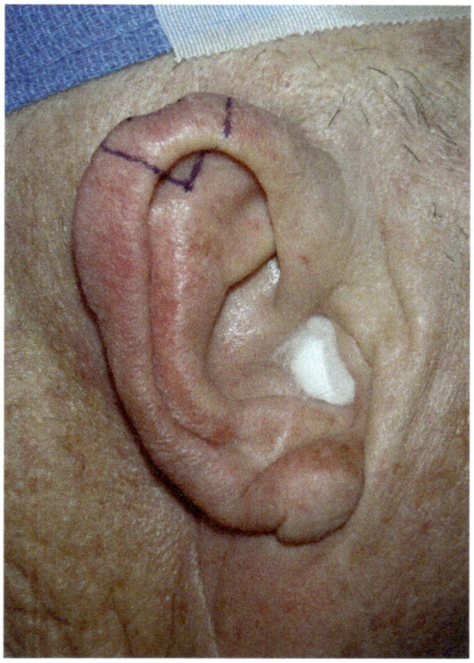

Fig. 21.8 Preparation for a V wedge excision of a helical lesion.

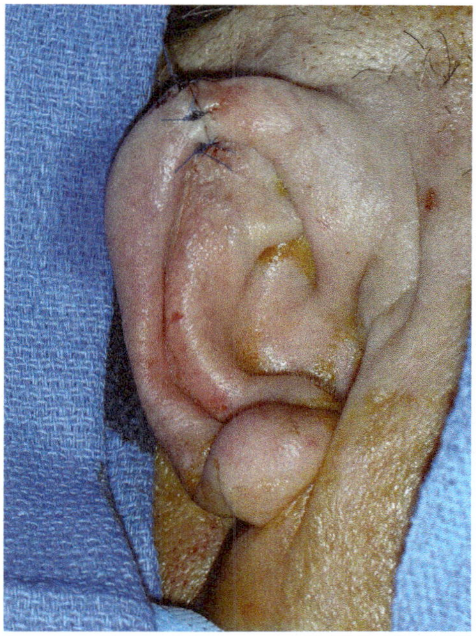

Fig. 21.10 Primary repair of the defect with minimal distortion of the ear.

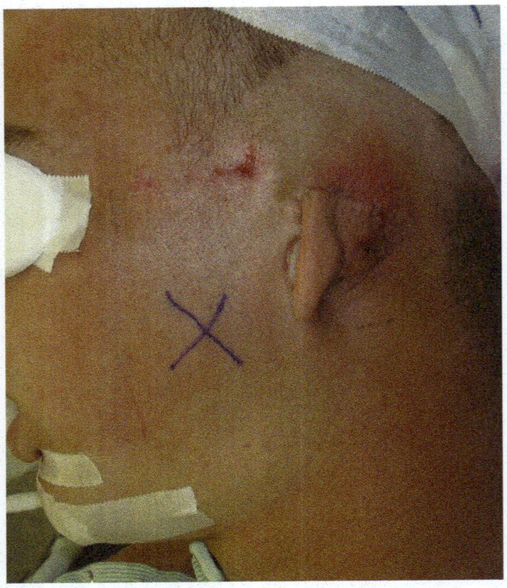

Fig. 21.11 Appearance of the left ear after previous trauma and burring of the ear in a soft tissue pocket.

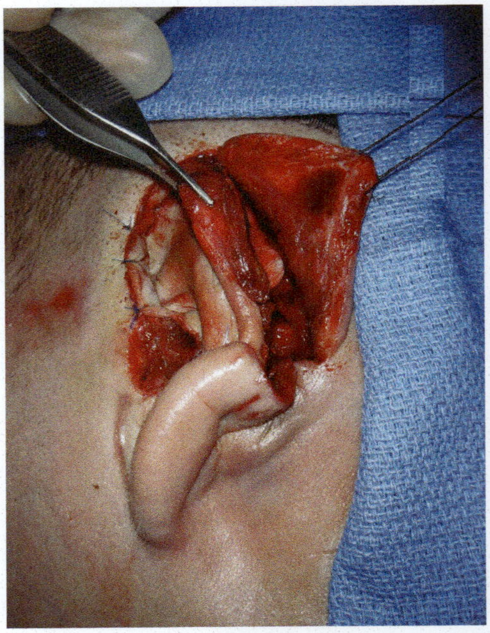

Fig. 21.13 Excellent appearance of the ear and development of the posterior ear flap to be replaced.

(Figures 21.12 to 21.16). The early postoperative appearance of the ear was satisfactory with good take of the graft and appearance (Figure 21.15).

Middle third

Case #4

A middle-aged African American male presented with a longstanding exophitic lesion located on the middle portion of the helix (Figure 21.17). The patient was taken to the operating room where a wedge excision and release incisions along the helix were performed (Figure 21.18). The final appearance of the ear on the early postoperative visit was acceptable without causing a deformity of the contour (Figure 21.19).

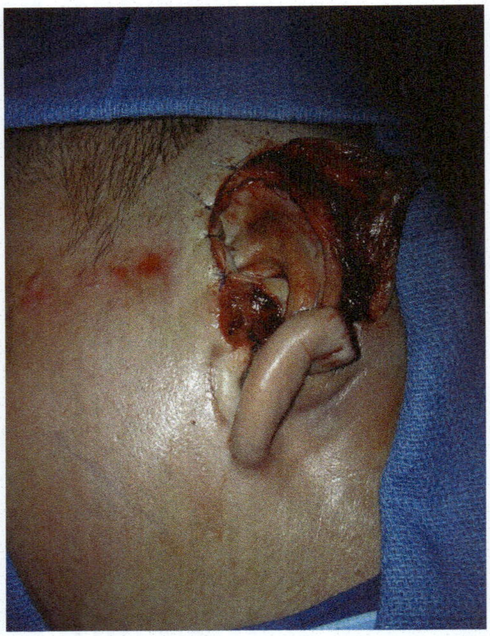

Fig. 21.12 Exposure of the buried ear; note the good vitality of the ear.

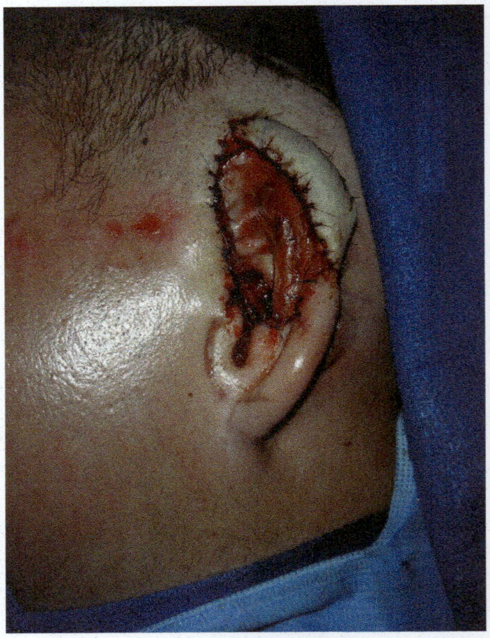

Fig. 21.14 Full-thickness skin graft of the helix and posterior aspect of the ear.

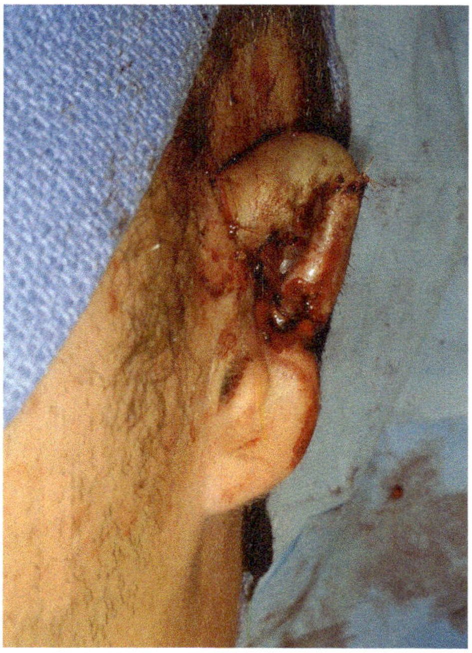

Fig. 21.15 Frontal view of the grafted ear.

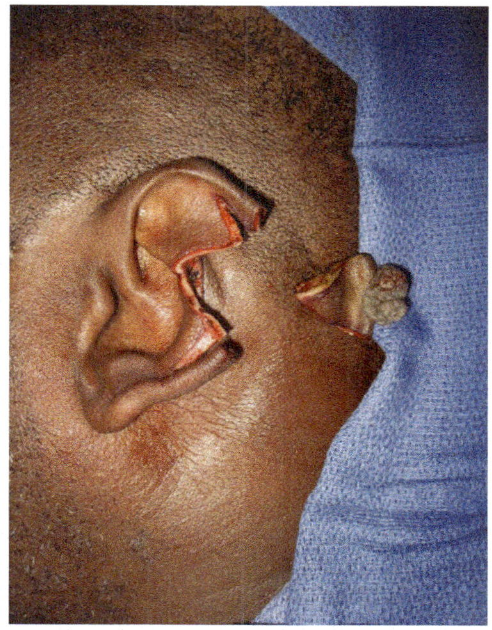

Fig. 21.17 View of a large resection of the ear with in a V-shaped design. Design for the advancement flap was done and the incisions performed.

Case #5

A 45-year-old male presented for excision of a malignant leasion located on the middle portion of the helical rim. The area was resected using a V excision and a superior and inferior releasing incision was performed (Figure 21.20). The helix was then mobilized to see if the defect could be closed primarily (Figure 21.21). The defect was then repaired in the usual way without any deformity of the external ear (Figure 21.22).

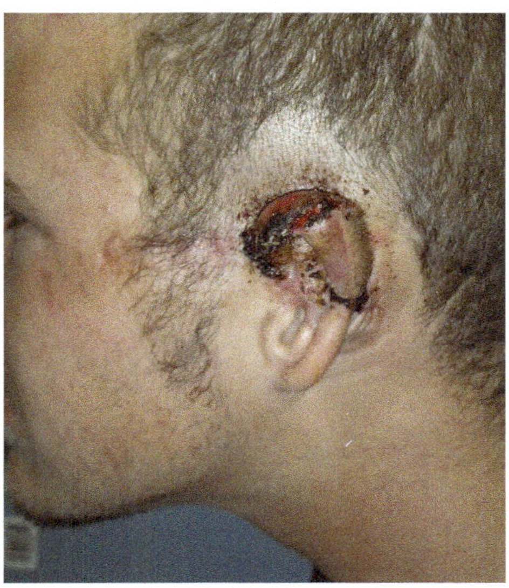

Fig. 21.16 Early postoperative appearance of the replanted ear, note the hair growth on the skin graft site.

Lower third

Case #6

An 18-year-old teenager presented for the reconstruction of a partial right ear defect, which had occurred secondary to a motor vehicle accident approximately 1 month earlier. Upon evaluation, it became evident that

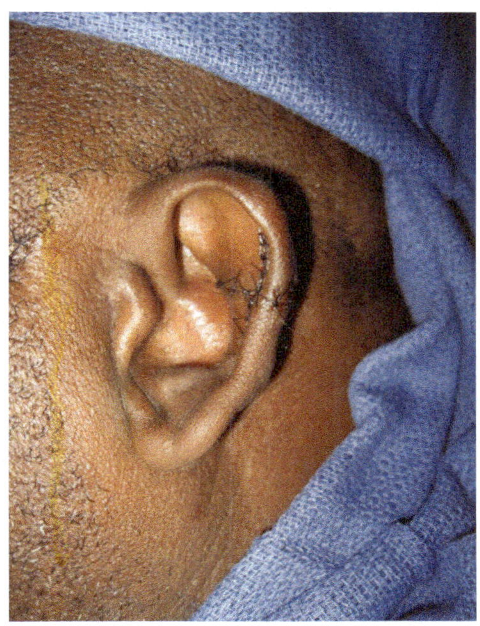

Fig. 21.18 Closure of the ear with preservation of the form.

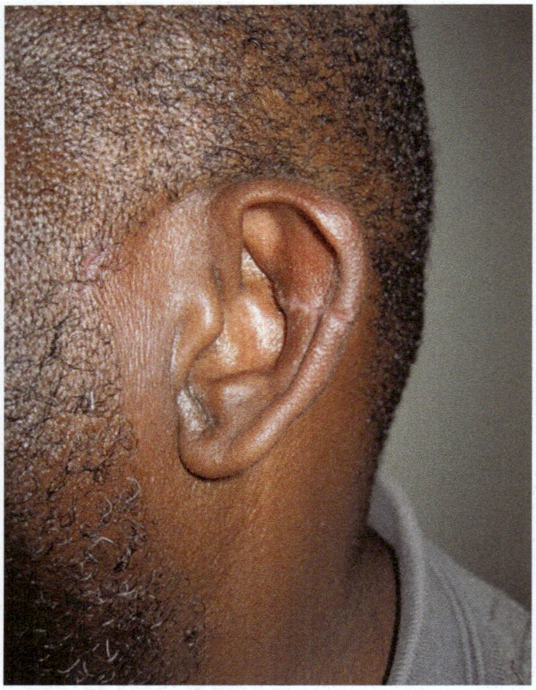

Fig. 21.19 Early postoperative healing revealing normal form of the ear without evidence of the large resection.

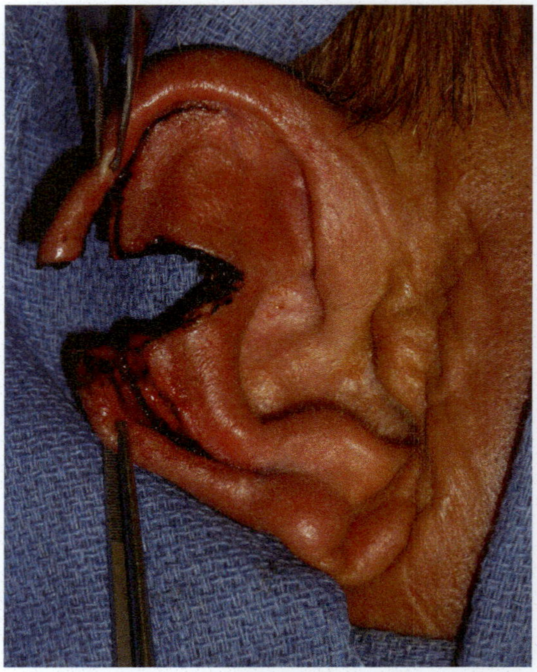

Fig. 21.21 Appearance of the helical flaps.

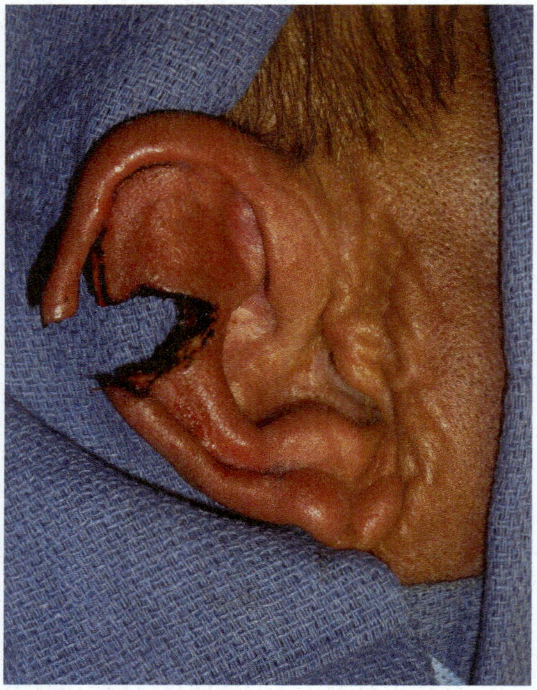

Fig. 21.20 Defect after excision of the ear lesion and developing of a helical flap to obtain primary repair.

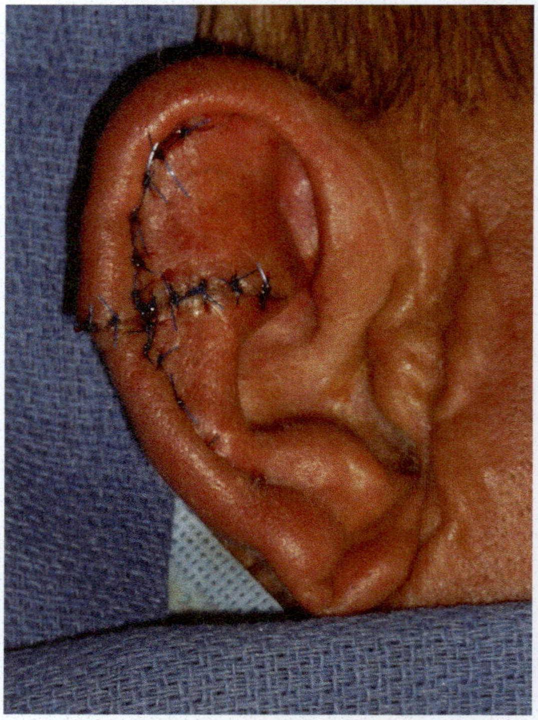

Fig. 21.22 Primary repair of the ear defect.

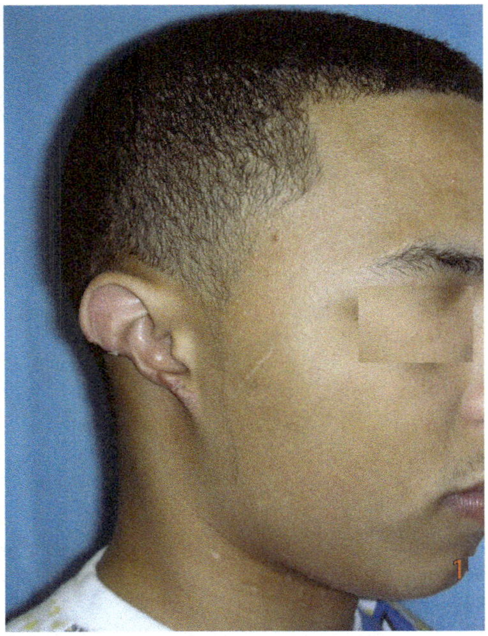

Fig. 21.23 Appearance of a large avulsive injury in a young man.

most of the right ear lobe and helix had been lost (Figures 21.23 and 21.24).

A plan was made for a staged reconstruction of the defect with a tubed flap (Figure 21.25). The tissue posterior to the ear was marked for the development of a tube flap. The tissue was elevated and then tubed into a flap with the adjacent tissue undermined and primarily closed (Figures 21.26 to 21.29). The tubed flap healed well (Figure 21.30). Approximately 3 weeks later, the patient was returned to the operating room and the superior portion of the flap was separated and transferred to the defect site, which had been prepared to receive the flap (Figures 21.31 and 21.32). The flap was once again allowed to heal for another 3 weeks when it was separated and the final inset performed (Figures 21.33 to 21.35).

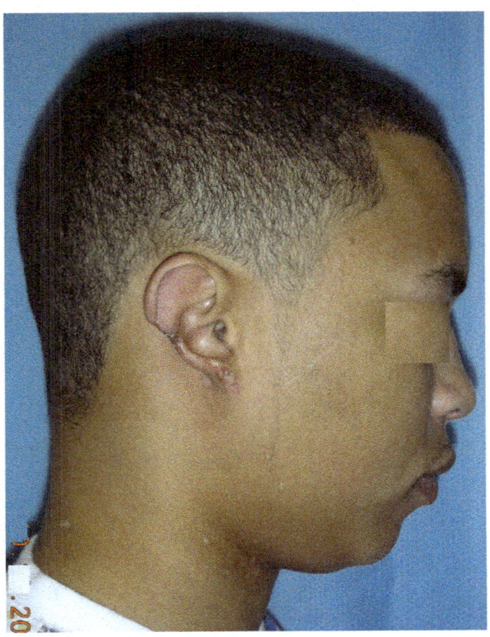

Fig. 21.24 Profile view revealing the amount of tissue loss.

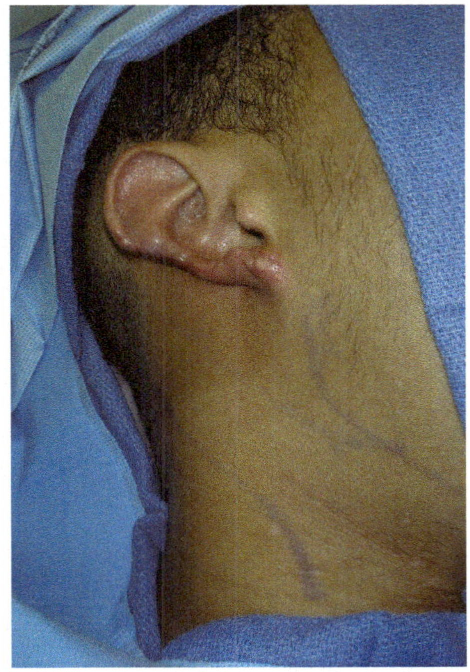

Fig. 21.25 Preparation for a stage one tube flap.

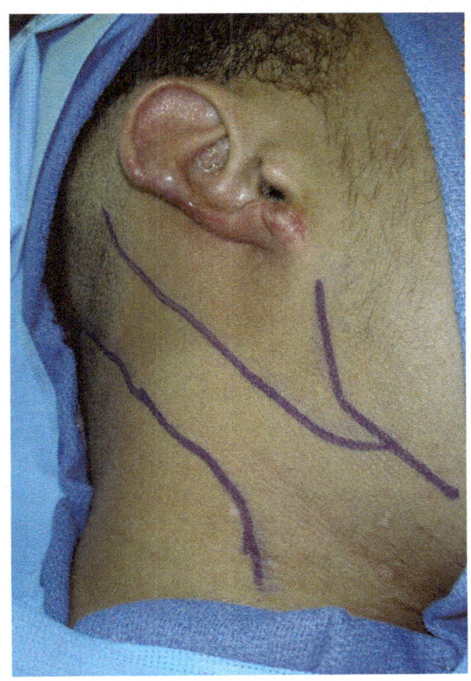

Fig. 21.26 Markings for the tube flap.

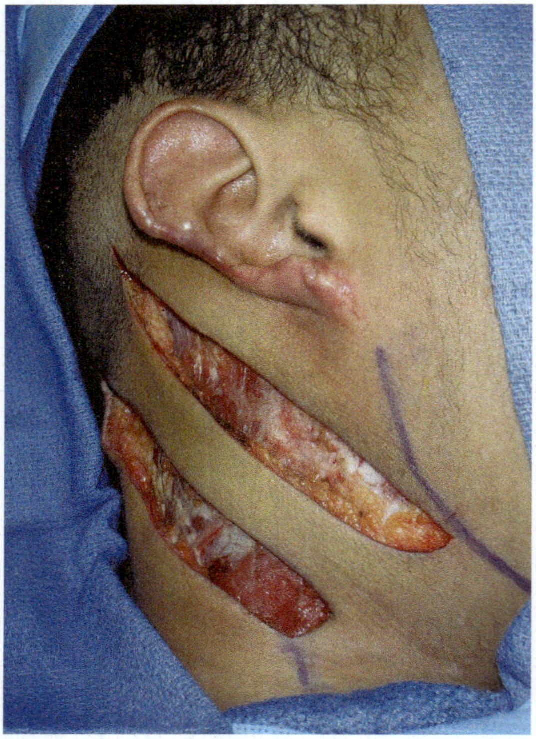

Fig. 21.27 Elevation of a bipedicled flap prior to tubing.

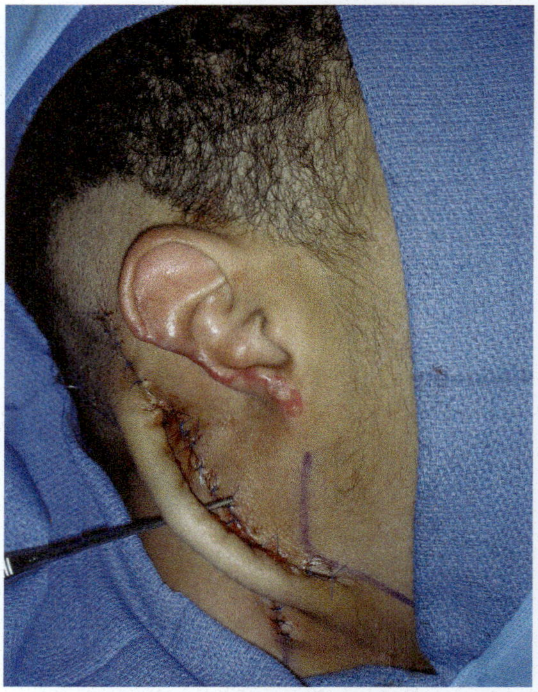

Fig. 21.29 Closure of the donor site.

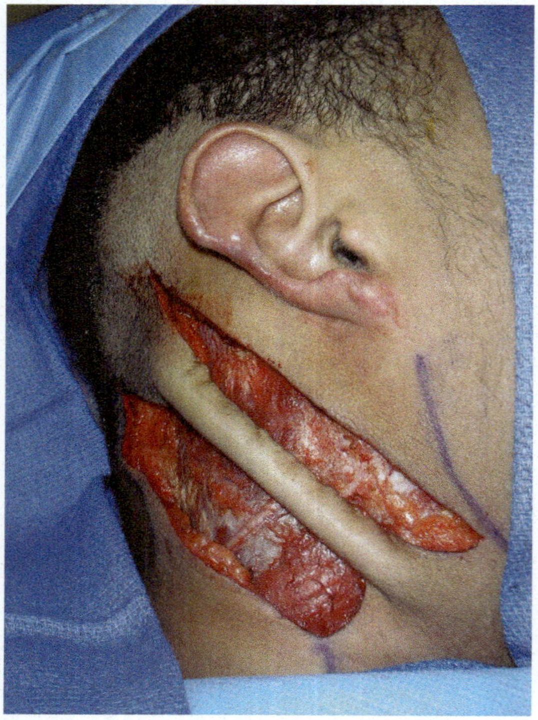

Fig. 21.28 Tubed flap.

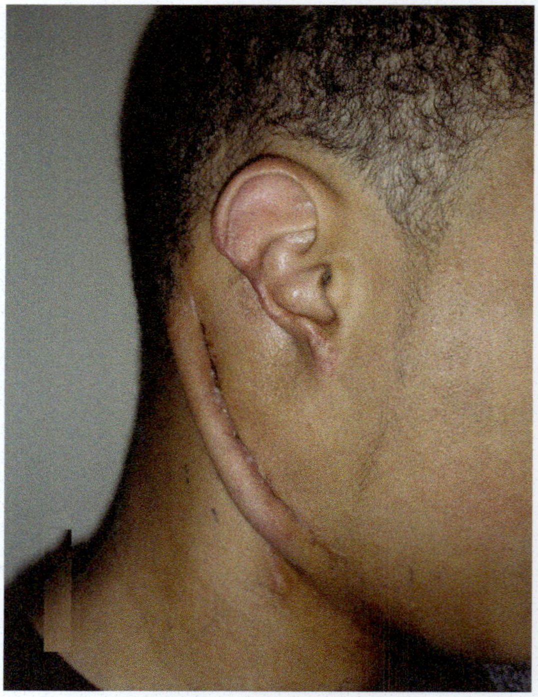

Fig. 21.30 Healed tubed flap prior to transfer.

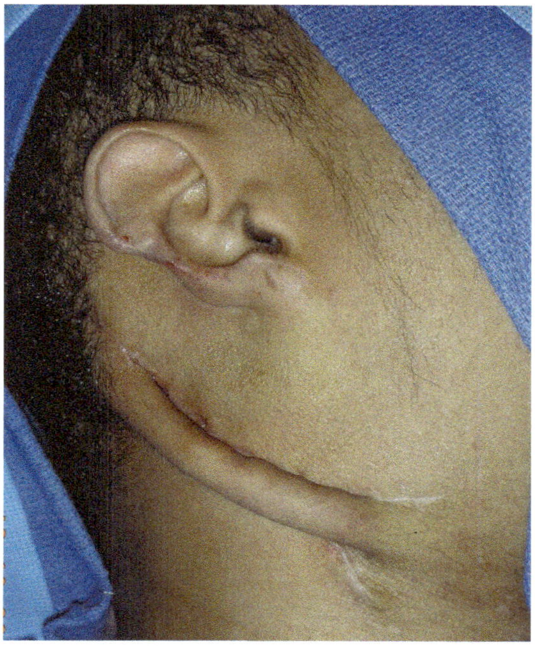

Fig. 21.31 Intraoperative view prior to separation of the tube.

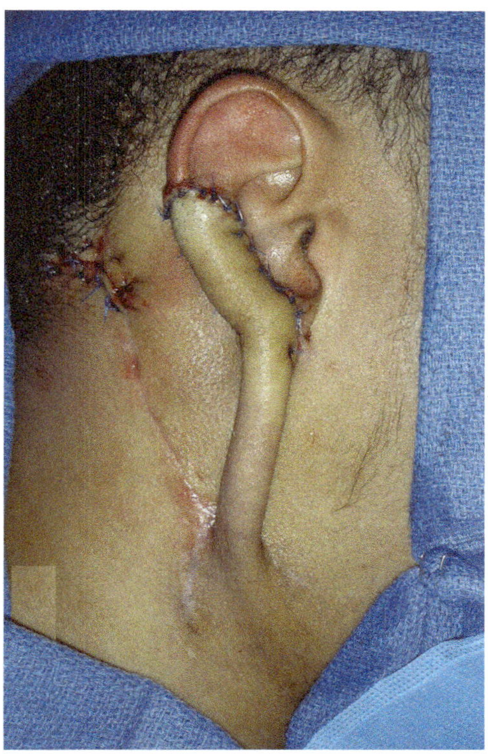

Fig. 21.32 Transfer of the superior portion of the tubed flap to recreate the missing lower portion of the ear.

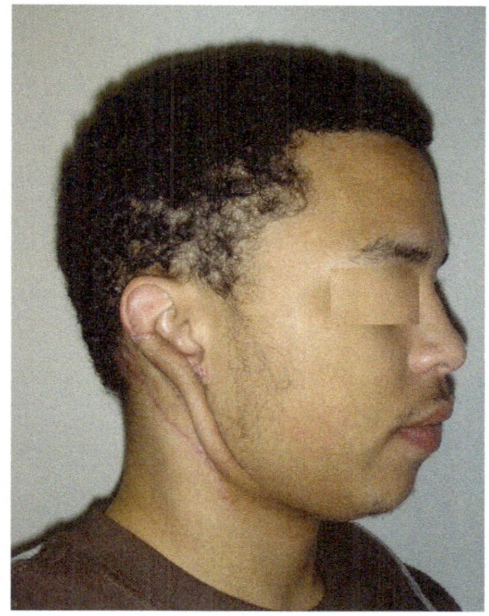

Fig. 21.33 Initial healing of the transferred flap.

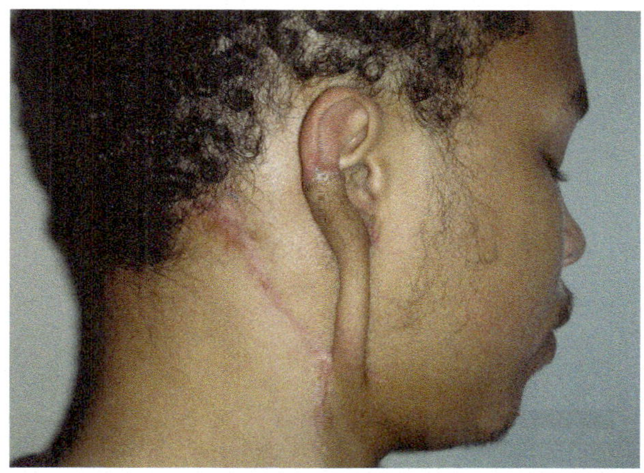

Fig. 21.34 Posterior aspect of the tubed flap.

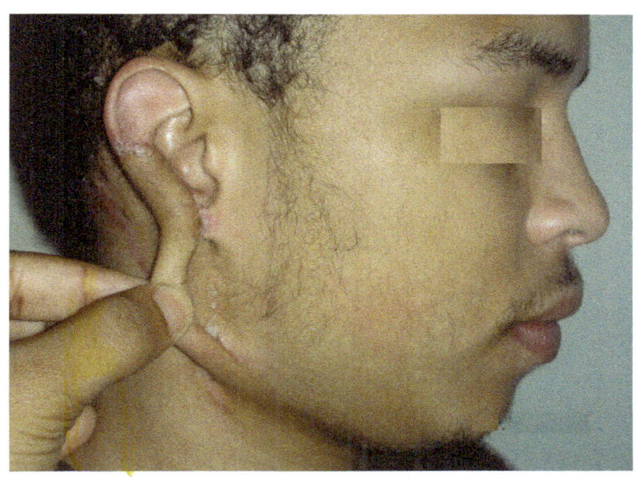

Fig. 21.35 Note that the flap is attached inferiorly in the neck and superior in the ear.

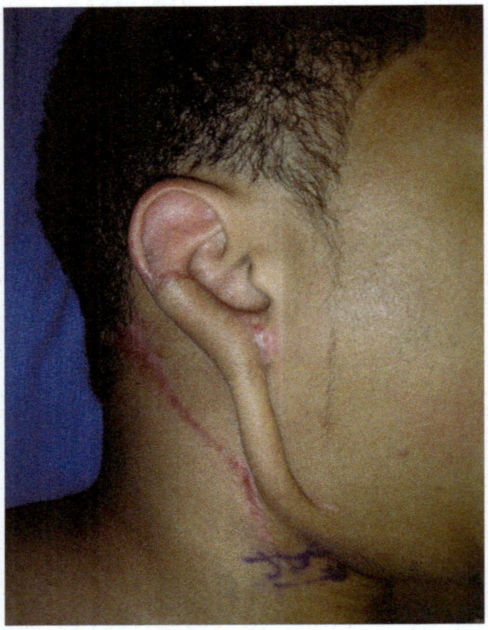

Fig. 21.36 Appearance prior to section of the flap.

For the final stage, the patient was once again brought back to the operating room and the inferior portion of the tube was sectioned and the lobule of the ear was reconstructed (Figures 21.36 and 21.37). The final appearance of the reconstructed ear was acceptable (Figure 21.38).

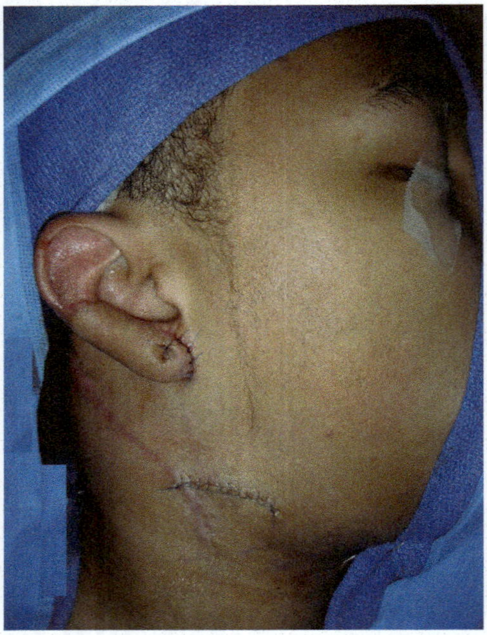

Fig. 21.37 Initial appearance of the reconstruction after sectioning and insetting of the tubed flap.

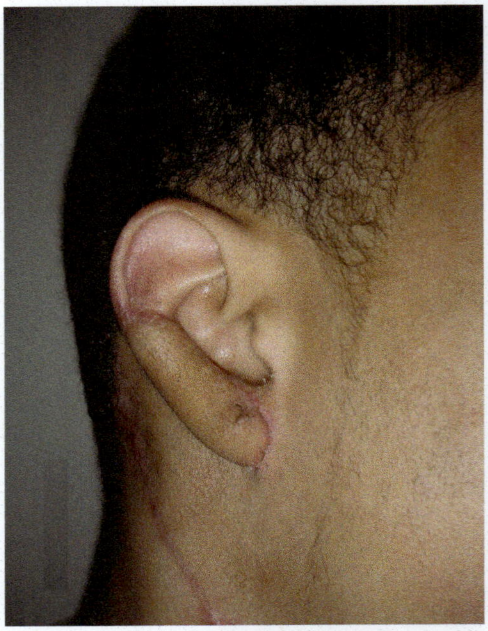

Fig. 21.38 Early postoperative healing of the reconstructed ear.

Total ear defect

Total or subtotal defects of the ear are usually the result of tumor excision. In these cases, the surgeon has to make a decision about if and when to reconstruct the defect. In some circumstances, the better option is to delay the reconstruction until after treatment of the underlying cause that may lead to the need for removing the ear.

Case #7

The patient is an older Caucasian male who presented with a large squamous cell carcinoma of the ear with evidence of nodal metastasis to the upper cervical nodes (Figure 21.39). The patient was taken to the operating room for a total auriculectomy and cervical lymphadenectomy (Figure 21.40). The resection was performed and the deep margins assessed to ensure that the tumor was completely resected (Figures 21.41 and 21.42). A pedicled flap was developed to repair the defect and cover the exposed mastoid bone (Figures 21.43 and 21.44). The flap was then inset taking care to maintain the patency of the external auditory canal (Figure 21.45).

The early appearance of the reconstructed defect was acceptable (Figure 21.46). The patient was then referred to radiation for the adjuvant treatment needed. He was evaluated soon after completion of his radiation therapy. The flap was intact with the exception of a few areas where he had some healing ulcers secondary to the radiation burn (Figure 21.47).

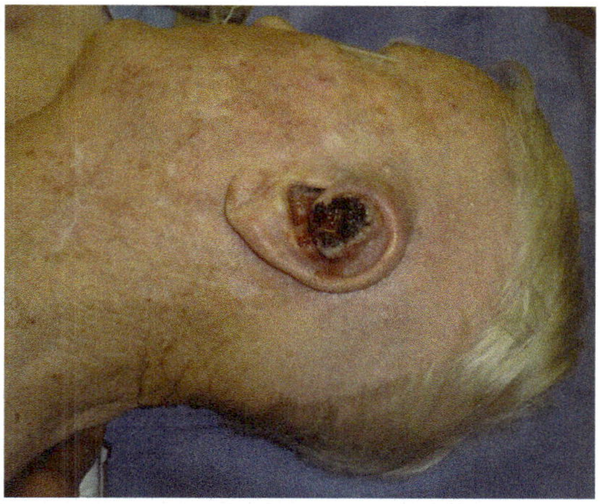

Fig. 21.39 View of the left ear with a large tumor filling the entire concha.

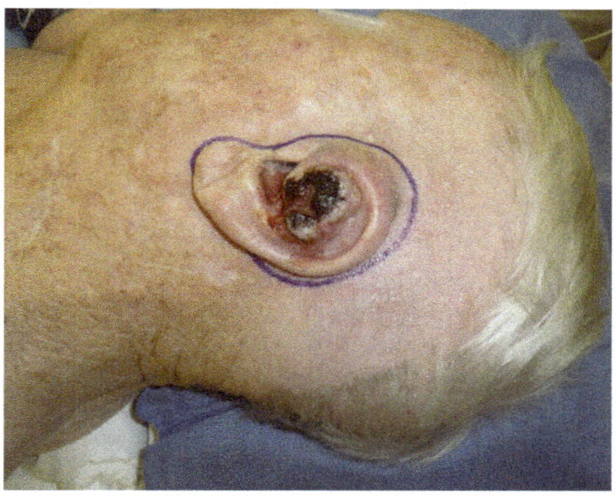

Fig. 21.40 Plan for a total auriculectomy.

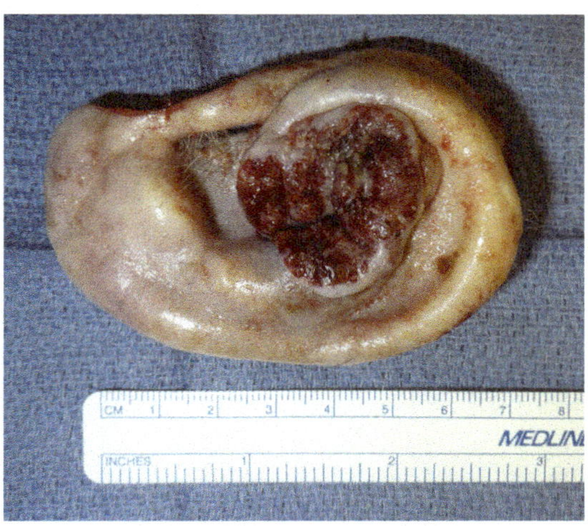

Fig. 21.41 View of the resected specimen.

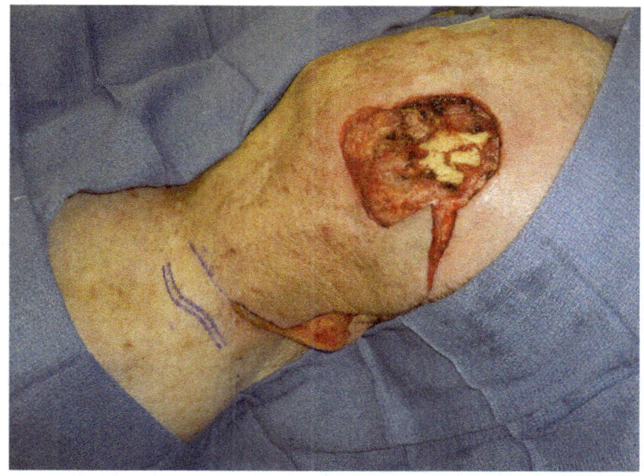

Fig. 21.42 View of the resection bed with incision made for a rotation flap to repair the defect.

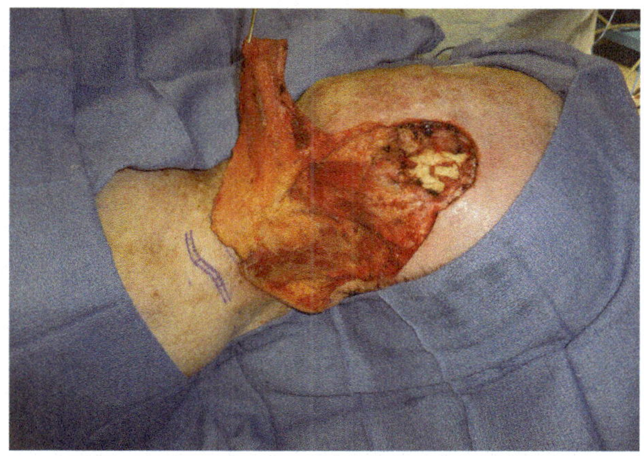

Fig. 21.43 Elevation of the flap prior to rotation and transfer.

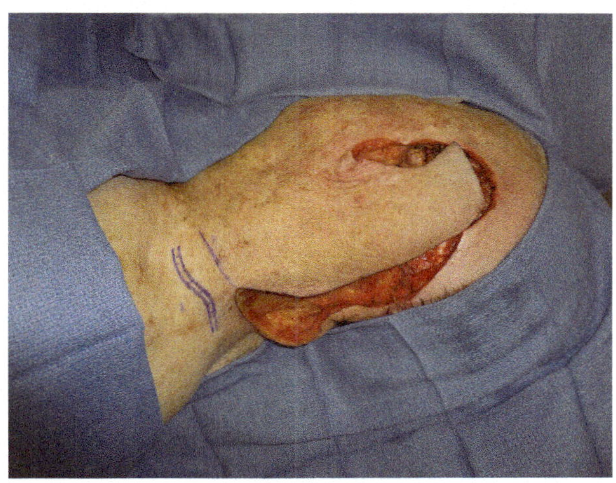

Fig. 21.44 Assessment of the rotation of the flap.

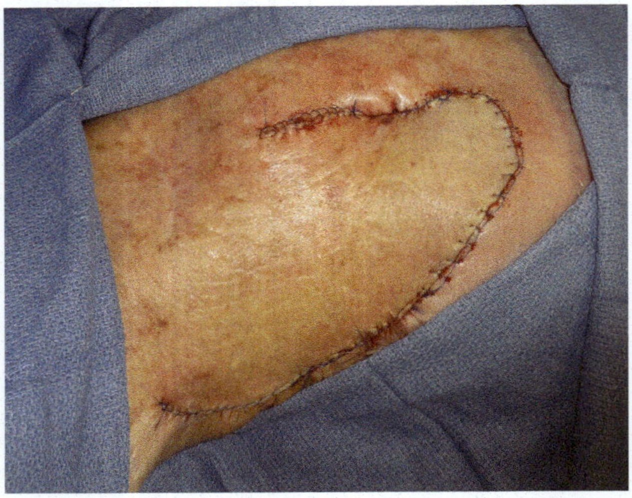

Fig. 21.45 Inset of the flap with repair of the auriculectomy defect.

Costal cartilage reconstruction

Ear reconstruction is an acceptable standard for the reconstruction of ear defects. The reason for this has been in large part due to the contributions of surgeons such as Tanzer,[3] Brent,[4] and Nagata.[5] The reconstruction of the microtic ear or acquired traumatic defect can be performed with the aid of rib cartilage as the support structure.

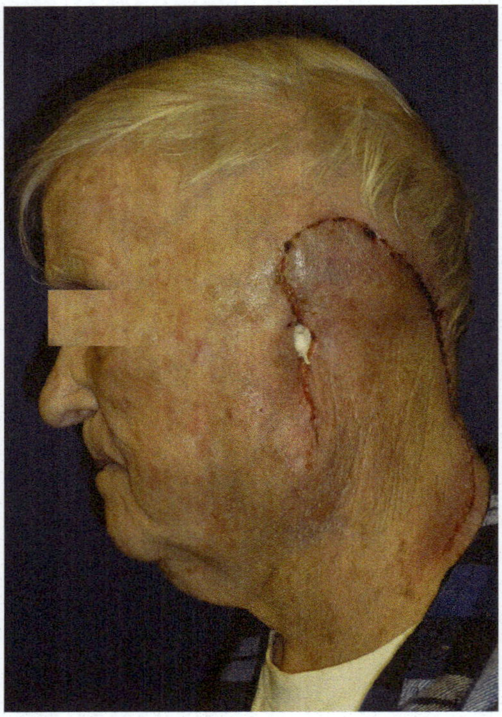

Fig. 21.46 Early postoperative view of the reconstruction.

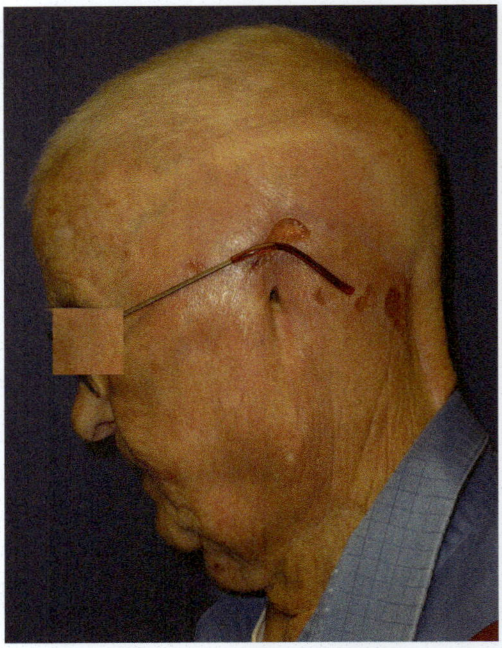

Fig. 21.47 Late postoperative view of the reconstruction after completion of radiation therapy. Note the areas of skin breakdown secondary to radiation treatment.

The cartilaginous rib graft can be harvested from the 6th to 9th ribs. The surgeon should seek to have adequate cartilage to allow for the harvest of the needed structures. In cases where there is a need to carve a total ear, the quantity of cartilage needs to be evaluated prior to harvest to be sure that it is of good quantity and quality for carving (Figure 21.48). Sometimes, using a template from the intact ear can be very helpful when harvesting the cartilage (Figure 21.49). Once the cartilage is harvested, it should be carved by the surgeon to fit the needs of the defect (Figures 21.50 and 21.51).

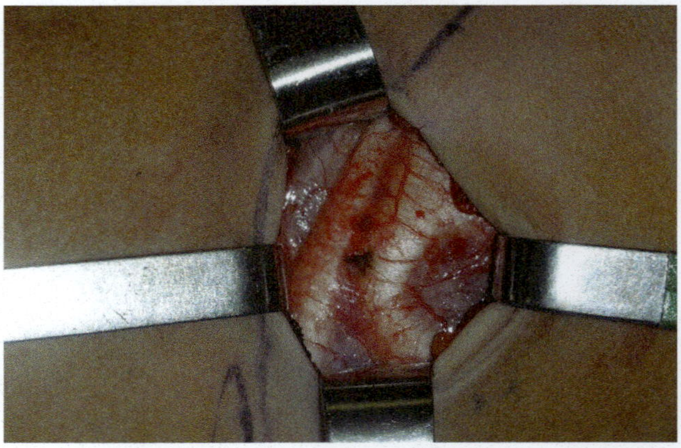

Fig. 21.48 View of the cartilage prior to harvest and carving.

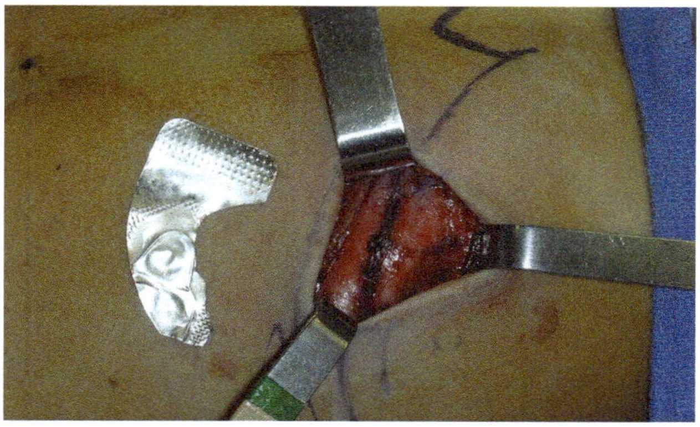

Fig. 21.49 Markings of the cartilage prior to harvest.

Alloplastic reconstruction

The most commonly utilized alloplastic reconstructive method for subtotal or total ear reconstruction uses porous polyethylene (Medpor, Porex Surgical, Newnan GA). The product is manufactured in two parts to allow for greater flexibility in sizing and positioning of the helical rim onto the base portion.[6] The use of the alloplast for support requires that the structure is wrapped with vascularized tissue. The options most commonly used are the temporoparietal fascial flap or a pre-expanded tissue.

Case #8

A young lady was involved in a car accident and suffered a near total loss of the helix and antihelix portion of the ear (Figure 21.52). A decision was made for the reconstruction of the missing ear with an alloplastic implant and a temporoparietal fascial flap. The temporoparietal fascial flap was developed to have enough quantity to wrap the prosthesis (Figures 21.53 and 21.54). Once the flap was elevated, the recipient bed was prepared, the prosthesis implanted, and the flap wrapped around the prosthesis (Figures 21.55 and 21.56). A skin graft was then used to cover the flap (Figure 21.57). The patient was then

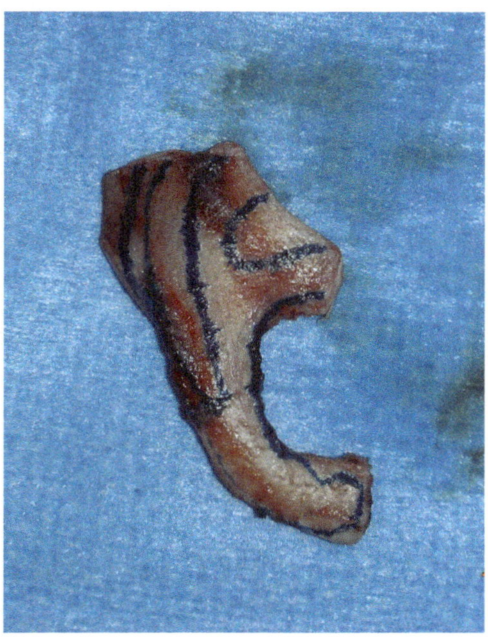

Fig. 21.50 Initial markings of the cartilage prior to carving.

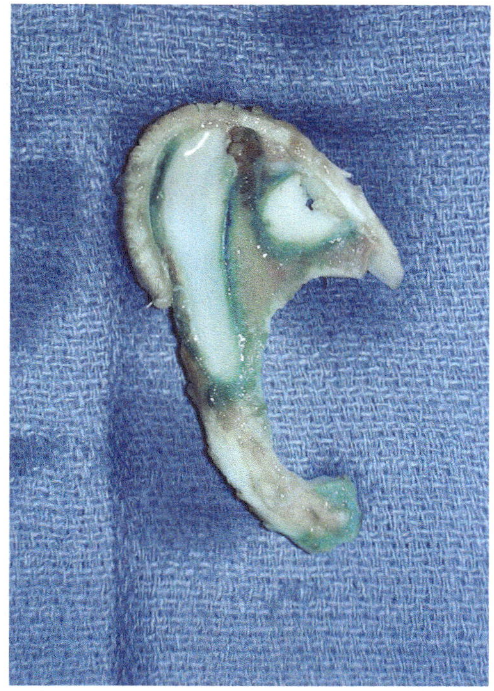

Fig. 21.51 initial construct of the cartilage graft construct.

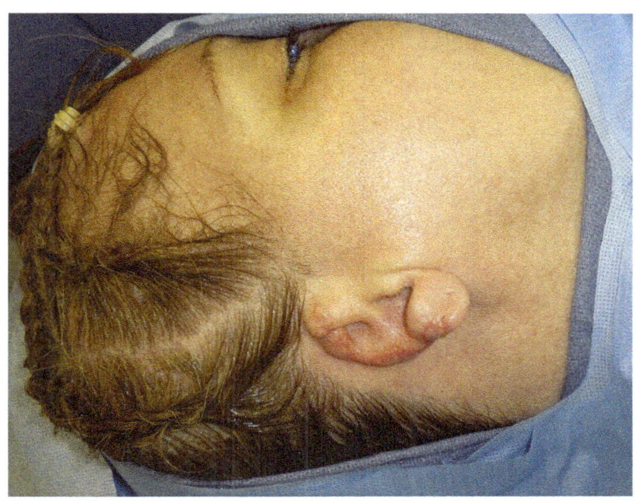

Fig. 21.52 View of the patient with loss a large portion of the ear secondary to a traumatic injury.

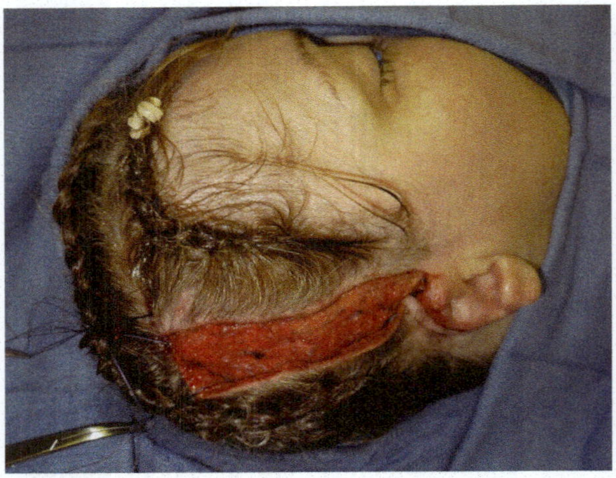

Fig. 21.53 Initial harvest of the temporoparietal fascia flap.

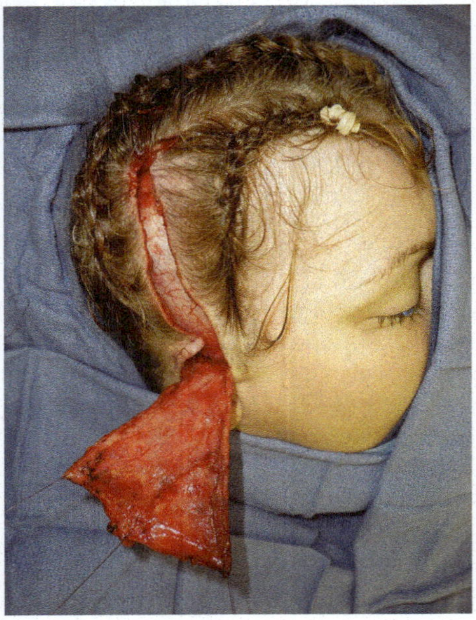

Fig. 21.54 Elevated temporoparietal fascia flap.

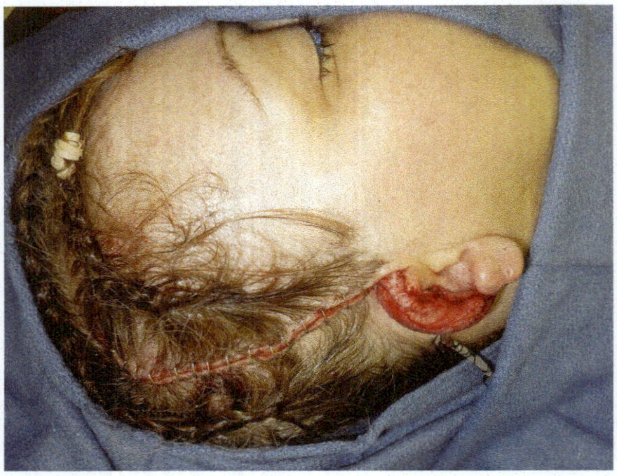

Fig. 21.55 Reconstruction of the ear with wrapping of the construct with the temporoparietal fascia flap.

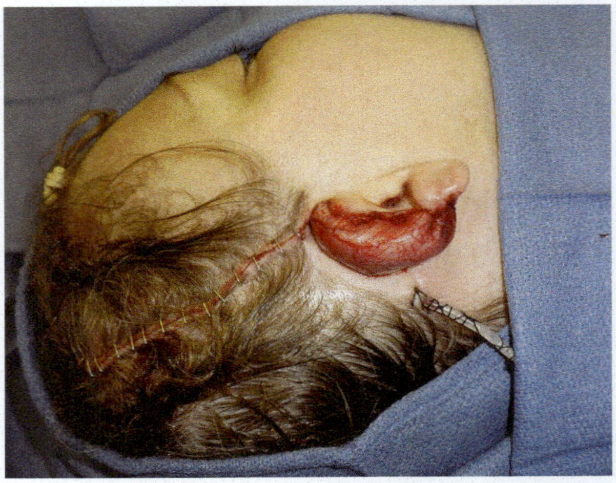

Fig. 21.56 Posterior view of the reconstruction.

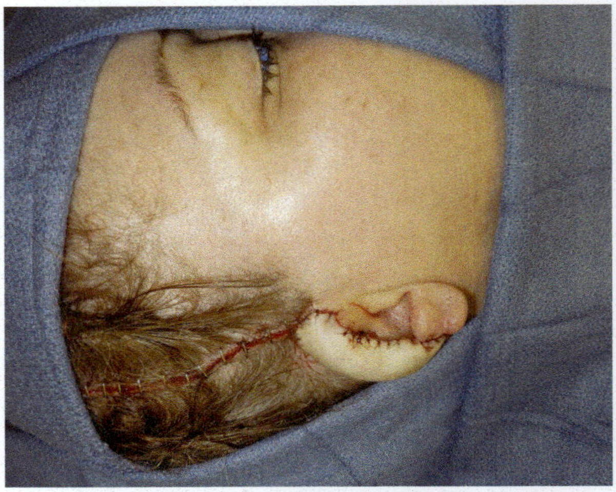

Fig. 21.57 View of the reconstruction after placement of a skin graft.

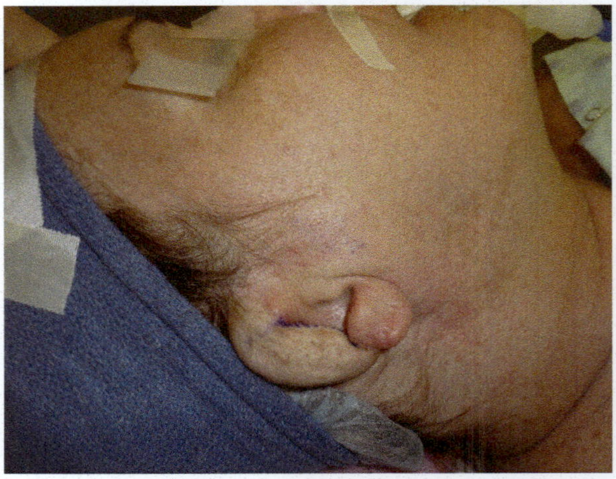

Fig. 21.58 Early appearance of the reconstruction prior to debulking.

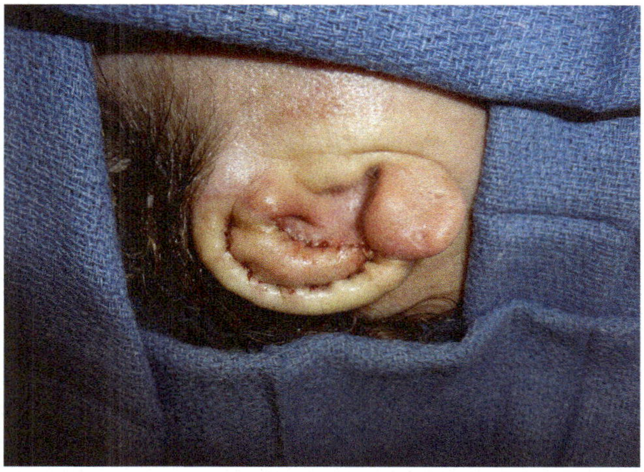

Fig. 21.59 Initial appearance of the reconstruction after debulking.

brought back to the operating room and the area was debulked and quilting sutures used to enhance the drape of the flap over the prosthesis (Figures 21.58 and 21.59). The early appearance of the patient was acceptable and she was content with the outcome (Figure 21.60).

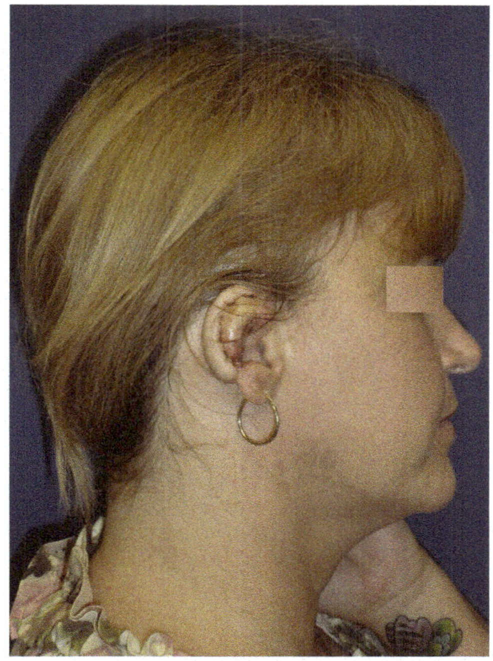

Fig. 21.60 Late appearance of the reconstructed ear.

Prosthetic reconstruction

An important consideration in total ear reconstruction is the use of a total prosthetic ear. When the surgeon is considering the use of maxillofacial prosthetics is critical to have a solid foundation for the prosthetic. In these cases, the rotational flaps used to prepare the bed have to be adequate enough to support the prosthesis and thin enough that if bone anchored implants are used; the tissue also will need to be of appropriate thickness to allow for the emergence of the implants. The use of prosthetic ear will not be covered in this text.

The above examples illustrate various reconstructive examples based on defect locations. There are a number of other options in addition to the ones covered on this chapter.

References

1. da Silva Freitas R, Sánchez ME, Manzotti MS, Baras F, Ono MC, de Oliveira e Cruz GA. Comparing cephaloauricular and scaphaconchal angles in prominent ear patients and control subjects. *Aesth Plast Surg* 2008; 32:620–623.
2. Eppley BL. Auricular reconstruction after oncological resection. *Oper Techn Plast Reconstr Surg* 1999; 6:275–283.
3. Tanzer RC. Total reconstruction of the external ar. *Plast Reconstr Surg* 1959; 23:1–15.
4. Brent B. Technical advances in ear reconstruction with autogenous rib cartilage grafts: personal experience with 1200 cases. *Plast Reconstr Surg* 1999; 104:319–334.
5. Nagata S. A new method of total reconstruction of the auricle for microtia. *Plast Reconstr Surg* 1993; 92:187–201.
6. Renner G, Lane RV, Auricular reconstruction: an update. *Curr Opin Otolaryngol Head Neck Surg* 2004; 12:277–280.

Chapter 22
Lip reconstruction

Introduction

The lips along with the eyes are the two most expressive structures in our face. The lips are able to convey a myriad of minute expressions and emotions. Additionally, the lips are critical in eating and speaking. Because of its role, the need to properly repair lip defects is very important to the reconstructive surgeon. The challenge increases proportionally with the size and location of the defect. Over the years, many surgeons have tackled this challenge with numerous approaches.

The most commonly encountered lip defects are those resulting from excision of lesions affecting the lower lip. Because of the lower lips' prominence and exposure to sunlight, it is affected nearly nine times more than the upper lip. Conversely, traumatic defects occur more often in the upper lip. This is particularly more so in bite incidences.

Traditionally, the approaches to reconstruction of lip defects have followed a simple algorithm of defect size. This approach takes into account the differences in shape, size, and pliability of the lower lip compared to the upper lip. When using the traditional approach, defects of the lower lip less than one-third of the total lip size can be repaired by primary closure. Defects greater than one-third but less than two-thirds can be reconstructed with a variety of local flap techniques. Defects greater than to two-thirds or total lip defects are often addressed with free tissue transfer. A similar approach can be used for upper lip defects with a simple caveat that smaller defects can be closed primarily; this percentage is usually around 25% of the upper lip.

Anatomy

The surface anatomy of the upper and lower lip are different. The upper lip is divided into four subunits: the central philtral, the two lateral units, and the mucosal subunit. The lateral units extend lateral to the philtral column and medial to the melolabial fold. The surface anatomy of the lower lip is composed of two subunits: the mucosal and the central.

The lip is composed of a circular muscle, the orbicularis oris, which forms the oral sphincter. The orbicularis is responsible for maintaining oral competence and seal. Attached to the orbicularis, the levators and depressors of the lips are entrusted with the fine movements of the lip and for helping to convey many of our emotions through facial expressions emanating from this area. The lateral condensation of these muscles forms the modiolus.

The inner aspect of the orbicularis muscle is lined by the oral mucosa while the skin covers the muscle. Interposed between the muscle and the mucosa are numerous minor salivary glands. The vermillion is the mucosal extension from the inner lip extending to the external aspect to meet the skin and form the vermillion cutaneous junction often referred to as the white line or white roll.

The blood supply to the lip emerges from the facial artery as it travels superiorly over the mandible towards the lip and gives off a branch to perfuse the lower lip. This branch is the inferior labial artery. The facial artery continues its superior migration lateral to the modiolus, and gives off another branch that travels medially to perfuse the upper lip. This branch is the superior labial artery. Veins bearing the same name and travelling alongside

Local and Regional Flaps in Head & Neck Reconstruction: A Practical Approach, First Edition. Rui Fernandes.

Companion website: www.wiley.com/go/fernandes/flapsreconstruction

the arteries supply the venous drainage to the upper and lower lips.

The lips receive motor innervation from branches of the seventh cranial nerve. The buccal branches innervate the upper lip while the lower lip is innervated by the marginal mandibular branches. The sensory innervation is supplied by the fifth cranial nerve. The upper lip is supplied by the second division while the lower lip is supplied by the third division.

Defect assessment

Upper lip defects

Defects less than 25%

Small defects of the upper lip can be readily addressed by ensuring freshening of the lateral borders of the defect (in traumatic cases) and reapproximation of the mucosa, muscular, and skin layers. The outcome of these defects is often pleasing without much evidence of the surgical intervention.

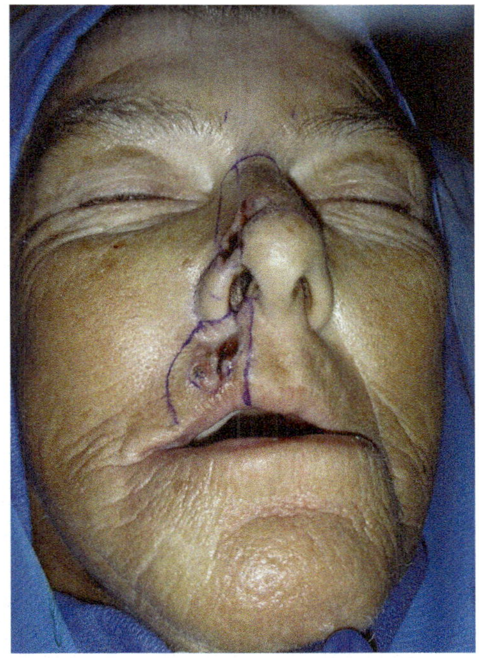

Fig. 22.1 View of a patient with an upper lip carcinoma with markings made for the resection.

Defects greater than 25%

Abbe flap

In cases where the defect size is greater than what could be closed with a simple advancement and closure, an Abbe flap may be used to repair the defect. The initial description of the Abbe flap is attributed to Dr. Robert Abbe based on his publication in 1898.[1] Recent attention has been given to the accuracy of this attribution; some authors feel that the procedure had been previously described, albeit in different language[2,3].

The flap is designed by borrowing a composite from the lower lip and transferring it to the upper lip. This is carried out in stages. The initial assessment is made after removing the lesion from the upper lip and then assessing the width and height of the defect (Figures 22.1 to 22.3). The defect measurement or template is then transferred to the lower lip. The width of the flap should be less than that of the defect (about half) while the height should remain the same (Figure 22.4). A decision should be made as to what side the flap should be pedicled from, this is done from the side that would allow easiest of transfer to the defect without kinking the pedicle and compromising the flap (Figure 22.5). The flap is then rotated to the defect (Figure 22.6). The inset should be done with care to reapproximate each of the three layers, i.e. the mucosa, the orbicularis, and the skin. Particular attention should be taken to the reapproximation of the white roll from the flap and each recipient side (Figure 22.7). The flap is allowed to heal for 2 to 3 weeks. During this time period, the flap will develop enough collateral flow that will allow for the takedown of the flap and ligation of the inferior labial artery (Figures 22.8 and 22.9). The adequacy of the collateral blood flow to the flap can be assessed prior to separation of the flap by ligating the pedicle with a rubber band and evaluating the flap for perfusion and congestion (Figure 22.10). Once the

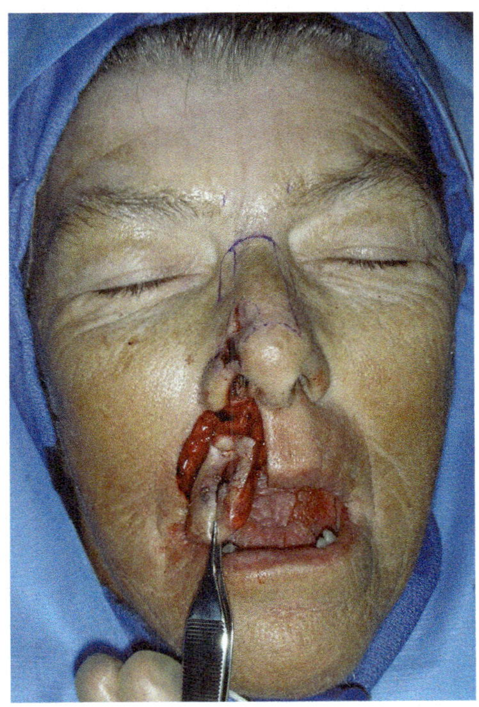

Fig. 22.2 Incision of the lesion.

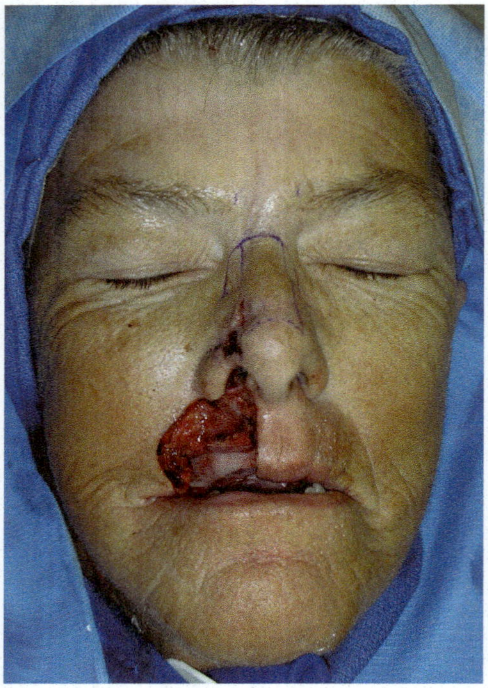

Fig. 22.3 View of the resection and area to be reconstructed.

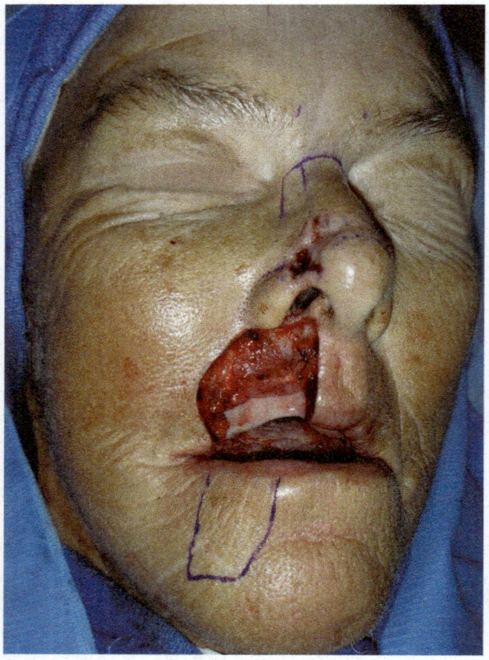

Fig. 22.4 Markings for a transposition flap in the form of an Abbe flap.

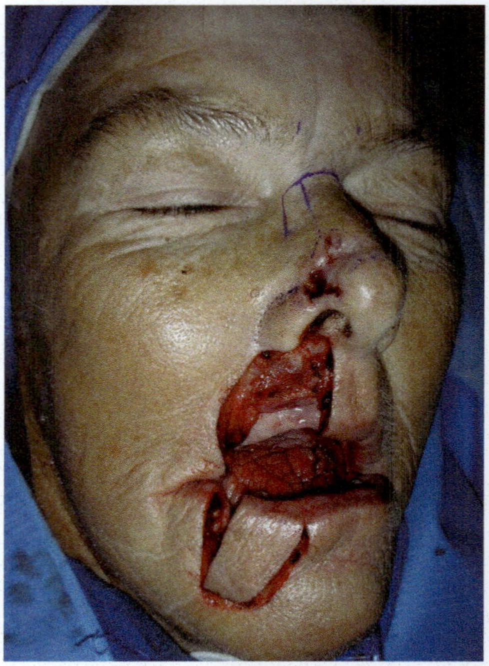

Fig. 22.5 Incision of the Abbe flap with the pedicle located on the upper left portion of the lip.

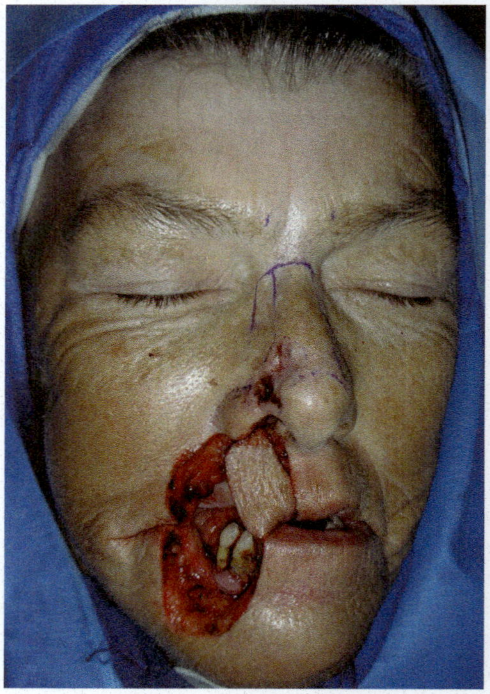

Fig. 22.6 Rotation of the Abbe flap prior to inset.

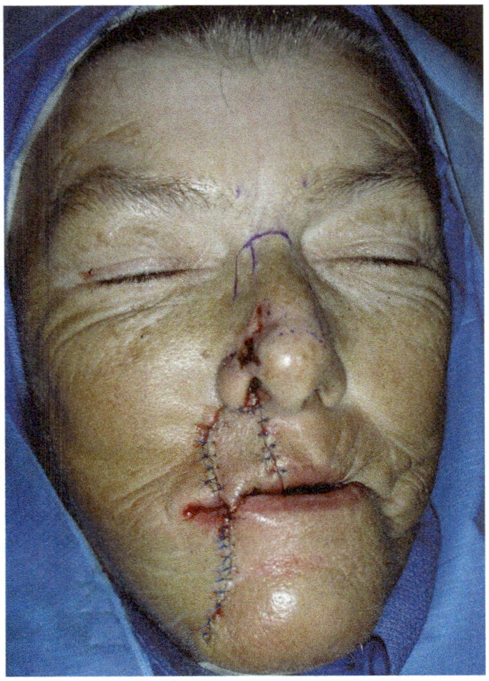

Fig. 22.7 Inset of the flap with the pedicle coming in from the lower lip.

perfusion is determined to be adequate, the flap is separated and the mucosa and superior aspects of the muscle are reapproximated to establish a normal lip contour (Figure 22.11).

V–Y advancement flap

The V–Y technique is described in Chapter 8. The technique can be used throughout the head and neck. In the reconstruction of upper lip it can be used in conjunction with other local flaps to repair very large defects. The

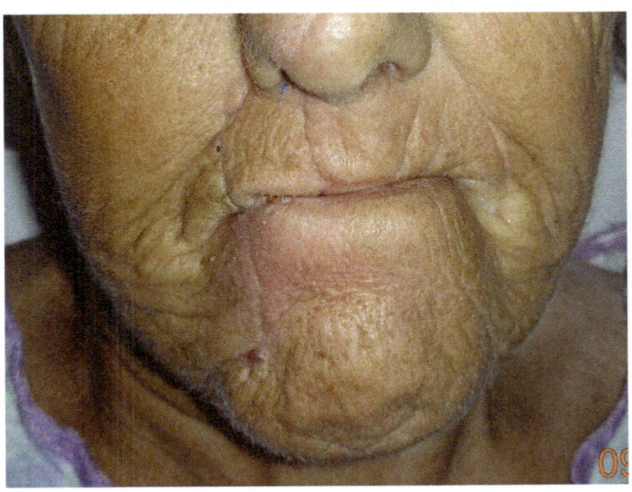

Fig. 22.8 Appearance of the reconstructed lip prior to takedown of the pedicle.

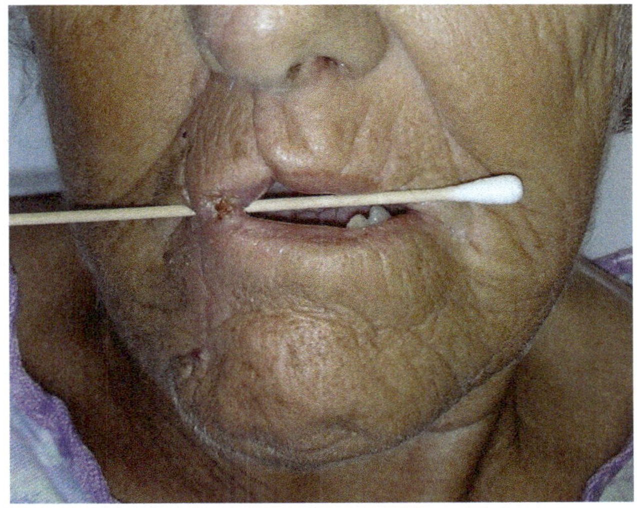

Fig. 22.9 View of the pedicle prior to resection.

patient in this example was referred from a mental institution for evaluation of a longstanding basal cell carcinoma of the left upper lip with extension to the cheek (Figure 22.12). The lesion was marked for resection with the anticipation of reconstructing the defect with local tissue (Figure 22.13). The defect was found to extend to the cheek and encompass nearly half of the upper lip (Figure 22.14). A combination of a V–Y flap based on the perforators from the facial artery and a cheek advancement flap was planned (Figure 22.15. The flap was elevated and mobilized while taking care not to injure the perforators to the skin flap (Figures 22.16 to 22.18). The flap was then mobilized along with a perialar crescentic flap from the

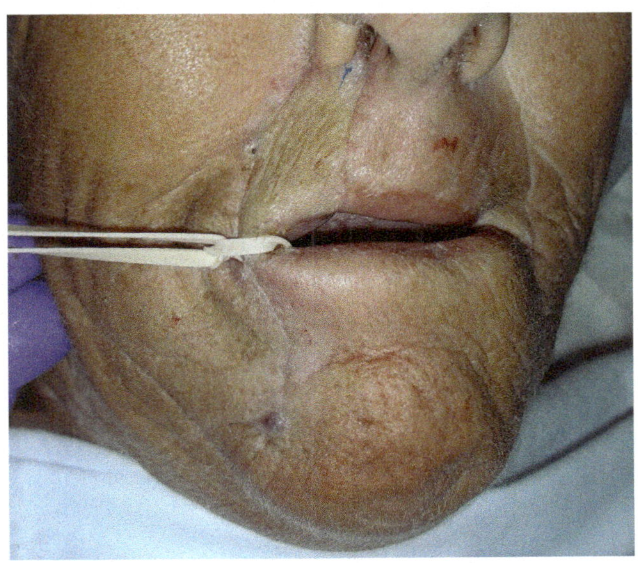

Fig. 22.10 Assessment of perfusion of the flap from the collateral supply by occlusion of the pedicle.

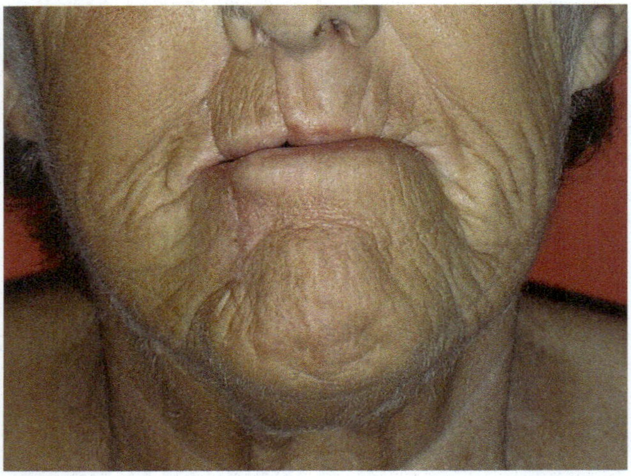

Fig. 22.11 Appearance of the final reconstruction.

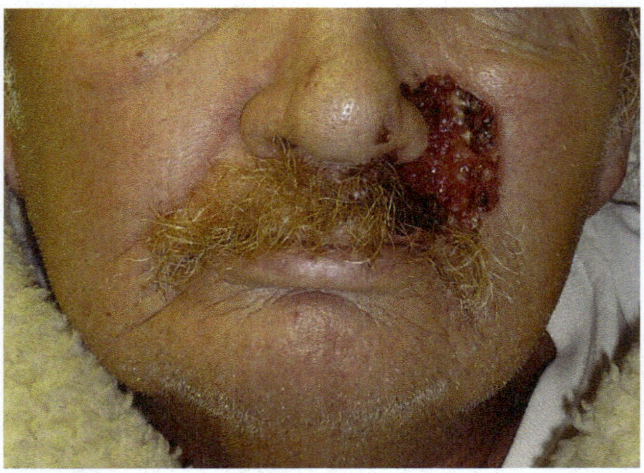

Fig. 22.12 View of a patient with a large neglected malignancy on the left upper lip extending to the cheek.

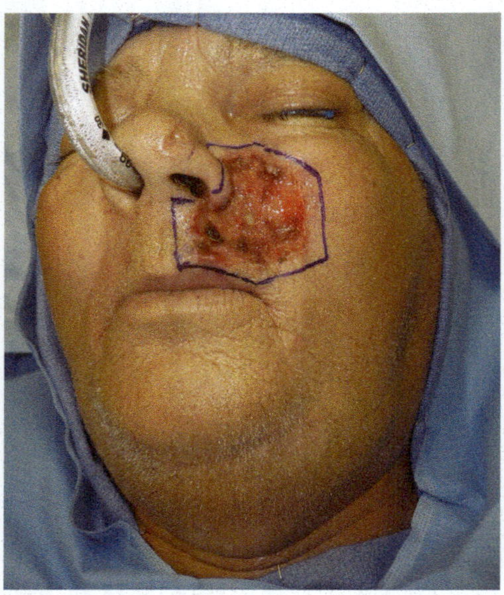

Fig. 22.13 Outline for the planned resection; note the very large outline.

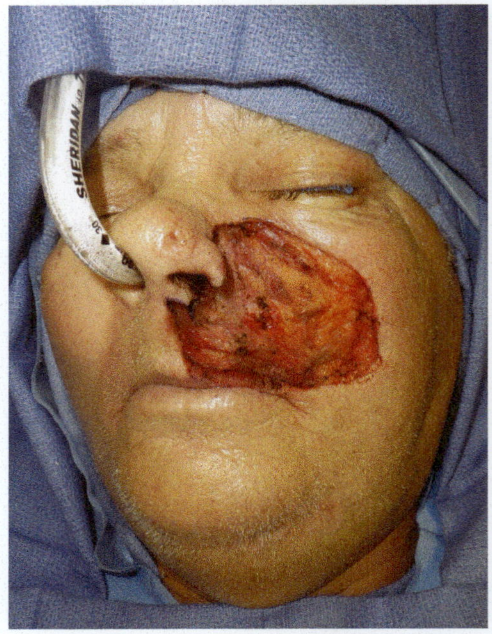

Fig. 22.14 View of the defect with greater than half of the upper lip missing as well as a large portion of the cheek.

contralateral side and the cheek advancement flap from the ipsilateral side to repair the defect with minimal distortion (Figures 22.19 and 22.20).

The final appearance of the patient was acceptable overall (Figure 22.21). This case illustrates the use of combining the V–Y flap with other techniques to repair very large upper lip defects.

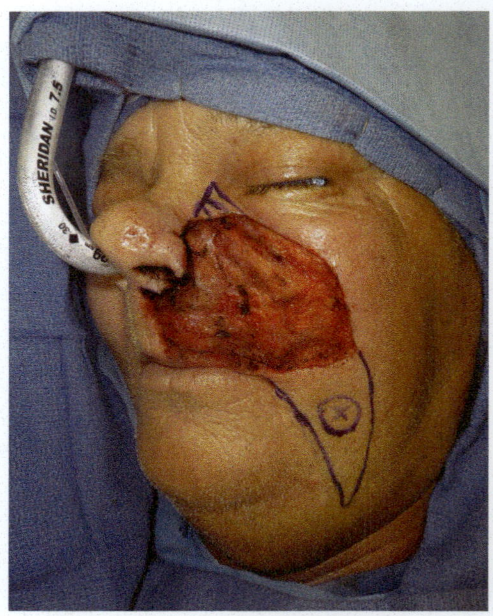

Fig. 22.15 Plan for the use of a facial artery perforator flap and a cheek advancement.

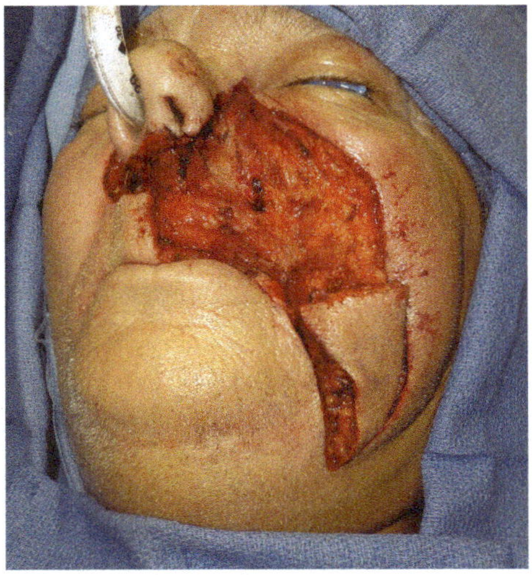

Fig. 22.16 Incision of the planned flap prior to transfer.

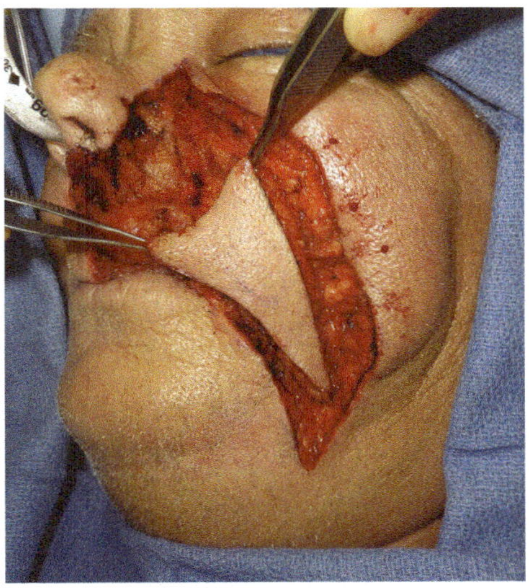

Fig. 22.17 Assessment of the advancement of the flap into the defect.

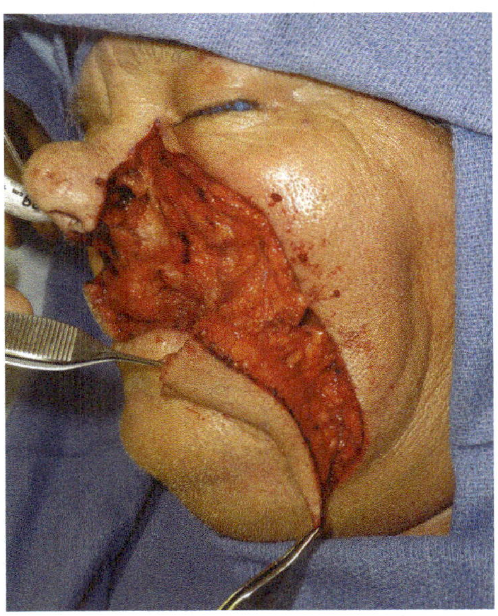

Fig. 22.18 View of the underside of the flap where the perforators are gaining access to the flap.

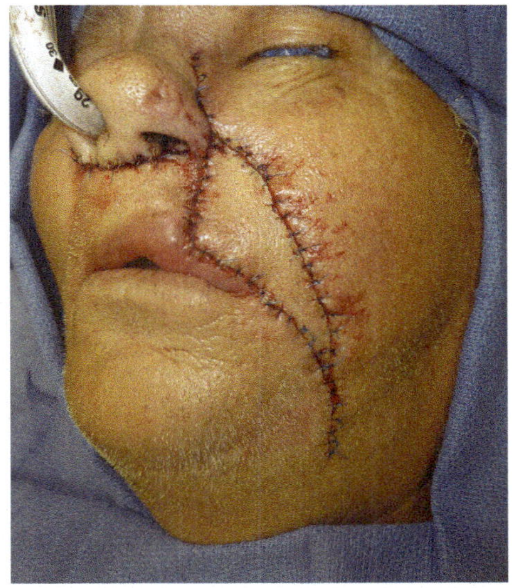

Fig. 22.19 Advancement and inset of the facial perforator flap and cheek advancement. Note that there is no distortion of the lip in this very large repair.

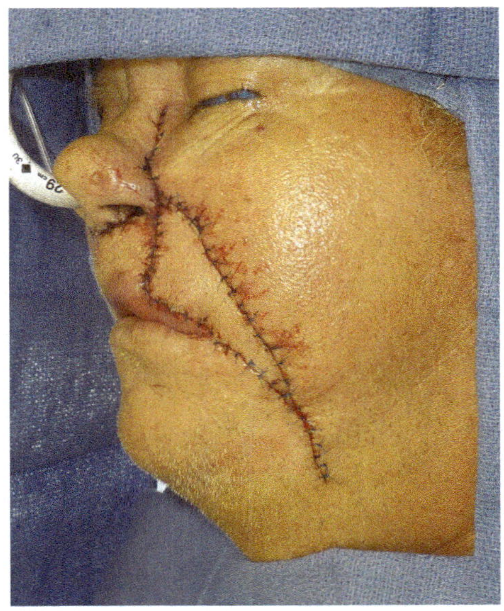

Fig. 22.20 Lateral view of the reconstruction.

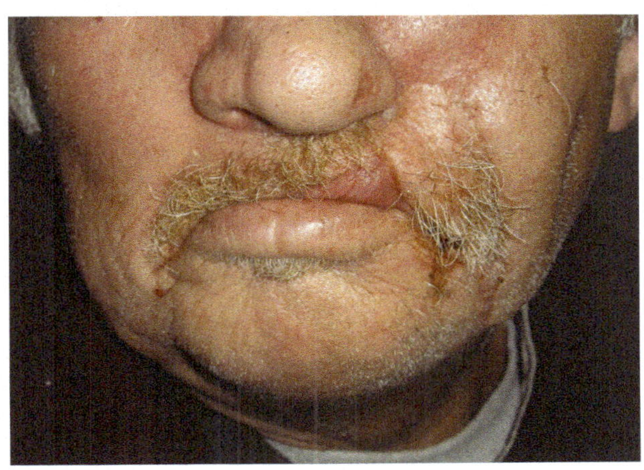

Fig. 22.21 Postoperative view of the reconstructed lip again showing little deformation of the upper lip.

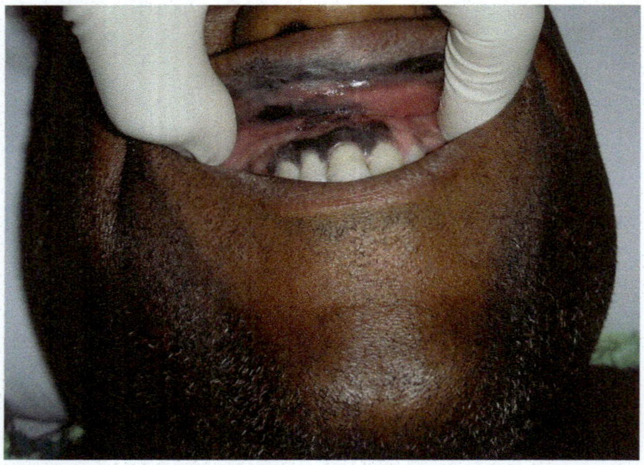

Fig. 22.22 View of the upper lip and pre-maxilla revealing a large mucosal melanoma.

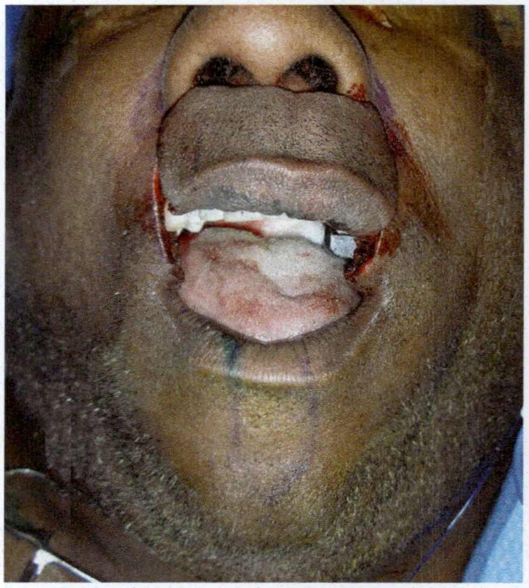

Fig. 22.24 Incision of the upper lip prior to resection.

Perialar crescentic flap

The perialar crescentic flap allows for the reconstruction of upper lip defects by mobilizing the tissues inward towards the defect. The perialar crescentic flap can be used in combination with another flap in order to repair large defects of the upper lip. The following case illustrates the use of such a combination. The patient was diagnosed with a mucosal melanoma of the upper lip, which extended towards the gingiva of the anterior maxilla (Figure 22.22). The anticipated defect would require a combination of flaps to restore the oral sphincter. The planned excision involved a near total upper lip resection and an anterior maxillectomy. The planned reconstruction was for bilateral perialar crescentic flap advancement and an Abbe transfer from the central lower lip (Figure 22.23). The resection of the upper lip and anterior maxilla was carried out as planned (Figures 22.24, 22.25, and 22.26a–c). The markings for the perialar crescentic flap were made in order to decrease the defect to about half of its original size (Figure 22.27). The skin excision was performed allowing for the advancement of the flap (Figures 22.28 and 22.29). With the size of the defect reduced to nearly 50% of its original size, the Abbe flap was marked, elevated, and transferred to repair the defect (Figure 22.30). The patient did well from the reconstruction.

Free tissue transfer

In some circumstances, the defect in the upper lip is too large to be effectively reconstructed with local or

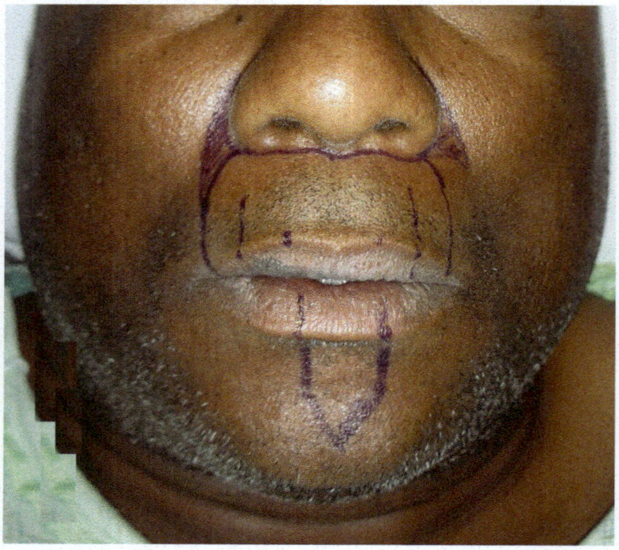

Fig. 22.23 Outline for a total upper lip resection and a midline Abbe flap in conjunction with bilateral crescentic flap.

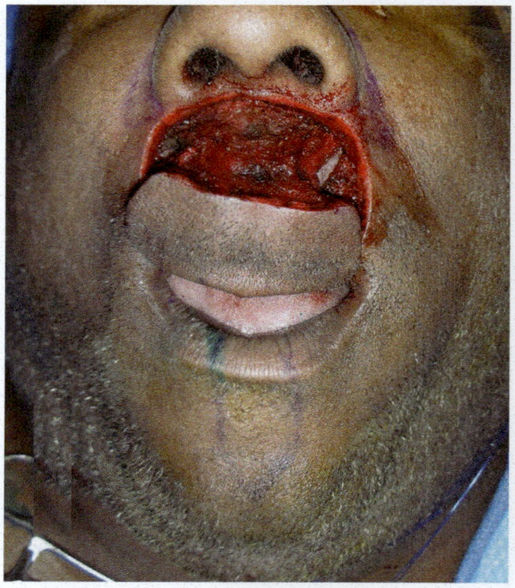

Fig. 22.25 Mobilization of the upper lip prior to resection.

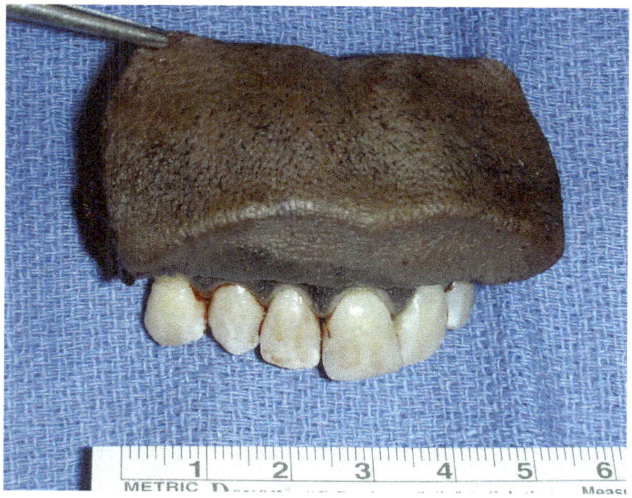

Fig. 22.26a View of the resected composite upper lip and premaxilla.

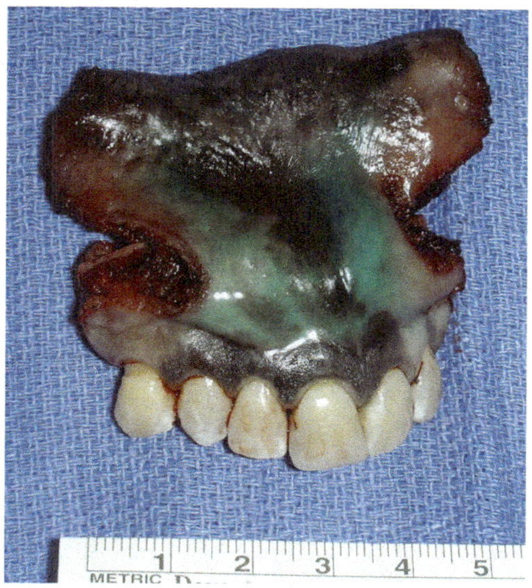

Fig. 22.26b View of the resected lip and maxilla.

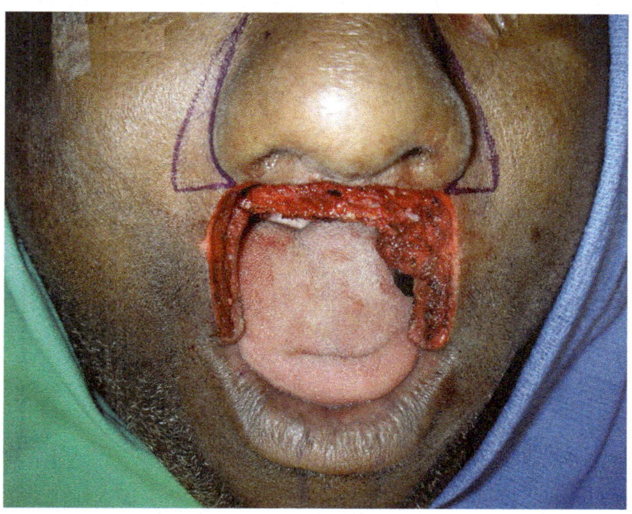

Fig. 22.27 Defect after resection with markings for the bilateral crescentic flaps.

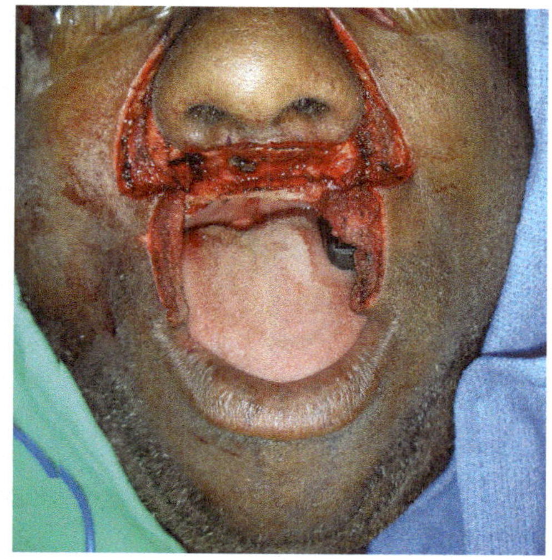

Fig. 22.28 Incision of the crescentic flap prior to advancement.

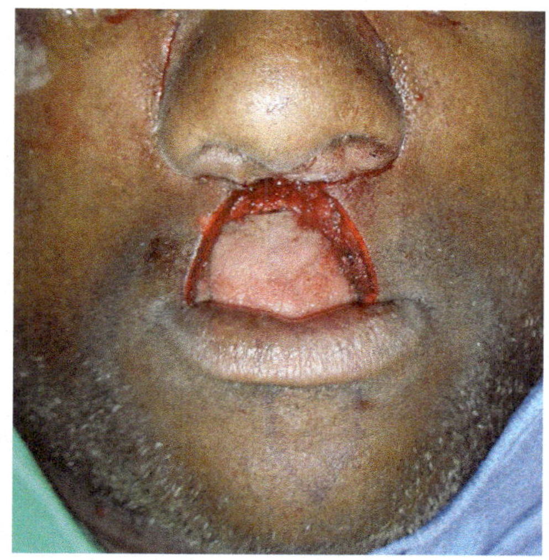

Fig. 22.29 Advancement of the crescentic flaps with a significant reduction of the defect size.

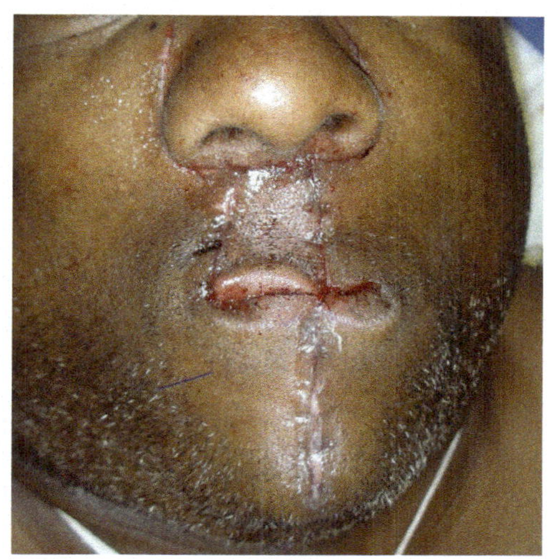

Fig. 22.30 View of the transferred Abbe flap to finish the reconstruction.

regional flaps. In these situations, the reconstructive surgeon should contemplate the use of free tissue transfer. Attempts at repairing very large defects encompassing extended total lip defects with local flaps often leads to an unacceptable decrease in oral opening and significant distortion of the face. The free tissue options for reconstructing lip defects are limited due to the demands of the site as the flap needs to be thin, pliable, and able to be contoured and suspended to the defect. The flap that most fits these demands is the radial forearm free flap. The main disadvantage of reconstructing a lip defect with fasciocutaneous free flaps is the loss of dynamic function of the lip, i.e., the maintenance of the oral sphincter. The other downsides of these reconstructions are the poor color match and the difference in texture. In spite of these drawbacks, there is still a role for free tissue transfer in lip reconstruction. The typical case for consideration of free tissue transfer is reconstruction of large, neglected lip cancers (Figure 22.31).

The planned resection is carried out based on the oncologic needs but also taking into consideration the esthetic subunits of the lip (Figure 22.32). The defect is then evaluated and a template is created to aid in the design of the flap (Figure 22.33). The radial forearm flap is marked and elevated based on the previously template design (Figures 22.34, and 22.35). The flap is transferred and inset into the defect site and the anastomosis is carried out as per routine (Figures 22.36 and 22.37. Early postoperative results show good contour of the reconstructed lip (Figure 22.38.

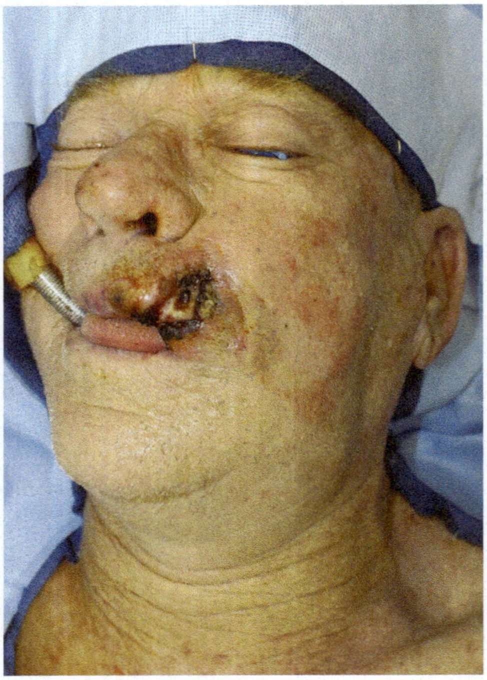

Fig. 22.31 View of a patient with a large upper lip malignancy.

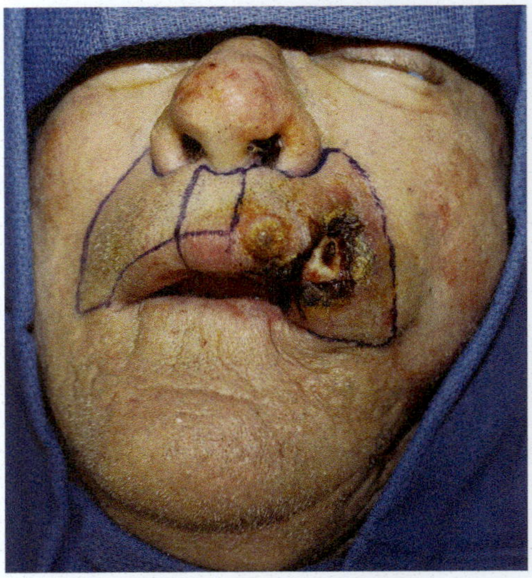

Fig. 22.32 Subunit markings of the upper lip prior to resection of the lip malignancy.

Lower lip defects

Defects less than 33%

Vermillionectomy with mucosal advancement

The vermillionectomy is a procedure carried out when the lesion affecting the lip is superficial and involves only the mucosal aspect of the vermillion. Removing the mucosa and the underlying tissue up to the muscle bed makes up the excision of the vermillion. The resultant defect extends from one commissure to the other. Anteriorly, it extends to the lip skin (white roll) and posteriorly to the inner lip mucosa or the wet line (Figure 22.39). The mucosa advancement is performed to advance the inner lip mucosa to the skin edge of the lip. To accomplish this,

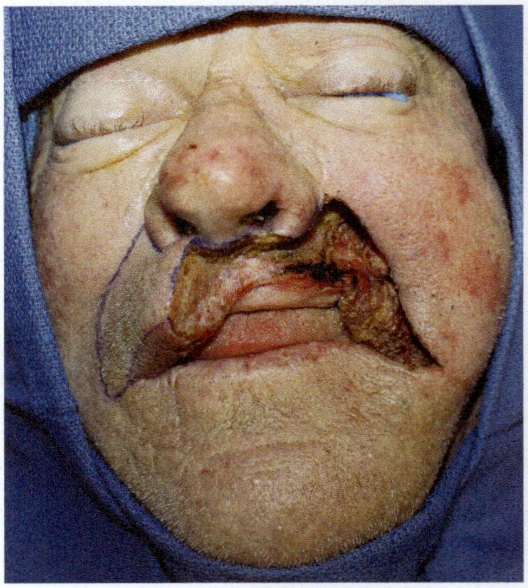

Fig. 22.33 View of the resected upper lip tumor. Note the very large defect.

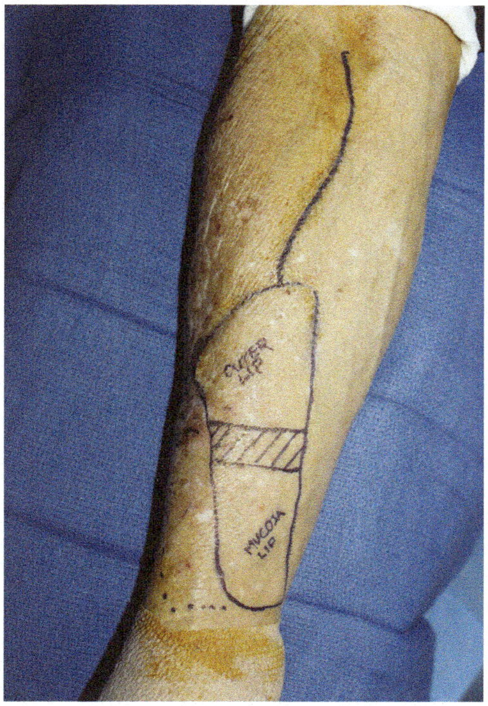

Fig. 22.34 Markings for a radial forearm free flap to repair the lip defect.

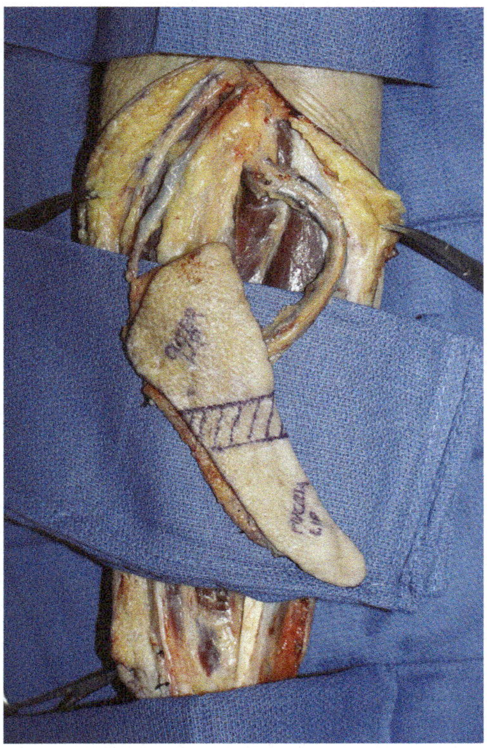

Fig. 22.35 Raised radial forearm flap prior to transfer.

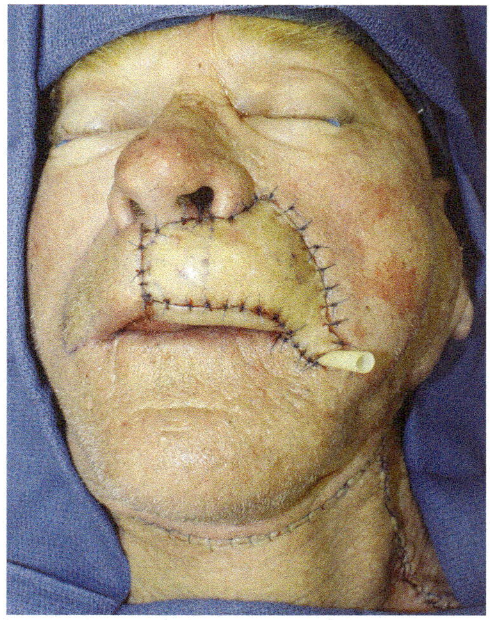

Fig. 22.36 Inset of the flap in the upper lip reconstructing the pre-tumor form.

the mucosa should be undermined with care not to cause a hematoma, which may lead to the loss of the mucosa at that site once it is transferred. Equally, the minor salivary glands that will be encountered should be removed to prevent the appearance of submucosal nodules at the final reconstruction. The advancement should allow for a passive closure of the mucosa flap to the skin edge

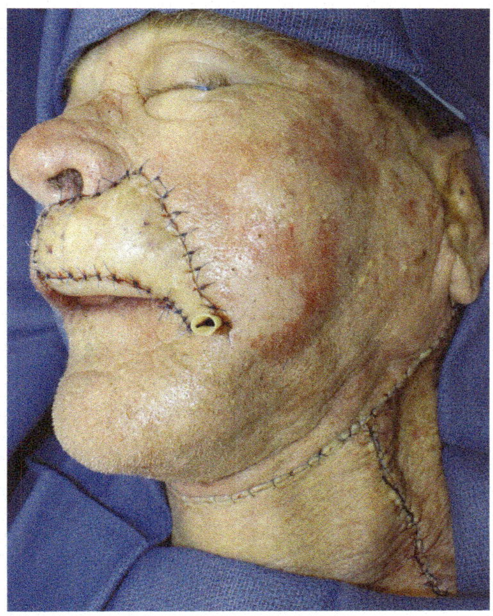

Fig. 22.37 Lateral view of the reconstructed upper lip with a radial forearm flap.

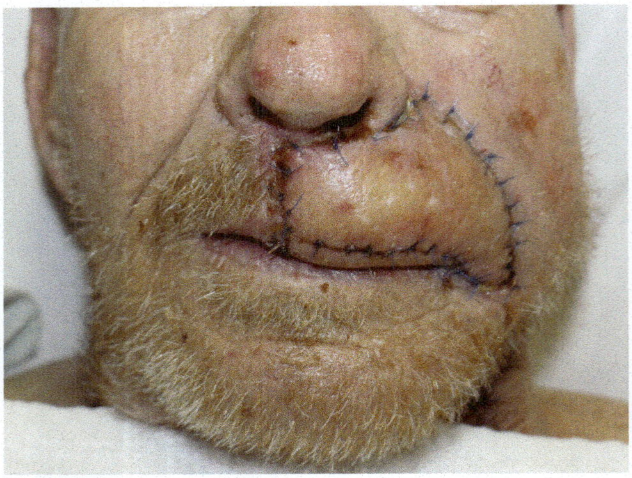

Fig. 22.38 Early postoperative appearance of the lip reconstruction.

(Figure 22.40). If the advancement is found to cause tension, a lower sulcular incision should be made from the depth of the vestibule from one commissure to the other; this maneuver will modify the mucosa advancement to bipedicled advancement. The mucosa release allows for ease of closure without a resultant inversion of the lip and loss of the lip vermillion. Although this complication may seem to be insignificant, it results in the loss of satisfaction in female patients as they no longer will have adequate vermillion to apply lipstick, and in males the hair growth along the edge of the skin and mucosa will turn upwards and cause irritation to the upper lip (Figure 22.41).

Wedge resection

Small defects of the lower lip resulting from the excision of small malignancies are often easily addressed with a wedge resection in the form of a W (Figures 22.42 to

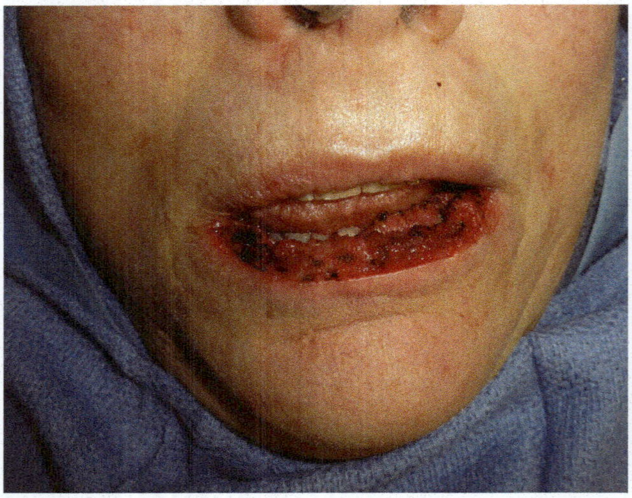

Fig. 22.39 View of the lower lip after a vermillionectomy.

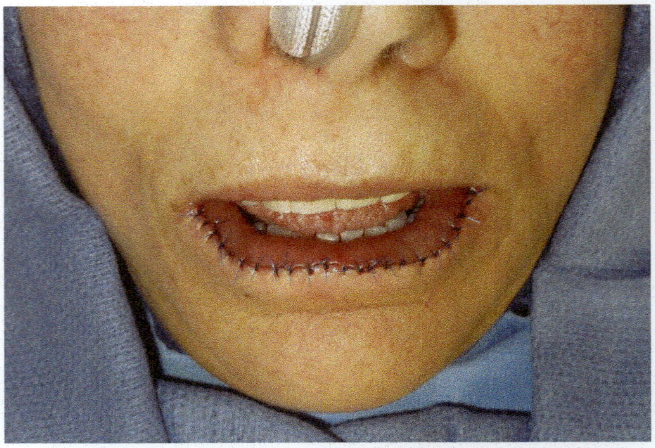

Fig. 22.40 Appearance of the lower lip after mucosal advancement flap reconstruction.

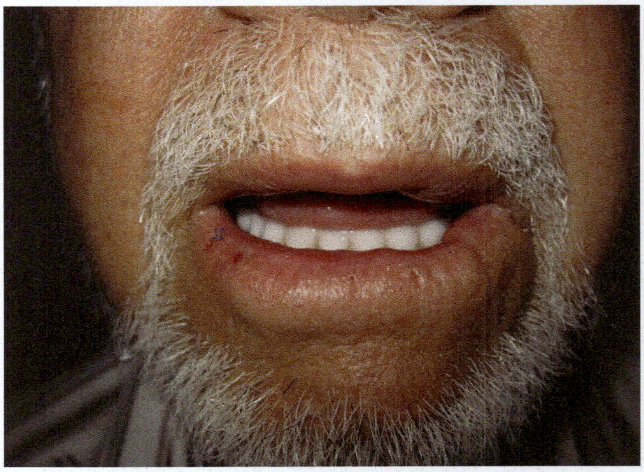

Fig. 22.41 View of a male patient with early on after a mucosal advancement flap for a vermillionectomy defect.

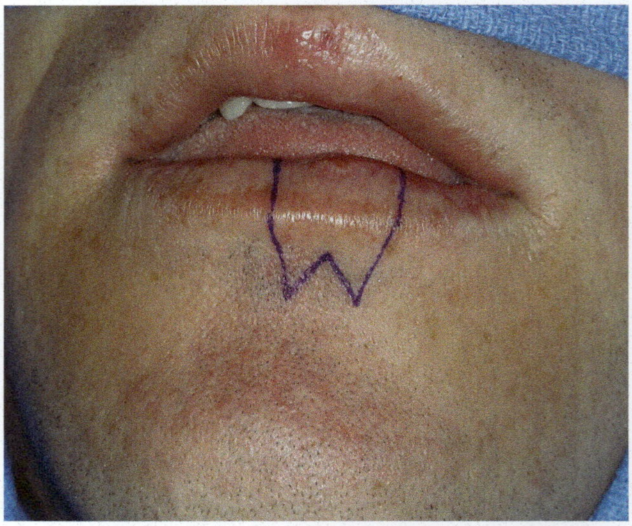

Fig. 22.42 Markings for a wedge incision of a lower lip lesion, the excision is planned as a W.

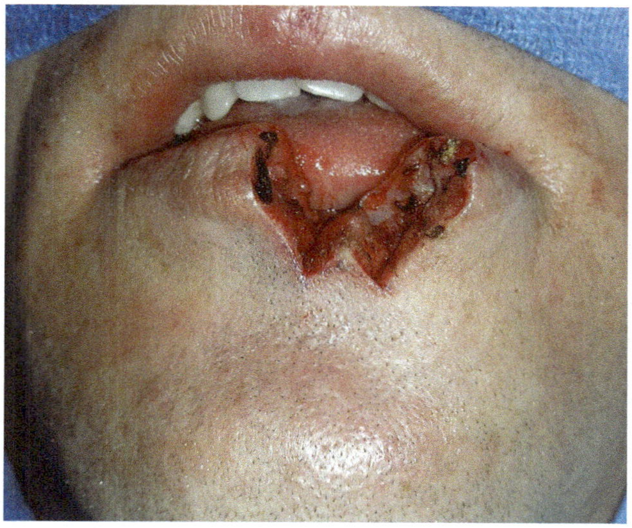

Fig. 22.43 Defect after the W excision.

22.45). The V excision is another form of simple lip resection (Figures 22.46 to 22.48). These various resections are often less than a third of the width of the lip and therefore enable the advancement of the two edges of the defect and reapproximation of the muscle followed by the mucosa and skin. The closure of the vermillion cutaneous junction should be performed carefully to insure that the two sides are exactly aligned or it will result in a readily apparent flaw in the repair once the lip is healed. The lip vermillion closure should also be carried out carefully to prevent clefting. This can be prevented by having a proper reapproximation of the underlying muscle, and sometimes using horizontal sutures to evert the mucosa in the area.

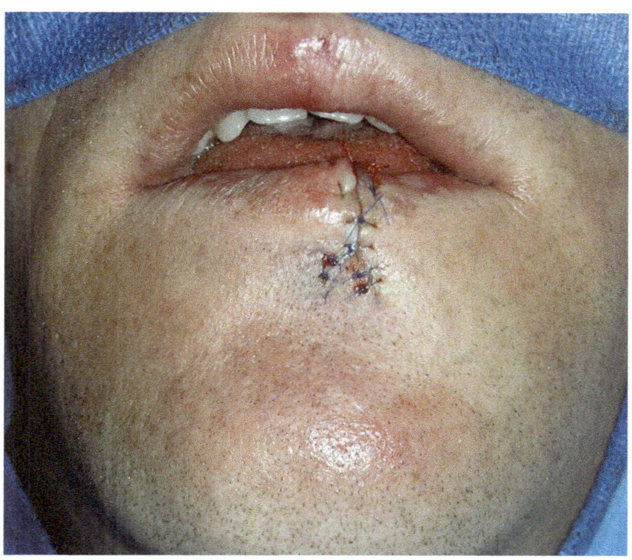

Fig. 22.44 Closure of the defect.

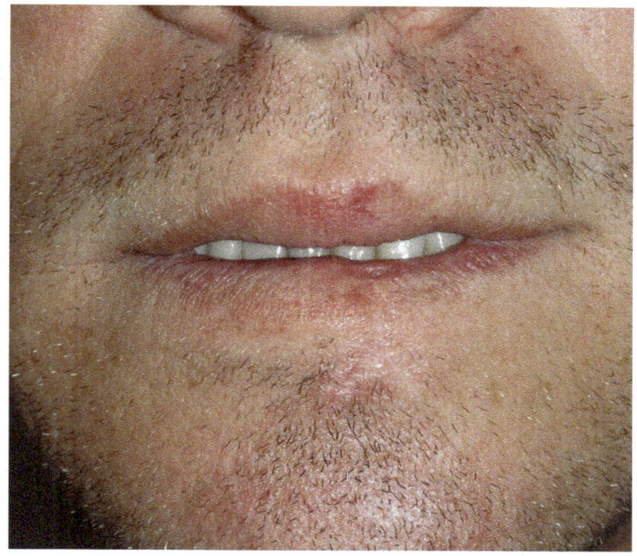

Fig. 22.45 Late postoperative view of the reconstructed lower lip.

Defects greater than 33%

Bernard Webster flap

The Bernard Webster flap allows for the reconstruction of large lower lip defects where remnants of the lower lip remain.[4] The flap advances the cheek and the remaining lower lip to repair the defect. In order to gain the necessary advancement, Burrow's triangles are removed from the upper lip and when necessary also from the lower lip. This design gives the Bernard Webster flap the appearance of a jumping man (Figure 22.49). The flap

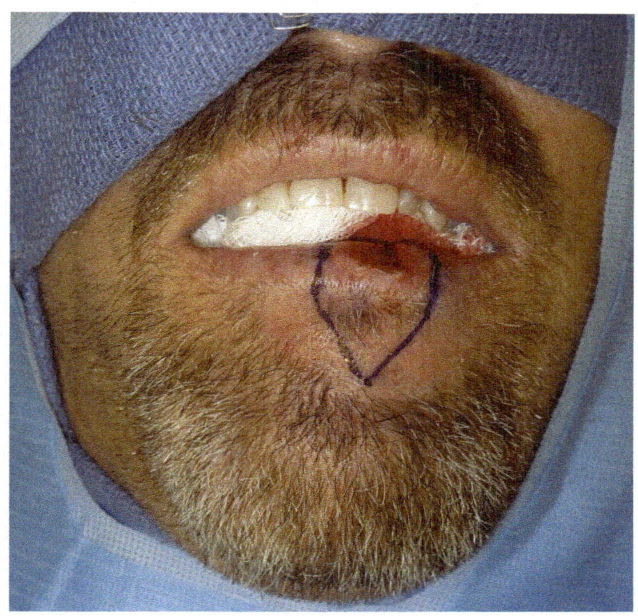

Fig. 22.46 Plan for a shield excision of a lower lip lesion.

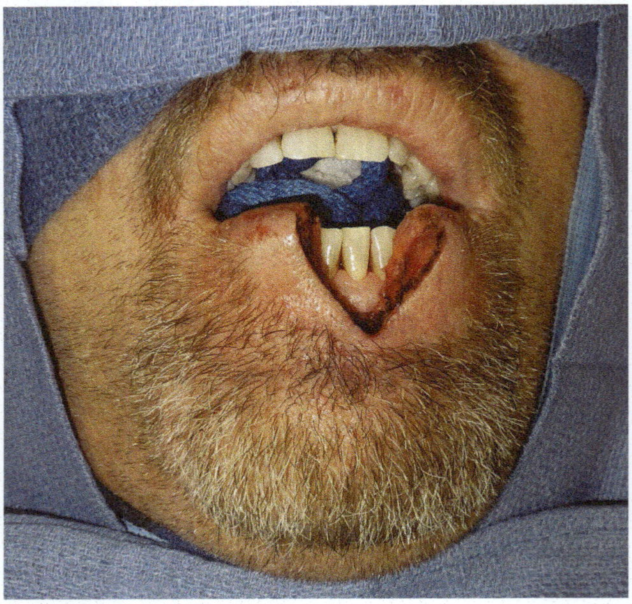

Fig. 22.47 Defect after the shield excision.

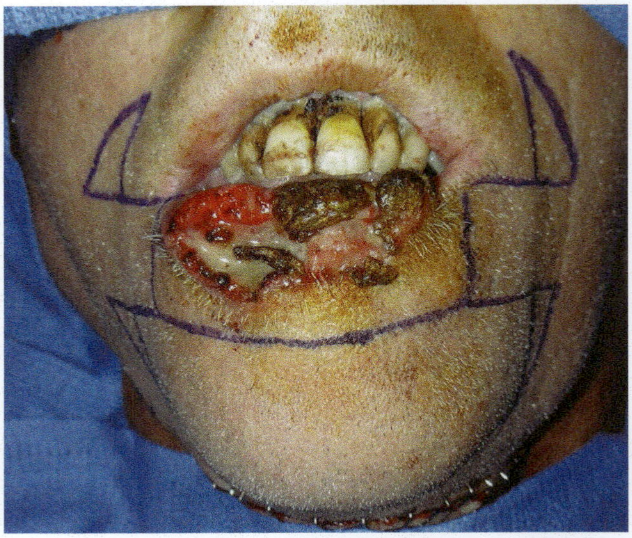

Fig. 22.49 Markings for a large lower lip resection with immediate reconstruction with a Bernard Webster flap.

incorporates the mucosal reconstruction by rotating the mucosa over the denuded advanced muscle and cheek. The added mucosa is obtained by making the horizontal mucosal incision higher than the skin incision by roughly the width of the vermillion (Figure 22.50).

The main downside of this reconstructive option is the final appearance of the lip. The lip takes on a very typical appearance of a tight lower lip with the upper lip draping over it with a resultant loss of the lower lip vermillion (Figure 22.51).

Karapandzic flap

The Karapandzic flap has long been utilized for the reconstruction of larger lip defects.[5] The flap is particularly useful in repairing defects of the lower lip that approach

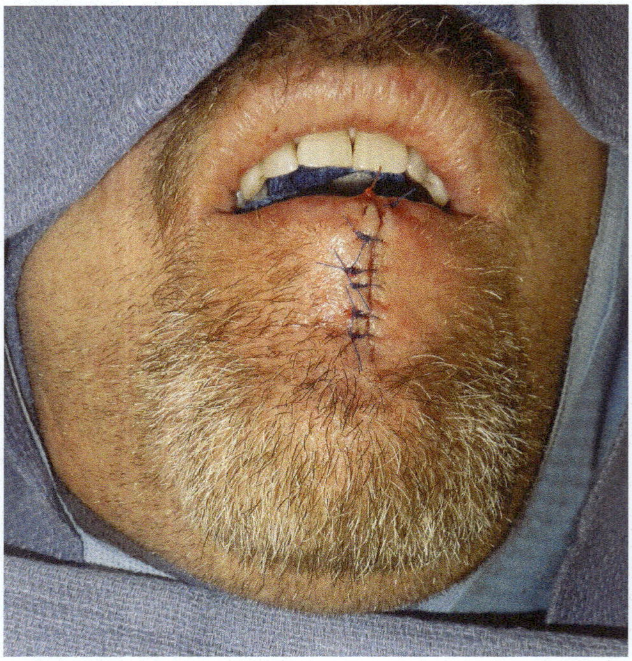

Fig. 22.48 Primary repair of the lip defect.

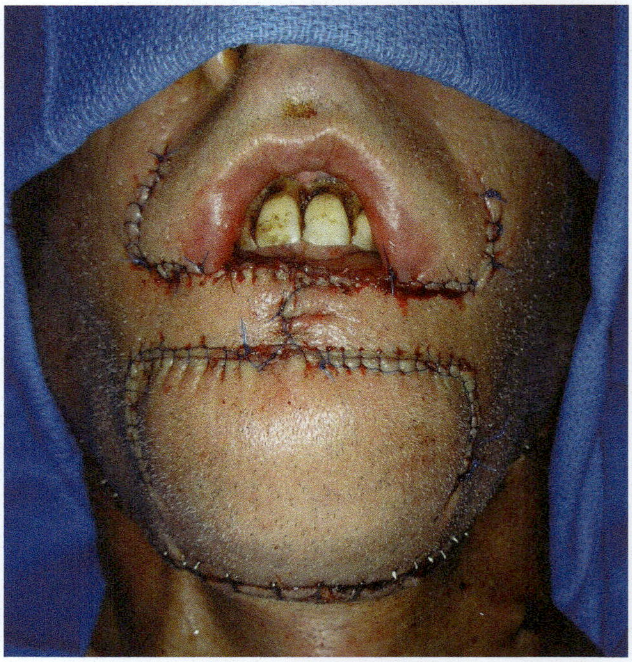

Fig. 22.50 View of the immediate reconstruction.

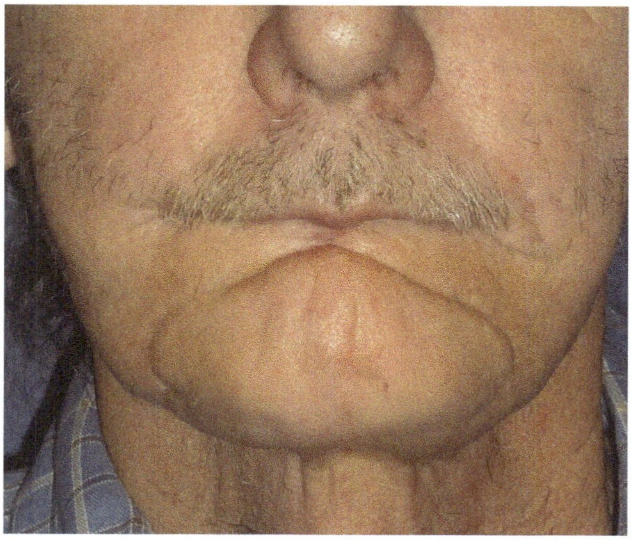

Fig. 22.51 Late postoperative view of the lower lip reconstruction with flattening of the lip.

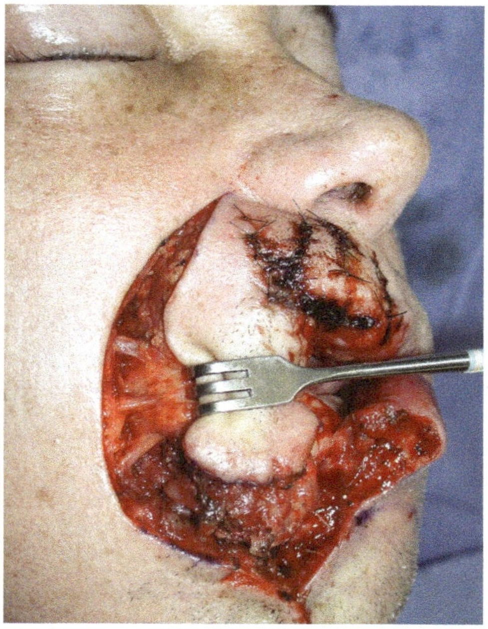

Fig. 22.53 Dissection of the neurovascular branches to the lip.

total defect. The flap is a rotation of the adjacent tissues remaining in the lower lip and around the commissure extending along the nasolabial groove towards the ala of the nose (Figure 22.52). The dissection of the flap requires that the vasculature and the innervation of the upper lip remain intact (Figure 22.53). The preservation of the neurovascular bundle is critical in order to take advantage of the use of the additional benefit of the flap, which is to reestablish the oral sphincter. The main disadvantage of the flap is that it inevitably results in a significant microstomia (Figure 22.54).

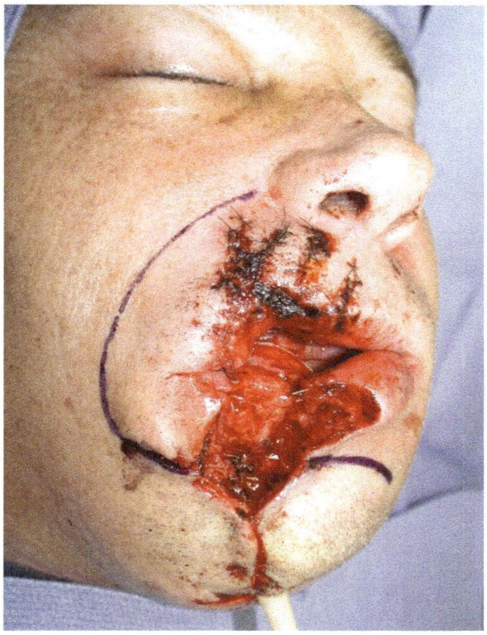

Fig. 22.52 Appearance of a traumatic lip defect with markings for a Karapandzic flap.

Crescentic flap

The crescentic flap approach to the reconstruction of the lower lip takes advantage of the curvature created at the junction of the lower lip central subunit and the mental subunit.[6] The flap can be utilized in defects where a primary closure would lead to deformation of the lip. The width of the defect is measured. Then a line is drawn from the labiomental crease extending laterally towards the mental crease (Figures 22.55 and 22.56). A crescent

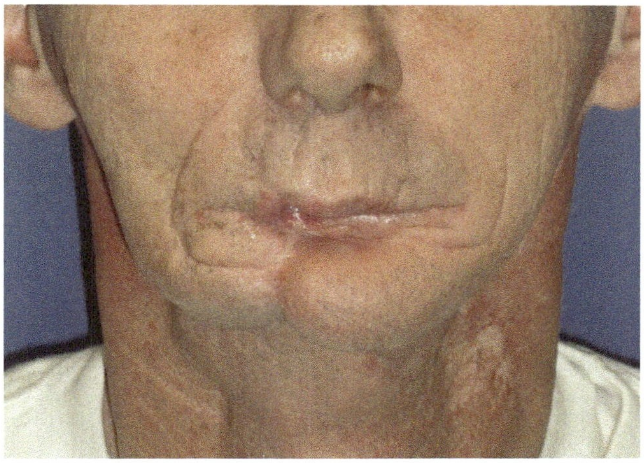

Fig. 22.54 Postoperative appearance of the reconstructed lower lip.

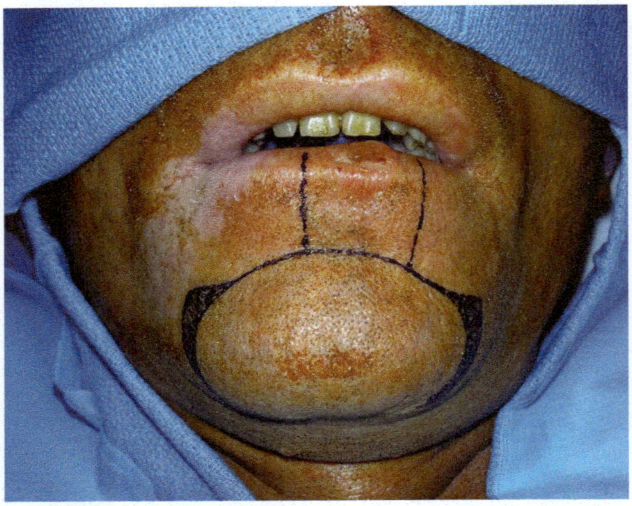

Fig. 22.55 Markings for a resection of a lower lip lesion with planning for immediate reconstruction with bilateral lower lip crescentic flaps.

measuring half the width of the defect is drawn along the lateral curvature of the labiomental crease. The marked crescent is removed to include the skin and underlying tissues and the incision is extended along the crease to meet the defect along the labiomental crease (Figure 22.57). Another incision is made along the depth of the vestibule of the lip and extended laterally toward the commissure (Figure 22.58).

The lateral lip and cheek flap is then mobilized and advanced medially to reconstruct the defect (Figures 22.59 and 22.60).

The closure of the defect is carried out in layers. Reconstruction of a lip defect making up to 50% of the lower lip can be performed using this simple technique with good predictable results (Figure 22.61).

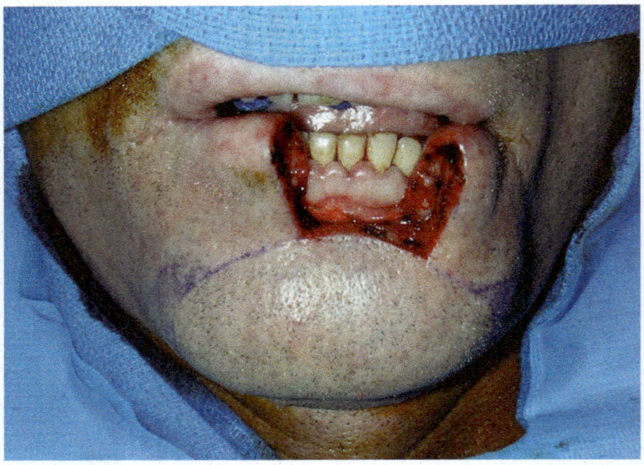

Fig. 22.56 View of the defect prior to reconstruction.

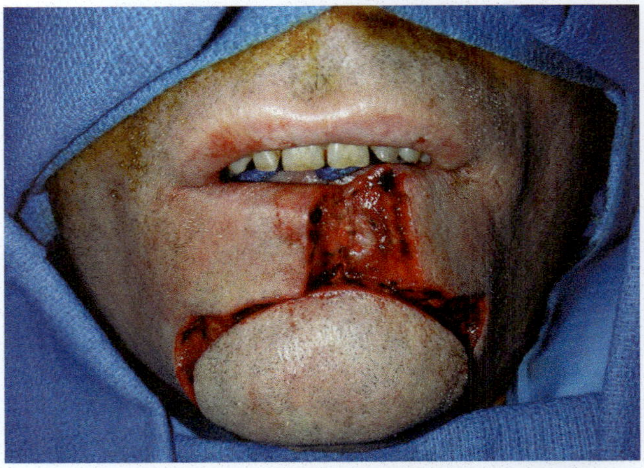

Fig. 22.57 View of the defect prior to advancement of the flap.

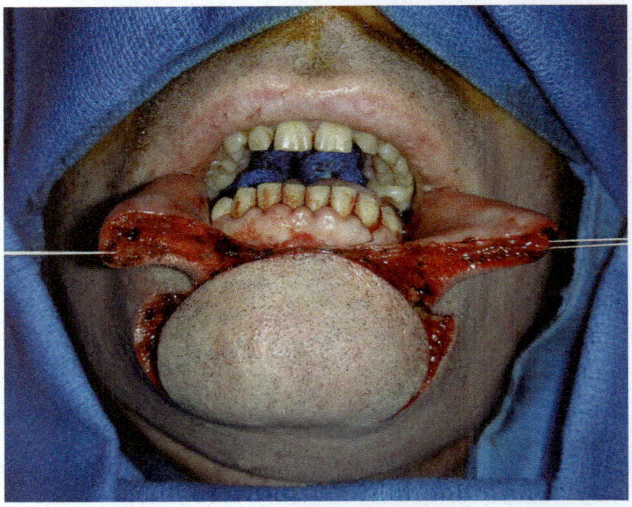

Fig. 22.58 Assessment of the flaps prior to advancement.

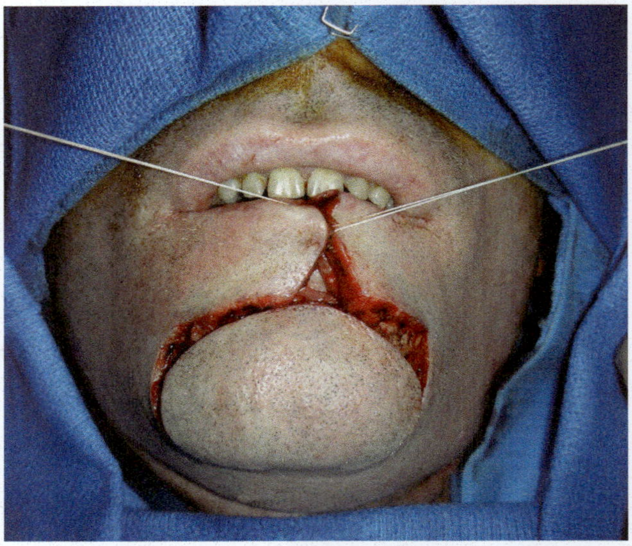

Fig. 22.59 Confirmation of the reach of the flaps prior to inset.

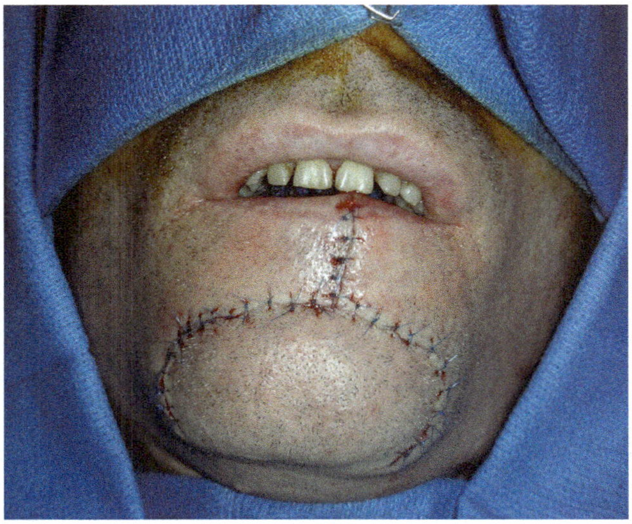

Fig. 22.60 Inset of the flap with placement of the scar along the facial grooves.

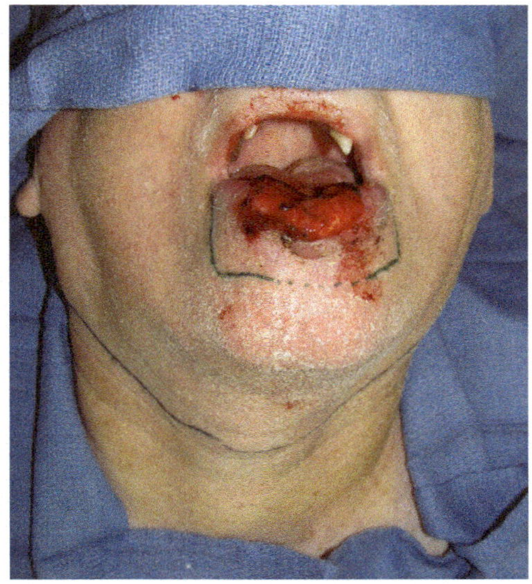

Fig. 22.62 View of a patient with a large lower lip malignancy, markings for a total lower lip resection and bilateral neck dissections.

Free tissue transfer

Free tissue transfer is more commonly employed in the reconstruction of lower lip defects that are near total or total, or lip defects extending to another subunit such as the buccal mucosa, the mandible, or the mental region. As already described in the section on reconstruction of upper lip defects, the radial forearm is the most commonly utilized free flap for the repair of total lip defects. The use of free tissue in lower lip reconstruction has to anticipate and prevent sagging of the reconstruction. If sagging is not anticipated it will often result in the loss of oral seal and drooling. To prevent sagging of the reconstructed lip, the surgeon has to incorporate a form of flap suspension. When using the radial forearm flap, the palmaris longus tendon is transferred and the fasciocutaneous flap is draped over the flap and suspended along the commissure in an upward and lateral vector.

Free tissue transfer enables the reconstruction of very complex lip defects as illustrated in the following case. A 69-year-old male with a biopsy-proven melanoma of the lower lip was referred for management (Figure 22.62). The resection of the entire lower lip was performed with simultaneous bilateral neck dissection (Figure 22.63). The measurements from the defect were transferred to the forearm and marked for the reconstruction with the anticipated transfer of the palmaris longus tendon (Figures 22.64 and 22.65). The flap was then transferred to the

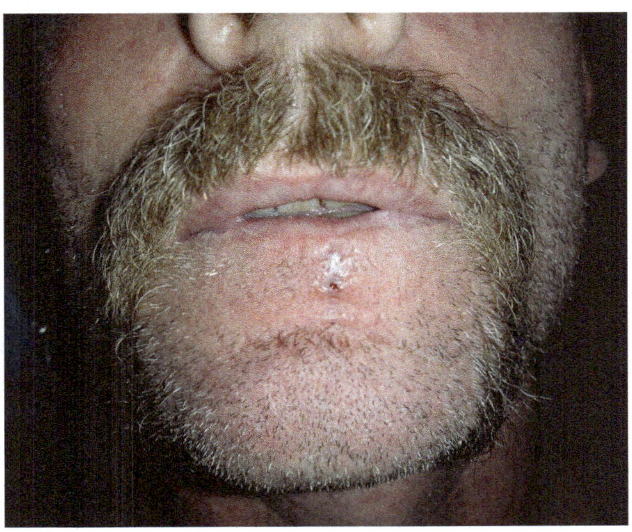

Fig. 22.61 Early postoperative appearance of the reconstructed lip.

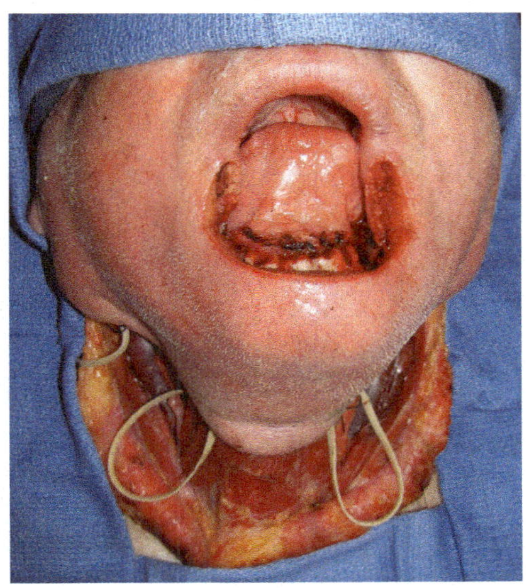

Fig. 22.63 View of the defect after resection.

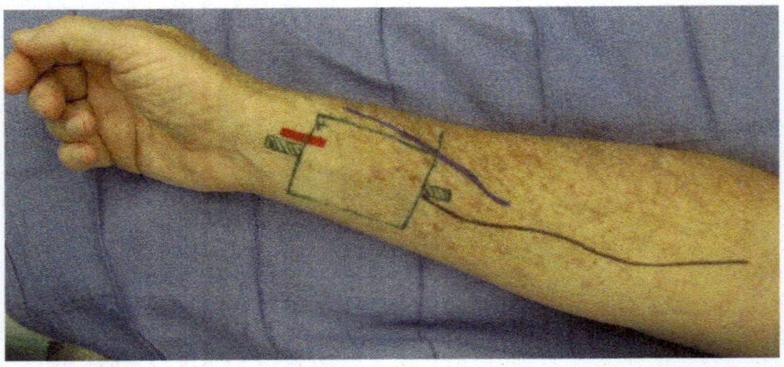

Fig. 22.64 Planning for a radial forearm free flap with palmaris longus tendon for the reconstruction of the lower lip.

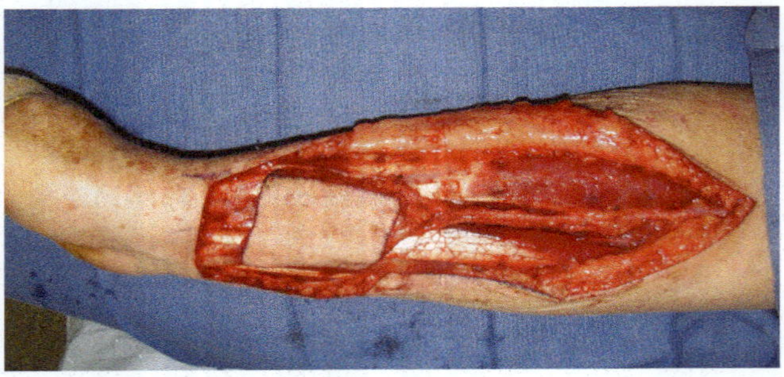

Fig. 22.65 Elevated forearm flap prior to transfer.

defect and the inset was performed along with the vascular anastomosis (Figure 22.66). The final appearance of the reconstruction was acceptable with good oral competence (Figure 22.67).

Another example of the use of the radial forearm free flap for the reconstruction of a complex lip defect is illustrated in the next case.

The patient had an extensive resection of an upper, lower, and commissure squamous cell carcinoma resulting in a large complex defect (Figures 22.68 and 22.69).

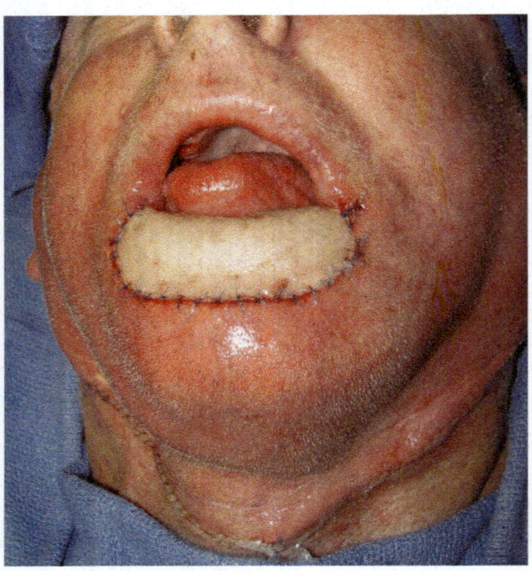

Fig. 22.66 Inset of the lower lip reconstruction.

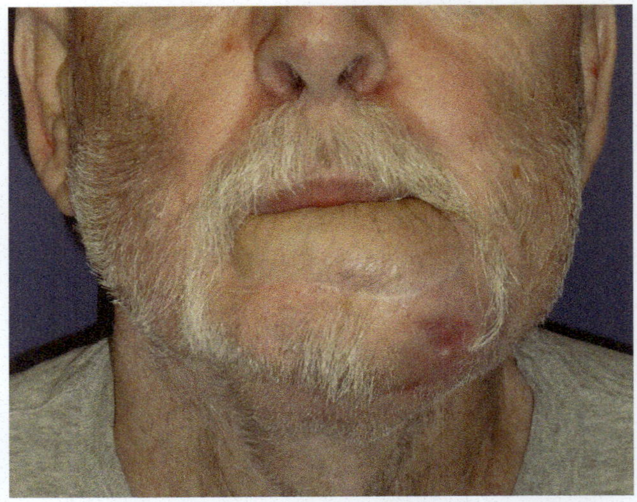

Fig. 22.67 Appearance of the reconstructed lower lip.

A template was designed and transferred to the forearm, and the flap was then elevated and folded to recreate the defect (Figures 22.70 and 22.71). The flap was then inset into the defect with immediate restoration of the lip form (Figure 22.72).

Commissure defects

Estlander flap

Defects of the upper or lower lip involving the commissure of the mouth, bring with them a higher level of complexity. When repairing defects that involve the corner of the mouth, the reconstructive method chosen will impact

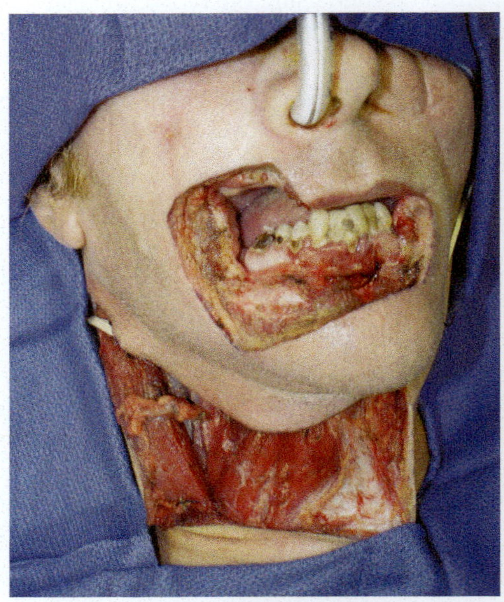

Fig. 22.68 View of a near total lower lip resection with commissure and a third of the upper lip.

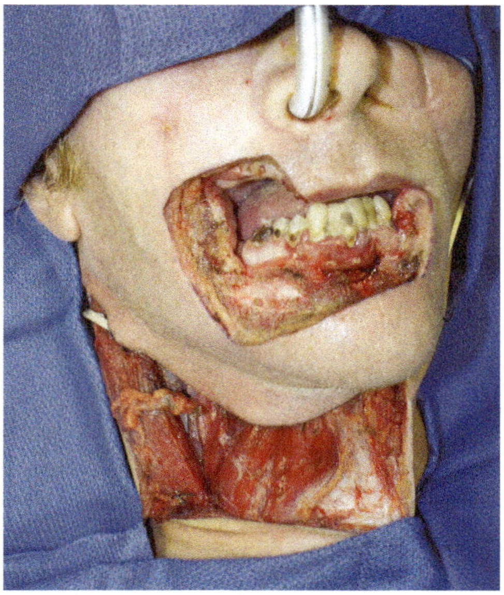

Fig. 22.69 View of the resected specimen.

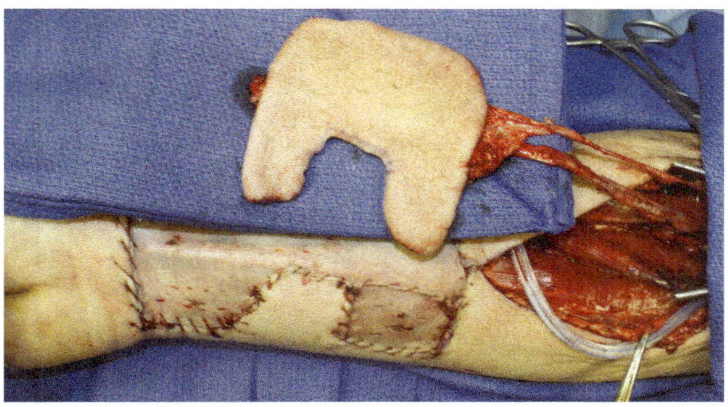

Fig. 22.70 Raised radial forearm flap design for the reconstruction of the lip defect.

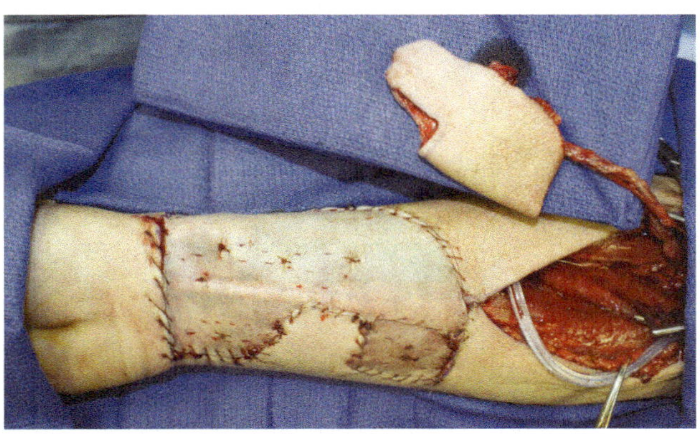

Fig. 22.71 Folding of the forearm flap prior to transfer.

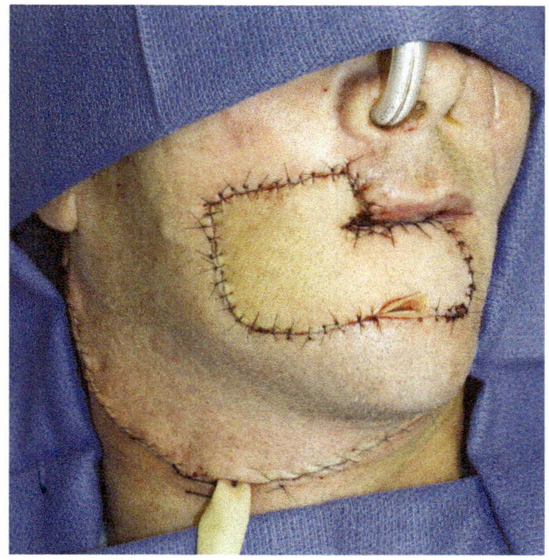

Fig. 22.72 Inset of the flap into the defect with restoration of the lip form.

on the final appearance of the lip. The Estlander flap is a method of transposition of tissue from one lip to the other when the defect encompasses the commissure; it was described in 1968.[7]

The use of this flap, unlike the Abbe flap, is carried out in a single stage without the need for sectioning the pedicle.

Commissuroplasty

The recapitulation of the natural shape of the oral commissure is perhaps the most difficult aspect in lip reconstruction. The normal shape and appearance of the commissure is that of a soft triangle with the obtuse angle at its most lateral aspect where the upper and lower vermillion connects. Blunting and or rounding of the commissure are encountered when the lip is advanced to repair a large defect or when the defect involves the commissure and therefore the reconstruction addresses the site.

Several options exist to address the commissure. The method used by most surgeons is one that attempts to recreate this anatomy by excising the cutaneous skin area and advancing and rotating the mucosa to recreate the shape of the lip.

The technique to achieve a more balanced look begins by taking a measurement from the midpoint of the cupids bow to the lateralmost area of the commissure on the intact side. The measurement is transferred from the same point in the midline at Cupid's bow to the involved side. A line is drawn from the marked point to the nearest cutaneous junction with normal appearing upper and lower vermillion. The resultant triangle of skin delineates what needs to be excised. A line is next drawn from the apex of the triangle to the midpoint of the base of the triangle. This point usually corresponds to the junction of the upper and lower lip. The excision is made through

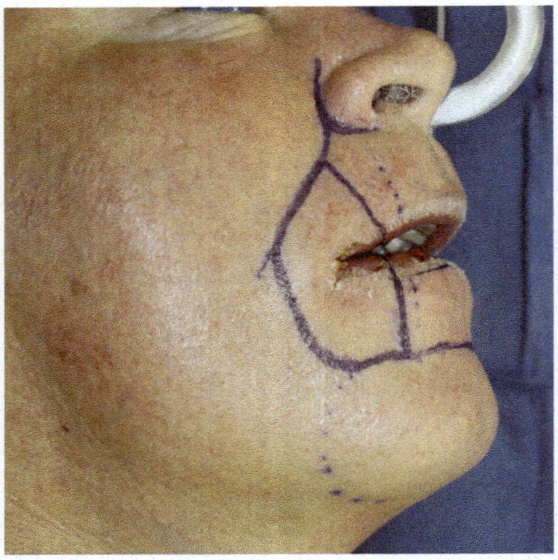

Fig. 22.73 View of a planned complex resection of a buccal carcinoma with extension to the commissure and dermis.

the skin through to the mucosa. The upper and lower skin and the muscle triangle are excised but the mucosa is left intact. The mucosa is then rotated and trimmed and moved to the defect to recreate the proper commissure shape.

In cases where a previous microvascular flap was used to reconstruct the buccal mucosa and the missing skin at the commissure site, a staged approach is taken to recreate the normal lip form (Figures 22.73, 22.74a and b, 22.75). Once an appropriate time has elapsed since the initial reconstruction, the external skin component should be assessed for the planned excision and advancement of local tissues or for serial excisions and advancement (Figure 22.76). The goal of these excisions is to render the

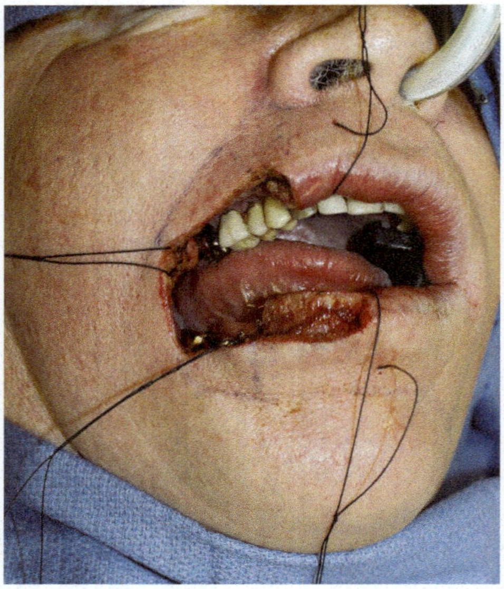

Fig. 22.74a View of the defect showing defect of the upper, lower, and commissure defect.

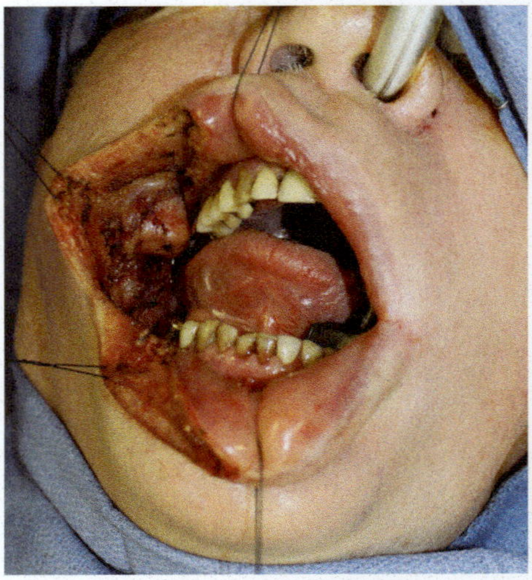

Fig. 22.74b View of the large buccal mucosal defect.

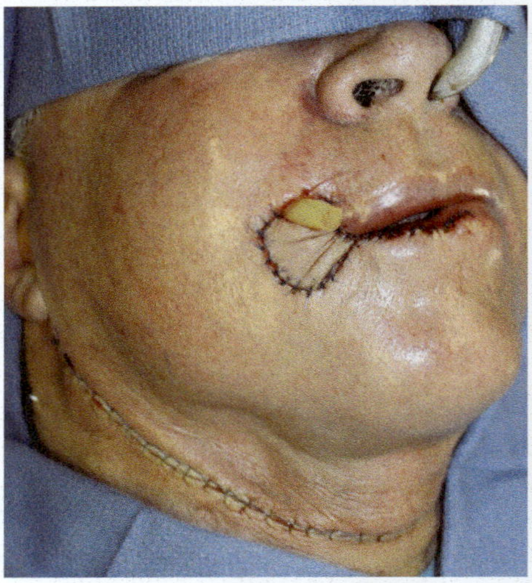

Fig. 22.75 View of the reconstruction with portion of the radial forearm folded to recreate the commissure and skin defect.

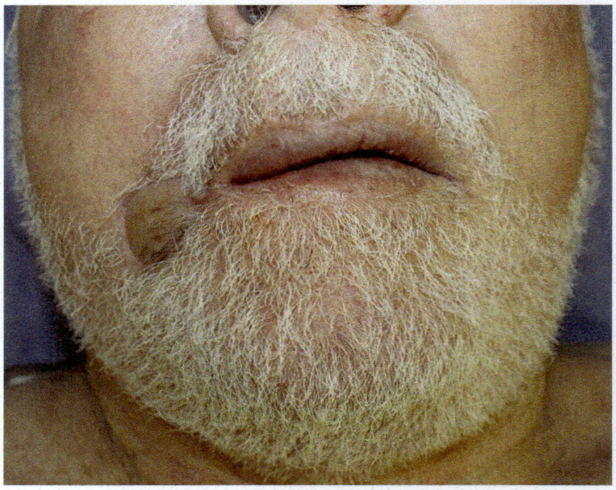

Fig. 22.76 View of the healed reconstruction with the skin mismatch on the right commissure.

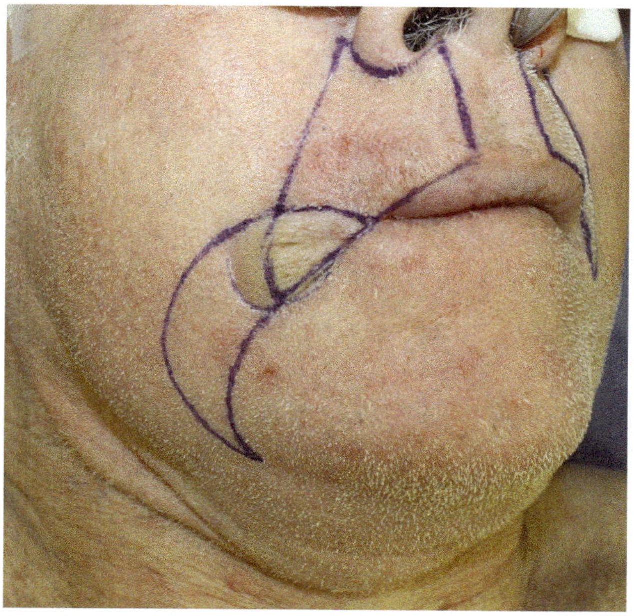

Fig. 22.77 Markings of the lip subunit with plan for the excision of the skin from the forearm.

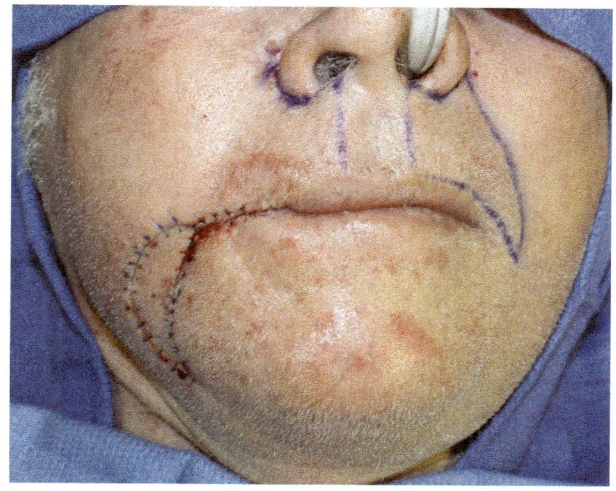

Fig. 22.79 Advancement and inset of the flap.

patient free of any vestiges of the previous surgical intervention. This plan is not only to excise the donor skin but also to repair the lip in a manner that is least conspicuous to others (Figures 22.77 to 22.79). Doing so allows for a better long-term appearance (Figure 22.80).

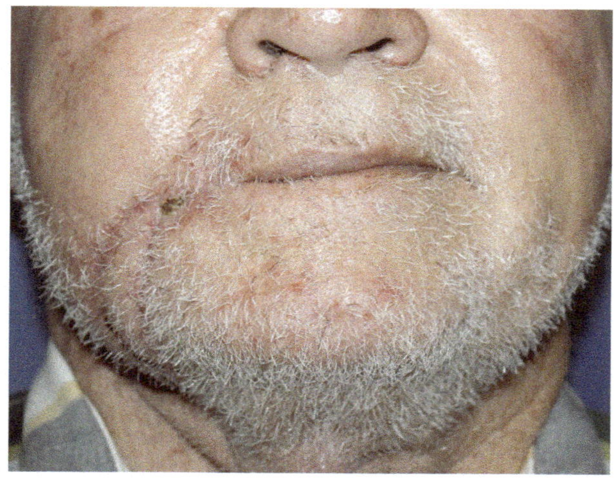

Fig. 22.80 Early postoperative view of the final reconstructed lip.

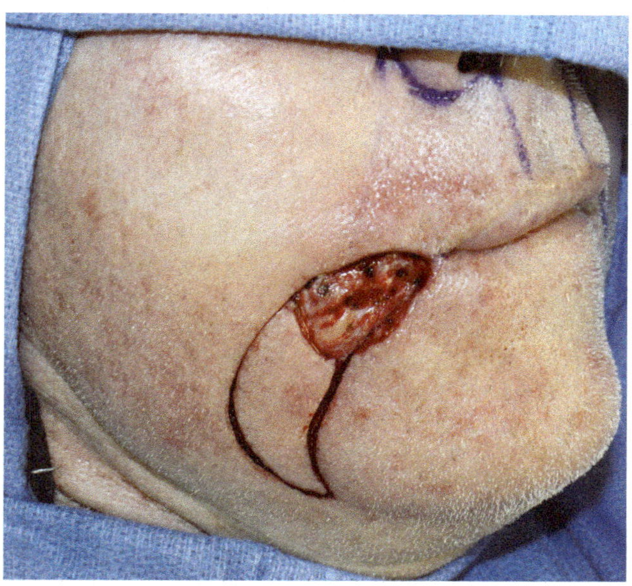

Fig. 22.78 Excised skin with incision for the advancement of the facial flap to repair the defect.

References

1. Abbe RA. New plastic operation for relief of deformity due to double harelip. *Med Rec* 1898; 53:477.
2. Agostini T. The Sabattini–Abbe flap: a historical note. *Plast Reconstr Surg* 2009; 123:767.
3. Al-Benna S, Steinstraesser L, Steinau HU. The cross-lip flap from 1756 to 1898. Reply to "The Sabattini–Abbe flap: a historical note". *Plast Reconstr Surg* 2009; 124:666–667.
4. Webster RC, Coffey RJ, Kelleher RE. Total and partial reconstruction of the lower lip with innervated muscle-bearing flaps. *Plat Reconstr Surg Transpl Bull* 1960; 25:360–371.
5. Karapandzic M. Reconstruction of lip defects by local arterial flaps. *Br J Plast Surg* 1974; 27:93–97.
6. Pirgousis P, Fernandes R. Reconstruction of subtotal defects of the lower lip: a review of current techniques and a proposed modification. *J Oral Maxillofac Surg* 2011; 69:295–299.
7. Estlander JA. A method of reconstructing loss of substance in one lip from the other lip (reprint). *Plast Reconstruc Surg* 1968; 42:361–369.

Chapter 23
Nasal reconstruction

Introduction

The nose takes on a prominent role in our face and is one of the principle contributors to our facial appearance. Aside from its role in facial appearance, the nose also serves an important functional role in filtering and humidifying the air that we breathe. Given its role as both a functional and esthetic unit, defects of the nose have the potential to affect both our respiratory function as well as our psyche (Figure 23.1).

The reconstruction of nasal defects dates back several hundred years to the Indian continent. Various methods are available to reconstruct nasal defects. The option for which flap or technique to use will be directly related to the size and composition of the defect. The focus of the nasal defect evaluation should not be simply a determination of size, it should be an evaluation of the layers of tissues that are missing. The assessment of the missing tissue should determine the status of the nasal lining, the structural support (i.e., the cartilage), and finally, the skin component.

Anatomy

The external nasal anatomy can be approached based on the subunit analysis as was described by Gonzales-Ulloa in 1957.[1] Many years later, in 1985, Burget and Menick further developed this concept, focusing on nasal reconstruction.[2] In their manuscript, they divided the nose into six subunits and advocated the excision of the entire subunit in order to achieve the best esthetic result. The nose was divided into the following subunits: dorsal subunit, the nasal sidewalls, the soft triangle, the ala, the columella, and the nasal tip. The nasal sidewalls, ala, and soft triangle are paired subunits; when this is taken into account, the nose can be subdivided into 9 subunits.

The bony and cartilaginous framework of the nose provides the support for the nasal cover and its arrangement is reflected in the contour of the skin.[3] The structural composition of the nose is made up by the nasal bone, which extends from the nasofrontal suture until it meets the upper lateral cartilage. Extending caudally from the upper lateral cartilage is the lower lateral cartilage (alar cartilage).

The midline support is formed by the bony and cartilaginous septum. The bony component is formed by the perpendicular plate of the ethmoid, and the vomer.

The blood supply to the nose is formed by the contribution of both the internal as well as the external carotid system. The nasal sidewalls and dorsum are supplied by the dorsal nasal and angular branches of the ophthalmic artery as well as the infraorbital artery, a branch of the maxillary artery. The nasal cavity is supplied by the anterior and posterior ethmoidal arteries, the sphenopalatine artery, and the septal branch from the superior labial artery.

Defect assessment

Nasal defects are most often encountered due to excision of either benign or malignant tumors. Other causes of nasal defects are traumatic and due to degenerative diseases such as Wegner's granulomatosis. Traumatic defects can present secondary to motor vehicle collisions, interpersonal violence (Figure 23.2), and animal bites (Figure 23.3). The major difference between defects resulting from trauma vs. tumor excision is the ability to design and plan the defect.

Menick advocates that the reconstructive surgeon ask the following set of questions: What is missing anatomically? What is missing esthetically (e.g., the facial landmarks, practically described as regional subunits)? Is the

Local and Regional Flaps in Head & Neck Reconstruction: A Practical Approach, First Edition. Rui Fernandes.

Companion website: www.wiley.com/go/fernandes/flapsreconstruction

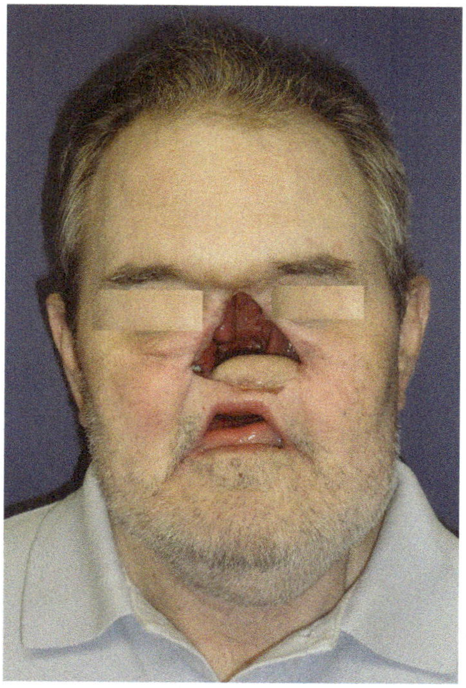

Fig. 23.1 View of a patient post rhinectomy with reconstruction of the oral nasal defect with a free tissue transfer.

underlying disease process controlled? Are donor sites available or depleted or devascularized by prior injury or surgery? Does the patient's health limit surgical stages, anesthesia, materials, or techniques?[4]

Once the defect is analyzed, whenever possible the surgeon should utilize the intact contralateral subunit to

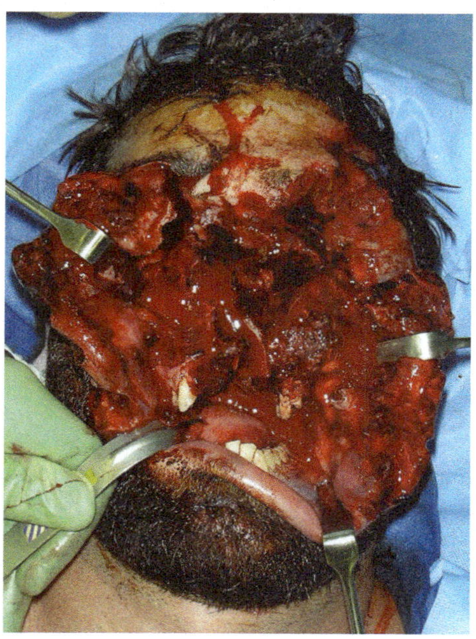

Fig. 23.2 View of a horrific defect secondary to a self-inflicted gunshot wound to the face.

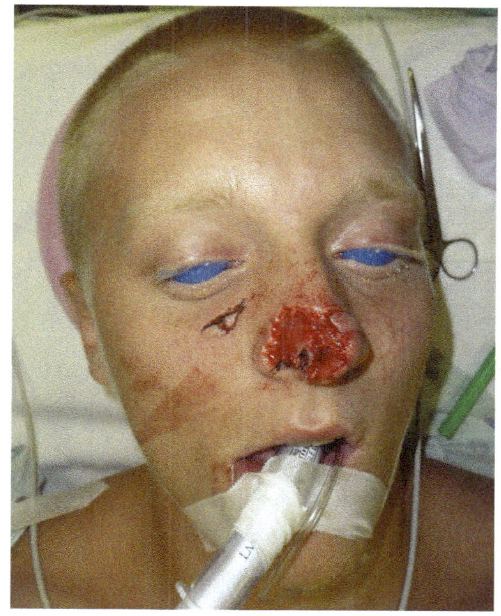

Fig. 23.3 View of a nasal defect after avulsive injury from a dog bite.

make a precise template which can be transferred to the defect site and, if needed, the remainder of the affected subunit can be excised. The use of the contralateral intact subunit gives a more precise reconstruction.

Site and size oriented approach to reconstruction

As previously stated, the location of the defect is only one of the considerations for nasal reconstruction. The surgeon should critically assess the composition of the defect as it will play a critical factor in the choice of reconstruction. The complexity of the reconstruction increases with the layers involved in the resection. Defects affecting the skin will be easier to reconstruct compared to those involving the skin and underlying cartilage and that in turn is easier than defects affection all the layers.

Resurfacing the nose

Small defects

Small size defects may occur in any of the subsites of the nose. The location of the defect will often dictate the choice of reconstruction. Defects measuring less than 1.5 cm can be reconstructed with a variety of techniques ranging from healing by secondary intention, full thickness skin grafts (Figure 23.4), or various local tissue transpositions (Figures 23.5 to 23.10).

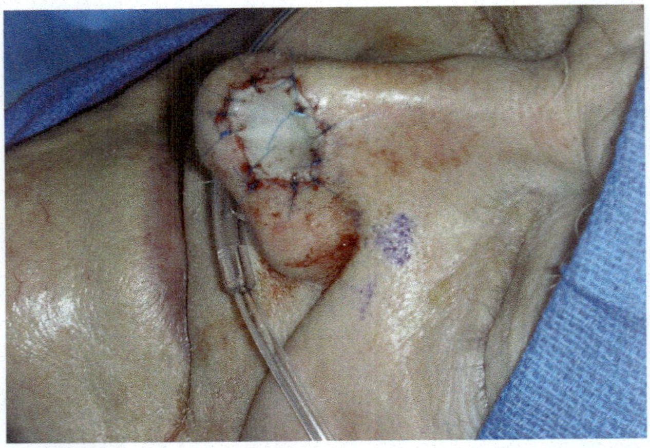

Fig. 23.4 Appearance of a full-thickness skin graft to the nasal defect.

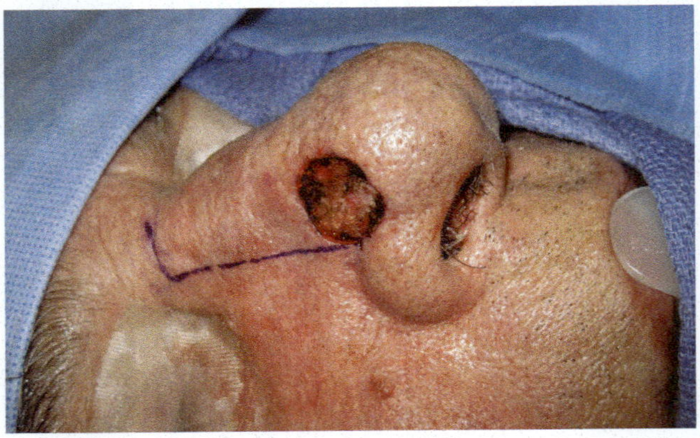

Fig. 23.5 Defect of the lateral nasal wall with markings for a repair with a sliding nasal flap.

Medium defects

Larger defects will typically extend beyond a single subunit to encompass multiple subunits. The approach to these defects should be made with the final appearance in mind. A commonly accepted approach has been to

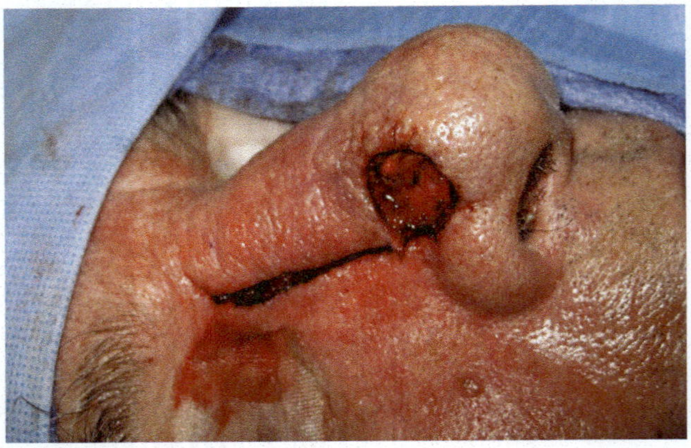

Fig. 23.6 Incision of the nasal flap prior to advancement.

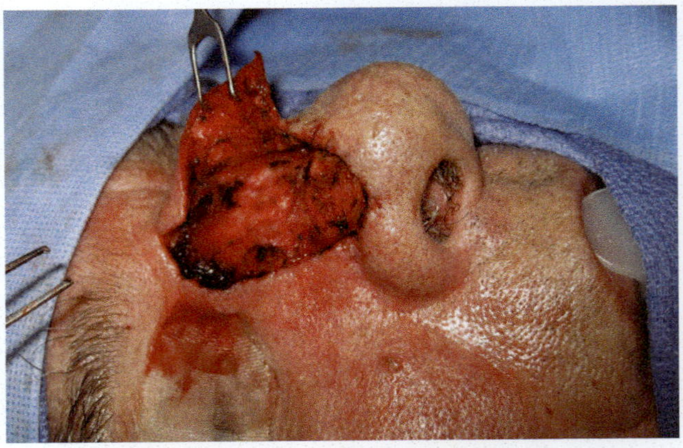

Fig. 23.7 Elevation and undermining of the flap.

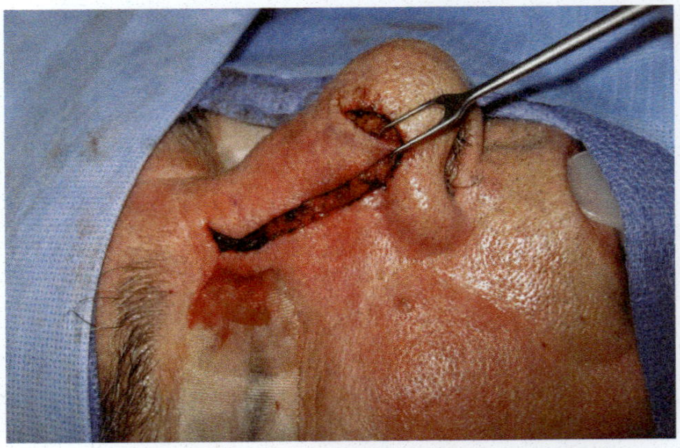

Fig. 23.8 Confirmation of the passive reach of the sliding nasal flap.

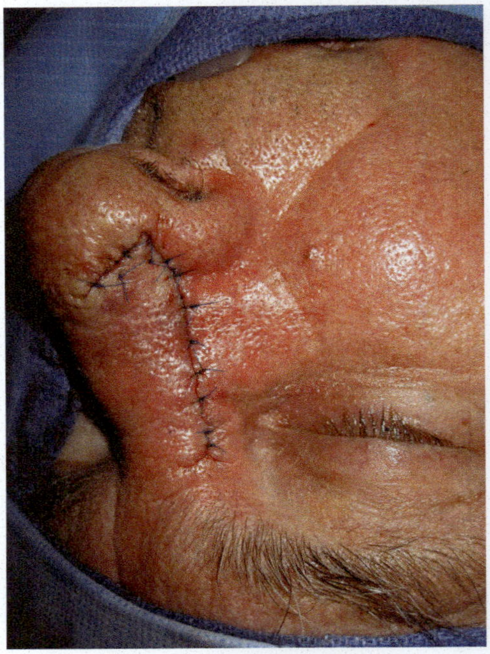

Fig. 23.9 Primary repair of the defect with the sliding flap.

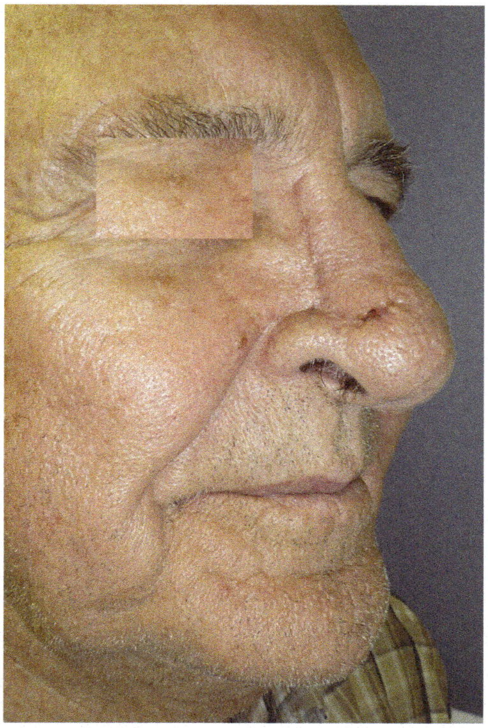

Fig. 23.10 Early postoperative appearance of the nasal reconstruction.

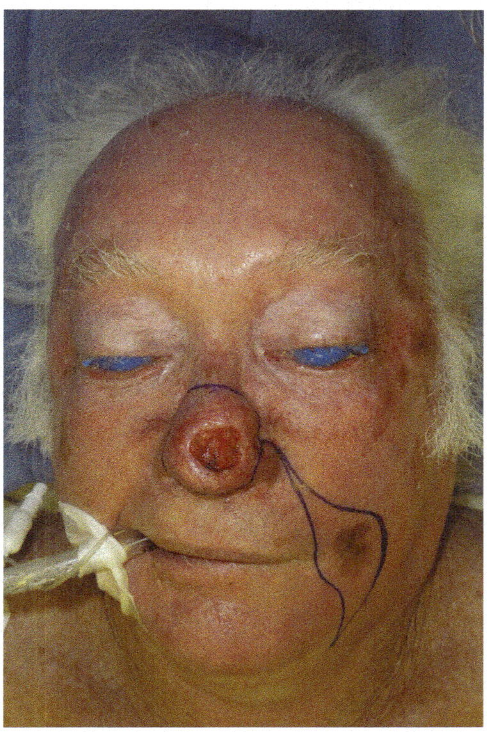

Fig. 23.11 Appearance of a patient with markings for resection of a large nasal lesion as well as a cheek lesion.

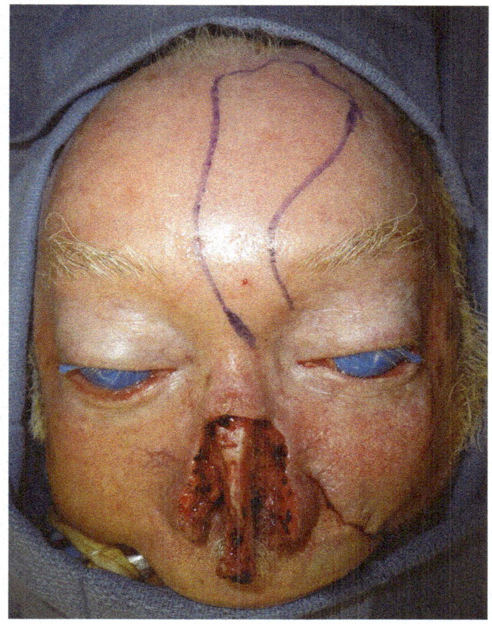

Fig. 23.12 Defect after complex resection and frozen section assessment; markings for a paramedian flap reconstruction.

examine the involved units and to carry out a complete subunit excision where the defect is greater than 50% of the subunit. Although this approach will result in a greater soft tissue defect, the resurfacing of the nose with a single flap gives a better final outcome of the reconstruction. When resurfacing a larger area of the nose, the most commonly utilized flap is the paramedian forehead flap.

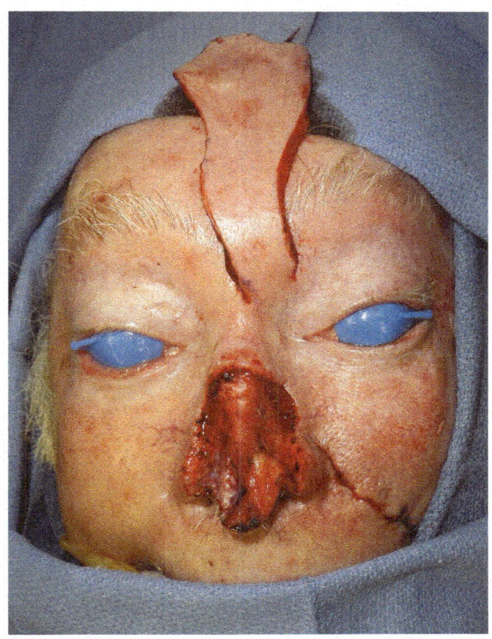

Fig. 23.13 Elevated paramedian flap prior to transfer.

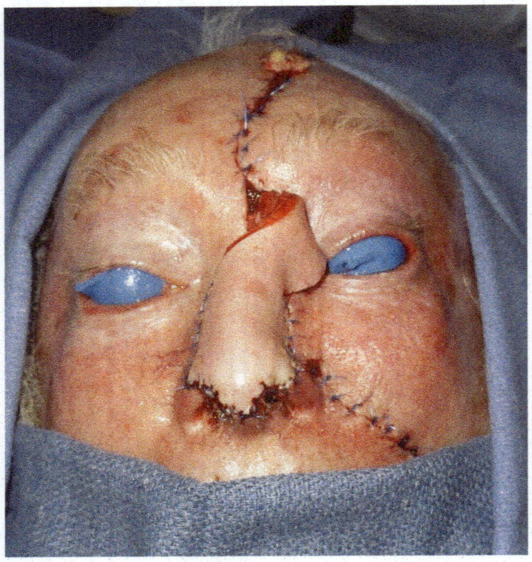

Fig. 23.14 Inset of the paramedian forehead flap.

The flap, as described previously, allows small defects to be resurfaced in areas such as the ala as well as resurfacing of the entire nose. An example of the need to resurface several subunits can be seen in the case of an 80-year-old Caucasian male who was referred for reconstruction of two neglected squamous cell carcinomas of the face, one located on the nose and the other on the left face (Figure 23.11). The resection of the nasal lesion resulted in a large defect (Figure 23.12). The paramedian forehead flap was utilized to resurface the nose as a two-stage procedure (Figures 23.13 to 23.15). The final appearance after take-down of the pedicle was acceptable to the patient and he declined any further revisions (Figure 23.16).

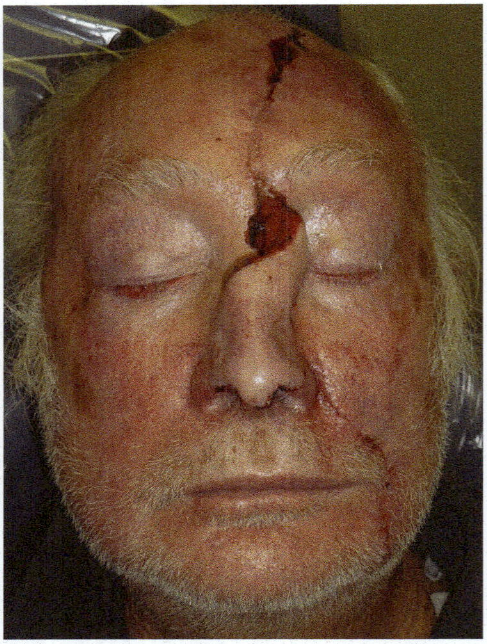

Fig. 23.15 Early postoperative view of the reconstructed nasal defect with the paramedian flap prior to second stage.

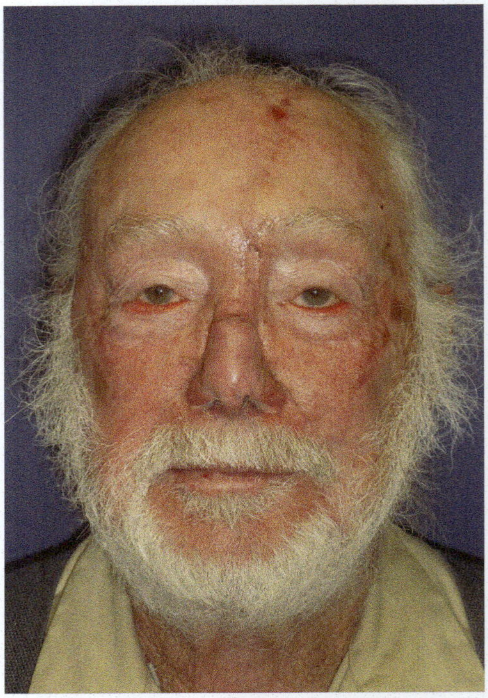

Fig. 23.16 Early view of the final nasal reconstruction without any revision.

Composite defects

Hemirhinectomy defects

Defects that result in the loss of half of the nose tend to be most often due to the excision of malignant skin tumors. As such, these defects are complex and typically involve all of the layers, i.e., skin, cartilage, and mucosal lining. The most important factor in these cases is the margin assessment. In cases where there is concern for the potential of a positive margin, it is better to delay the reconstruction until clear margins can be ascertained. The reconstruction of these defects will inevitably require the use of multiple flaps to recreate the missing layers. A common combination in these cases is the use of a septal mucosal flap, structural support with ear or septal cartilage, and skin resurfacing with the forehead flap. Another option is the combination of the septal mucosa flap and nasolabial flap for lining, with support and coverage as stated earlier. Examples of these combined approaches to hemirhinectomy defects can be seen in Chapter 6.

Total rhinectomy defects

One of the biggest challenges in craniofacial reconstruction is the total nasal defect. These defects are almost entirely caused by the resection of malignant tumors affecting the nasal dorsum and extending to the mucosa. The spread of disease often necessitates the excision of the entire nose. Infrequently, a total rhinectomy defect may be seen in the traumatic setting. In these cases, they are usually due to a self-inflicted gunshot wound and as such the defect not only encompasses the nose but often the upper and lower lip, the mandible, and the anterior maxilla.

In these complex defects, the first priority is to re-establish mandibular and maxillary continuity as well as to seal the oral cavity from the nasal cavity. The surgeon has to establish the platform for the nose irrespective of whether the nasal reconstruction will be performed using the patient's tissues or a prosthetic.

Most surgeons opt for the reconstruction of these defects with the collaboration of a maxillofacial prosthodontist rather the necessary staged approach with autogenous methods. A common problem is that the prosthesis does not meet the patient's expectations (Figure 23.17).

The challenges encountered in the reconstruction of these defects with autogenous means are numerous. The surgeon needs to re-establish the nasal height, projection, and form while recreating the lining, support, and finally the skin coverage. Prior to embarking on this complex reconstructive journey, both the surgeon as well as the patient must be committed to the number of surgeries and revisions that will be necessary to accomplish the goal. The main advantages of this reconstructive method are self-explanatory; no need to remove the prosthesis, patients own tissues, and better color and texture match to name a few.

To illustrate the inherent difficulties with this approach, two cases will be presented; a traumatic reconstruction and a postoncologic reconstruction.

Case #1: Posttraumatic reconstruction of a total rhinectomy defect

A 20-year-old Caucasian male was the unfortunate victim of multiple gunshots wounds in a work-related incidence. He presented with numerous injuries through the body as well as a major facial wound with the loss of maxilla and soft tissues of the midface (Figure 23.18). The patient was initially reconstructed by a colleague with local tissue flaps as well as paramedian forehead flap. Due to the lack of proper midface projection, and reconstruction of the missing layers of the nose, the reconstruction was not ideal (Figures 23.19 to 23.21). The patient was referred for further reconstruction. The initial injury to the midface region was reopened to recreate the necessary anterior maxillary arch form and to provide the proper platform for the staged nasal reconstruction (Figures 23.22 and 23.23). A composite fibula osteocutaneous flap was used to reconstruct the maxillary defect (Figures 23.24 to 23.26). A bony strut from the fibula was used to provide the proper nasal projection. The bone was placed under the previously utilized paramedian forehead flap.

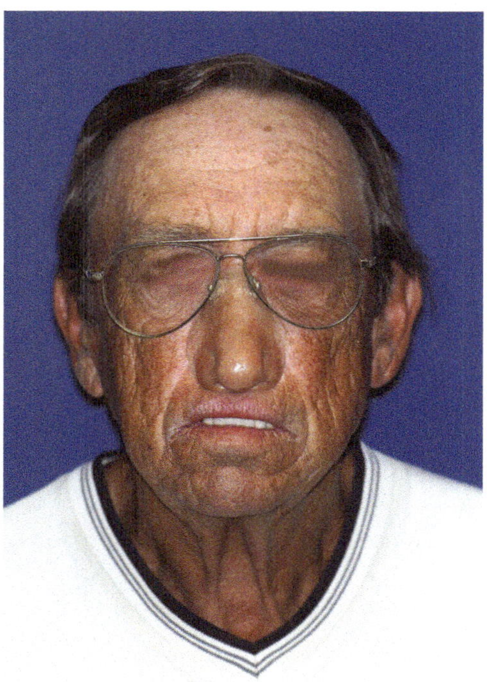

Fig. 23.17 View of a patient with a total rhinectomy using a prosthesis connected to the eyeglass.

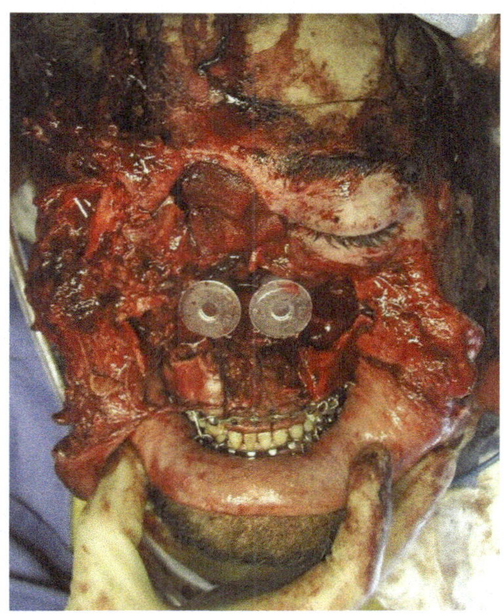

Fig. 23.18 View of a large midface defect with significant defect secondary to a gunshot injury.

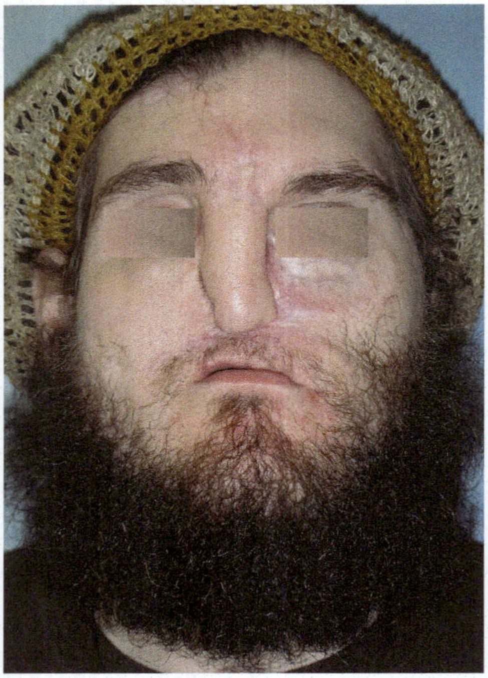

Fig. 23.19 View of poor result after reconstruction of the nasal defect without proper shape or projection.

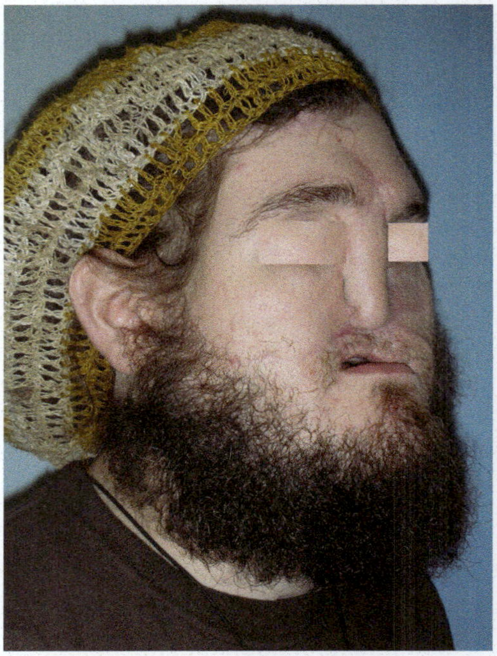

Fig. 23.21 Three-quarter view of the patient's profile.

At a later stage, a tissue expander was used to create the forehead tissue needed for another paramedian forehead flap. The flap was elevated on a wide base and transferred to the defect. A turn-in flap was performed using the skin from the previous flap to create a simulation of the nostrils (Figure 23.27). The forehead flap was then elevated and transferred (Figures 23.28 to 23.30). The initial postoperative appearance prior to the second stage was acceptable to the patient (Figure 23.31) and at second stage procedure (Figure 23.32). The final appearance for the patient reveals an acceptable nasal reconstruction

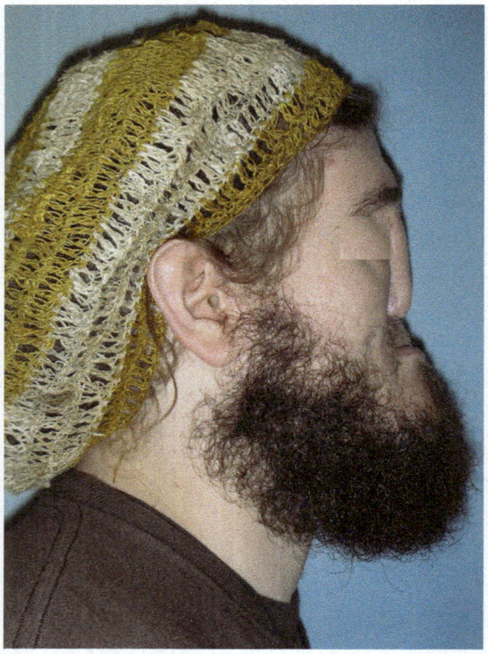

Fig. 23.20 Profile view of the patient demonstrating lack of projection and collapse of the midface.

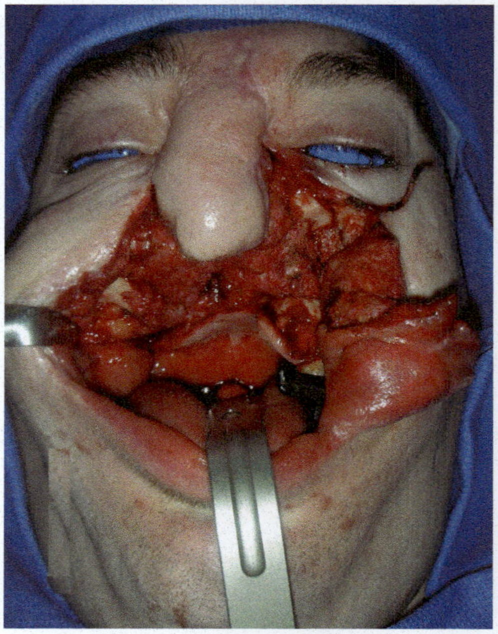

Fig. 23.22 Recreating the midface defect prior to reconstruction.

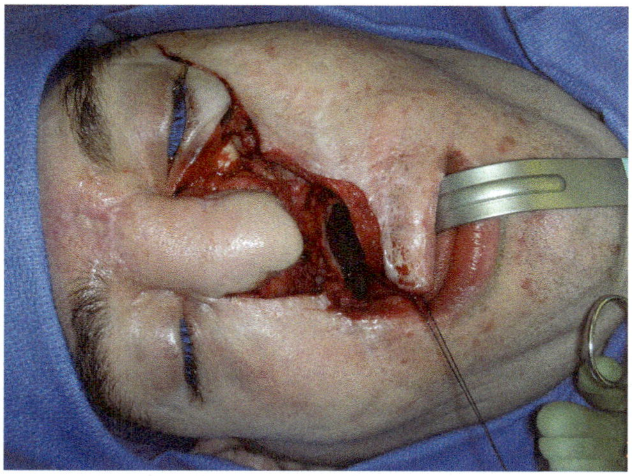

Fig. 23.23 Release of the upper lip revealing the needed tissue for the reconstruction.

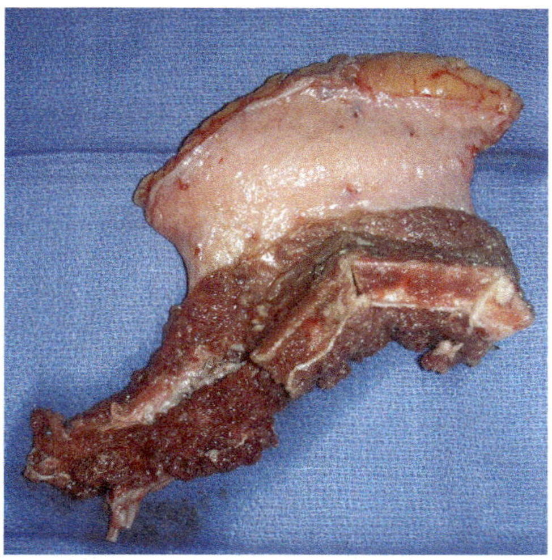

Fig. 23.24 Composite fibula flap to recreate the midface and skin paddle to recreate the palate and missing upper lip tissue.

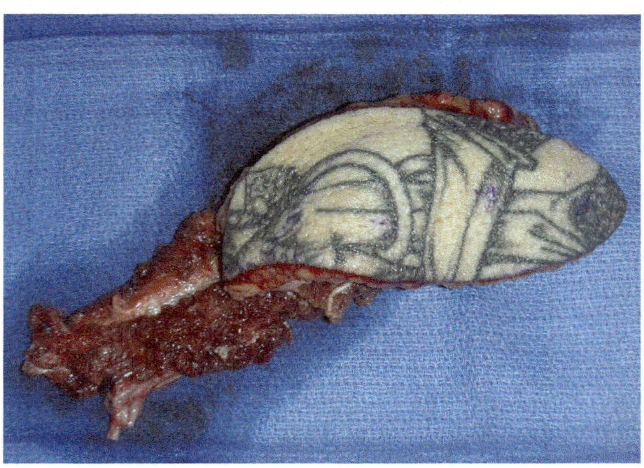

Fig. 23.25 Another view of the fibula flap prior to transfer.

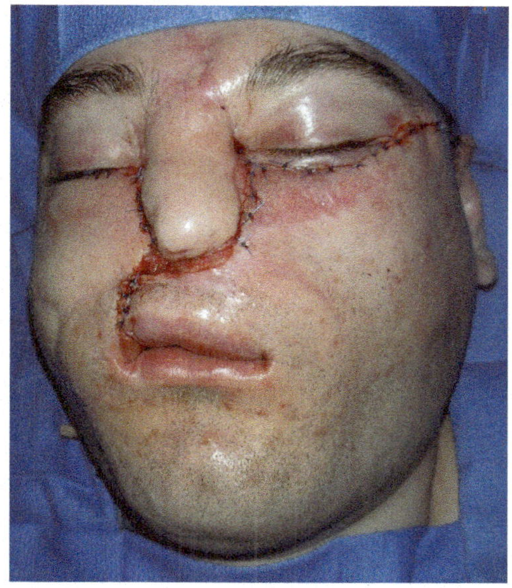

Fig. 23.26 Immediate appearance of the reconstruction of the midface and restoring the lip length.

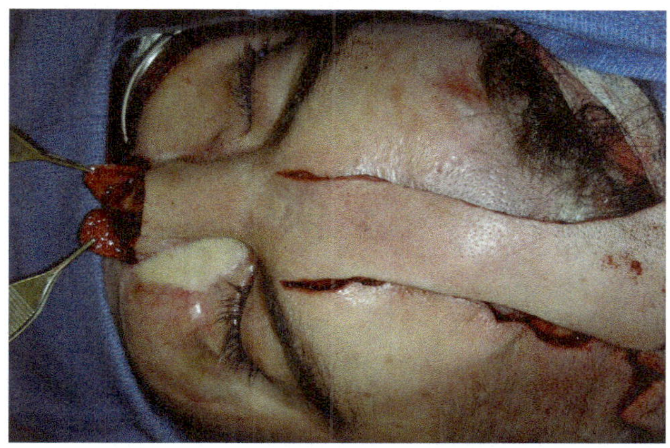

Fig. 23.27 Preparation of the nasal form prior to reconstruction with another paramedian flap and use of a portion of the fibula bone for nasal projection.

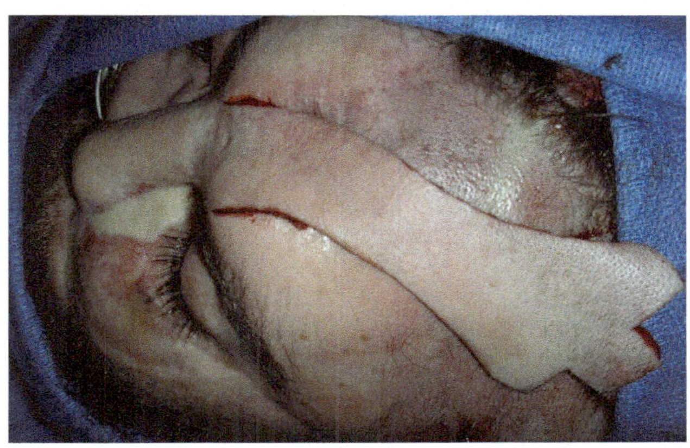

Fig. 23.28 Close up view of the paramedian forehead flap.

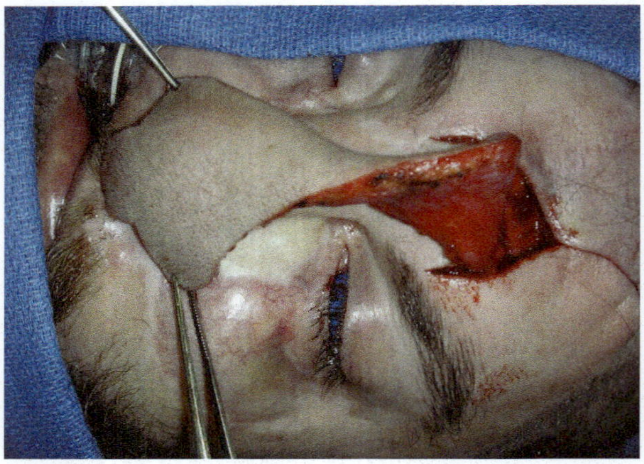

Fig. 23.29 Rotation of the forehead flap to check for adequate and passive reach.

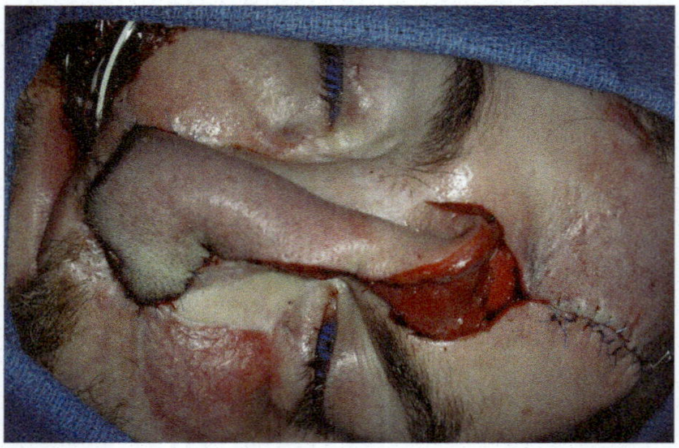

Fig. 23.30 Inset of the forehead flap to reestablish the correct nasal form.

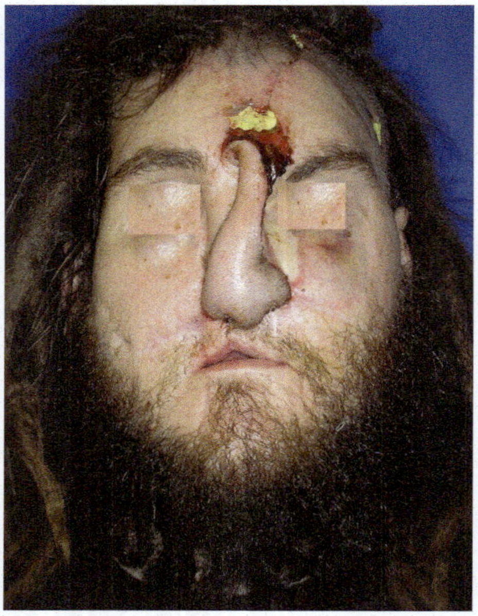

Fig. 23.31 Early postoperative view of the nasal reconstruction with the paramedian forehead flap.

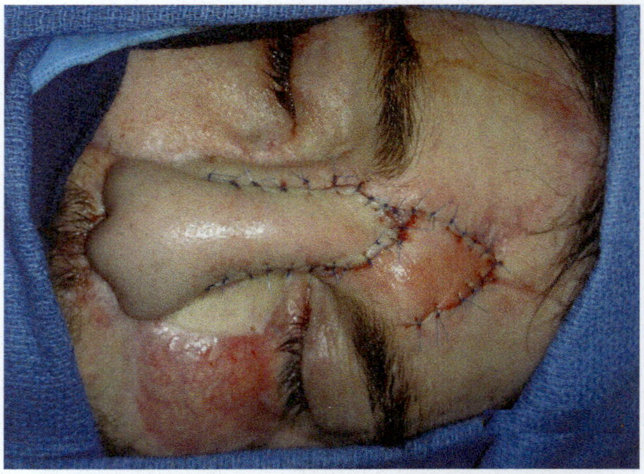

Fig. 23.32 Second stage nasal reconstruction with the takedown of the forehead flap.

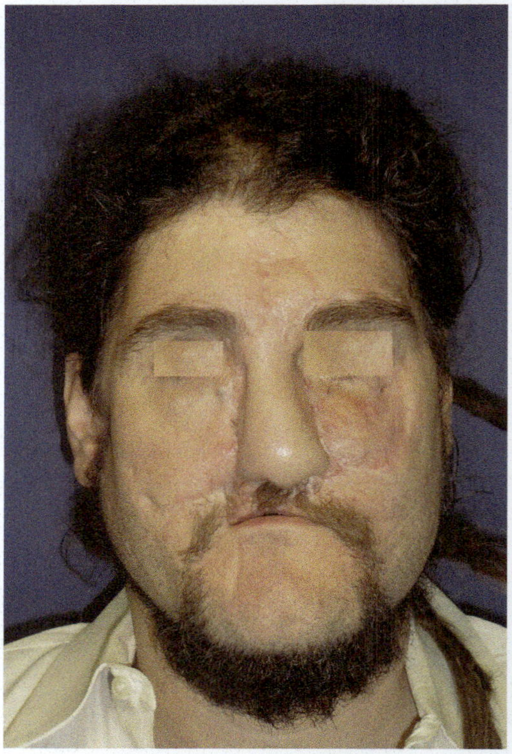

Fig. 23.33 Late postoperative view of the reconstructed nose.

with near normal midface projection (Figure 23.33 and 23.34).

This case highlights the difficulties encountered in reconstructing these complex defects. It also emphasizes the need to employ multiple reconstructive techniques to provide a better reconstructive outcome.

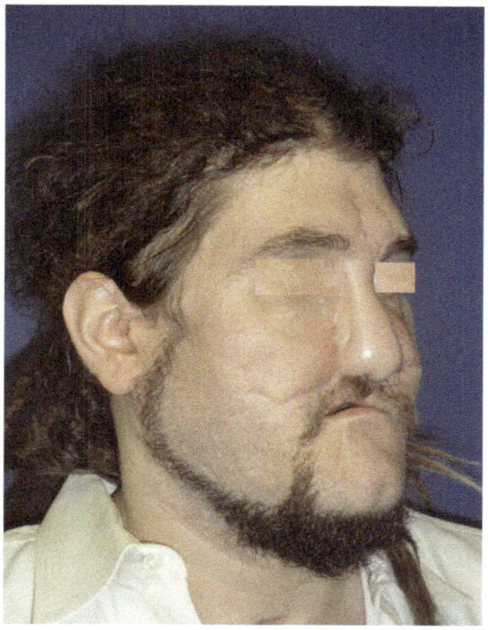

Fig. 23.34 Three-quarters view of the nasal reconstruction.

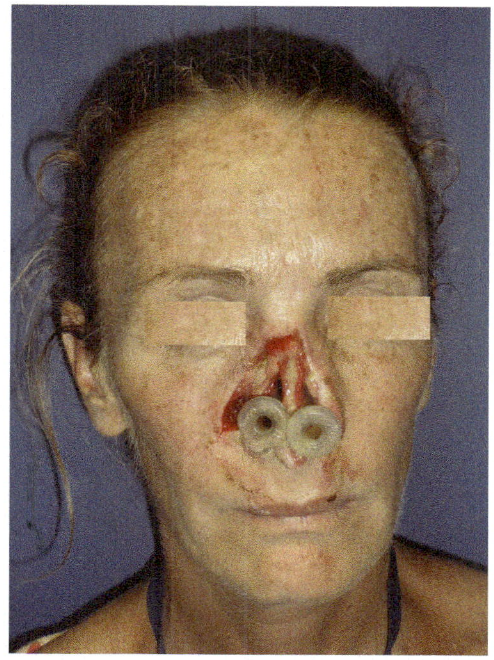

Fig. 23.36 Appearance of a rhinectomy defect after confirmation of clear margins.

Case #2: Postoncologic reconstruction of a total rhinectomy defect

A 43-year-old Caucasian female was referred for surgical treatment of an advanced squamous cell carcinoma with significant subcutaneous extension (Figure 23.35). The patient underwent a near total rhinectomy with plans for delayed reconstruction upon margin clearance (Figures 23.36 to 23.39). The patient had a temporary prosthesis made while awaiting the reconstruction. She was later brought to the operating room for evaluation of the defect and reconstruction of the defect with a septal pivot flap and a radial forearm free flap (Figures 23.40 to 23.45). The immediate postoperative result was typical for a formless reconstruction without any projection (Figures 23.46 and 23.47). She was later brought to the operating room for the reconstruction of the support layer and the nasal resurfacing (Figure 23.48). The reconstruction was carried out by performing turn-in flaps using the portions of the skin from the radial forearm free flap (Figure 23.49) and using bilateral ear cartilage to establish support (Figures 23.50 to 23.52). The nasal resurfacing was performed using a paramedian forehead flap (Figures 23.53 to 23.57).

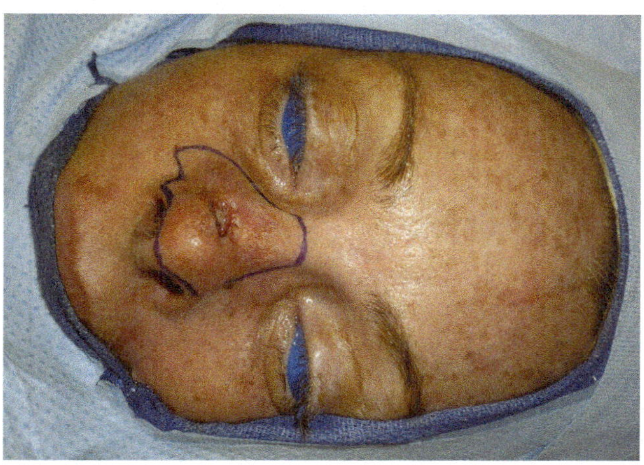

Fig. 23.35 Markings for a large nasal resection of a multiply recurrent carcinoma.

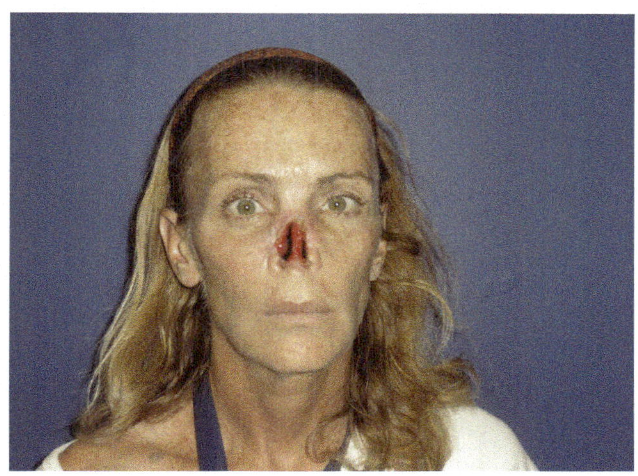

Fig. 23.37 Late view of the rhinectomy defect.

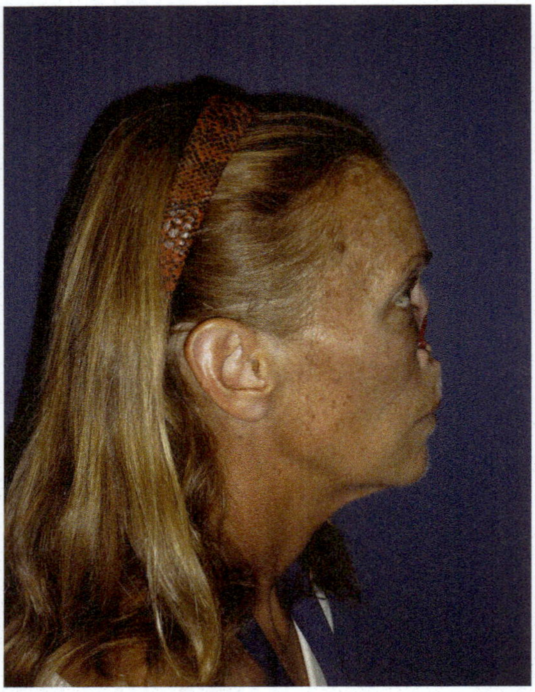

Fig. 23.38 Profile view of the rhinectomy defect.

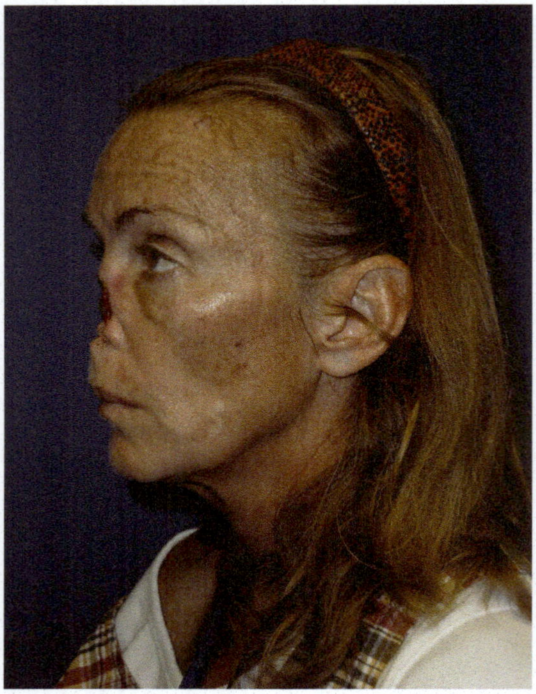

Fig. 23.39 Contralateral profile view of the rhinectomy defect.

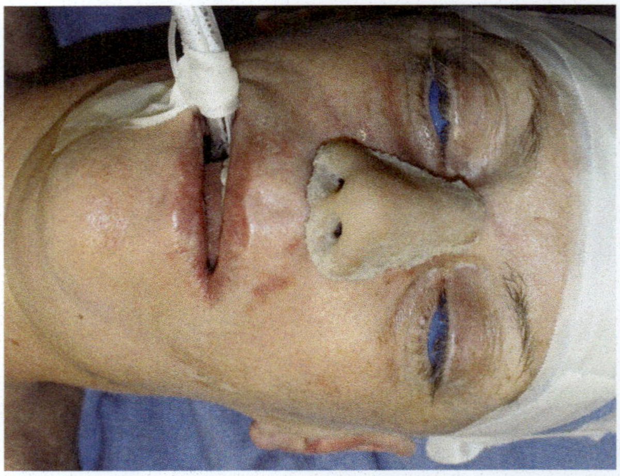

Fig. 23.40 Intraoperative view of a poorly constructed prosthesis.

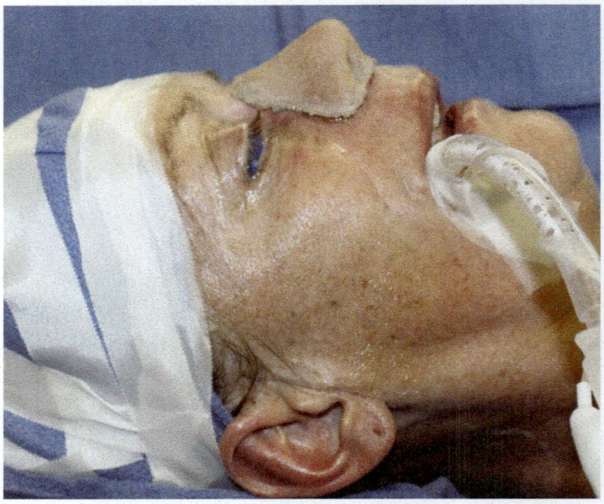

Fig. 23.41 Profile view of the nasal prosthesis.

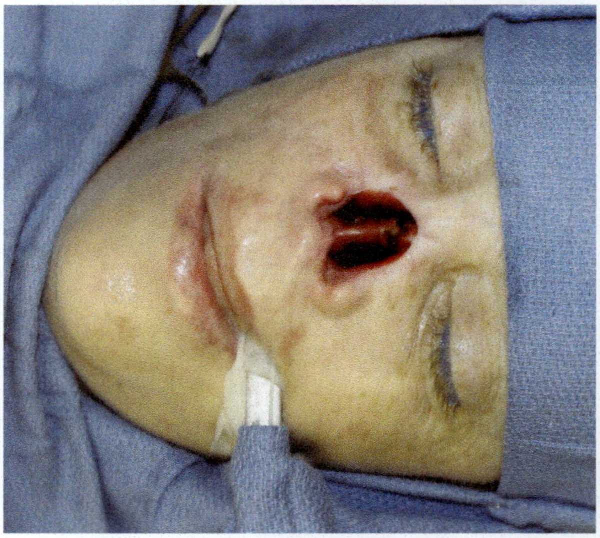

Fig. 23.42 Intraoperative view of the nasal defect.

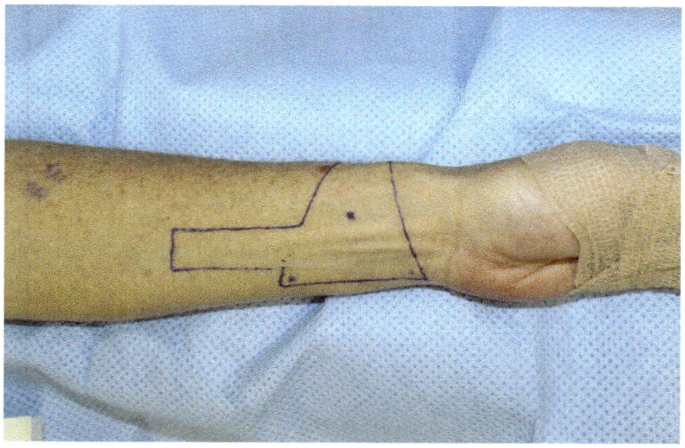

Fig. 23.43 Markings for the radial forearm flap to recreate the nasal lining.

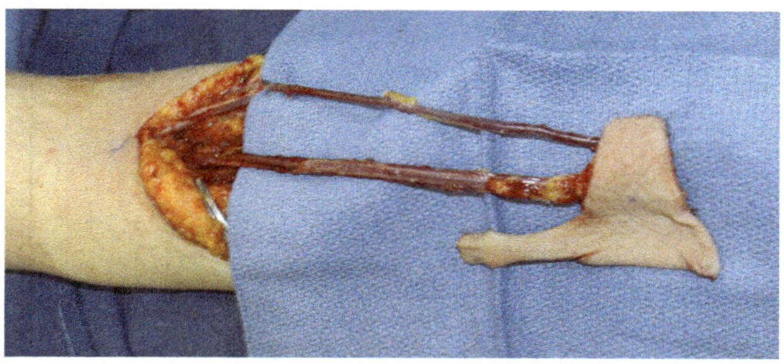

Fig. 23.44 Elevated forearm flap prior to transfer to the nasal cavity.

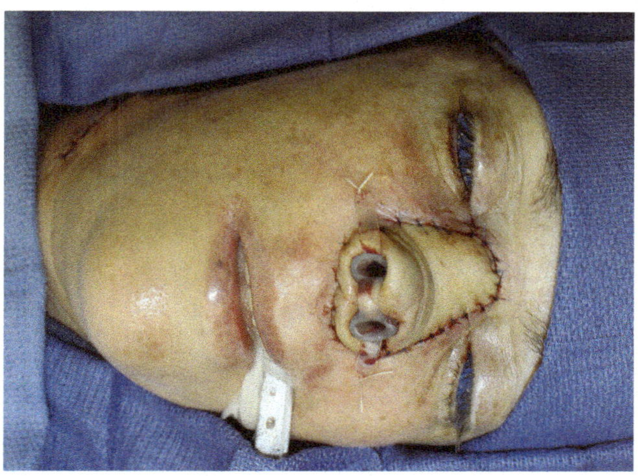

Fig. 23.45 Inset of the forearm flap to create the first stage in the nasal reconstruction.

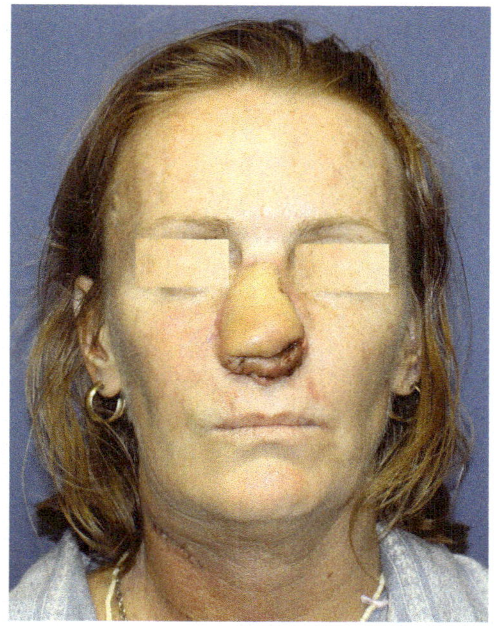

Fig. 23.46 Early postoperative view o the reconstruction.

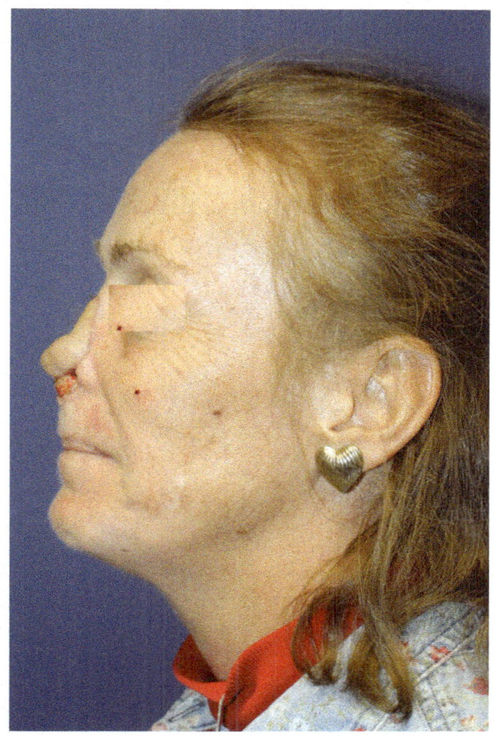

Fig. 23.47 Profile view of the nasal reconstruction.

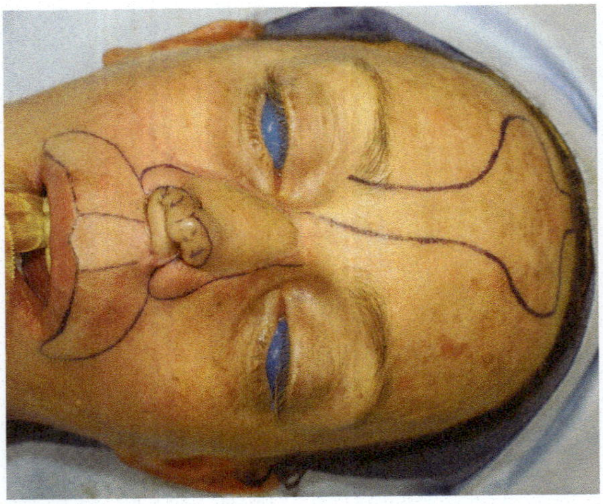

Fig. 23.48 Markings for a second stage reconstruction of the nose.

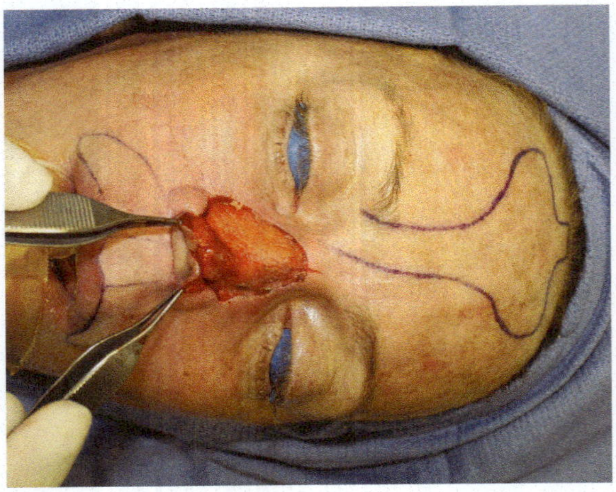

Fig. 23.49 Using the skin from the previous reconstruction as a turn in flap for the lining.

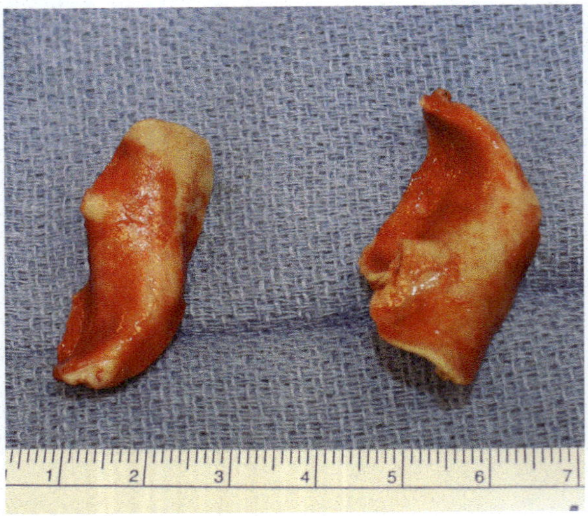

Fig. 23.50 Harvested ear cartilage to use as structural form prior to the paramedian flap.

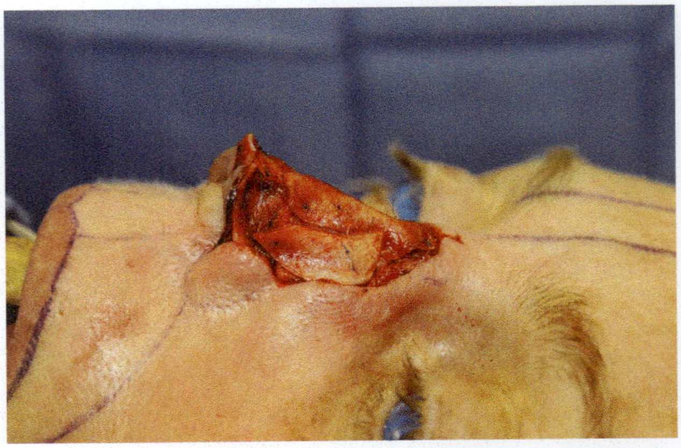

Fig. 23.51 View of the cartilage placement to create the nasal shape.

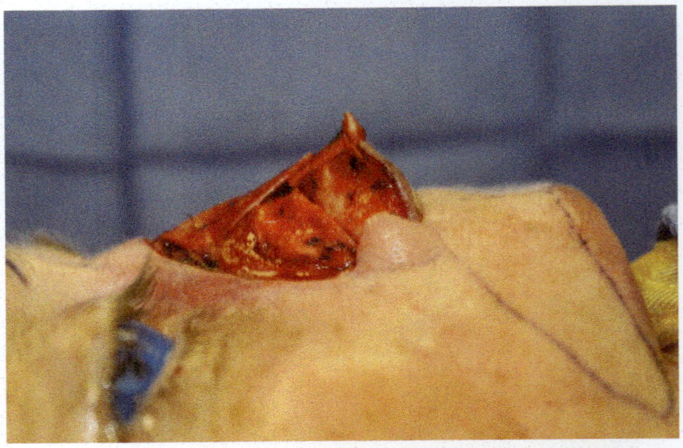

Fig. 23.52 Contralateral view of the nasal profile after cartilage grafting.

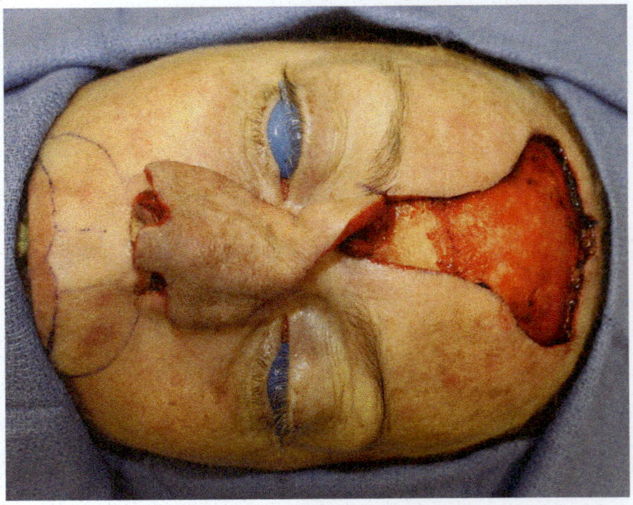

Fig. 23.53 Assessment of the reach of the forehead flap prior to inset.

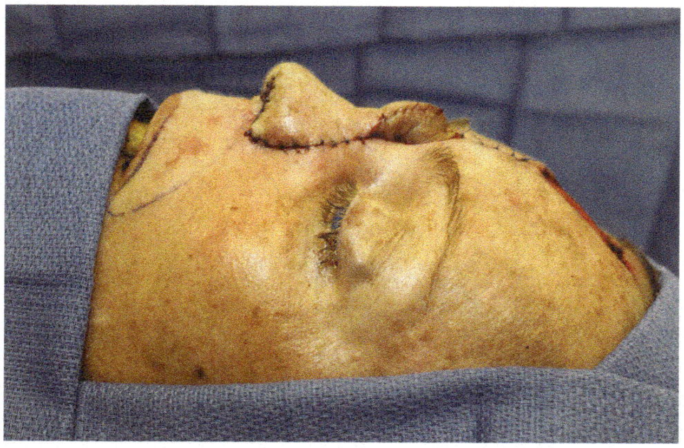

Fig. 23.54 Profile view of the inset of the paramedian flap.

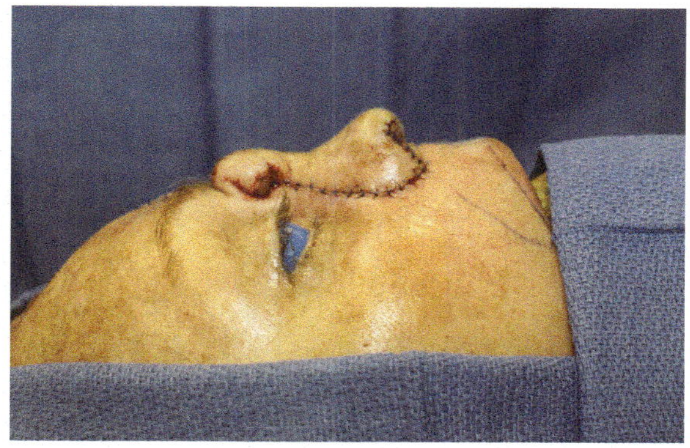

Fig. 23.57 Contralateral profile view of the inset.

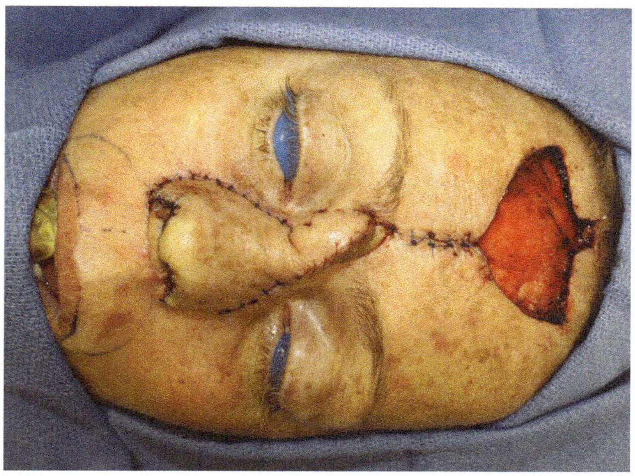

Fig. 23.55 Frontal view of the inset of the flap.

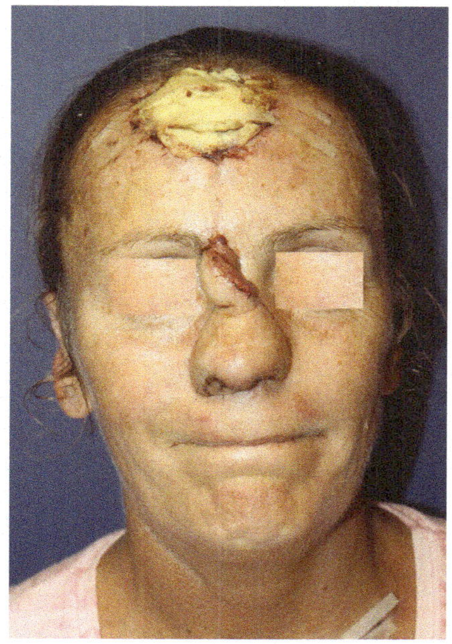

Fig. 23.58 Early postoperative view of the reconstruction prior to takedown of the pedicle.

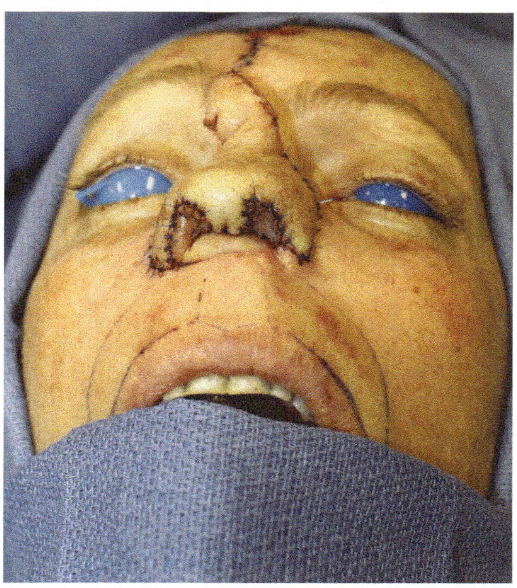

Fig. 23.56 Inferior view of the nostril form.

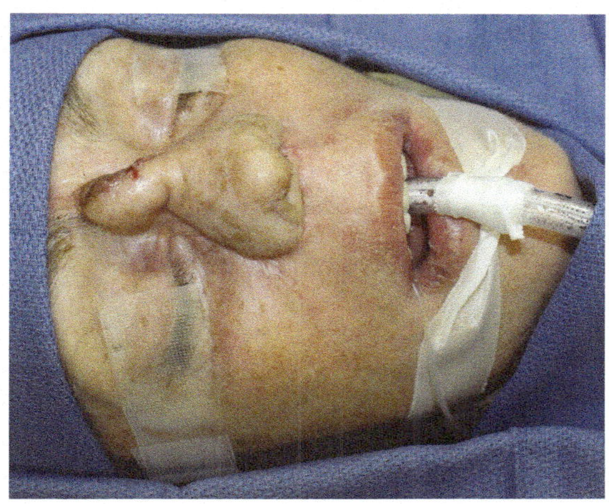

Fig. 23.59 Close-up view of the reconstruction prior to debulking.

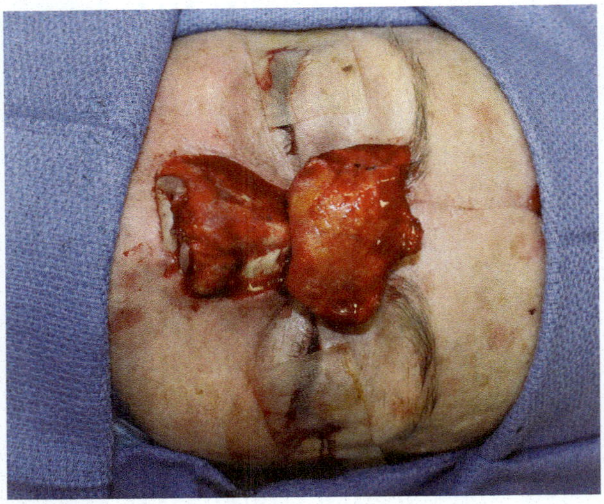

Fig. 23.60 Elevation of the flap and thinning of the construct.

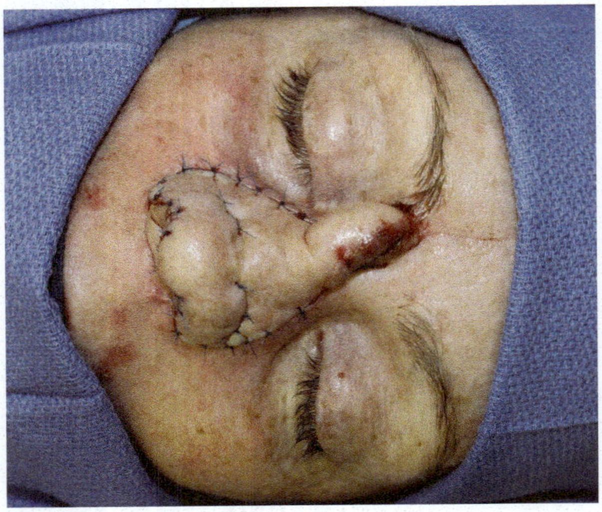

Fig. 23.61 Placement of quilting sutures after debulking.

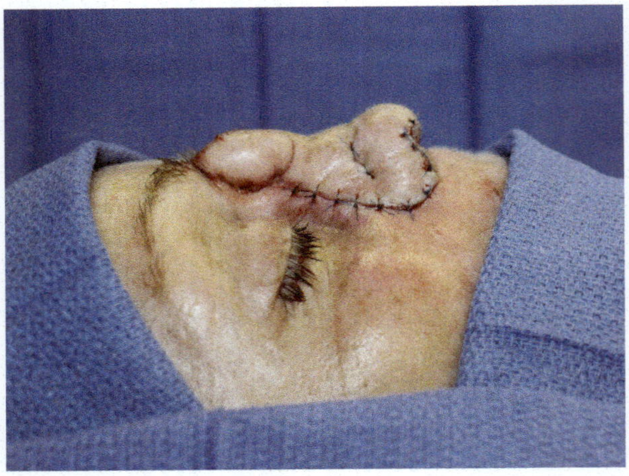

Fig. 23.62 Profile view of the quilting sutures.

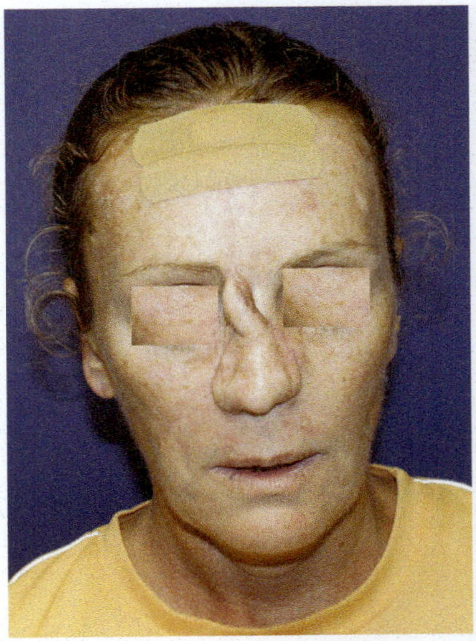

Fig. 23.63 View of the nasal form after flap debulking.

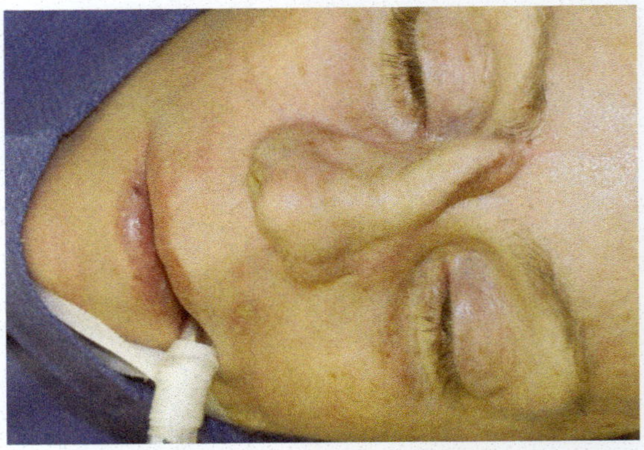

Fig. 23.64 Frontal view of the reconstruction prior to takedown of the pedicle.

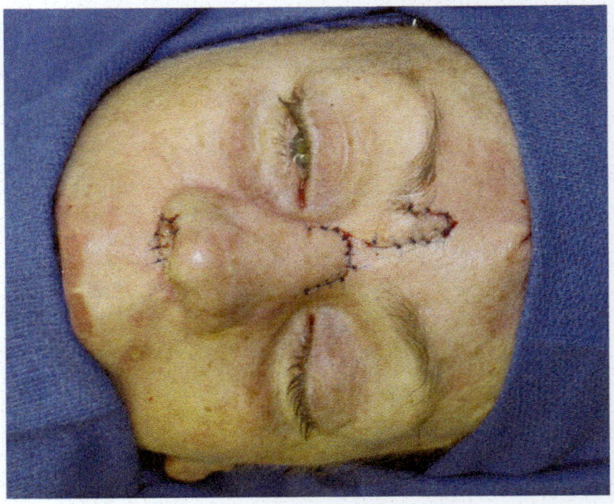

Fig. 23.65 Immediate view of the inset.

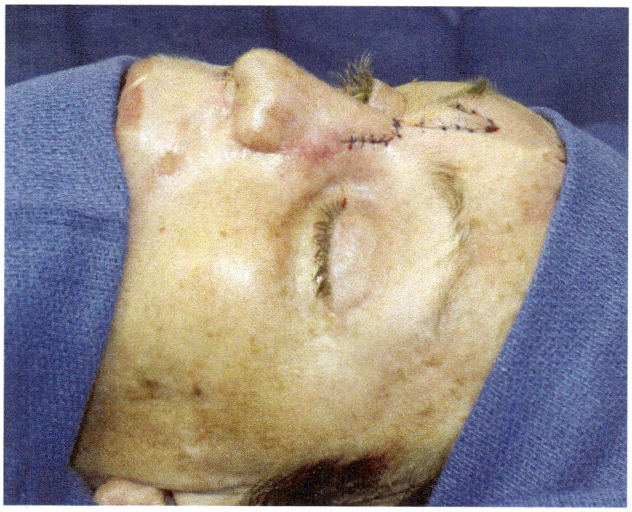

Fig. 23.66 Profile view of the inset after takedown of the pedicle.

The postoperative appearance from the second stage was pleasing to the patient and her family and served as an encouragement for continued progression with the reconstruction (Figure 23.58). The patient was brought back to the operating room for debulking of the flap and

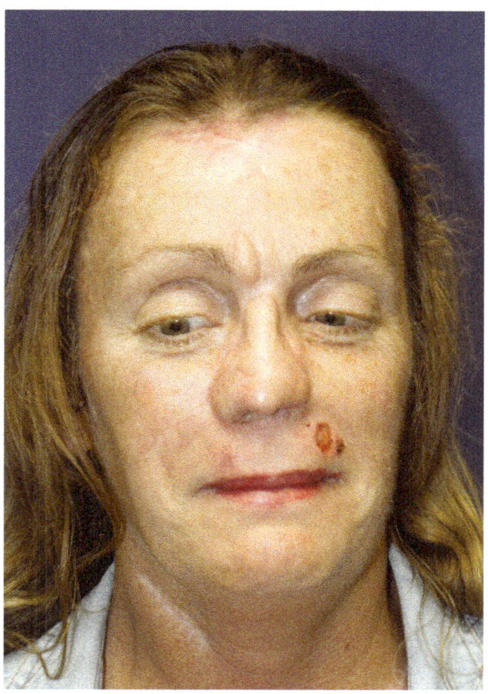

Fig. 23.67 View of the final reconstruction of the total rhinectomy reconstruction.

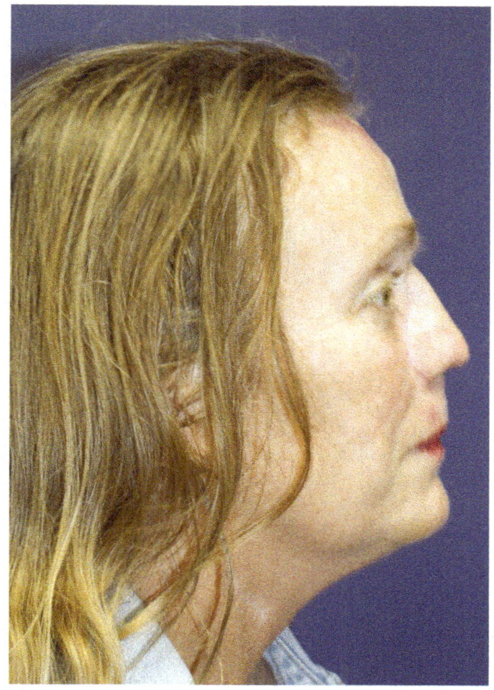

Fig. 23.68 Profile view of the nasal projection after final reconstruction.

to sculpt the nasal form with the aid of selective defatting and quilting sutures (Figures 23.59 to 23.62). The nasal appearance following the third procedure revealed good nasal form and proper projection (Figure 23.63). The last stage was the final takedown of the paramedian forehead pedicle (Figures 23.64 to 23.66). The final nasal reconstruction was acceptable to the patient and she opted to delay any further retouching procedures (Figures 23.67 and 23.68).

Case #2 illustrates the necessary commitment needed by the patient and the surgeon in order to reach an acceptable total nasal reconstruction.

References

1. Gonzales-Ulloa M. Selective regional plastic restoration by means of esthetic units. *Rev Bras Cir* 1957; 33:527–533.
2. Burget GC, Menick FJ. The subunit principle in nasal reconstruction. *Plast Reconstr Surg* 1985; 76:239–247.
3. Michelotti B, Mackay D. Nasal reconstruction. *Clin Anat* 2012; 25:86–98.
4. Menick FJ. Nasal reconstruction. *Plast Reconstr Surg* 2010; 125:138e

Chapter 24

Scalp reconstruction

Introduction

The reconstruction of scalp defects can be very challenging. The location and size of the defect can influence the degree of complexity for the surgeon. Defects of the scalp are most often encountered due to the presence of malignant lesions (Figures 24.1 and 24.2), after radiation (Figure 24.3), and occasionally due to trauma (Figure 24.4). The inherent challenges in the reconstruction of scalp defects is the status of the remaining scalp tissue as it relates to the existing blood supply and previous exposure to radiation therapy.

Many authors have described their approaches to scalp reconstruction. A name commonly associated with scalp reconstruction is Orticochea. Dr. Mario Orticochea made significant contributions to the reconstruction of scalp defects with his description of the four-flap[1] reconstruction and later the three-flap technique reconstruction, which improved the vascularity of the elevated flaps and the success of the reconstruction.[2] His contributions have come to be referenced to as the banana peel flaps. Since then others have incorporated newer techniques such as the use of tissue expanders to aid and at times improve the overall reconstruction of complex scalp defects.[3,4] Equally, the addition of microvascular techniques has increased our ability to reconstruct scalp defects that would previously have been deemed inoperable.[5]

The reconstructive surgeon involved in scalp reconstruction has to pay particularly close attention to the location of the hairline and the use of flaps so the normal hairline is not disrupted. Successful scalp reconstruction often requires intraoperative use of the intrinsic viscoelastic properties of skin, specifically, stress relation and creep.[8]

Anatomy

The skin of the forehead, scalp, and nape of neck constitute a single anatomic subunit.[6]

The layers of the scalp can be remembered according to the mnemonic SCALP: S skin, C subcutaneous tissue, A aponeurotic layer, L loose areolar tissue, and P pericranium.[7] The galea aponeurosis, the strength layer of the scalp, is contiguous with the paired frontalis muscles anteriorly, the paired occipitalis muscles posteriorly, and the temporoparietal fascia laterally.[8] The ability to move the scalp is gained by the loose areolar plane.

The scalp has a very rich blood supply, which it receives from both the internal as well as the external carotid systems. The blood supply to the anterior scalp is from the paired supraorbital vessels and the supratrochlear vessels. The lateral supply comes from the superficial temporal vessels. The posterior blood supply to the scalp comes from the occipital vessels which supply the territory above the nuchal line and from perforators from the trapezius and splenius capitus.

The scalp can be divided into tight and loose regions based on the underlying tissue. In areas where no muscle or fascia is present, the scalp is tight (centrally), whereas in areas where these components are present, the scalp is loose (peripherally).[6]

Defect assessment

Site and size oriented approach to reconstruction

The approach to the reconstruction of scalp defects can be broken down into its basic components as falling into one

Local and Regional Flaps in Head & Neck Reconstruction: A Practical Approach, First Edition. Rui Fernandes.

Companion website: www.wiley.com/go/fernandes/flapsreconstruction

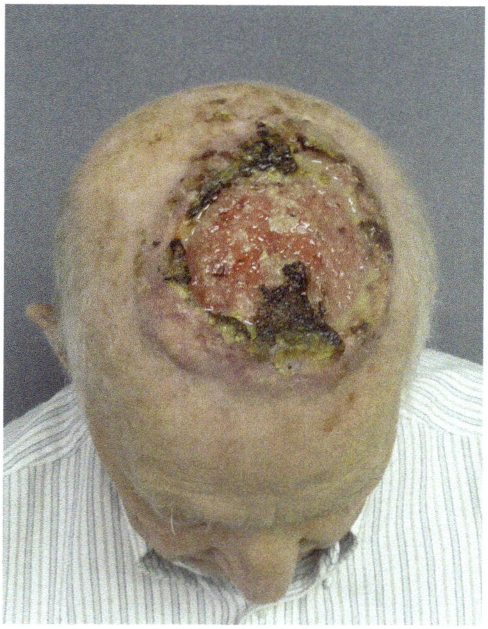

Fig. 24.1 View of a large neglected scalp malignancy.

of the following categories: primary closure, healing by secondary intention, skin grafting, local or regional flaps, and lastly, microvascular reconstruction. The next sections will develop each category and provide case examples to substantiate each option. When discussing each option, the pros and cons of the particular reconstructive technique will be highlighted.

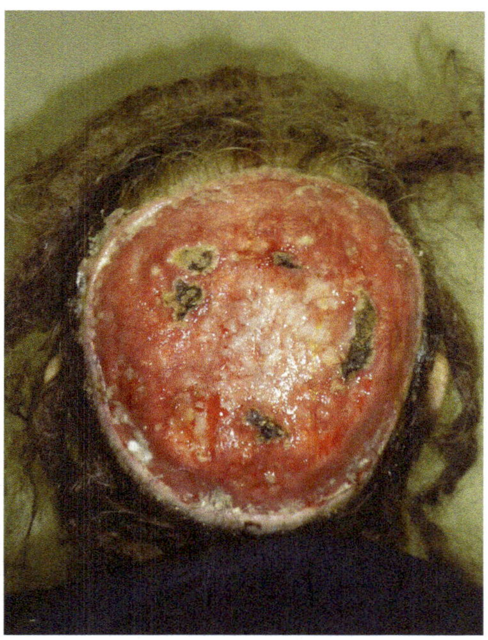

Fig. 24.2 Appearance of a very large scalp malignancy with destruction of the calvarium.

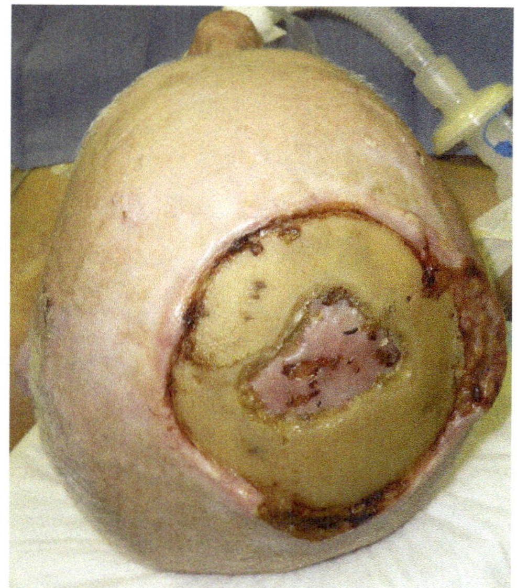

Fig. 24.3 View of a large exposed calvarium after previous radiation therapy to the scalp. Note recurrent disease on the right lateral aspect.

Primary wound closure

Scalp defects amenable to primary closure may result from the resection of small tumors or more commonly from trauma. Traumatic scalp defects are often misdiagnosed during the primary assessment as missing significant amount of tissues. The reason for this common misdiagnosis is due to the resultant contraction of the scalp (Figure 24.5). Upon closer inspection, it becomes evident

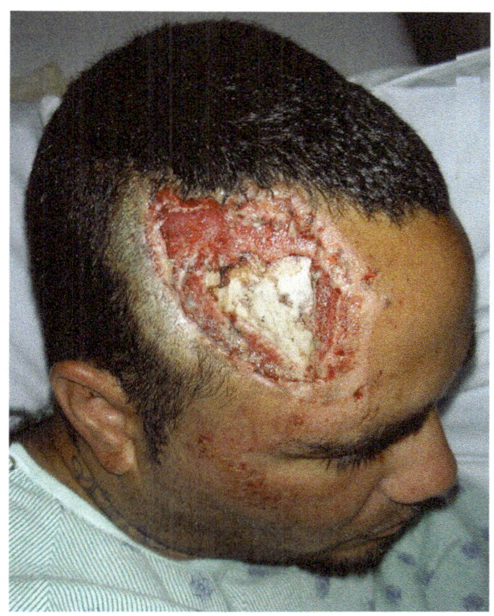

Fig. 24.4 View of a large avulsive injury of the forehead and scalp with exposed cranium.

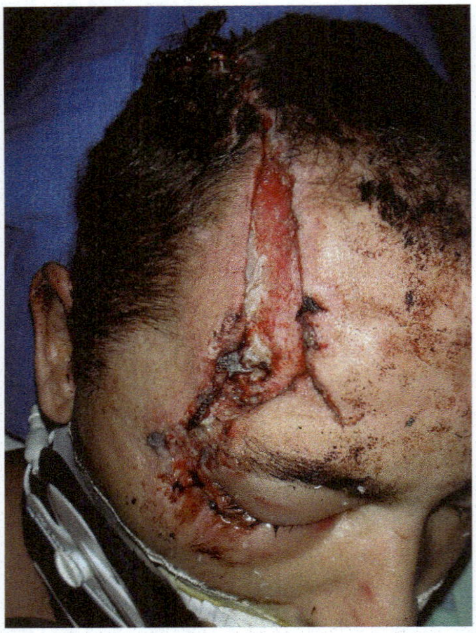

Fig. 24.5 Appearance of a large laceration of the scalp extending from the frontal region to the occipital region.

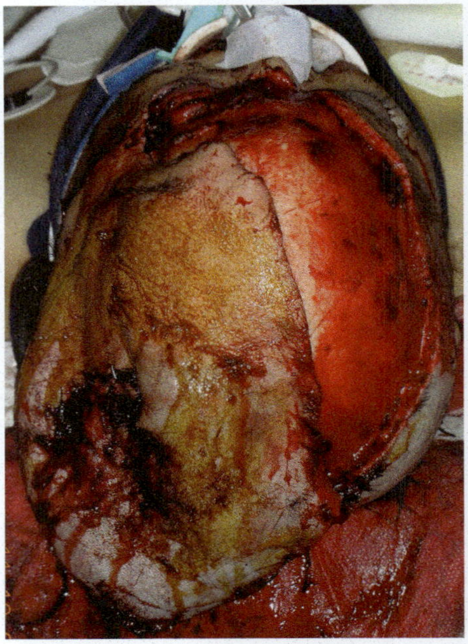

Fig. 24.6 View of a scalp avulsion pedicled on a small portion of the left posterior scalp.

that the tissues are not missing and that there is adequate tissue for primary repair of the scalp.

Defects originating from ablative procedures that would be amenable for primary closure are typically very small. The defects that would fall into this category are usually not referred to the reconstructive surgeon. They are often repaired by the ablative surgeon.

Case #1

A middle-aged Caucasian female was involved in a motor vehicle accident and suffered significant injuries. One of her injuries was a near scalp amputation (Figures 24.6 and 24.7). The patient was taken to the operating room where there scalp was thoroughly irrigated and all debris were removed (Figure 24.8). The scalp was then evaluated for vascularity and overall integrity. The scalp was then repaired with primary closure over suction drains (Figure 24.9). The appearance of the patient several months after the injury shows an acceptable repair of the near total scalp avulsion with normal hair growth (Figure 24.10).

Skin grafts

The use of skin grafts to reconstruct scalp defects is generally relegated to patients with significant medical comorbidities that would preclude them from more complex reconstructions, or to those patients in whom a staged reconstruction is contemplated. When staging the reconstruction with a skin graft, it is usually anticipated that the patient will have a tissue expander put in place and

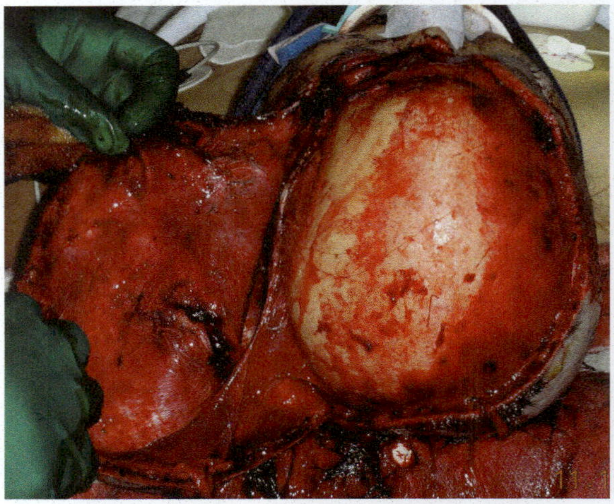

Fig. 24.7 Exposure of a large scalp laceration pedicled on the left.

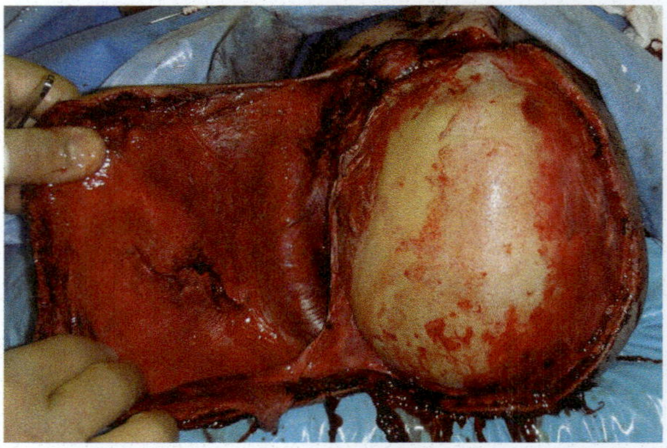

Fig. 24.8 Appearance after washout and debridment in the operating room.

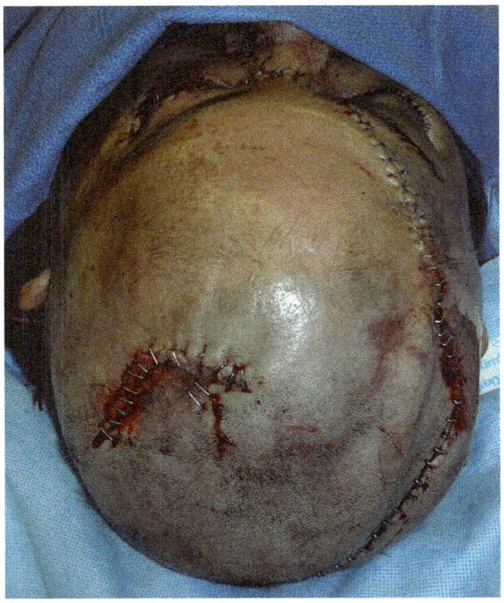

Fig. 24.9 Repaired scalp.

the expanded tissue used later to repair the original defect with hair-bearing scalp tissue (Figures 24.11 and 24.12).

When contemplating the use of a skin graft for scalp reconstruction, the ablative surgeon should preserve the pericranium whenever possible. The successful take of the skin graft is significantly increased when the recipient tissue bed is composed of a vascularized soft tissue.

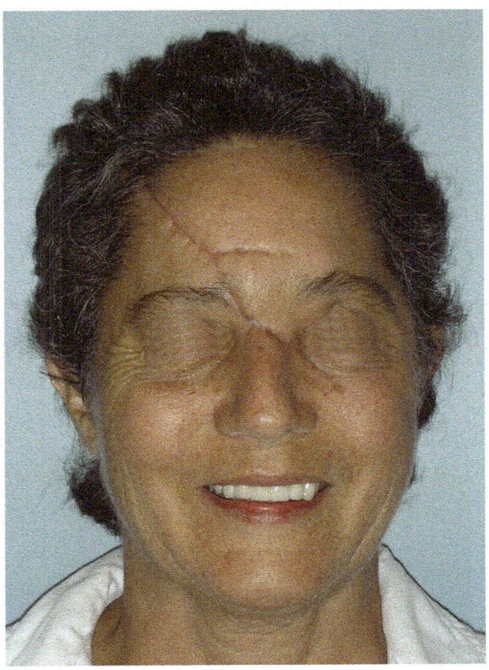

Fig. 24.10 Postoperative appearance of the repaired scalp.

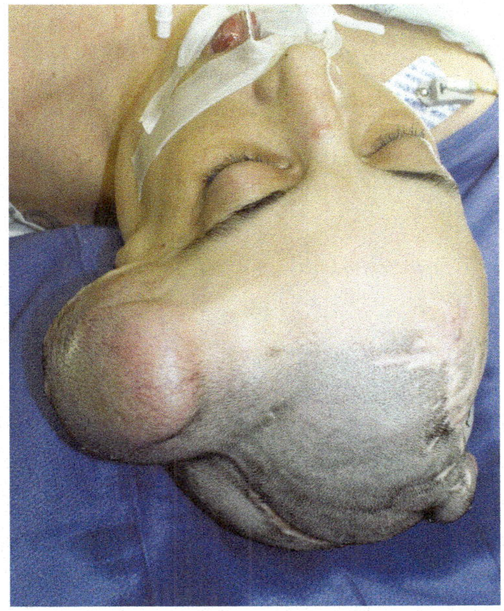

Fig. 24.11 View of a tissue expander placed on the left scalp prior to takedown and scalp reconstruction.

The use of skin grafts should be avoided in patients with a history of radiation therapy to the scalp or in those patients where the skull is barren. In these situations the likelihood of graft take is significantly less than in those cases where these issues are not present. If circumstances mandate an attempt at skin grafting the denuded skull, small drill holes should be made to bring bleeding points to the bed in the hope of improving the take of the graft. The skin graft should be a split graft with fenestrations.

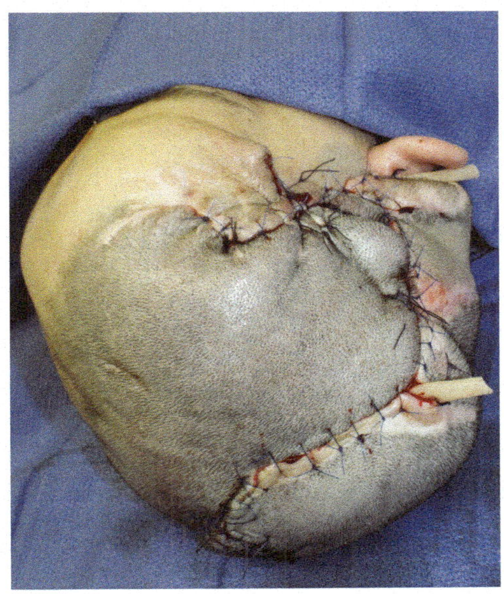

Fig. 24.12 Repair of the scalp after advancement and rotation of the expanded scalp.

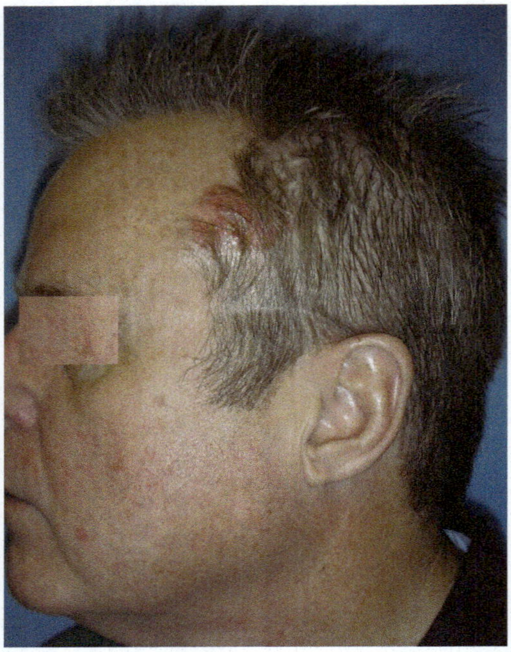

Fig. 24.13 Appearance of a left scalp malignancy which extends slightly to the forehead.

Case #2

A 49-year-old Caucasian male presented with a biopsy-proven squamous cell carcinoma of the anterior lateral scalp region (Figure 24.13). The area for resection was marked and the lesion was removed with frozen section margin assessment (Figures 24.14 and 24.15). A split thickness skin graft was then harvested and grafted to the defect and a bolster dressing was placed (Figure 24.16). The patient was pleased with his final reconstructive appearance (Figure 24.17).

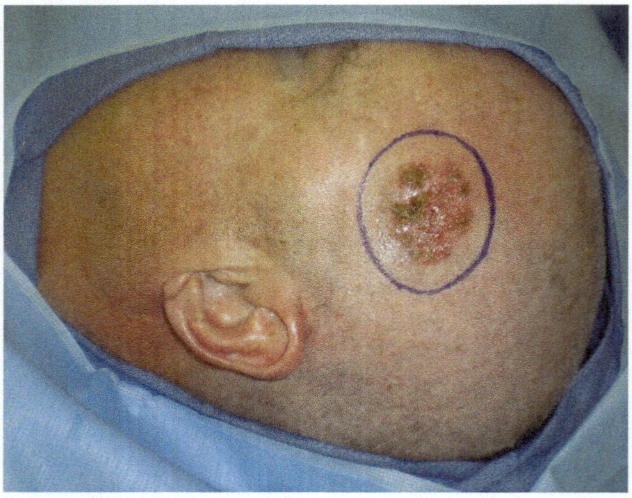

Fig. 24.14 Markings for the excision of the lesion.

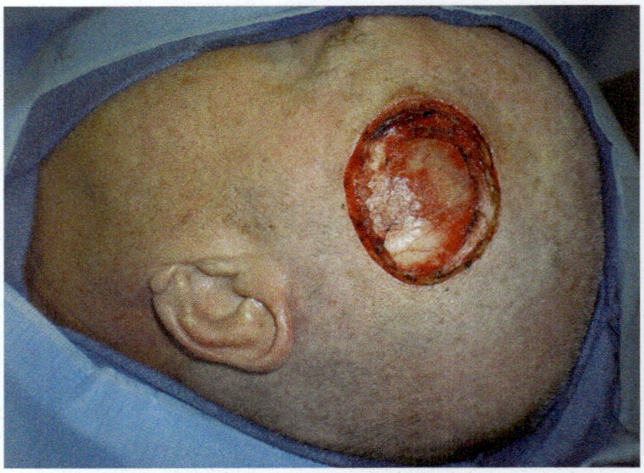

Fig. 24.15 Appearance of the defect after resection of the tumor.

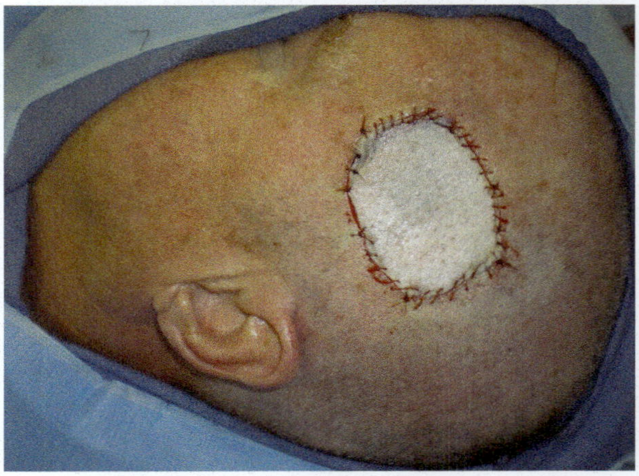

Fig. 24.16 Skin graft reconstruction of the scalp defect.

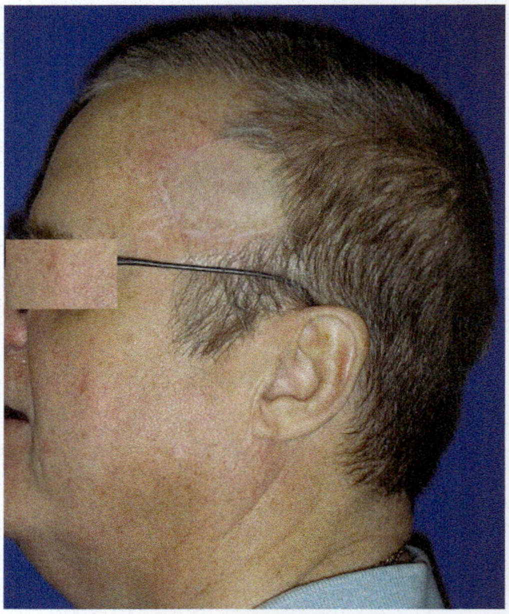

Fig. 24.17 Late appearance of the reconstruction of the defect with a skin graft.

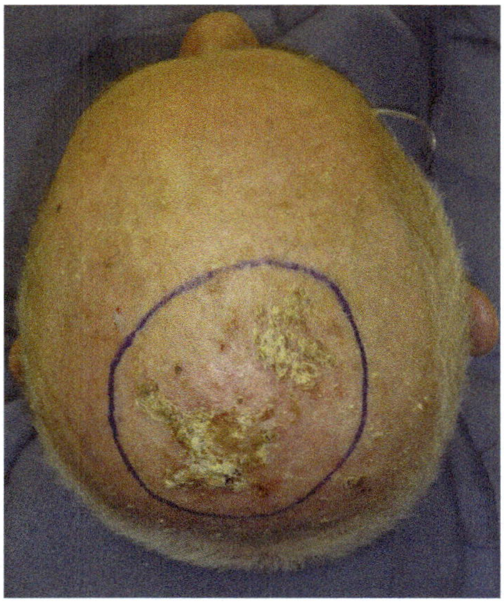

Fig. 24.18 Markings for a large scalp resection of a squamous cell carcinoma.

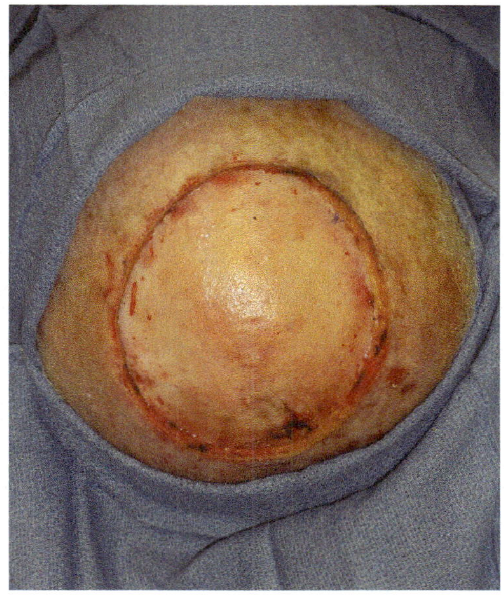

Fig. 24.20 View of the defect and scalp bed prior to repair with a skin graft.

Case #3

An 87-year-old Caucasian male with multiple comorbidities was referred for the management of a biopsy-proven squamous cell carcinoma of the scalp vertex (Figure 24.18). Due to the patient's overall poor health status, a decision was made for a resection and immediate reconstruction with a split thickness skin graft. This decision was felt to be the quickest way to get the patient reconstructed and off the operating table in the hope of minimizing operative and perioperative complications. The lesion was resected with a wide margin (Figures 24.19 and 24.20). The pericranium was left intact to increase the take of the graft. A large skin graft was harvested and grafted to the defect site (Figure 24.21). A large bolster dressing was made and wrapped with a petroleum-based dressing and secured in place with circumferential staples (Figures 24.22 and 24.23). The final appearance of the reconstructed scalp was acceptable with a complete take of the skin graft (Figure 24.24).

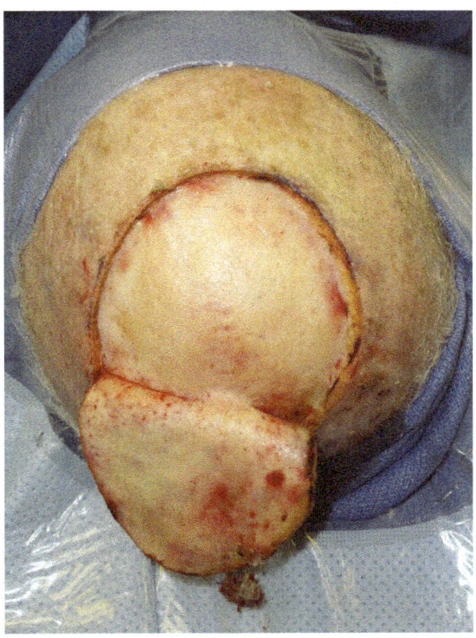

Fig. 24.19 Excision of the tumor.

Local flaps

A comprehensive understanding of the vasculature of the scalp and the inherent properties of scalp tissue

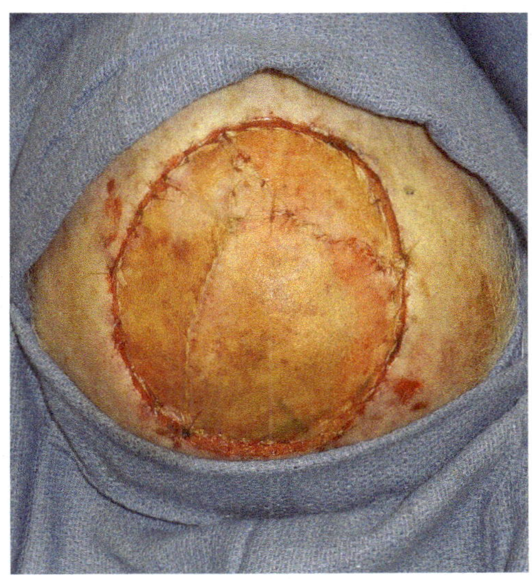

Fig. 24.21 Skin graft repair of the scalp defect.

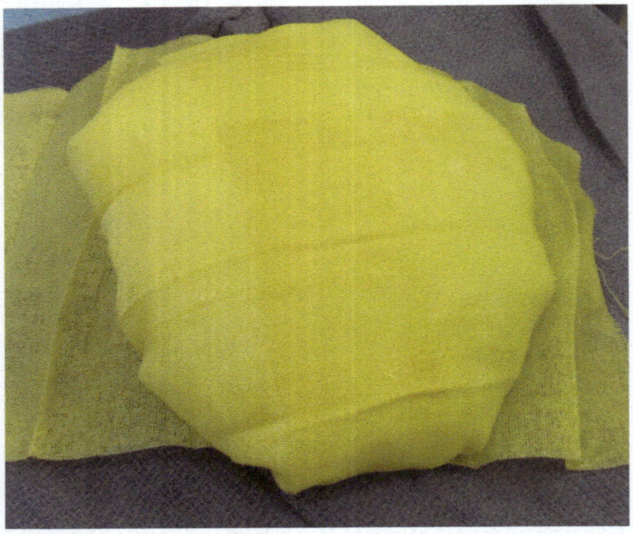

Fig. 24.22 Making of a bolster dressing to be used in the scalp.

allows for numerous local flap options in the reconstruction of various scalp defects. The use of transposition flaps, rotational flaps, and various other combinations can be routinely used to repair moderate to large scalp defects.

The options for the reconstruction of moderate to large scalp defects include the use of multiple rhomboid flaps as previously described in Chapter 4, use of the hatchet flap as described by Emmett in 1977,[9] or rotational flaps such as the pin wheel or Ying Yang flap.

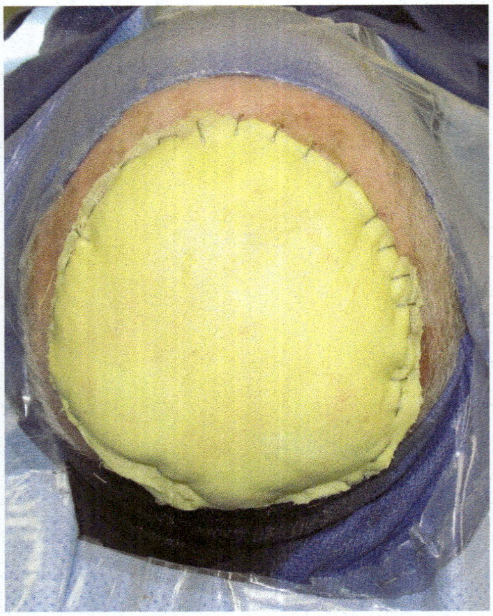

Fig. 24.23 Placement of the bolster dressing to secure the skin graft in the scalp.

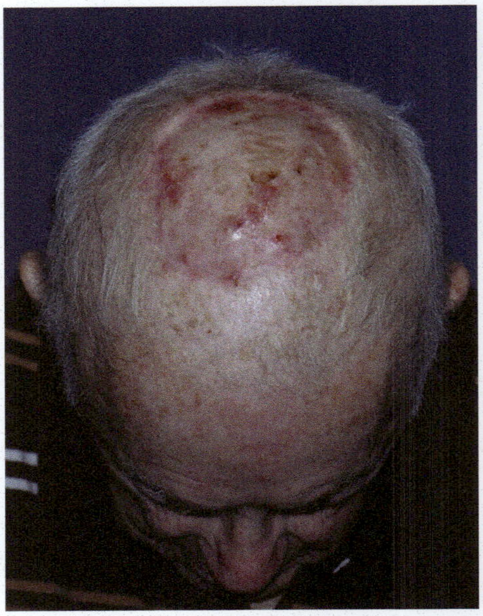

Fig. 24.24 Postoperative appearance of the reconstructed scalp with the skin graft.

Case #4: Multiple rhomboid flap

The use of the rhomboid flap to reconstruct various defects including the scalp was discussed in Chapter 4. This case illustrates the use of multiple rhomboid flap in a patient with a moderate size scalp defect. The patient was a 73-year-old African American male with a lesion on the vertex of the scalp (Figure 24.25). The lesion was removed and markings for various rhomboid flap

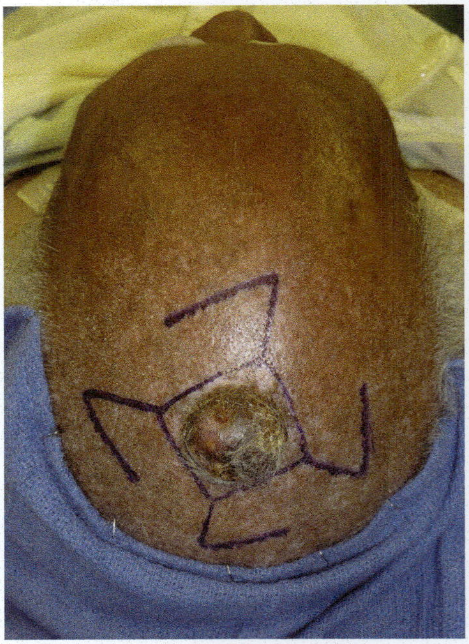

Fig. 24.25 Markings for a wide local excision of a scalp malignancy with possible options of rhomboid flaps.

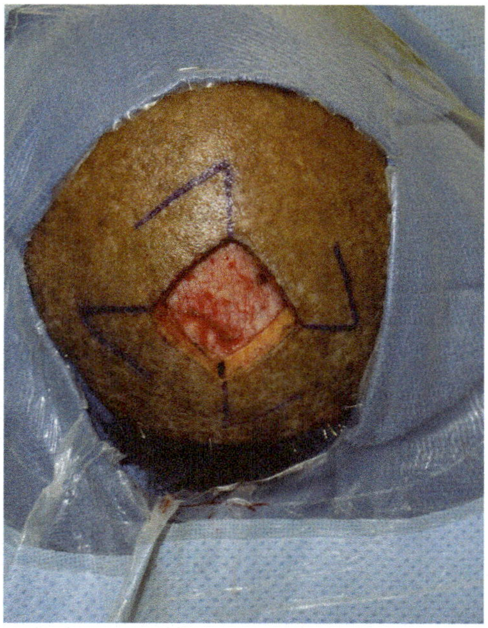

Fig. 24.26 View of the defect and flap options.

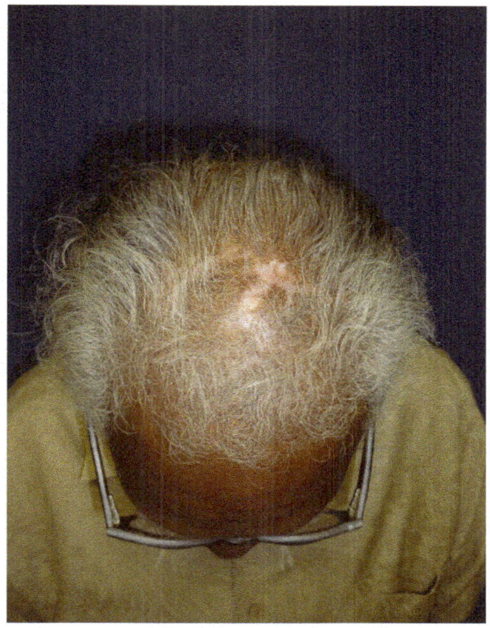

Fig. 24.28 Late postoperative view of the reconstruction.

options were marked (Figure 24.26). Two flaps were elevated and rotated to reconstruct the defect in a tension-free manner (Figure 24.27). The final appearance of the reconstruction was pleasing to the patient and preserved hair growth (Figure 24.28).

Case #5: Hatchet flap

The hatchet flap is a triangular local rotation flap with a greater or lesser degree of advancement and with a back cut at the base of the flap, through which it derives its vascular supply[10]. The shape of the flap does not have to be a precise triangle but can be a curvilinear shape with the back cut allowing for the perfusion to the flap.

The following case illustrates the use of this technique. The patient had a remote history of a craniotomy for evacuation of a hematoma. She states that within a week of the surgery she developed a dehiscence of the incision with exposure of the underlying titanium mesh. The patient stated that the surgeon believed that the site would eventually heal by secondary intention and did not want to intervene. Nine years later, she was seen by another neurologist and encouraged to have the area repaired (Figure 24.29). The previous mesh was removed and the area was debrided and the flap edges were incised

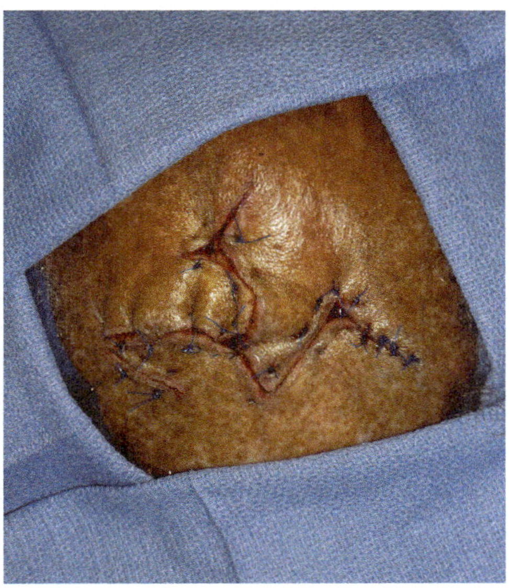

Fig. 24.27 Repaired defect with rhomboid flaps.

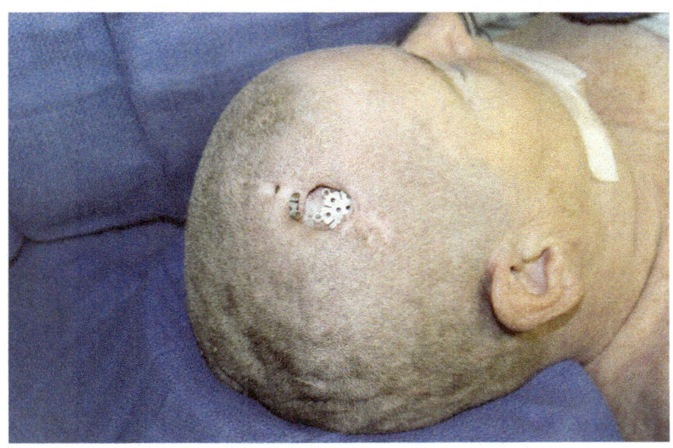

Fig. 24.29 View of an exposed titanium flap which had been used for the coverage of a burr hole.

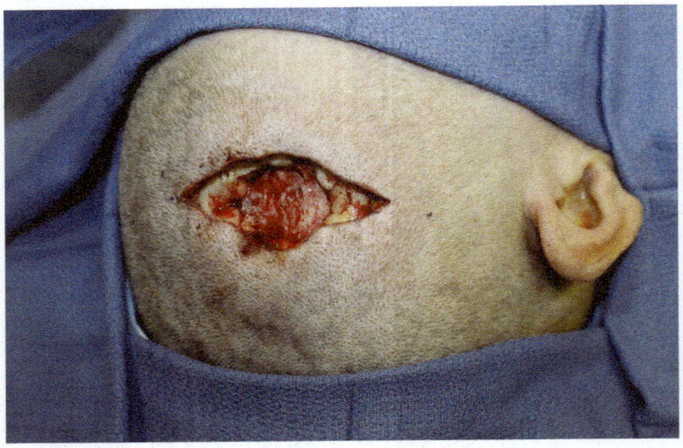

Fig. 24.30 Defect after removal of the hardware and debridment.

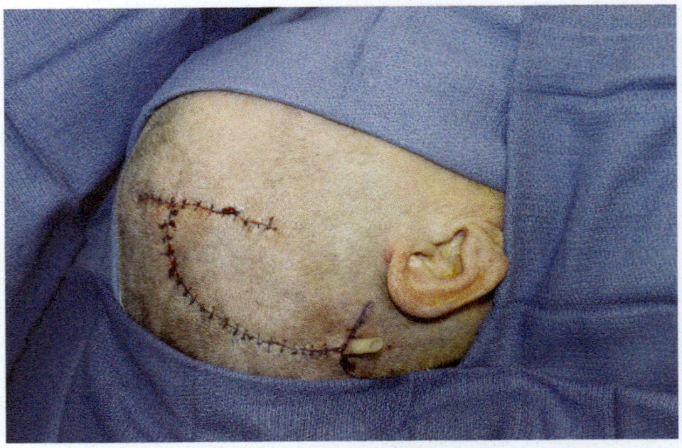

Fig. 24.32 Closure of the defect with a hatchet flap.

(Figure 24.30). Another titanium mesh was used to repair the skull defect (Figure 24.31). A hatchet-type flap was designed and rotated to repair the defect (Figure 24.32). The initial postoperative appearance was acceptable with good repair of the initial defect (Figure 24.33).

Case #6: Pinwheel flap
The use of the pinwheel flap design was described by Vecchione in 1978[11]. The design is based on the creation of four flaps radiating away from the defect at approximately 90 degree intervals and to about twice the diameter of the initial defect. This technique distributes tension along the various flaps with minimal undermining. The following case illustrates the pinwheel concept with the use of three flaps and skin grafting to the graftable site. The patient was a 74-year-old male with a large squamous cell carcinoma of the scalp referred for surgical management (Figure 24.34. The lesion was excised with the involved pericranium with drilling of the outer cortex of the cranium (Figure 24.35. A design was marked for a pinwheel rotation of three flaps to repair this large

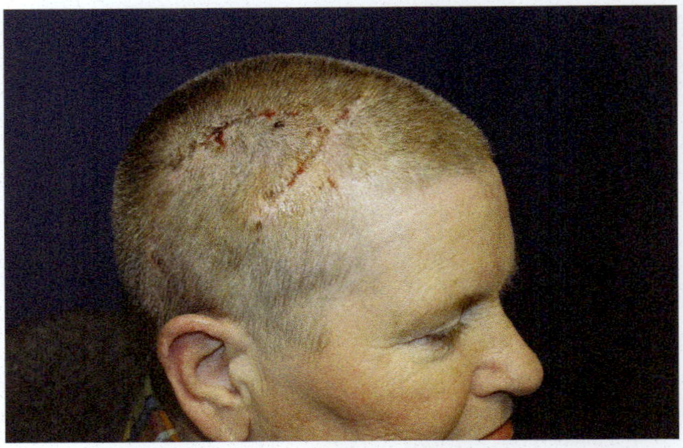

Fig. 24.33 Healed reconstruction of the scalp defect with the hatchet flap.

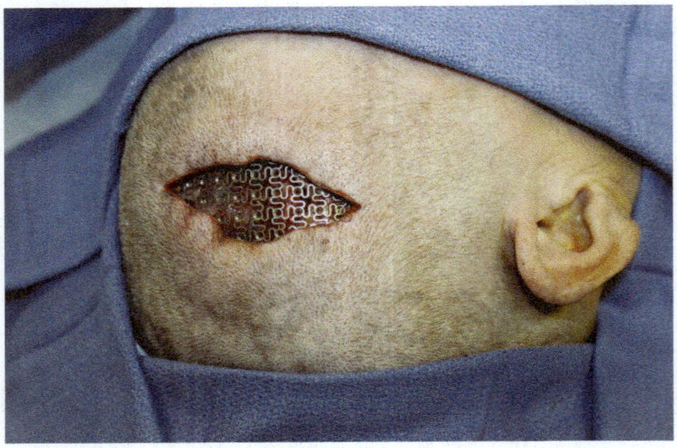

Fig. 24.31 Placement of a new titanium mesh prior to repair.

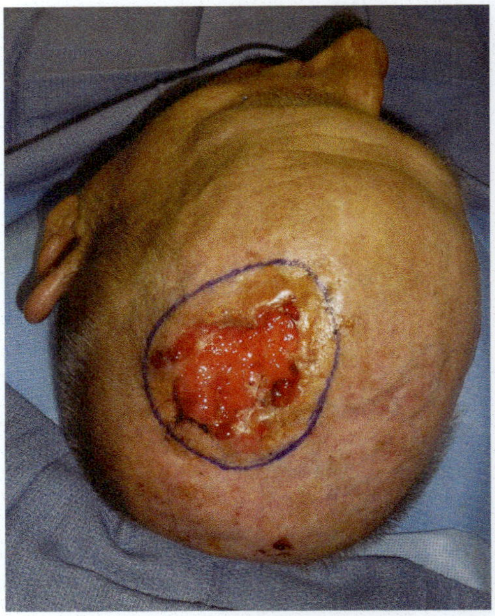

Fig. 24.34 View of a large scalp tumor with markings for the resection.

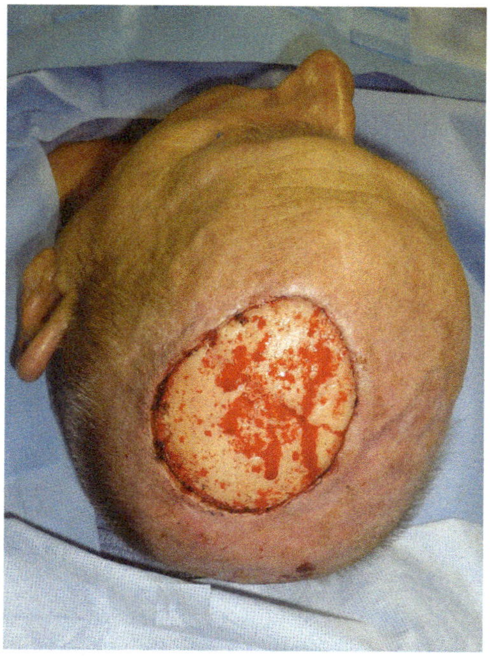

Fig. 24.35 Appearance of the defect after resection.

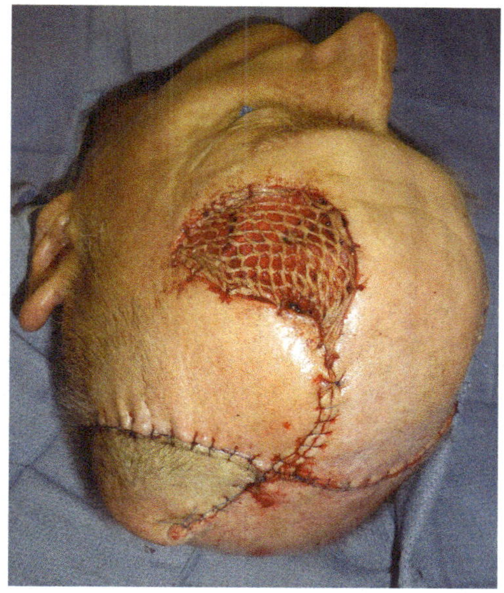

Fig. 24.37 Repair of the defect with flap transposition and a skin graft over the anterior temporalis and frontal muscle.

defect (Figure 24.36). The flaps were elevated, undermined, and rotated to repair the defect; an anterior lateral defect overlying the temporalis muscle was grafted with a split thickness skin graft (Figure 24.37).

The use of the pinwheel concept can be modified by using two flaps rather than four or three as previously described. The design of the flaps is dependent on the location of the defect and the available tissue surrounding the defect. The following case illustrates the use of the technique when there is a limitation by the location of the defect. The patient is a 55-year-old Caucasian female with melanoma of the right parietal scalp (Figure 24.38). The lesion was removed with a portion of the defect over the temporalis muscle and the other half over bare cranium (Figure 24.39). The markings for two rotation flaps in a pinwheel design was planned (Figure 24.40). The two flaps were elevated and the area was undermined and checked for passive advancement to the defect

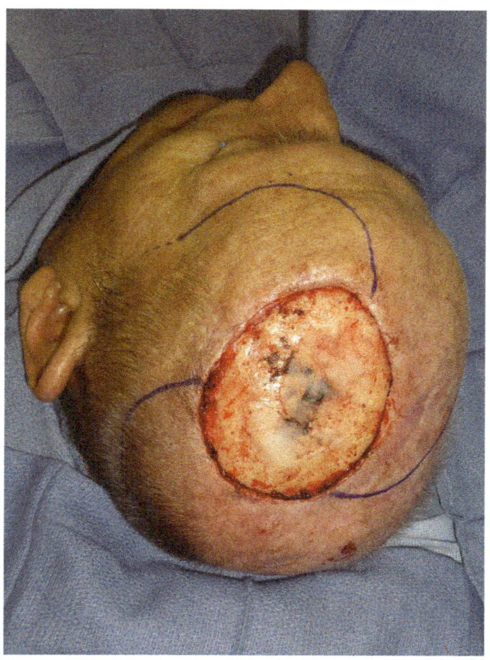

Fig. 24.36 Markings for pinwheel reconstruction of the defect.

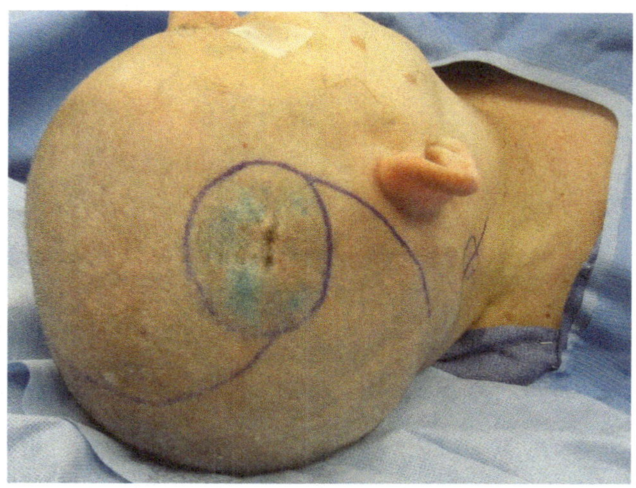

Fig. 24.38 View of a scalp melanoma after sentinel node dissection and markings for flap transposition.

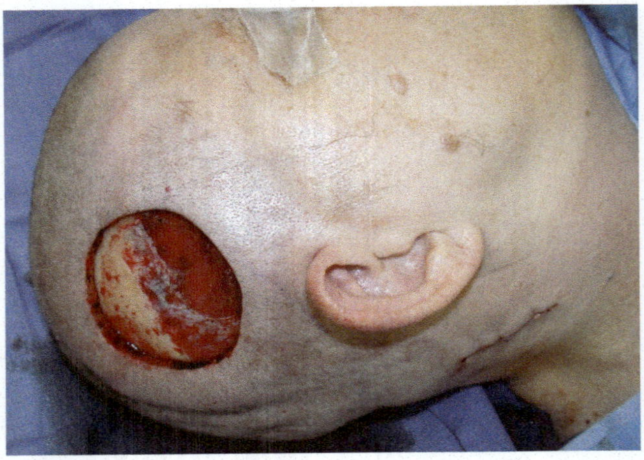

Fig. 24.39 Defect after resection of the lesion.

(Figure 24.41 and 24.42). The flaps were then advanced and the defect repaired (Figure 24.43).

Case #7: Yin Yang flap

The concept of the Yin Yang flap design is based on the use of two opposing semicircular flaps around the diameter of the defect. The design is a very simple one but is dependent on the design of each flap having a sufficient base to allow adequate perfusion to the tip of the flap. Once elevated, the flap will often need to have fasciotomies performed to increase the reach to repair the defect. The following two cases illustrate the use of the technique to repair vertical and occipital defects.

The initial case illustrates the use of the technique in a patient who had previously been diagnosed with a sebaceous carcinoma of the scalp. Markings for a wide local excision surrounding the scar at the previous biopsy site and the design for the rotation transposition flaps were made (Figure 24.44). The lesion was removed deep to the pericranium (Figure 24.45). The two opposing flaps were

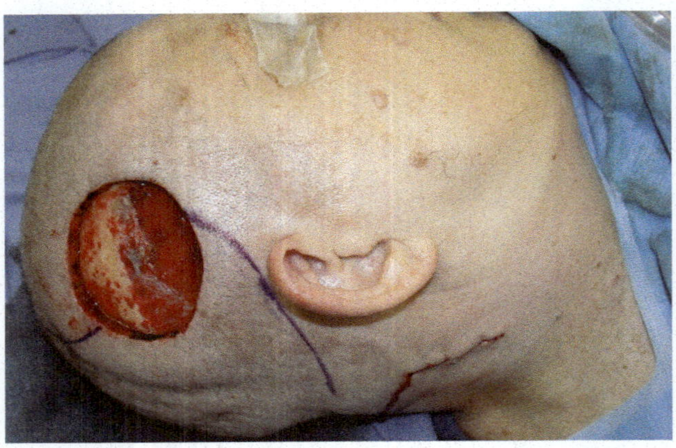

Fig. 24.40 Markings for the reconstruction.

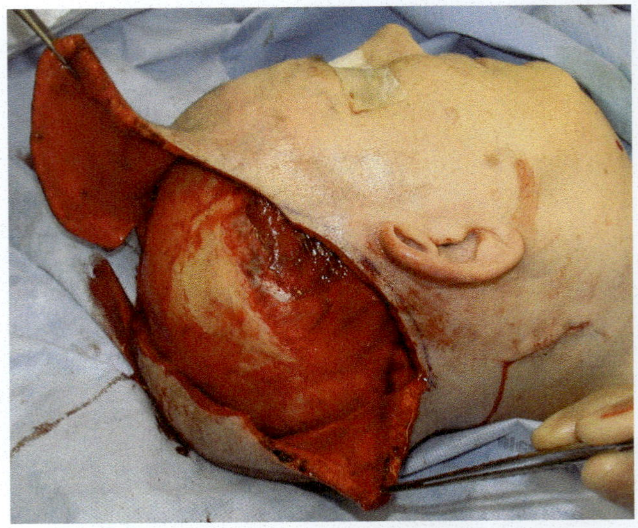

Fig. 24.41 Elevation of the scalp flaps prior to rotation and transfer.

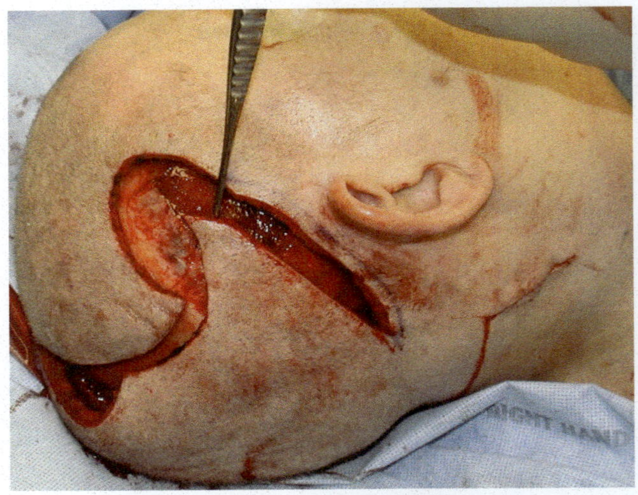

Fig. 24.42 Assessment of the reach of the flaps into the defect.

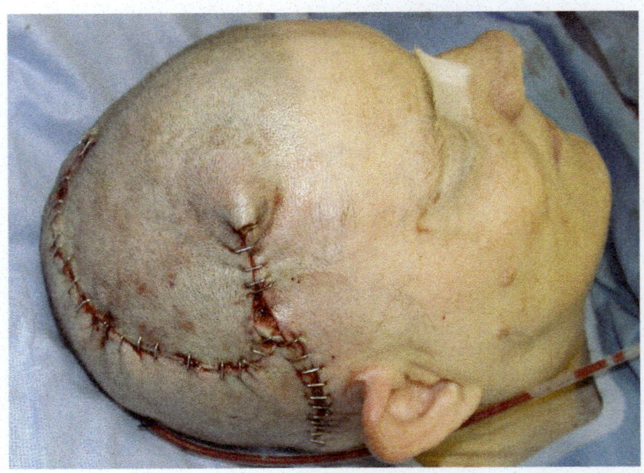

Fig. 24.43 Repair of the scalp defect.

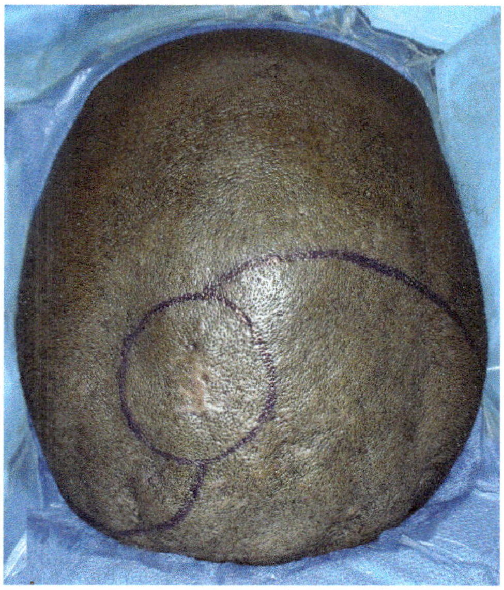

Fig. 24.44 Planning for a wide local excision of a scalp malignancy with markings for bilateral rotational advancement flaps.

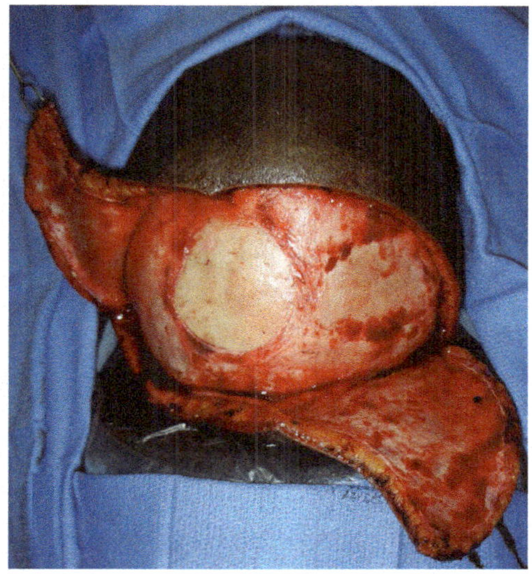

Fig. 24.46 Elevation of bilateral scalp flaps prior to rotation.

elevated and galeotomies performed to aid in the rotation and advancement of the flaps to the defect (Figures 24.46 and 24.47). The flap was then inset into the defect without tension and the patient had an uneventful postoperative healing course (Figure 24.48).

A 59-year-old male was referred for the surgical management of a scalp malignancy which had been refractory to primary treatment with radiation therapy (Figure 24.49). Given the location of the lesion and the fact that the area was previously radiated, the plan was for immediate reconstruction with rotational flaps. The patient was positioned on the operating table in the prone position (Figure 24.50) and the area for a wide excision was marked. The excision gave a large occipital defect in a radiated bed (Figure 24.51). A design was made for the elevation of two opposing Yin Yang flaps which were then elevated (Figure 24.52). Several galea-releasing incisions were made to aid in the advancement of the flap. The flap was then rotated into the defect and the site repaired (Figure 24.53). The final appearance a few weeks postoperatively revealed a healed defect with an acceptable cosmetic result (Figure 24.54).

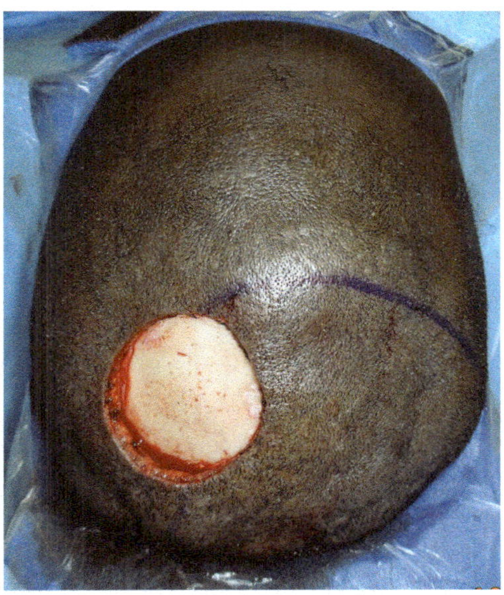

Fig. 24.45 Scalp defect after resection of the tumor.

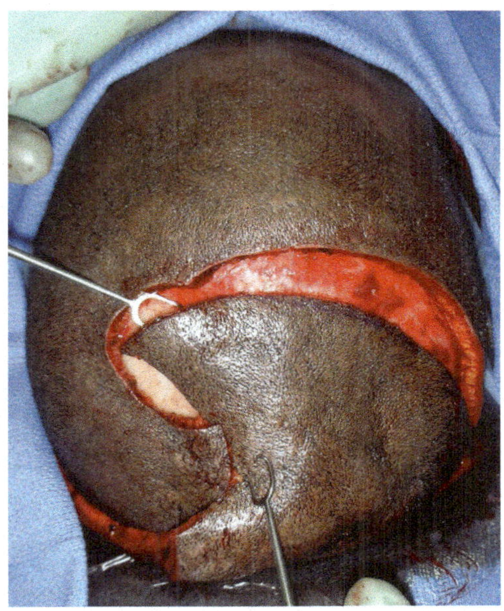

Fig. 24.47 Confirmation of the reach of the flaps into the defect.

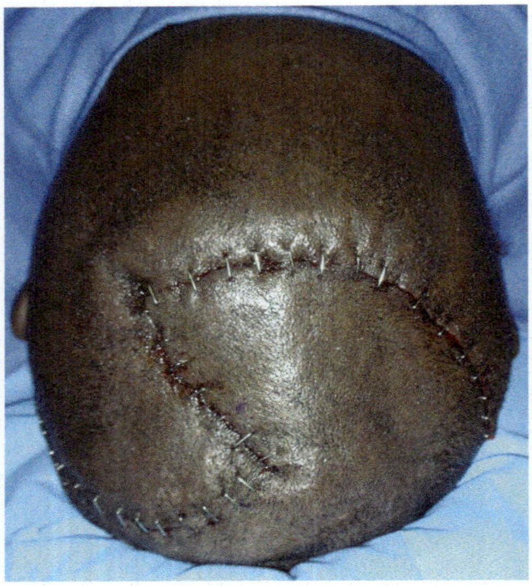

Fig. 24.48 Closure of the defect after transposition of the flap.

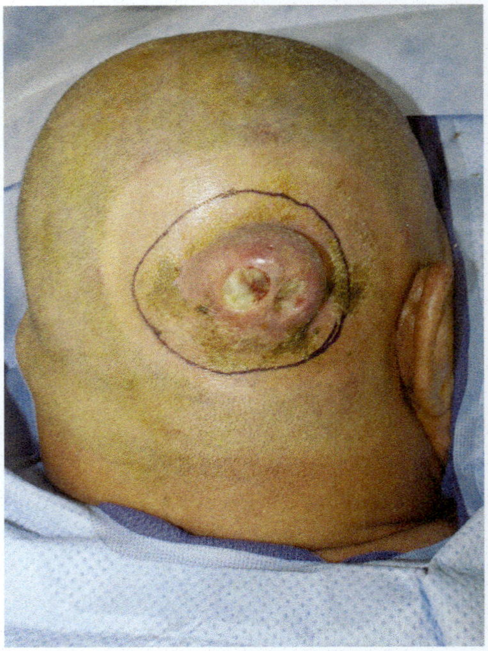

Fig. 24.50 Markings for a wide local excision of the lesion.

Microvascular flaps

The best technique for the reconstruction of total or near total scalp defects is the use of microvascular tissue transfer. The technique is also the most predictable option for the reconstruction of moderate to large defects in the heavily radiated scalp. The available recipient vessels along with the quantity of tissue needed for the reconstruction will often dictate the flap selection. Commonly used free flaps in scalp reconstruction are the radial forearm free flap, the anterior lateral thigh flap, and the latissimus dorsi flap.

The initial approach in reconstructing scalp defects after previous failed attempts is to determine the availability of recipient vessels. The arterial assessment can be done in the office with a handheld Doppler to determine the presence of the superficial temporal artery or other potential recipient vessels. The previous operative notes should be reviewed if at all possible.

The use of the radial forearm free flap in scalp reconstruction is often relegated to small to moderate size defects in radiated patients. These cases will often present to the reconstructive surgeon after multiple failed attempts at repair. Because of the history of radiation

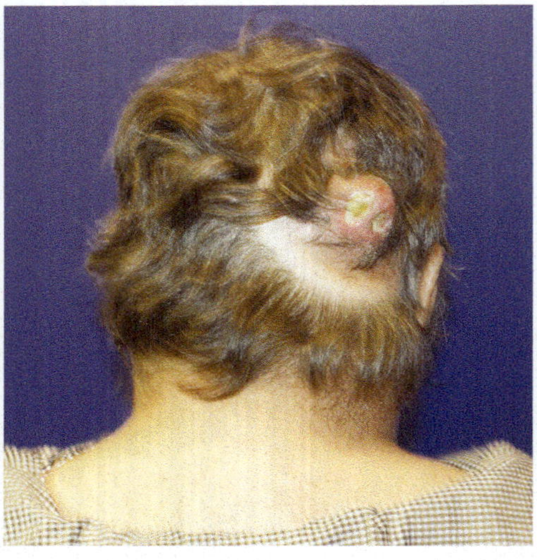

Fig. 24.49 View of a large scalp malignancy after failed radiation therapy.

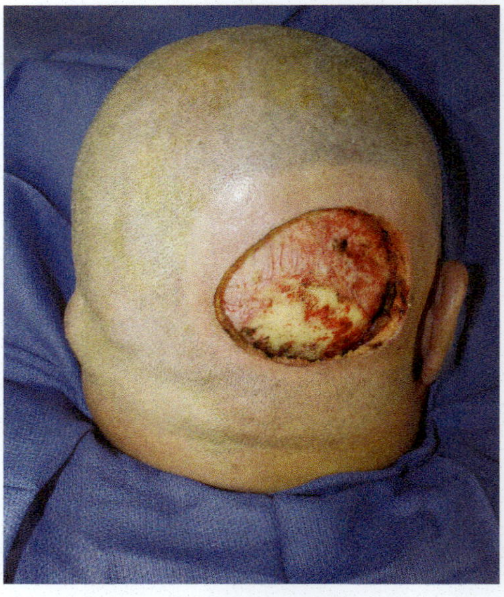

Fig. 24.51 Defect after resection of the malignancy.

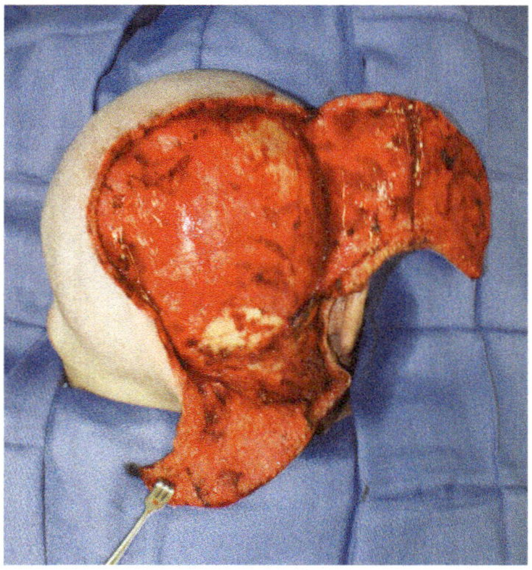

Fig. 24.52 Elevation of two wide flaps prior to reconstruction.

and failed reconstructive attempts, the calvarium is often exposed, desiccated, and with areas of necrosis, all consistent with osteoradionecrosis. The thickness of the radial forearm is an advantage in the reconstruction of partial scalp defects in that is does not result in a bulky reconstruction.

The radial forearm has the added advantage of possessing a long pedicle length, which can be used in instances where the superficial temporal vessels are not available for anastomosis. The pedicle length can easily reach the facial vessels for anastomosis.

Case #8

A 65-year-old Caucasian male was referred for the surgical management of a scalp melanoma (Figure 24.55).

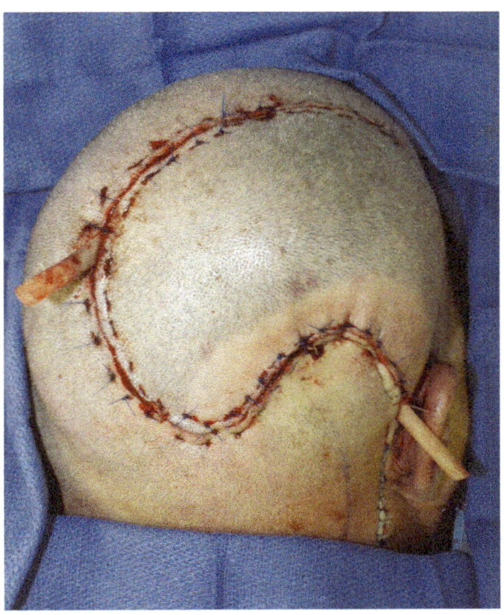

Fig. 24.53 Final appearance of the reconstruction after inset of the flaps.

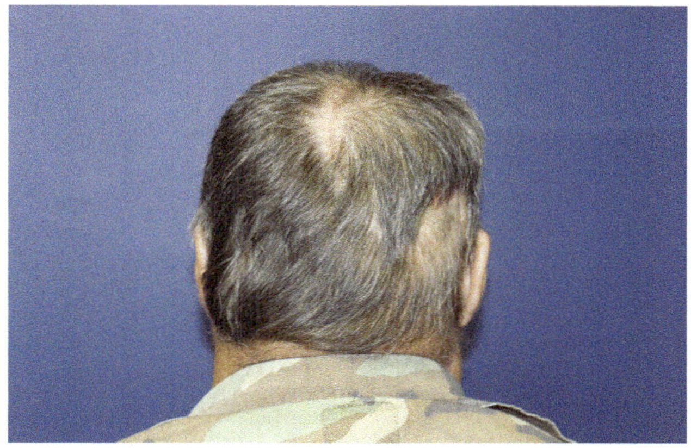

Fig. 24.54 Postoperative appearance of the reconstruction.

The area for the excision was marked and circumferential incision was made prior to excision of the lesion (Figure 24.56). The defect was deep to the cranium (Figure 24.57). The size of the defect was transferred to the right forearm and the flap was elevated (Figures 24.58 and 24.59). The superficial temporal artery and vein were prepared as the recipient vessels (Figure 24.60). The flap was inset into the defect and the postoperative healing was uneventful with an acceptable cosmetic appearance (Figures 24.61 and 24.62).

Case #9

A 66-year-old Caucasian female was referred for reconstruction of a persistent right scalp defect with exposed

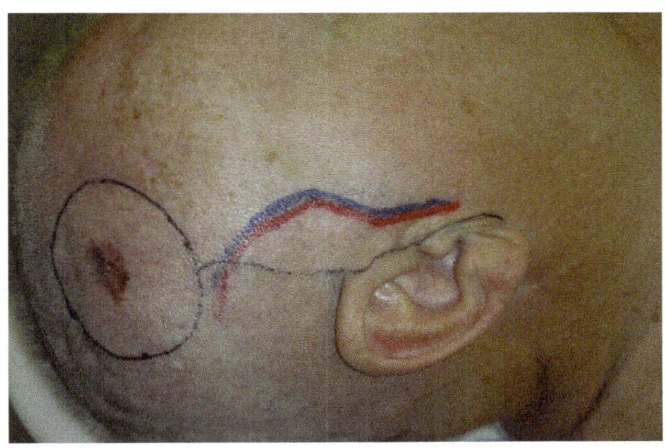

Fig. 24.55 Markings for a wide resection of a biopsy-proven melanoma of the scalp.

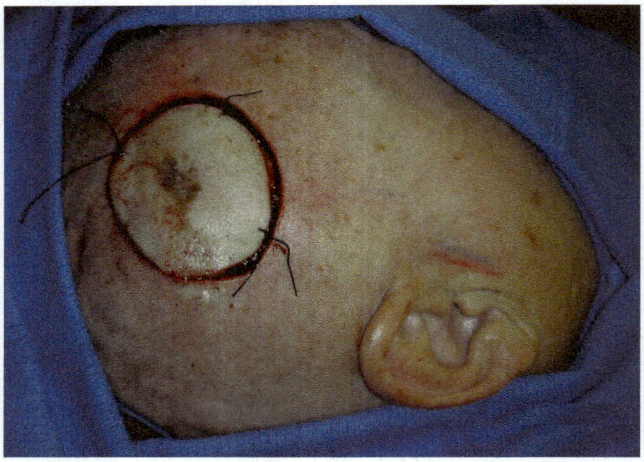

Fig. 24.56 Incision and markings of the resection.

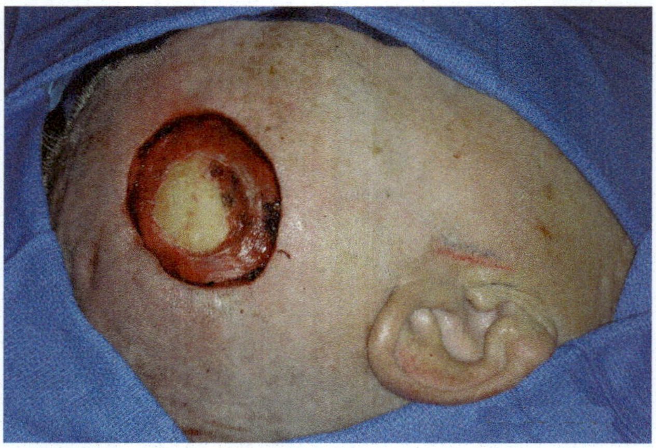

Fig. 24.57 Defect after removal of the tumor.

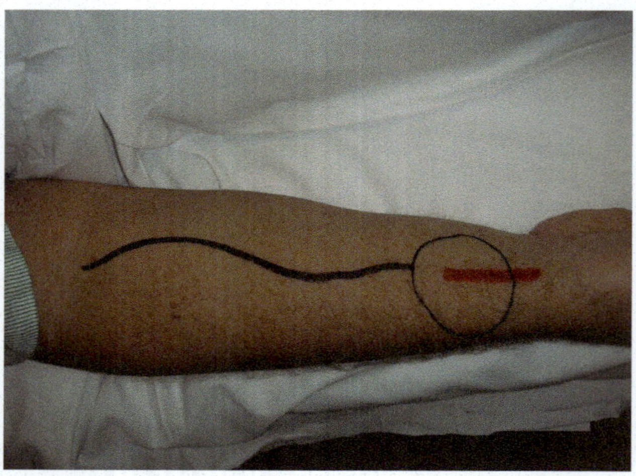

Fig. 24.58 Markings for the transfer of a radial forearm flap to repair the scalp defect.

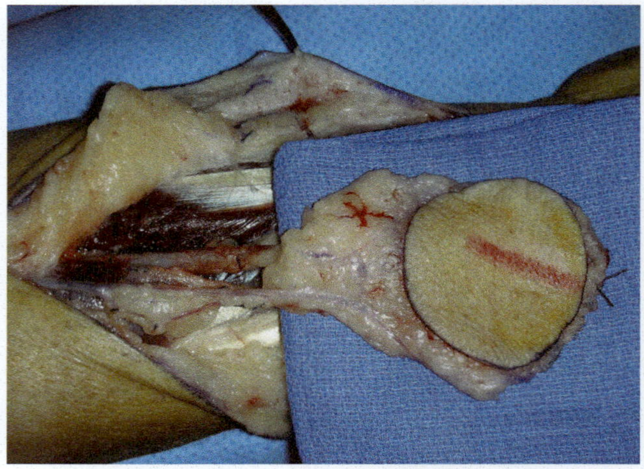

Fig. 24.59 Elevated forearm flap prior to transfer to the scalp.

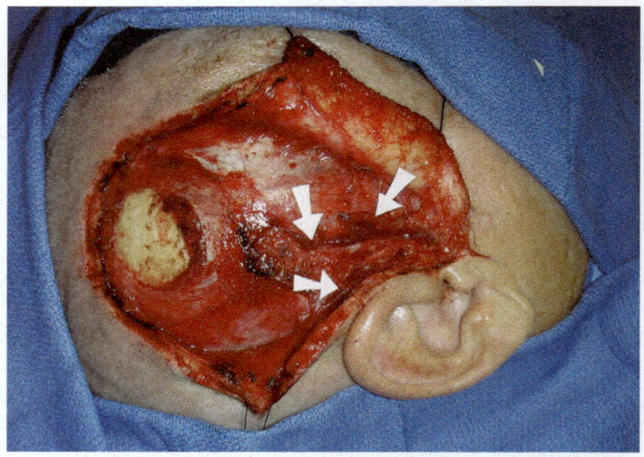

Fig. 24.60 View of the superficial temporal vessels for the anastomosis.

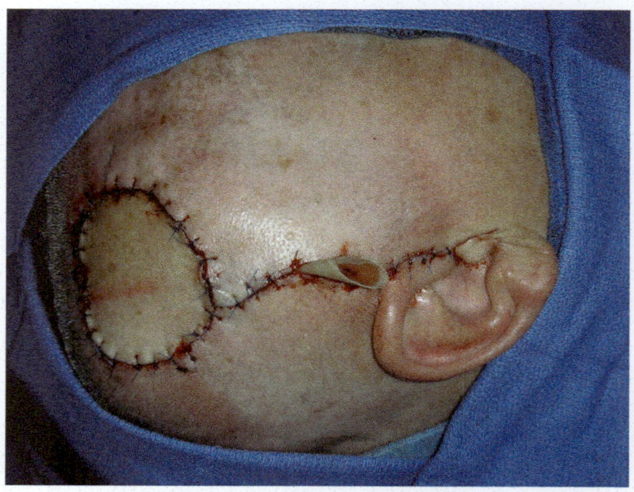

Fig. 24.61 Inset of the forearm flap.

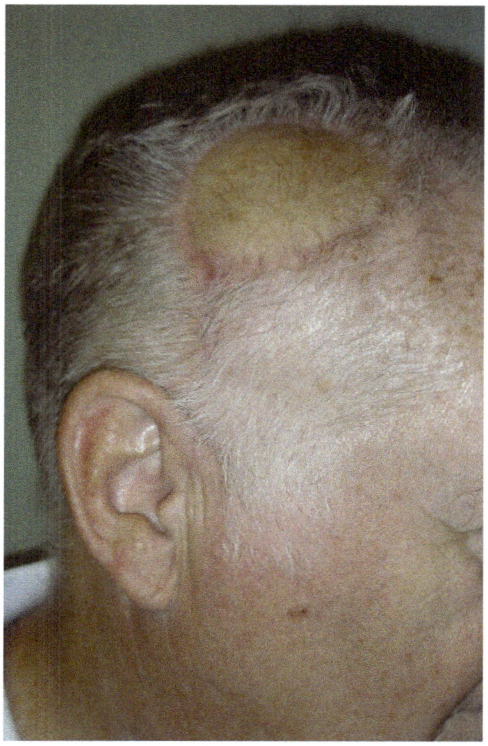

Fig. 24.62 Late postoperative view of the reconstructed scalp.

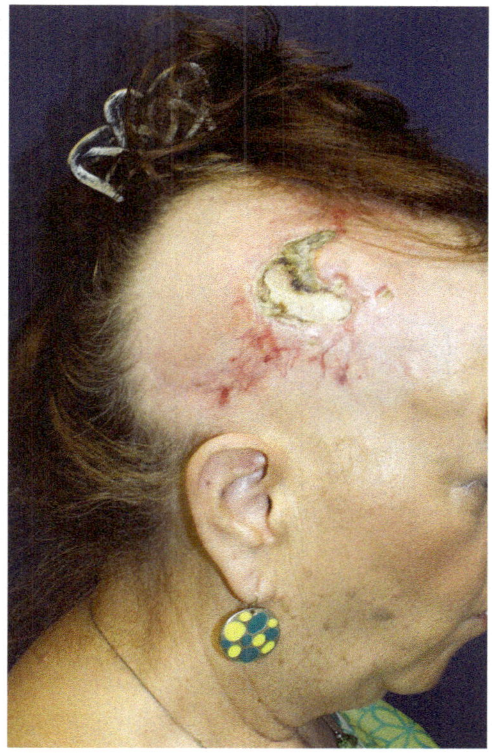

Fig. 24.63 Patient with an osteoradionecrosis of the skull and unstable skin after radiation therapy to the scalp for a scalp malignancy.

cranium. The patient reported a history of squamous cell carcinoma treated with radiation therapy with eventual exposure of the underlying cranium and loss of hair in the area. She had undergone several attempts at repair of the defect with skin grafts and local tissue rearrangements, all of which had failed (Figure 24.63). The patient was brought to the operating room with a plan for excision of the unstable skin surrounding the defect, removal of the exposed bone, and reconstruction of the defect with a radial forearm free flap (Figures 24.64 and 24.65). The superficial temporal artery and vein were dissected and found to be of good caliber for anastomosis (Figure 24.66). The radial forearm flap was elevated and a long pedicle was dissected (Figure 24.67). The flap was inset and anastomosed to the previously prepared temporal vessels (Figure 24.68). The postoperative appearance was acceptable with closure of the skull defect (Figures 24.69 and 24.70).

Case #10

The patient was referred for the excision of a biopsy-proven angiosarcoma of the left scalp region (Figure 24.71). A wide excision was performed and the superficial temporal vessels were prepared as recipient vessels for the microvascular anastomosis (Figures 24.72 and 24.73). The flap was transferred to the defect site and inset (Figure 24.74). The appearance of the reconstruction after

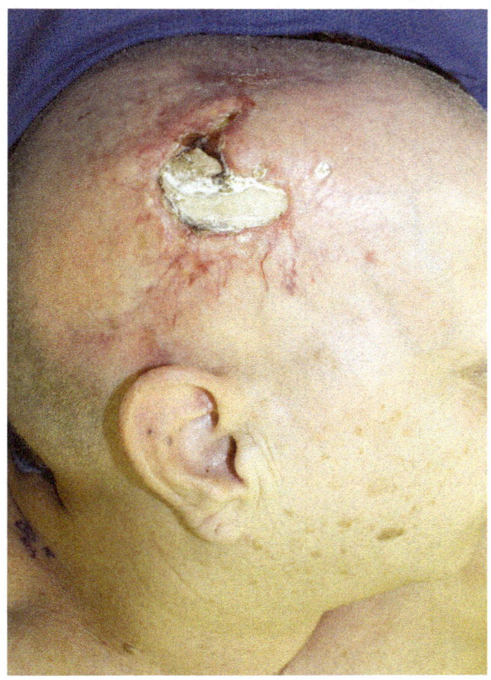

Fig. 24.64 View of the prepared scalp prior to debridment and removal of the unstable skin.

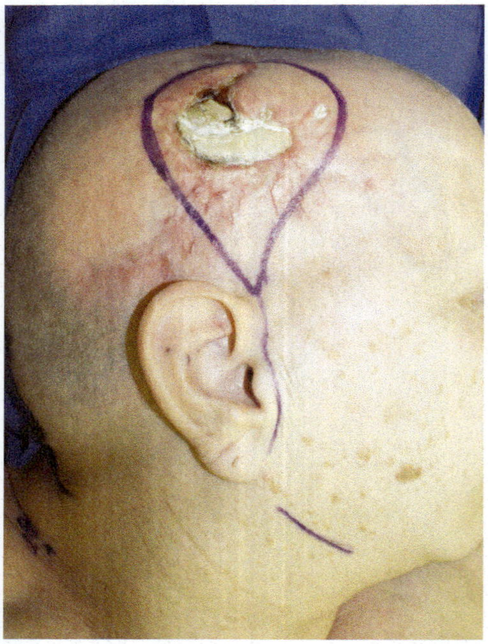

Fig. 24.65 Planned resection area and exposure of the recipient vessels.

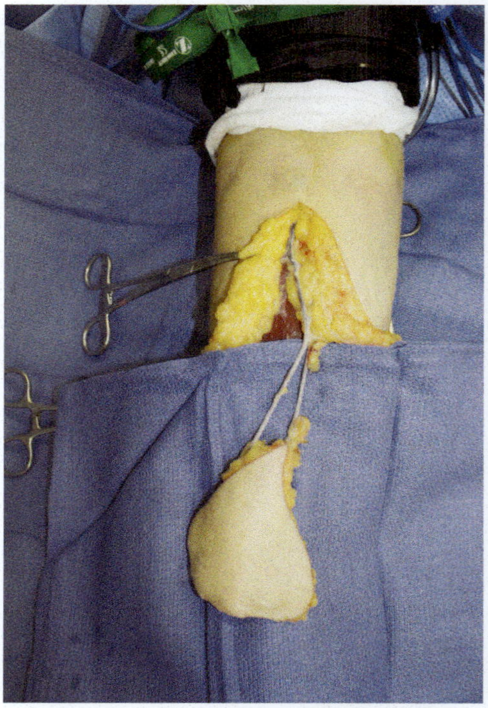

Fig. 24.67 Elevated radial forearm flap prior to transfer.

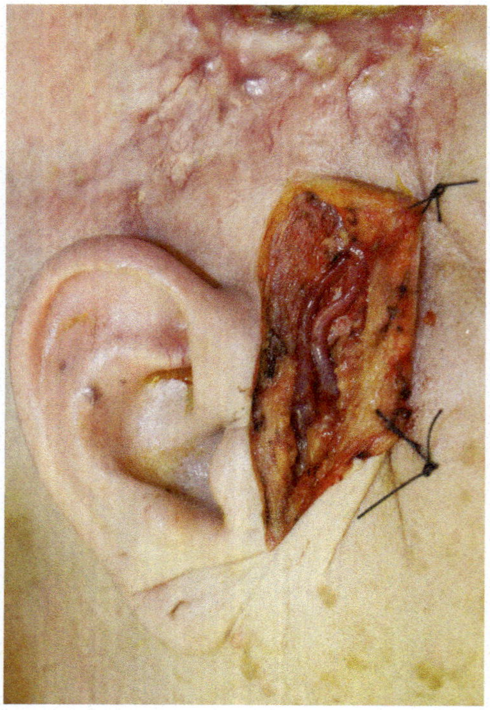

Fig. 24.66 Exposed superficial temporal vessels.

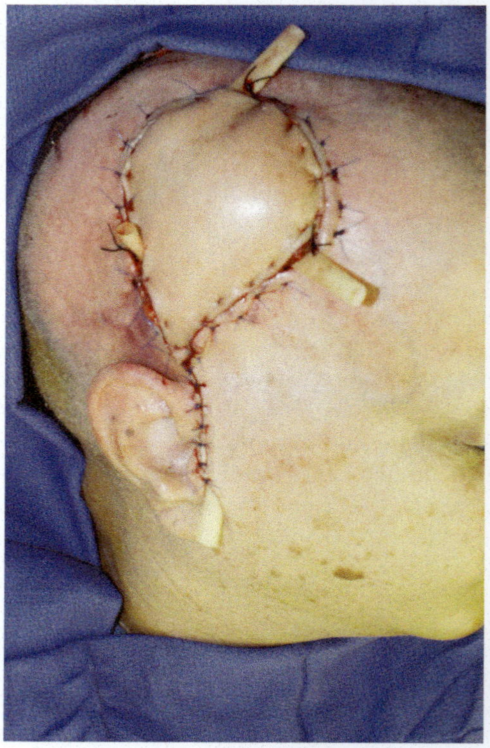

Fig. 24.68 Inset of the flap with anastomosis to the superficial temporal vessels.

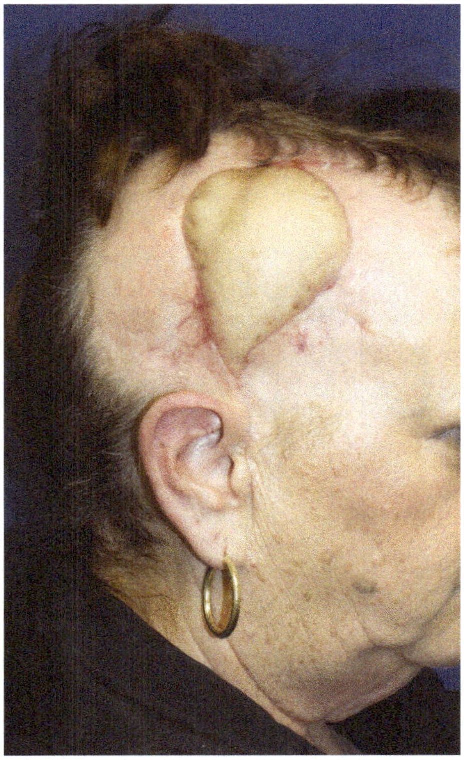

Fig. 24.69 Early postoperative appearance of the reconstructed scalp.

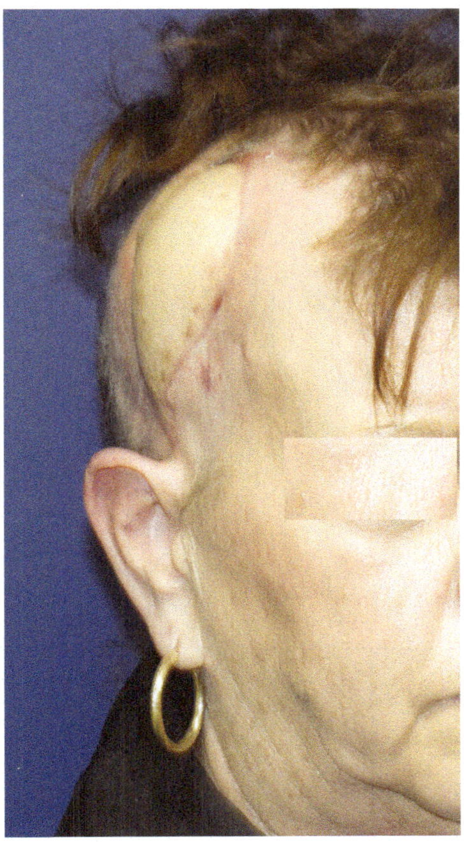

Fig. 24.70 Frontal view of the reconstructed scalp.

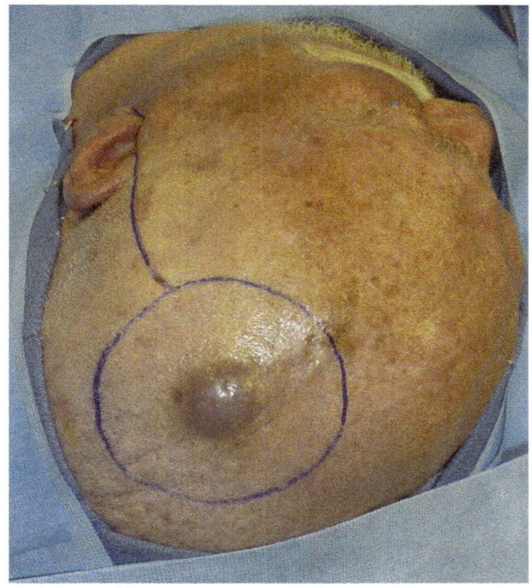

Fig. 24.71 Markings for the resection of a scalp malignancy.

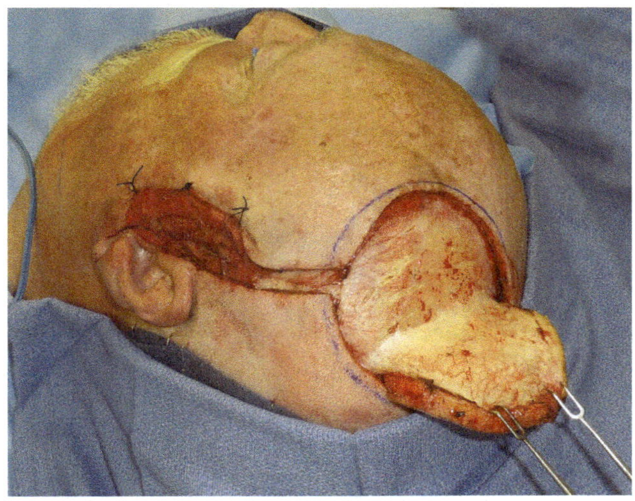

Fig. 24.72 Exposure of the vessels and elevation of the scalp flap.

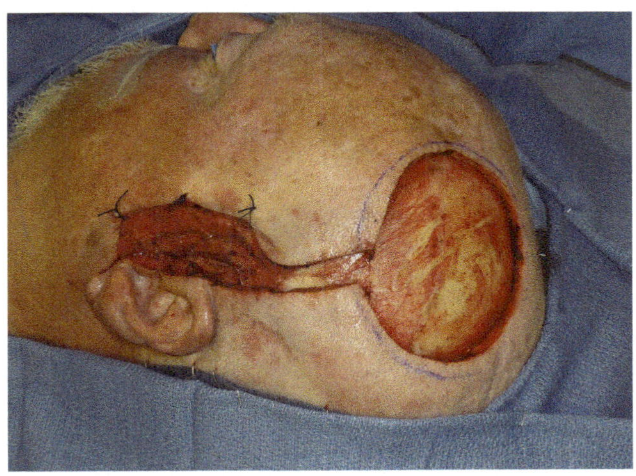

Fig. 24.73 Appearance of the resection bed and recipient vessels prior to reconstruction.

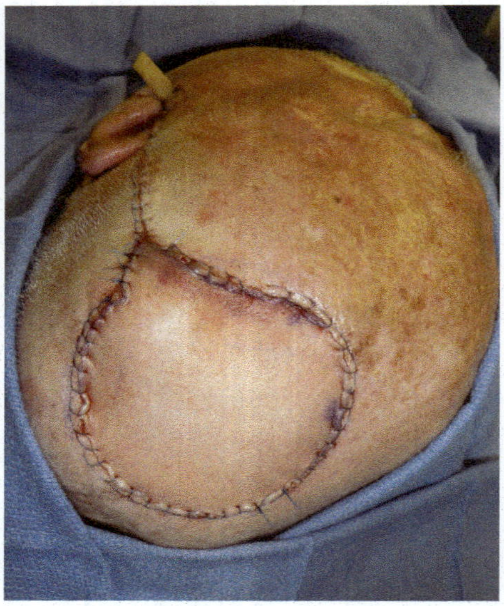

Fig. 24.74 Inset of the free flap transfer to repair the scalp defect.

the completion of the adjuvant radiotherapy was very acceptable with an excellent contour and an acceptable color match (Figure 24.75).

The anterolateral thigh flap (ALT) was first described by Song *et al.* in 1984.[12] The use of the flap for scalp reconstruction was first reported by Koshima in 1993.[13] The ALT enables the harvest of large quantity of fasciocutaneous flap with a good pedicle length that permits an easy reconstruction of the scalp defect. Additional advantages of the ALT are the ability to have a two-team approach, which enables preparation of the defect site at the same time as harvest of the flap. The disadvantages of the flap are the color mismatch and the potential for a large adipose component of the flap, which complicates the harvest as well as the inset and overall cosmesis. The final disadvantage is common to all microvascular flaps, that is, the lack of adequate hair growth. The amount and quality of hair that may grow even in hirsute males is not enough to camouflage the missing hair.

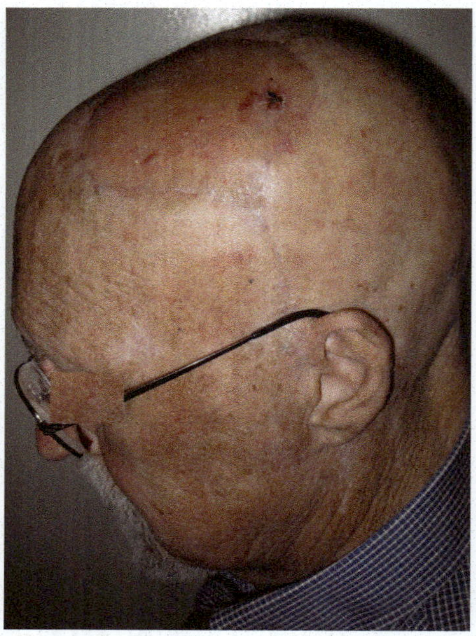

Fig. 24.75 Late appearance of the reconstructed scalp with the free tissue transfer.

Several other possible perforator flaps can be used in the reconstruction of scalp defects. Two other perforator flaps routinely used in scalp reconstruction are the thoracodorsal perforator flap and the deep inferior epigastric flap.

Case #11

An older Caucasian male with a history of Merkel cell carcinoma of the scalp treated with radiation therapy was referred for the management of a large osteoradionecrosis of the scalp with areas of exposed dura (Figure 24.76). A plan was made to use an ALT for the reconstruction of the large defect (Figure 24.77). The necrotic tissues were removed with neurosurgery, performing a large craniotomy, and reconstructing the defect with a large titanium mesh (Figure 24.78). The ALT flap was elevated and transferred to the defect. The appearance of the flap 2 weeks postoperatively was very good (Figure 24.79).

The last type of microvascular flap commonly used in scalp reconstruction is the latissimus dorsi flap. The latissimus dorsi can be used in the reconstruction of total or near total scalp defects. The flap can be elevated as a muscle-only flap or as a myocutaneous flap.

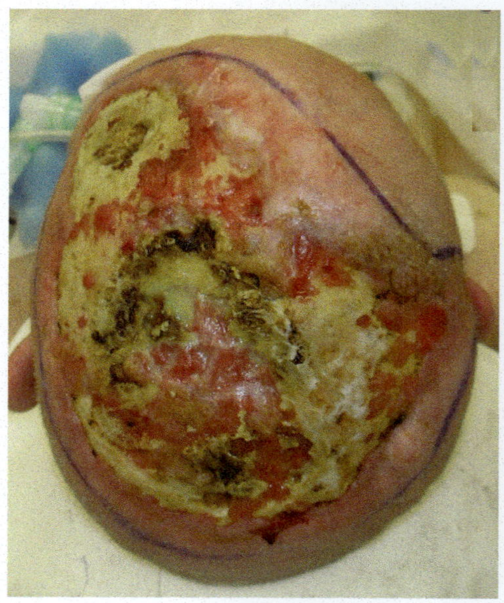

Fig. 24.76 View of a large scalp ORN with markings for resection.

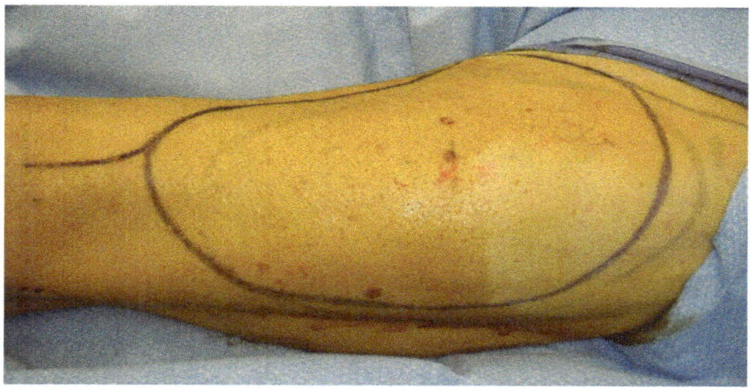

Fig. 24.77 Markings for the harvest of a large anterolateral thigh flap.

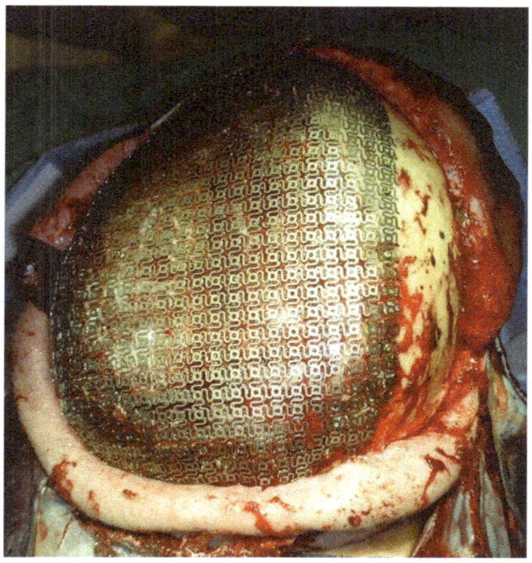

Fig. 24.78 Resected ORN and reconstruction of the skull with a large titanium mesh.

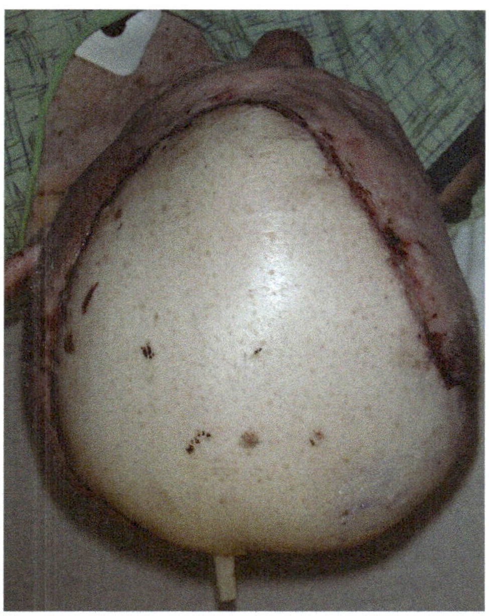

Fig. 24.79 Early view of the reconstructed scalp with the ALT flap.

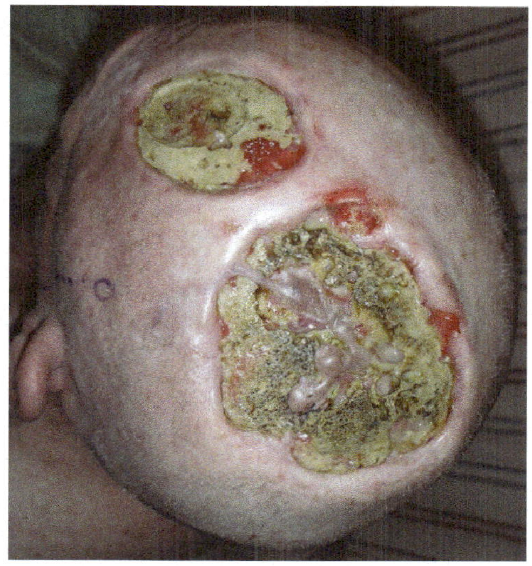

Fig. 24.80 View of ORN of the skull.

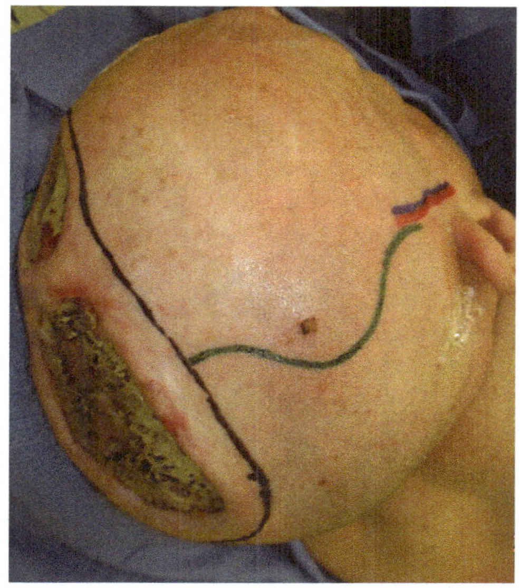

Fig. 24.81 Planned for reconstruction with free tissue transfer and reconstruction to the superficial temporal vessels.

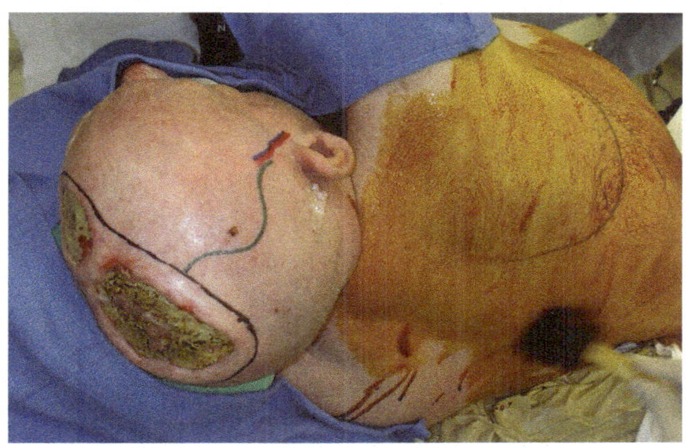

Fig. 24.82 View of the positioning of the patient for the harvest of the flap and simultaneous resection.

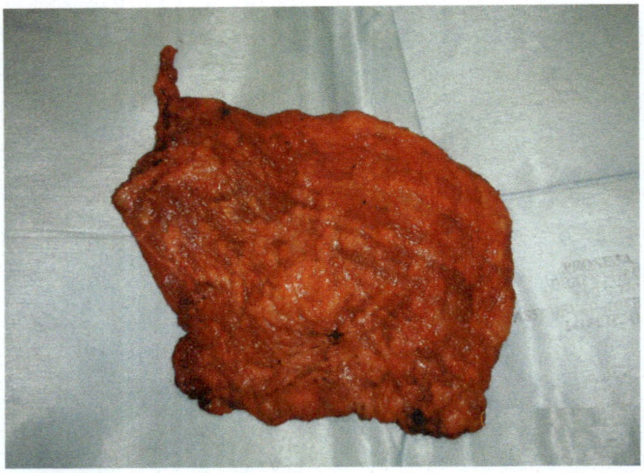

Fig. 24.83 Raised latissimus dorsi flap prior to transfer.

When used as a muscle-only flap, a skin graft is used to cover the muscle.

Case #12

A patient was referred for the management of a large scalp osteoradionecrosis and unstable skin (Figure 24.80). The necrotic tissues to be removed were marked and the recipient bed was prepared for the transfer of a latissimus free muscle flap (Figures 24.81 and 24.82). A muscle-only latissimus dorsi flap was raised and the vessels prepared for anastomosis (Figure 24.83). The flap was then transferred and the anastomosis was performed (Figure 24.84). The latissimus dorsi flap was then reconstructed with a series of split thickness skin grafts (Figure 24.85).

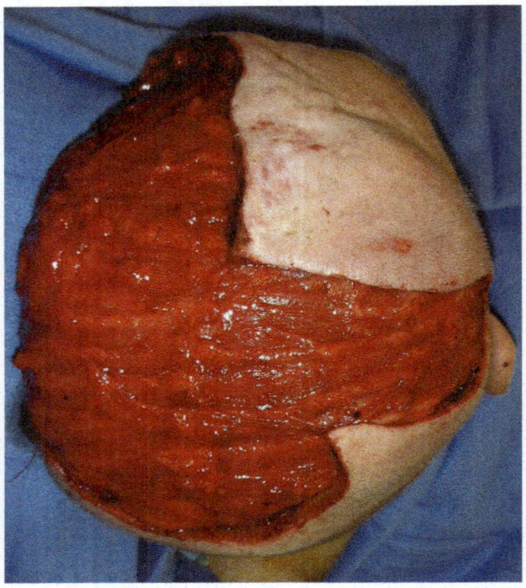

Fig. 24.84 inset of the latissimus dorsi flap prior to skin grafting.

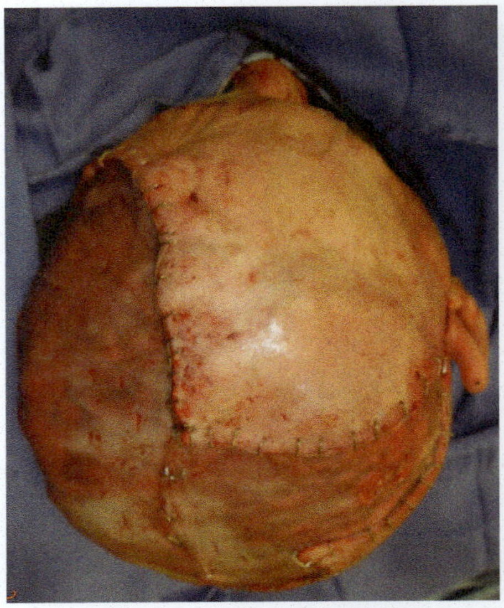

Fig. 24.85 Skin grafted latissimus dorsi flap reconstruction of the scalp defect.

References

1. Orticochea M. Four-flap scalp reconstruction technique. *Br J Plast Surg* 1967; 20:159–171.
2. Orticochea M. New three-flap reconstruction technique. *Br J Plast Surg* 1971; 24:184–188.
3. Radovan C. Tissue expansion in soft tissue reconstruction. *Plast Reconstr Surg* 1984; 74:482.
4. Manders EK, Schenden MJ, Furrey JA, Hetzler PT, Davis TS, Graham WP 3rd. *Plast Reconstr Surg.* 1984 Oct 74(4): 493:507.
5. Lutz B S, Wei FC, Chen HC, et al. Reconstruction of scalp defects with free flaps in 30 cases. *B. J Plast Surg* 1998; 51:186–190.
6. Earnest LM, Byrne PJ. Scalp reconstruction. *Facial Plast Surg Clin N Am* 2005; 13:345–353.
7. Tolhurst MD, Carstens MH, Greco RJ, Hurwitz DJ. The surgical anatomy of the scalp. *Plast Reconstr Surg* 1991; 87:603–612.
8. Leedy JE, Janis JE, Rohrich RJ. Reconstruction of acquired scalp defect an algorithmic approach. *Plast Reconstr Surg* 2005; 116:54e–74e.
9. Emmett AJ. The closure of defects by using adjacent triangular flaps with subcutaneous pedicles. *Plast Reconstr Surg* 1977; 59:45–52.
10. Fernandes-Calderon M, Casado-Sanchez C, Cabrera-Perez C. Versatility of hatchet flaps for the repair of scalp defects. *Actas Dermosifiliogr* 2012; 103(7):629–631.
11. Vecchione TR, Griffith L. Closure of scalp defects by using multiple flaps in a pinwheel design. *Plast Reconstr Surg* 1978; 62:74–77.
12. Song YG, Chen GZ, Song YL. The free thigh flap: a new free flap concept based on the septocutaneous artery. *Br J Plast Surg* 1984; 37:149–159.
13. Koshima I, Fukuda H, Yamamoto H, Moriguchi T, Soeda S, Ohta S. Free anterolateral thigh flaps for reconstruction of head and neck defects. *Plast Reconstr Surg* 1993; 92:421–430.

Index

Local and Regional Flaps in Head & Neck Reconstruction: A Practical Approach, First Edition. Rui Fernandes.

Companion website: www.wiley.com/go/fernandes/flapsreconstruction